Mereness' essentials of psychiatric nursing

Mereness'

essentials of psychiatric nursing

Cecelia Monat Taylor, R.N., Ph.D.

Professor of Nursing,
Syracuse University,
Syracuse, New York

TWELFTH EDITION

Illustrated

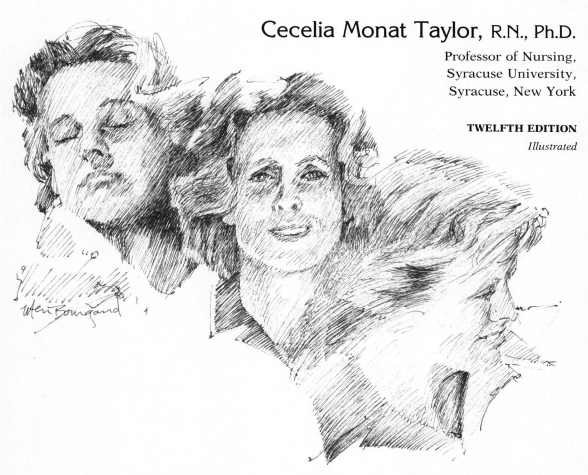

The C. V. Mosby Company

St. Louis · Toronto · Princeton   1986

To the **Deans and Directors** of Schools of Nursing
who have worked tirelessly for the advancement of nursing
education, thereby making a major contribution to the
improvement of nursing care of all persons

MOSBY

A TRADITION OF PUBLISHING EXCELLENCE

editor: Nancy L. Mullins
assistant editor: Maureen Slaten
manuscript editor: Jean Babrick
design: Nancy Steinmeyer
production: Jeanne A. Gulledge

TWELFTH EDITION

Previous editions copyrighted 1940, 1944, 1949, 1953, 1958, 1962, 1966,
1970, 1974, 1978, 1982

Printed in the United States of America

The C.V. Mosby Company
11830 Westline Industrial Drive, St. Louis, Missouri 63146

Library of Congress Cataloging in Publication Data

Mereness, Dorothy A.
  Mereness' Essentials of psychiatric nursing.

  Includes bibliographies and index.
  1. Psychiatric nursing.   I. Taylor, Cecelia Monat.
II. Title.   III. Title: Essentials of psychiatric
nursing.   [DNLM: 1. Psychiatric Nursing.   WY 160 M559e]
RC440.M38   1986   610.73'68   85-21718
ISBN 0-8016-4895-5

C/VH/VH   9 8 7 6 5 4 3 2 1   03/B/316

foreword to the eleventh edition

1940-1982 the evolution of a textbook

This text has played an important role in my life throughout my entire professional career. It was first published by The C.V. Mosby Company in the spring of 1940 and carried the title *Psychiatry for Nurses*. The major author was Dr. Louis J. Karnosh, Professor of Nervous Diseases at the medical school of Western Reserve University (now Case Western Reserve University) and Clinical Director of the Psychiatric Division of Cleveland City Hospital (now Cleveland Metropolitan General Hospital). Miss Edith Gage, Director of Nursing at the Psychiatric Division of City Hospital, was the nurse co-author.

This book was one of the earliest psychiatric texts for nurses. It became available just as I began a student experience in psychiatric nursing at City Hospital. Dr. Karnosh, who was interested in improving the nursing care of the mentally ill, always gave a series of lectures to each group of student nurses. He was a fascinating speaker who was a favorite of students. I was intrigued by the lectures, the new textbook, and the psychiatric nursing experience. Unfortunately, Dr. Karnosh was shot at his home and severely wounded by a distraught individual 2 weeks after the course began. He was able to give only two lectures to my student group. After 6 months he was able to return to work, but this was long after my experience at City Hospital had been concluded.

I was distressed because I had missed so many of Dr. Karnosh's lectures. Thus it was arranged at the University Hospital in Cleveland that I could be free on the day of his lectures to travel across the city by public transportation to hear the entire series. My classmates commented that I all but stood up and cheered during those lectures.

Edith Gage died about a year after the first edition of *Psychiatry for Nurses* had become available. Her position was filled by the instructor of psychiatric nursing. This created a vacancy about 6 months after I had completed the nursing curriculum at Western Reserve University. Dr. Karnosh suggested that I fill this vacancy. Although I had been a teacher before becoming a student nurse, and held a baccalaureate degree from a teachers' college, I knew nothing about teaching psychiatric nursing. The opportunity of working with Dr. Karnosh and learning more about psychiatric nursing overpowered my better judgment and I accepted the position in November 1941. Within a month the United States declared war on Japan. I was declared an essential worker and frozen in my position. This began a 4-year stint of teaching an ever-growing student body without an assistant or vacations.

Because of the epidemic of mental illness that the experience with the Armed Forces precipitated among American youth, and because so few nurses at that time had had any experience in psychiatric nursing, our students were a precious commodity. Many of them were made head nurses and supervisors of psychiatric units as soon as they were inducted into the U.S. Nurse Corps.

It was not until the third edition of *Psychiatry for Nurses*, which appeared in 1949, that I was involved in a revision of the text. My name was included in the flyleaf as the collaborator. In that edition I was allowed to add only a few comments concerning nursing care at the end of each chapter. Dr. Karnosh wrote in the preface of the third edition that psychiatric nursing had come into its own following World War II. This revision emphasized the shock therapies. A long chapter on syphilis of the central nervous system was included, and a new chapter on psychosomatic disorders was added.

The illustrations were pictures of actual patients, many of whom were unpleasant looking. Some purchasers of the text objected to these pictures. Since that time, a continuing effort has been made to identify meaningful illustrations for this text.

The fifth edition was published in 1958. My name appeared

for the first time on the outside cover of the book. A chapter on psychopharmacology and a glossary were added.

The seventh edition appeared in 1966. My name was given the position as major author with Dr. Karnosh becoming the collaborator. The name of the text was changed to *Essentials of Psychiatric Nursing,* and the book was enlarged. This edition emphasized self-understanding on the part of the nurse and the development of psychiatric nursing skills. In 1968 this edition was published in the Philippines.

In 1970 the eighth edition was published. It carried me as the only author. Chapters on children and adolescents, individuals with faulty intellectual development, and community psychiatry were added. Additional case histories were included in each chapter and discussed from the standpoint of the implications for nursing. Each chapter was concluded with a list of important concepts that the content of the chapter had covered. Finding appropriate illustrations continued to be a challenge. In the eighth edition pictures of nurses actively involved in patient activities were included.

The ninth edition, which appeared in 1974, introduced Cecelia Monat Taylor as the second author. Mrs. Taylor completed the master's curriculum in Psychiatric Mental Health Nursing, which I developed and directed at New York University from 1955 to 1965. She and I had similar beliefs about psychiatric nursing and we worked together harmoniously. Mrs. Taylor was actively involved in psychiatric nursing at Syracuse University at the time I had left the field to become the Dean of the School of Nursing at the University of Pennsylvania. In this edition the philosophy was revised, the entire content was reorganized, much of the book was rewritten, and all of it was updated. We attempted to emphasize the fact that a great deal of the treatment in psychiatry was being given outside an institution.

In the tenth edition, published in 1978, the word *patient* was discarded in favor of *client* or *individual.* Again the book was enlarged. Emphasis was placed on understanding the psychodynamics of observed behavior and the use of the nursing process.

In 1982 the eleventh edition of this text will not carry my name as one of the authors. This entire revision has been the work of Cecelia Monat Taylor. For the first time this book will be accompanied by a workbook, the author of which is Carol Lofstedt.

During the past 25 years I have spent many summers, weekends, and Christmas vacations searching for new, appropriate articles to be added to each chapter's bibliography, reading all of the competing texts, doing background reading in current journals, writing and rewriting chapters that were being revised or being added, trying to develop more appropriate illustrations, and desperately trying to meet the publisher's deadlines.

In a sense, the development of this text, which has been published continuously for 40 years and has proved to be the most durable in the field, is the story of the development of psychiatric nursing itself.

Dorothy A. Mereness
Philadelphia, Pennsylvania

foreword to the twelfth edition

what does the future hold for psychiatric nursing?

No one has a crystal ball in which to catch a glimpse of the future. However, inferences can be drawn about the future prospects for psychiatric nurses by studying the years since the 1946 Mental Health Act was passed by the U.S. Congress. That act was a direct result of the impact of the mental illness developed by many soldiers after serving in the Armed Forces during World War II. There was a paucity of professional workers to provide therapeutic approaches to the needs of those ill soldiers. When World War II ended, the Congress set about to rectify this serious weakness. Thus the Mental Health Act provided financial resources for the education of the members of the psychiatric team—psychiatrists, psychologists, psychiatric social workers, and psychiatric nurses. In the fall of 1947, six universities provided programs in psychiatric nursing for nurses interested in this field. The National Institute of Mental Health provided funding for these universities and the students recruited by them. This funding was increased as time progressed, and many more universities were added to the list of those which originally provided graduate programs in psychiatric nursing. NIMH continued to supply educational funding until today, although the amount of assistance has been dramatically curtailed in recent years. In the future, funding for psychiatric nurses from governmental sources will probably be nonexistent.

Since the passage of the Mental Health Act, many psychiatric nurses have developed clinical knowledge and expertise in teaching psychiatric nursing and in providing therapy for mentally distressed clients. Some of these nurses were able to complete a doctoral degree. Eventually, many of the educational leaders in the schools of nursing in this country were originally trained in psychiatric nursing. This fact will undoubtedly have an impact on the education of nurses and on the future practice of nursing. One can expect a continuing emphasis on recognizing and dealing therapeutically with the emotional needs of all clients.

NIMH also funded programs in schools of nursing that emphasized the integration of mental health concepts in all aspects of nursing. Thus the focus of nursing education on the psychosocial needs of patients was increased by this movement. These concepts were viewed as essential to the nursing care of all patients, regardless of the primary health problem. Unfortunately, in some current nursing education programs with integrated curriculums, study of psychopathology and the nursing care of psychiatric patients has disappeared entirely.

As a result of this lack of emphasis on psychiatric nursing at the undergraduate level, the number of applicants to graduate programs in psychiatric nursing is declining. If leadership in the field is to be continued, undergraduates must have educational experience in psychiatric nursing to awaken their interest and encourage them to pursue graduate study in this area.

About 30 years ago, while many nurses were being prepared

as clinical specialists in psychiatric nursing, a new understanding developed about the impact of long-term care in large public institutions. Professional workers came to realize that long-term institutionalization was increasing the illness of many clients rather than improving their mental health. When this idea became widely understood among those responsible for long-term care, many clients who had been institutionalized for years were discharged.

Deinstitutionalization occurred without adequate planning, monitoring, or funding. The result was a lack of follow-up care and a high potential for the abuse of the mentally ill who were discharged into the community.

Many discharged patients were not able to cope at all and returned again and again to the institution that discharged them, thus creating what was known as "the revolving door." Some individuals managed to live away from the institution more or less satisfactorily. A third group did not return to the institution, would not live with relatives or in group homes, and refused to accept any type of help. This group of homeless, destitute, emotionally ill people began living on the streets of many large cities and became known as the "street people." Their presence has been distressing to the public, but no real solution to this sociological problem has developed. It may be that in the not too distant future, the public will demand that facilities be provided for the physical and psychological care of these individuals.

Eventually, this attempt to change the pattern of hospitalization from large, impersonal, long-term care in public institutions resulted in the development of many smaller units in general hospitals and in small private agencies. All of these units provide intensive therapy and short-term hospitalization. In addition, smaller specialized units have begun to develop for the treatment of clients with special problems; examples include units for the treatment of emotionally disturbed children or for clients with alcohol or drug-related problems. Since people are living longer than in the past, a new specialty, geropsychiatry, has developed, which focuses on the treatment of the psychiatrically ill older client.

Despite these positive changes, the mental health system today is burdened with large numbers of both young and elderly patients with chronic psychiatric problems. The needs of this population place increasing demands on society to provide institutional, community mental health, and psychiatric nursing home facilities. There continue to be few programs for the chronically mentally ill, few funds for community services, and severe fragmentation of the system of delivering psychiatric care. Psychiatric nurses must become more involved in health policy planning to develop well-coordinated inpatient and outpatient supportive services for these clients.

Many psychiatrically ill clients are living in the community in group homes or in single occupancy situations. This provides an opportunity for some psychiatric nurses who are skilled in working with the chronically ill to offer specialized services for these individuals.

Psychiatric liaison nursing is another new area of specialization. These nurses work with medically ill patients and the staff members who are providing general patient care. The psychiatric liaison nurse assists the staff with planning care, serves as a role model for therapeutic intervention, and works with groups of staff members to help them deal with stressful situations.

Independent practice appeals to many psychiatric nurses who have successfully established offices and have been able to support themselves by providing a therapeutic relationship for troubled individuals. The passing of legislation has made third-party payment available for nurses in several states and has made independent practice a realistic goal for some nurses. Initially, independent practice is expensive and uncertain, but when satisfied clients begin to refer friends and acquaintances to the nurse, independent practice can become personally rewarding.

The broadened role of the psychiatric nurse is reflected in the 1982 American Nurses Association *Standards of Practice for Psychiatric/Mental Health Nursing*, which defined two levels of psychiatric nursing: the generalist and the specialist. Certification for both levels of practice, available through the ANA, is becoming increasingly popular as nurses attempt to demonstrate their competency and legitimize their practice. Peer review, another method of validating competency in practice, is being used by clinical specialists and nurses in private practice.

The skillful psychiatric nurse may choose to seek a position in a small treatment unit in a general hospital or one in a private specialized hospital. The role of the nurse clinician may involve providing group or individual therapy for selected clients or working with clients in a variety of innovative ways. Nurse clinicians may also function in units where treatment is provided specifically for children, for adolescents, for older clients, or for individuals who are hospitalized because of alcohol or drug abuse.

Other psychiatric nurses find the role of teacher in a school of nursing to be rewarding and fulfilling. It is reasonable to anticipate that for the foreseeable future schools of nursing will continue to seek psychiatric nurses to assist in the educational process.

Many psychiatric nurses find unique and innovative ways of using their talents and skills. This includes working with children in preparation for hospitalization or in sex education, working with couples in marriage counseling, helping groups of clients recovering from heart attacks to cope with anxiety and fear, or helping new mothers with feelings of inadequacy about their mothering skills.

Although the health care system is changing rapidly and dramatically, it is reasonable to believe that in the foreseeable future there will continue to be many calls for the special skills of the psychiatric nurse. It is for this reason that a learning experience in psychiatric nursing is essential for all students of nursing and that a textbook such as this is designed.

Dorothy A. Mereness, R.N., Ed.D., F.A.A.N.
Philadelphia, Pennsylvania

preface

This twelfth edition of *Mereness' Essentials of Psychiatric Nursing* has been prepared at a time when the practice of psychiatric nursing is being scrutinized as never before for its clinical effectiveness and cost efficiency. In addition, the number of nurses who are choosing to work in mental health settings is decreasing while the need for quality nursing care is as great as ever. Consequently, this book is designed to introduce the student nurse to the knowledge necessary to provide effective care for the mentally ill while presenting the parameters of the field in a challenging and realistic manner.

As with any new edition of a major textbook, this book represents a reorganization and revision, with the student's educational needs and the current and anticipated future practice of psychiatric nursing used as criteria. I continue in the belief that all nurses should have sound theoretical and experiential preparation in the care of the emotionally ill. At the same time it is important to emphasize that students of nursing who are preparing for beginning professional practice should not be expected to become psychiatric nursing specialists. Instead they should be encouraged to use knowledge learned during earlier learning experiences and in turn to apply skills gained during the psychiatric nursing experience to the care of all persons. As a result, this edition retains material on concepts basic to psychiatric nursing, which includes topics such as personality development and the process of communication, the understanding of which is integral to the effective practice of nursing in any setting and with any client.

It is my belief that an understanding of the history of psychiatric nursing is necessary to fully appreciate its current practice and influence its future course. However, I am fully aware that most students find the history of any profession irrelevant. Consequently, a major change in this edition is the deletion of a separate chapter about the history of psychiatric nursing and the inclusion of an opening section to each chapter entitled "Historical Perspective" where the historical background of the subject of the chapter is covered.

Each chapter that discusses clinical issues now includes a detailed case study that is analyzed in terms of the nursing process. All chapters begin with learning objectives and end with concluding statements designed to succinctly summarize significant content as directed by the learning objectives. Finally, every chapter is opened by a drawing by Meri Bourgard; many of these illustrations were created specifically for this text. The artist's sensitive depiction of the content of each chapter provides more than an aesthetic touch; it also conveys a feeling tone not possible to project through the written word.

New material includes Chapter 3—General Systems Theory and Stress and Adaptation: A Conceptual Framework; Chapter 12—The Nursing Process, which includes a list of selected nursing diagnostic categories and etiologic factors as approved by the Fifth National Conference on Nursing Diagnoses; and Chapter 19—Populations at Risk: Adolescents, which includes coverage of common eating disorders and adolescent suicide. The chapters devoted to the subjects of the nurse's self-awareness, psychotropic agents, substance dependence, antisocial behaviors, and the elderly all have been markedly enlarged and revised.

Dr. Dorothy Mereness, the collaborator and major author of this text from its fifth to tenth editions and whose name now appears in its title, has graciously written the foreword to this twelfth edition. I am grateful for her willingness to continue to share her observations of the current state of psychiatric nursing and her educated guesses about its future. The foreword she authored for the eleventh edition is included in this edition as well, since it conveys much significant information about the evolution of the oldest psychiatric nursing textbook still in print.

The plan of suggesting sources of additional information from easily obtained books and periodicals has been maintained. Thus foreign periodicals or relatively unknown ones have not been cited. In addition, references of several years ago have been retained when they are classics or still contain much currently valid information.

An attempt has been made to delete evidence of sexism in the language of this text; however, this has not always been possible. Therefore, for expediency and clarity, the client is often referred to in the third person, masculine gender, and the nurse is often referred to in the third person, feminine gender. Pronouns in quoted materials have not been changed.

The *Learning and Activity Guide* that accompanied the eleventh edition has been totally revised by its author, Carol Ruth Lofstedt, and continues to be a welcome and useful adjunct to this text. For the first time, an instructor's guide and a test bank (QUESTBANK) of questions correlated to each chapter will be available. I believe that the use of these additional materials, particularly the *Learning and Activity Guide*, will greatly enhance students' learning in a manner not possible within the constraints of a textbook.

No revision of a textbook is ever accomplished without the indirect and direct support and assistance of many others. The experience I have had over the last two and one-half decades working with students and clients as they interact has proven invaluable in enabling me to develop increasing awareness of the therapeutic needs of clients and the learning needs of students. I thank them! Professional colleagues have consistently provided support and interest in this project, whether they were psychiatric nurses or not. I thank them! Some have gone "the second mile" by offering specific information and insights. Specifically, Linda Beeber, M.A., R.N., a faculty colleague, has developed an understanding of the role of the nurse in regard to the use of psychotropic agents that is rare. She has been willing to share this with me, thus indirectly contributing to the chapter on psychotropic agents. Marianne (Mandy) Miles, M.S., R.N., a former student and now a doctoral student at the University of Rochester, has cheerfully worked endless hours on revising the bibliographies and sharing her expertise on the subject of adolescent eating disorders. I thank both of these women! Finally, Diane Piriano deserves more than mere acknowledgment for her willing cooperation in typing many drafts of manuscript and, rather than complaining, declaring that she had learned something! I thank her!

Dr. Mereness wishes to acknowledge the support and assistance of Margery (Peggy) Garbin, Ph.D., R.N., a friend and colleague who has provided invaluable personal and professional assistance since Dr. Mereness has lived in Philadelphia. We thank her!

Those of you who have used this textbook over the years have indirectly followed the progress of my daughter, Corliss, who is now 15 years old. Two pictures of her when she was 3 years old appeared as illustrations in the ninth, tenth, and eleventh editions of this textbook. They do not appear in this twelfth edition, reflecting the passage of professional as well as personal time. Corliss has never known life without the existence of this textbook and has demonstrated constant love and understanding through its several revisions. I thank her!

It is my hope that this text will make a meaningful contribution to the education of nursing students and that they in turn seize the opportunity to engage in sustained human contact with clients through which both are given the opportunity to grow.

Cecelia Monat Taylor

contents

xvii

section I

the context
of psychiatric
nursing practice

chapter one

the mental health
delivery system

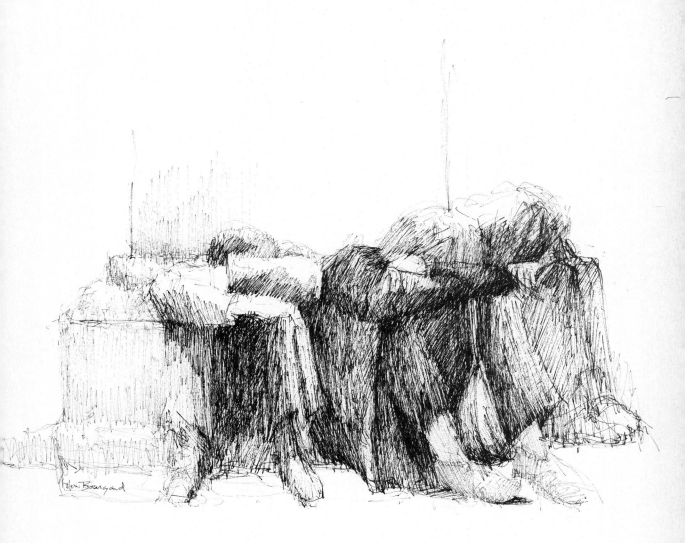

LEARNING OBJECTIVES

After studying this chapter the student will be able to:

1 State the primary mode of mental health treatment during key periods from prehistoric times to the present.

2 Identify the advantages and the disadvantages of the state mental hospital delivery system of the late nineteenth and early twentieth centuries.

3 Discuss the major pieces of legislation that led to the establishment of comprehensive community mental health centers as the system of mental health delivery.

4 List the characteristics of a comprehensive community mental health center.

5 Discuss the accomplishments and problems of the contemporary mental health delivery system.

Human beings have always been concerned with those of their members whose behavior is deviant from the norms of the society in which they live. The source of this concern has varied, at times stemming from compassion, at other times stemming from fear. Concomitantly, the label applied to those who behave in a deviant manner has varied throughout the ages and includes such terms as "sinner," "lunatic," "insane," and "mentally ill." The systems devised by the society to care for these afflicted have been strongly influenced by the prevailing beliefs about the cause and nature of the deviance. The responsibility for the provision of care has shifted among the various subsystems of the society, ranging from the family to the community as a whole, to specialized agents of the society such as the religious, political, and legal subsystems. The factors influencing this evolution are multiple and complex, but include such variables as population density, availability of resources, religious beliefs and social practices, and the prevailing body of knowledge about human behavior.

The following is a brief history of the treatment of the mentally ill, which is presented in the belief that the contemporary system of mental health care delivery can be understood best if there is an appreciation of its historical roots.

HISTORICAL PERSPECTIVE

The treatment of the mentally ill during prehistoric times can be inferred from the study of contemporary primitive peoples and their attitude toward mentally ill individuals. It seems likely that the victim of mental illness in the dim past was subjected to tribal rites designed to effect a cure. If these measures proved unsuccessful, the individual was simply abandoned to die quickly of starvation in a barren waste or to be devoured by animals in the wilderness. Critics of the contemporary practice of deinstitutionalization point to the large number of mentally ill persons left to fend for themselves on the streets and in single-room occupancy dwellings of large cities as reflecting a slightly more sophisticated parallel to the measures used by primitive peoples of ancient times.

In recorded ancient history, such as that of the Eastern Mediterranean civilizations, there are references to mental disorders. In later Egyptian civilization, particularly during the Alexandrian era, sanatoriums known as the temples of Saturn were operated for the care of those who were mentally afflicted.

The Golden Age of Greece was noted for its humane regard for the sick. The Greeks used as hospitals temples that had an abundance of fresh air, pure water, and sunshine. Theatricals, riding, walking, and listening to the sound of a waterfall were all recommended as methods to divert the melancholic. With this amazingly humane attitude, there were, however, instances when the treatment was not always free of its vicious aspects; even in the best of the Greek temples, starving, chains, and flogging were advocated "because with these it was believed that when those who refused food began to eat, frequently the memory was also refreshed thereby."

There is a surprising paucity of data about the Roman era in reference to mental illness. Galen, a Greek who practiced in Rome, based his treatment on the teachings of his Greek predecessors. Other physicians of the Roman era treated mental illness by bleeding, purging, and sulfur baths.

With the collapse of Greek and Roman civilization, medicine, along with other cultural developments, suffered an almost complete eclipse. The treatment of mental illness was left to priests, and every sort of superstitious belief flourished. The insane were flogged, fettered, scourged, and starved in the belief that the devils that possessed them could be driven out by these means.

A few bright spots in this tragic picture were some monasteries or shrines where this technique of "exorcising" the evil spirit was performed by the gentle laying on of hands instead of the whip. Members of the nobility, self-appointed ascetics, and holy men of varying degrees of sincerity practiced this art, which at least was not physically cruel.

Out of this tradition and belief in the "holy" or "royal touch" arose several great shrines, of which the one at Gheel in Belgium is most famous. The legend behind the beginnings of this colony is worth telling. Sometime in the dim past there lived a king in Ireland who was married to a beautiful woman and who became the father of an equally beautiful daughter. The good queen developed a fatal illness, and at her deathbed the daughter dedicated herself to a life of purity and service to the poor and the mentally bereft. The widowed king was beside himself with grief and announced to his subjects that he must at once be assuaged of sorrow by marrying the woman in his kingdom who most resembled the dead queen. No such paragon was found. But the devil came and whispered to the king that there was such a woman—his own daughter. The devil spurred the king to propose marriage to the girl, but she was appropriately outraged and fled across the English Channel to Belgium. There the king overtook her and, with Satan at his elbow, slew the girl and her faithful attendants. In the night an angel came, recapitated the body, and concealed it in the forest near the village of Gheel. Years later five lunatics chained together spent the night with their keepers at a small wayside shrine near this Belgian village. According to the legend, all the victims recovered overnight. Here indeed must be the place where the dead girl, reincarnated as St. Dymphna, was buried, and here was the sacred spot where her cures of the insane were effected.

In the fifteenth century, pilgrimages to Gheel from every part of the civilized world were organized for the mentally sick. Many of the pilgrims remained in Gheel to live with the inhabitants of the locality, and in the passing years it became the natural thing to accept them into the homes. Thus the first colony for the mentally ill, and for that matter the only one that has been consistently successful, was formed. In 1851 the Belgian government took charge of this colony of mentally ill persons. It continues to exist to the present day. Some 1500 certified mentally ill individuals live in private homes, work with the inhabitants, and suffer no particular restriction of freedom, except to refrain from visiting public places and from the use of alcohol and to report regularly to the supervising psychiatrist. In spite of the success of the Gheel colony and its great humanizing value most attempts at duplicating it elsewhere have been total or partial failures. The community mental health movement in the United States is, in a sense, an attempt to capture some of the values of community involvement demonstrated in Gheel.

Although the treatment of the mentally ill in the Middle Ages had little to recommend it, the period that followed was in some respects a great deal worse. When the church and the monastery gave up the care of the insane, it was gradually taken over by the so-called almshouse, the contract house, and the secular asylum. The more violent persons were placed in jails and dungeons. In the sixteenth century Henry VIII officially dedicated Bethlehem Hospital in London as a lunatic asylum. It soon became the notorious "Bedlam" whose hideous practices were immortalized by Hogarth, the famous cartoonist. There keepers were allowed to exhibit the most boisterous of the patients for 2 pence a look, and the more harmless inmates were forced to seek charity on the streets of London as the "Bedlam beggars" of Shakespear's *King Lear.*

In those dark days, society was interested in its own self-security, not in the welfare of the insane. The almshouses were a combination of jail and asylum, and within their walls petty criminals and the insane were herded indiscriminately. In the seventeenth and eighteenth centuries the dungeons of Paris were the only places where the violently insane could be committed. Drastic purgings and bleedings were the favorite therapeutic procedures of the day, and "madshirts" and the whip were applied religiously by the cell keepers.

Superstition about mental disease took a horrible turn in the seventeenth century. God and Satan were still thought to be engaged in a ceaseless battle for possession of one's soul. The year after the *Mayflower* sailed into Plymouth Harbor, Burton published his classic work *Anatomy of Melancholy*, wherein he stated that "witches and magicians can cure and cause most diseases." To seek out and execute witches became a sacred religious duty. At least 20,000 persons were said to have been burned in Scot-

land alone during the seventeenth century. Small wonder that
Cotton Mather precipitated the witch mania in Salem, since he
was merely subscribing to the dogma of the day.

The political and social reformations in France toward the
end of the eighteenth century influenced the hospitals and jails of
Paris. In 1792 Philippe Pinel (1745-1826), a young physician who
was medical director of the Bicêtre asylum outside of Paris, was
given permission by the Revolutionary Commune to liberate the
miserable inmates of two of the largest hospitals, some of whom
had been in chains for 20 years. Had his experiment proved a
failure he might well have lost his head by the guillotine. Fortu-
nately he was right, since by his act he proved conclusively the
fallacy of inhumane treatment of the insane. The reforms instituted by Pinel were continued by his pupil Esquirol, who
founded no less than 10 asylums and was the first regular teacher
of psychiatry. The Quakers, under the Brothers Tuke, had at this
time established the York Retreat and effected the same epoch-
making reforms in England.

In America the Pennsylvania Hospital was completed in 1756,
under the guidance of Benjamin Franklin. One of the first two
patients admitted was described as a "lunatic." Soon, however,
the insane were relegated to the cellar but at least they were assured clean bedding and warm rooms. Benjamin Rush (1745-
1813), a prime humanitarian and the "father of American psychiatry," began his duties at the Pennsylvania Hospital in 1783.
Subscribing in part to the lunar theory of insanity and inventing
an inhuman restraining device called the "tranquilizer" but at
the same time insisting on more humane treatment of the mentally afflicted, he stands as a prominent transitional figure between the old era and the new.

Most of the states were still without special institutions for
mentally ill persons in the first quarter of the nineteenth century.
The poorhouse or almshouse was still popular, but it invariably
became a catchall for all types of offenders, and the mentally ill
received the brunt of its manifold evils. Most shocking to people
of today was the placing of the poor and the mildly demented on
the auction block, where those with the strongest backs and the
weakest minds were sold to the highest bidder, the returns from
the sale being assigned to the township treasury.

About 1830 a vigorous movement for the erection of suitable

state hospitals spread simultaneously through several states. The excellent results obtained by private institutions such as the Hartford Retreat, founded in 1818, probably served as an object lesson. Horace Mann took an enthusiastic interest in the plight of the mentally ill, and the advantages of a state hospital system were publicized to promote construction of such institutions. The first public psychiatric hospital in America was built in Williamsburg, Virginia, in 1773. Today it is known as the Eastern Psychiatric Hospital.

However, it remained for an asthenic, 40-year-old schoolteacher to expose the sins of the poorhouse. From that day in 1841 when Dorothea Lynde Dix (1802-1887) described the hoarfrost on the walls of the cells of the East Somerville jail in Massachusetts to the day when she retreated into one of the very hospitals she was instrumental in creating, she effected reforms that shook the world. She so aroused the public conscience that millions of dollars were raised to build suitable hospitals, and 20 states responded directly to her appeals. She played an important part in the founding of St. Elizabeth's Hospital in Washington, D.C., directed the opening of two large institutions in the maritime provinces of Canada, completely reformed the asylum system in Scotland and in several other foreign countries, and rounded out a most amazing career by organizing the nursing forces of the northern armies during the Civil War. A resolution presented by the U.S. Congress in 1901 characterized her as "among the noblest examples of humanity in all history."

The state hospital system that rapidly developed throughout many states was limited almost solely to large institutions built in remote rural areas of the state and designed according to architectural plans developed by Dr. Thomas Kirkbride. The location of these institutions was determined by a multiplicity of considerations. For example, it was believed that the tranquil environment of the country would be soothing to disturbed individuals; rural land was inexpensive to purchase; and the remoteness of the setting effectively protected the society from the inmates, both physically and emotionally.

The design of the institution resulted from a genuine desire to provide a homelike environment that would also be safe. However, because of the remoteness of the setting, such staff as there were had to live in adjoining quarters and the institution had to produce its own food, heat, and other necessities. What evolved was a self-contained community where patients who were able worked on the farm; in the kitchen, laundry, and machine shop; and on the grounds and units. For some patients, this responsibility proved therapeutic because it provided meaningful activity, thereby increasing their sense of self-esteem and group cohesiveness. In some state hospitals, selected patients were invited to share the Sunday dinner with the hospital superintendent. Many, if not all, were more comfortable than they would have been had they remained in their local community. On the other hand, there were abuses. At the very least, even the most able patient was exploited, since he was not paid for his labor.

By the middle of the nineteenth century the asylum, "the big house on the hill" surrounded by its landscaped park and topped by high turrets and cupolas, became a familiar landmark. Although such matters as management, housing, and feeding of mental patients were slowly attaining decent humanitarian standards, as late as 1840 there was no clear classification of mental disorders. A German teacher, Dr. Heinroth, was still advancing the theory that insanity and sin were identical. It was not until 1845 that the first authentic textbook on mental disease was published, aligning the treatment of mental illness with the treatment of other illnesses.

In addition to exploitation and perhaps not unrelated to it, another negative outcome of the state hospital system was the syndrome of *institutionalization*. Because of the remoteness of its location the state hospital was not accessible to the community and families soon gave up any attempt to remain in contact with their hospitalized member. Having no contact with the outside world these inmates adapted to their surroundings and their roles within the hospital to the extent that they resisted the few attempts made on their behalf to return them to their homes. Consequently, it was not uncommon for an individual, once admitted to the hospital, to spend the remainder of his life there.

This system of mental health delivery, with all its advantages and disadvantages, might well have continued endlessly had it not been for the unprecedented waves of immigrants to the United States in the mid-nineteenth century. The effect of this artificial population explosion was an enlargement of the cities so that the state hospitals were no longer so geographically remote. In addition, and perhaps more importantly, the system was confronted with huge numbers of individuals who were deemed to need mental health care. Because the cultural backgrounds and language of the mentally ill immigrants were sufficiently different from those of the mainstream, their behavior was poorly tolerated by the society and the census of the state hospitals swelled. This made it impossible to continue the humane treatment delivered at an earlier time, and by the twentieth century the state hospital system had turned into an inefficient, expensive, and inhumane system able to do little more than protect inmates from each other and from the society.

Overt change in the state hospital system of mental health care began in 1908 when Clifford Beers, a psychiatric patient who was hospitalized several times during an otherwise productive life, wrote a book entitled *A Mind That Found Itself.* Being of vivid colorful temperament, Mr. Beers had unlimited enthusiasm, which he directed to founding the National Committee for Mental Hygiene. Under the momentum of his aggressive leadership the movement became worldwide and now has ramifications in the form of child guidance, prison psychiatry, vocational guidance, and other practical activities that are important to all concerned people.

Simultaneously with the mental hygiene movement came the astounding contributions of Sigmund Freud (1856-1939), which revolutionized the orthodox concepts of the mind, proposed a new technique for exploring it, and brought the subject of human behavior to the attention of every intelligent man and woman. Psychiatry at last left the closed doors of the asylums and participated in everyday human activity.

One of the most forward-looking actions the nation has ever taken in relation to mental illness was the passage of the National Mental Health Act in 1946. Among other accomplishments was the establishment of the National Institute of Mental Health. A similar act was passed about the same time in Canada, and it had a similar effect in moving Canada into the forefront in the field of mental health. Both these acts provided for the financing of research and training programs. Through their enactment the governments expressed their belief that it was necessary to acquire more knowledge concerning the cause, prevention, and treatment of mental illness and that more professionally trained workers were needed to improve the care and treatment of the mentally ill. Financial support for the education of psychologists, psychiatric social workers, psychiatrists, and psychiatric nurses was provided in the United States for many years through the National Mental Health Act.

The National Mental Health Act grew out of the experiences the nation had during World War II when more men in the Armed Forces were disabled by mental illness than by all the other problems related to actual military action. The many soldiers who were incapacitated by acute and chronic mental illness alerted the nation to the need for many more trained professional workers in the field, for greater knowledge about the cause and prevention of mental illness, and for greatly improved treatment techniques.

During World War II the psychiatrists in the medical corps, led by Dr. William Menninger, learned the importance of early recognition of psychiatric problems and the significance of initiating treatment rapidly and close to the place where the difficulty occurred. They developed a method of crisis-oriented treatment that promoted adaptation and an early return to duty. To individuals in decision-making positions, they demonstrated the usefulness of consultation when issues that affected the mental well-being of soldiers were concerned.

Psychotropic drugs, particularly the antipsychotic agents, played a large role in fostering change in the mental health delivery system. They were first used experimentally in 1953. By 1956 the populations of the state mental hospitals were reported to have fallen slightly, instead of increasing as they had done for decades. This development was largely a result of the fact that, with the help of these medications, more individuals could control their behavior and thus could spend time outside the hospital in the community. Had it not been for these drugs, many individuals would never have been able to control their unusual behavior sufficiently to remain at home and receive continuing treatment on an outpatient basis.

In the late 1940s and early 1950s the large public institutions for the care of the mentally ill began to change significantly through the development of new methods for approaching and understanding human problems. Some of these new methods included family diagnosis, the introduction of short- and long-term treatment programs, and the advent of crisis-oriented therapy. At about the same time several new ideas were introduced into public psychiatric hospitals. Such developments as the therapeutic community concept, which attempted to alter certain sections of larger psychiatric institutions to provide clients with an opportunity for achieving a more constructive social adjustment, the concept described as milieu therapy, and the approach known as the open-door hospital were introduced and refined. Some of these ideas, especially the open-door hospital and the therapeutic community, came to the United States directly from experimentation in England.

In 1955 the Congress of the United States passed the Mental Health Study Act. This act provided funds for a 5-year study of the problem of mental illness in the United States. As a result of the act the Joint Commission on Mental Illness was established. On December 31, 1960, this commission submitted its final report to the Congress, to the Surgeon General of the Public Health Service, and to the governors of the 50 states. The published report was entitled *Action for Mental Health* and was available to the public in 1961. It was widely read, provided an impetus for developing more effective services for people in need of psychiatric help, and was the basis for additional legislation.

A milestone in the nation's developing awareness of the need for an improved approach to the problems of mental health and illness was reached on February 5, 1963, when President John F. Kennedy delivered his special message to the Congress on mental illness and mental retardation. In this speech he mentioned a few goals: "Central to a new mental health program is comprehensive community care. . . . The mentally ill can achieve . . . a constructive social adjustment. . . . The centers will focus on community resources. . . . Prevention as well as treatment will be a major activity." In that same year, 1963, the Community Mental Health Centers Act was passed, followed in 1965 by the Staffing Act for the Community Mental Health Centers. These acts made money available to build and staff the centers and were the impetus for the rapid development of many centers in a relatively short period of time. The first federally funded centers began operation in 1966.

In 1975 the Congress of the United States enacted the Community Mental Health Centers Amendments of 1975. This law provided for the continuation of federal funds to community mental health centers but also designated specific guidelines for services that must be provided. Specified in these guidelines is a full range of inpatient, outpatient, and emergency services. Certain population groups such as children and the elderly were targeted as particularly requiring services. Individuals suffering from drug and alcohol abuse and addiction and those persons being discharged from mental institutions also were included in the population groups given priority for services.

In 1977 President Jimmy Carter called for the development of a President's Commission on Mental Health, which was charged with identifying "the mental health needs of the nation." Nursing was represented on such a commission for the first time by Martha Mitchell, a nurse educator and clinical specialist in psychiatric-mental health nursing. The report of the 1977 Commission recommended the development of a new federal grant program designed to strengthen existent community efforts and to develop new initiatives to address the mental health needs of communities. Special emphasis was placed on meeting the needs of underserved and high-risk populations such as the elderly, children, the chronically mentally ill, cultural minorities, rural communities, and inner-city neighborhoods. The very timely issue of the economics of mental health care was addressed by a recommendation that mental health coverage be included in all health insurance and that this coverage not be limited to hospitalization. The Commission also recommended that evaluation of federally funded community mental health centers be centralized.

In October of 1980 Congress passed the Mental Health Systems Act of 1980. This legislation grew out of the Commission's recommendations and it addressed, among other topics, research and training priorities and client's rights.

With the election in 1980 of a conservative administration, federal funding for all health services, including mental health services, was dramatically reduced. Funds that were allocated were distributed to the states in the form of "block grants" in the belief that it is both the right and the responsibility of the state level of government to determine priorities for finite resources. The one exception has been the maintenance of federal funding for research, particularly biomedical research, into the causes and treatment of mental illness. It is too soon to postulate about

TABLE 1-1   locus of mental health care throughout history

	family/ community	religious orders	penal institutions/ almshouses	state mental hospitals	community mental health centers	?
Before recorded history	X					
Egyptian and Greek civilizations		X				
15th century	X					
16th, 17th, 18th centuries			X			
19th century				X		
20th century				X	X	
21st century						X

the long-term effect of this change in federal funding priorities. In the short term, however, it is clear that the innovative programming of mental health services and the training of mental health professionals have been seriously curtailed.

CHARACTERISTICS OF A COMPREHENSIVE COMMUNITY MENTAL HEALTH CENTER

Despite reduction in funding, the public mental health delivery system continues to be that of the comprehensive community health center. The comprehensive community mental health center is organized around a demographic unit with a population small enough to permit the development of comprehensive mental health services. It seeks to serve the people who reside in a specific geographic area of a city or a locality that is referred to as a *catchment area*. The workers in the center attempt to assist the community to improve its level of mental health and to help individuals and families who have developed emotional problems to maintain their ties with the community and, when hospitalization is necessary, to return to community living as soon as possible. To achieve these goals it becomes essential that all helping agencies share information freely and cooperate effectively.

Specific requirements for a fully developed comprehensive community mental health center were identified in the law that made government funding available. When fully developed a comprehensive community mental health center includes inpatient and outpatient services, day and night hospital units, crisis intervention centers, halfway houses, family therapy centers, rehabilitation centers, transitional facilities where individuals may receive board and care, and suicide prevention centers. In addition, the community mental health center is expected to offer services to the community that include consultation to community agencies and professional personnel, diagnostic services, and rehabilitative services including vocational and educational programs. Finally, the community mental health center is expected to provide training for professional and paraprofessional workers; to conduct research into the prevention, cause, and treatment of mental illness; and to evaluate the effectiveness of the program being carried forward.

Although inpatient services, outpatient services, and partial hospitalization were required, the government expected individual communities to identify those services that would be developed first, those services that would be emphasized most, and what the specific focus of the outreach centers would be.

The need for suicide prevention and crisis clinics was identified early in the development of some mental health services in some communities, whereas other communities concentrated on the development of day-care and night-care centers. Thus each comprehensive community mental health center developed somewhat differently, depending on the needs of the community it served, the philosophy of the professionals involved in the development of the services, and the relationship the community had with the center.

In spite of many differences there are some significant similarities in comprehensive community mental health centers. There are also departures from the more traditional approach to the treatment of psychiatric problems, including the following:

1. Treatment focuses on helping the individual through the use of groups of which he is a member rather than by relying entirely on the use of the individual one-to-one relationship. Thus the treatment focus may be on family ther-

apy, group therapy, the therapeutic community, or crisis intervention. The development of knowledge and skill in the use of the group process and in intervening therapeutically in crisis situations is essential for all professional workers who hope to be involved with comprehensive community mental health centers.

2. The services of individuals who are already working with the larger population of the catchment area are used. These individuals may include welfare workers, police, clergy, teachers, public health nurses, and other community leaders. Some community mental health centers have involved individuals identified as indigenous workers. These are people who may lack formal education but who have lived in the community and understand the unofficial community organization. They are aware of the real hopes, interests, and concerns of the people. In addition, they speak and understand the language commonly used by the people being served. With professional guidance the indigenous workers have been surprisingly successful in some community mental health centers because of their ability to relate in a meaningful way with the people seeking help and to offer it to them on a level that is acceptable and useful.

3. Role definitions are becoming blurred as the various representatives of the professional disciplines work in the interdisciplinary climate of the comprehensive community mental health centers. All disciplines share treatment responsibilities in these centers. The leadership of the team may be held by any one of its members, depending on the background, experience, interests, and abilities of the individual team members.

4. Prevention is a major focus in community mental health centers. Thus consultation and educational activities become as important in the centers as treatment. Many of the professional workers spend more time in the consultation and educational aspects of their work than in the treatment aspects. They seek to help mothers of children, schoolteachers, public health nurses, workers in the juvenile courts, and individuals employed in social agencies to understand the concepts of mental health and the contribution they

can make in the areas of prevention of mental illness and the promotion of mental health among the groups with whom they deal.

5. Planned social change is another focus of comprehensive community mental health centers. Professional workers are concerned not only with the individuals who seek help but also with the community itself, which is the incubator, in a sense of the word, of the mental health problems from which the population suffers. Thus the professional staff of the community mental health center works to improve the social systems that serve the population within the community, that is, the family, the churches, the schools, the hospitals, recreational facilities, the court system, housing, local government, industry, and so on.

6. Comprehensive and continuous service to the individual is emphasized in community mental health centers. The individual is seen immediately when he presents himself for help. No longer are individuals asked to wait for weeks or months for an appointment. Some clinics are crisis clinics. Others are called *coping clinics* to emphasize the fact that they are available to anyone who feels that he is in some kind of urgent difficulty or trouble and needs help in coping with the situation. Still others are called *walk-in clinics*. Many of these clinics have a psychiatrist available around the clock. Cooperation among agencies is basic if these centers are to offer a comprehensive program that can deal with the range of mental problems that arise in any community.

7. Research into the cause and treatment of mental illness is a part of every well-developed community mental health center.

CONTEMPORARY MENTAL HEALTH DELIVERY SYSTEM

The Community Health Centers Act sought to revolutionize the provision of mental health care by emphasizing prevention and decentralized, local "community treatment" as opposed to "institutional care" for even those persons who manifest severe psychiatric difficulties. There is much debate as to whether these goals are even beginning to be achieved.

It is a fact that the number of actual public mental hospitals has not significantly decreased, although the patient population has become markedly smaller. This phenomenon is thought to be the result of political and economic issues that were not clearly envisioned when the Community Mental Health Centers Act was passed. Because of their size, public mental hospitals are major employers of residents of the community in which they are located. Attempts to close these hospitals have been met by cries of outrage from citizens who would lose their means of livelihood if these institutions were closed. Furthermore, because these mental hospitals are publicly supported, their future is in the hands of elected officials who strongly consider the desires of their constituency. Another factor mitigating against the closure of these institutions is the continuing resistance of most neighborhood groups against having small treatment centers in their midst. Newspapers and television news reports give almost weekly accounts of neighborhoods organizing to prevent the establishment of day treatment facilities, halfway houses, or residential centers for the emotionally ill or the developmentally disabled.

.Despite the decrease in patient population in public mental institutions, the number of admissions to public mental hospitals has increased every year since 1955. This fact becomes somewhat alarming when one realizes that it includes a large number of readmissions. The current early discharge and rapid readmission phenomenon in public mental hospitals is called the *revolving door syndrome.* Although more individuals are now out of the institution and in the community than 25 years ago, there has been considerable public and professional concern regarding the quality of life experienced by many of these individuals. Critics have even suggested that individuals have simply been moved from the back wards of the hospitals to the back alleys of the community.*

The decrease in the size of the population of public mental hospitals may not be due entirely to the community mental health movement. The psychotropic drugs have been widely used since the mid-1950s and have made it possible for many individuals to return to life in the community because of their ability to control behavior with the assistance of the drugs. The growth of nursing homes has occurred over about the same period of time.

*Test, Mary Ann, and Stein, Leonard: Practical guidelines for the community treatment of markedly impaired patients, Community Ment. Health J. **12**:73-74, Fall, 1976.

These facilities have offered an alternative to hospitalization in the public mental hospitals for a large number of aged individuals. In addition, psychiatric units in general hospitals have been developed in many parts of the country. This alternate care facility, where hospitalization benefits are as applicable as for physical illness, has played a part in lowering the rate of admissions to public mental hospitals. Thus it is difficult to evaluate the effect on the public mental hospitals of the community mental health movement. However, the majority of individuals now in the community and being treated through the activities of day-care centers and working in sheltered workshops would probably be hospitalized in public mental institutions if treatment facilities were not available in the community.

Underlying the treatment philosophy of most community mental health centers is the belief that the disturbed behavior of mentally ill individuals responds positively when the person is maintained in the community because, as with all people, the environmental demands are powerful determinants of his behavior. Thus every effort is made to achieve early discharge for mentally ill individuals from short-term treatment centers or day-care facilities. As a result, however, many communities are distressed by the presence of individuals who appear to require 24-hour care.

It seems reasonable to believe that some clients will continue to need long-term treatment situations. Undoubtedly there will continue to be some chronically disturbed individuals of all ages who require close supervision and a rigidly structured environment. To recover, selected individuals need to be removed from their normal surroundings. When this need is not acknowledged and these individuals are hospitalized only for short periods, damage is done to the individual, the community, and the community mental health movement.

To date the community mental health movement has had limited success in treating those mentally ill individuals who are markedly impaired. According to some authorities community treatment of such individuals should focus primarily on the teaching of basic coping skills necessary to live as autonomously as possible. These learning needs include (1) daily living skills, (2) vocational skills, (3) leisure time skills, and (4) social and interpersonal skills. In some situations treatment has been most effective when "taken to the patient" in the individual's natural environment. It is also thought by some that a nonsheltered facility may be more therapeutic than a sheltered arrangement because greater expectations for appropriate, responsible behavior encourage socially acceptable responses.*

Thus far many individuals in this country who are poor and members of minority groups are relatively untouched by the programs provided by community mental health centers. Programs must be developed to meet the needs of these groups, who may not respond positively to therapeutic methods that focus primarily on the sharing of feelings. Instead, these clients often require treatment techniques that emphasize actions rather than words, that deal directly with the problems of living rather than with fantasies, and that provide immediate assistance in coping with emergencies when they arise. These clients respond to therapeutic intervention that assists them to find a job, make friends, improve their domestic relations, improve their physical well-being, and get along better with relatives.†

As time has passed, this nation has become increasingly concerned about human rights. The court system has become an advocate for the client. The individual who is in need of treatment of mental illness now has a legal right to adequate treatment that adheres to minimum professional standards and that is designed appropriately to assist him in solving his problems. Among other legal rights is the right to the least restrictive setting necessary to achieve the treatment he requires and a right to an understandable explanation of the treatment planned for him.

The community mental health approach has been successful in altering the detrimental effects of long-term treatment in public hospitals, in clarifying the legal rights of the mentally ill, and in promoting an enlightened community response to the problems of the mentally ill. Therefore this approach has revolutionized the delivery of mental health services and is here to stay. However, much more needs to be done to develop new treatment methods that will effectively serve clients in relieving psycholog-

---

*Test, Mary Ann, and Stein, Leonard: Practical guidelines for the community treatment of markedly impaired patients, Community Ment. Health J. **12:**73-74, Fall, 1976.

†Levy, Rona: Behavior therapy techniques as a fulfillment of community mental health ideology, Community Ment. Health J. **12:**417-418, Winter, 1976.

ical distress and in intervening in social stress. The preparation and supervision of the workers in many centers must be upgraded. Professional and paraprofessional workers need to work toward solving the conflicts that arise when treatment responsibilities are shared. A more systematic approach to treatment and research is necessary. The requirements of the original act for significant programs in primary prevention, consultation, public education, community planning, and development are all essential factors that need more attention if the goals in the 1963 Community Mental Health Centers Act are to be achieved. Finally, more effective techniques for achieving these goals must be developed.

CONCLUDING STATEMENTS

1. An appreciation of the history of the treatment of the mentally ill can aid in understanding the contemporary systems of mental health delivery.
2. In prehistoric times the mentally ill person was likely to be treated by tribal rites. If these measures were unsuccessful, the victim was abandoned.
3. With the collapse of the Greek and Roman civilizations the humane treatment of the mentally ill deteriorated markedly and patients were flogged, fettered, scourged, and starved in the belief that the devils possessing them could be driven out by these means.
4. In the Middle Ages the evil spirit believed to be causing the patient to behave oddly was "exorcised." Exorcism was performed by a laying on of hands.
5. In the fifteenth century many mentally ill persons traveled to Gheel, Belgium where they believed they would be cured through contact with St. Dymphna, a legendary princess. Many of these pilgrims remained in Gheel and were welcomed into local homes, the forerunner of the contemporary community mental health movement.
6. In England during the sixteenth century keepers of the "lunatic asylums," as they were called, were allowed to exhibit boisterous patients to the public for a small fee, and more harmless patients were forced to beg on the streets of London.
7. In Paris in the seventeenth and eighteenth centuries the insane were kept in dungeons.

8. In 1792 Philippe Pinel (1745-1826), director of the Bicêtre asylum outside of Paris, liberated miserable inmates of two of the largest hospitals for the insane, some of whom had been in chains for 20 years. This was the beginning of many reforms in the care of the mentally ill.

9. In 1756 the Pennsylvania Hospital in Philadelphia was completed. It provided good custodial care for insane patients.

10. Benjamin Rush (1745-1813), who is known as the father of American psychiatry, began work at the Pennsylvania Hospital in 1783.

11. About 1830 a movement to erect suitable hospitals for the mentally ill swept the United States.

12. The first public psychiatric hospital in America was built in Williamsburg, Virginia, in 1773 and is still being used today under the name of the Eastern Psychiatric Hospital.

13. Dorothea Lynde Dix (1802-1887) effected tremendous reforms in the care of the mentally ill in the United States. She played an important role in founding St. Elizabeth's Hospital in Washington, D.C.

14. Most of the state hospitals of the late nineteenth century were located in remote rural regions of each state. Although many patients were exploited for their labor they were usually afforded some degree of comfort. This fact, combined with their isolation led to the syndrome of *institutionalization*.

15. The rapid increase in the number of mentally ill persons hospitalized in state mental hospitals was due in large part to the waves of immigrants to the United States. By the twentieth century, the state hospital system had turned into an inefficient, expensive, and inhumane system.

16. In 1908 Clifford Beers, a former mental patient, wrote *A Mind That Found Itself*, which revolutionized thinking about prevention and early recognition of mental illness.

17. Clifford Beers founded the National Committee for Mental Hygiene, which spearheaded the mental hygiene movement and initiated child guidance, prison psychiatry, and vocational guidance.

18. Sigmund Freud (1856-1939) revolutionized thinking about the mind and brought the subject of human behavior to the attention of the public.

19. The National Mental Health Act of 1946 supported the first

broad-based national approach to the long-neglected problems of mental illness and the promotion of mental health.

20. In 1956 the first of the many psychotropic drugs, chlorpromazine (Thorazine), was adopted for use in the care of the mentally ill. Under the influence of psychotropic drugs the atmosphere of disturbed wards changed dramatically.

21. *Action for Mental Health,* a report of the Joint Commission on Mental Illness published in 1961, provided an impetus for developing more effective services for people in need of psychiatric help and was the basis for additional legislation.

22. The Community Mental Health Centers Act of 1963 shifted the focus of mental health care from large publicly supported institutions to community-based centers.

23. When fully developed, a comprehensive community mental health center includes inpatient and outpatient services, crisis intervention and suicide prevention centers, facilities for partial hospitalization, consultation and education services, diagnostic services, rehabilitation services, training for professional and paraprofessional workers, and a research program.

24. Each comprehensive community mental health center has developed differently, depending on the needs of the community it serves, the philosophy of the professional workers involved, and the relationship of the community to the center.

25. Treatment in the comprehensive community mental health center focuses on helping individuals through the use of a variety of group techniques.

26. Role definitions are becoming blurred as representatives of several professional disciplines work together in an interdisciplinary climate.

27. Comprehensive community mental health centers focus on (a) prevention, (b) planned social change, (c) comprehensive and continuous service to the client, (d) research into the cause and treatment of mental illness, and (e) consultation and community education.

28. Public mental hospitals have not disappeared, but their patient population has grown markedly smaller. Unfortunately a tremendous number of admissions are readmissions, reflecting the phenomenon of the *revolving door syndrome.*

29. It seems reasonable to believe that long-term treatment situations will be needed for selected clients for many years to come.
30. More effective treatment programs must be developed to provide the assistance required by the poor and by the members of minority groups, who respond best to action-oriented techniques.

SUGGESTED SOURCES OF ADDITIONAL INFORMATION

Classical

Angrist, Shirley S.: The mental hospital; its history and destiny, Perspect. Psychiatr. Care **1:**20-26, Dec., 1963.

Beers, Clifford: A mind that found itself, New York, 1948, Doubleday & Co., Inc.

Bulbuylan, Ann, Davidites, Rose Marie, and Williams, Florence: Nurses in a community mental health center, Am. J. Nurs. **69:**328-331, 1969.

Caplan, Gerald: An approach to community mental health, New York, 1966, Grune & Stratton, Inc.

Carty, Rita Cardillo, and Breault, Gretchen Clemento: Gheel: a comprehensive community mental health program, Perspect. Psychiatr. Care **5:**281-285, Nov.-Dec., 1967.

Elwell, Richard: Community mental health centers, and community mental health nursing, Am. J. Nurs. **70:**1014-1021, 1970.

Freed, Harvey M., et al.: Community mental health-second class treatment? Ment. Hyg. **56:**26-29, Summer, 1972.

Gorman, Mike: Community mental health: the search for identity. Community Ment. Health J. **6:**347-355, Oct., 1970.

Grinker, Roy R.: Mid-century psychiatry, Springfield, Ill., 1953, Charles C Thomas, Publisher.

Joint Commission on Mental Illness and Health: Action for mental health, New York, 1961, Basic Books, Inc., Publishers.

Marshall, Helen E.: Dorothea Dix, forgotten samaritan, New York, 1967, Russell Sage Foundation.

Margolin, Reuben J.: A concept of mental illness: a new look at some old assumptions, Community Ment. Health J. **4:**417-424, Oct., 1968.

Mereness, Dorothy: The potential significant role of the nurse in community mental health services, Perspect. Psychiatr. Care **1:**34-39, May-July, 1963.

Mistr, Virginia R.: Community nursing service for psychiatric patients, Perspect. Psychiatr. Care **6:**36-41, Jan.-Feb., 1968.

Ozarin, Lucy D.: The community mental health center: concept and commitment, Ment. Hyg. **52:**76-80, 1968.

Richards, Hilda: The role of the nurse in therapy of lower socioeconomic psychiatric patients. Perspect. Psychiatr. Care **5:**82-91, March-April, 1967.

Sheldon, Alan, and Hope, Penelope: The developing role of the nurse in a community mental health program, Perspect. Psychiatr. Care **5:**272-279, Nov.-Dec., 1967.

Stretch, John J.: Community mental health: the evolution of a concept in social policy, Community Ment. Health J. **3:**5-12, Spring, 1967.

Ujhely, Gertrud B.: The nurse in community psychiatry, Am. J. Nurs. **69:**1001-1005, 1969.

Zahourek, Rothlyn: Nurses in a community mental health center, Nurs. Outlook **19:**592-595, 1971.

Contemporary

Adler, Peter T.: The community as a mental health system, Ment. Hyg. **56:**29-32, Fall, 1972.

Ames, David: The limits of general hospital care: a continuing role for state hospitals, Hosp. Community Psychiatry **34:**145-150, Feb., 1983.

Anchor Mental Health Association: Community support services for adult psychiatric outpatients, Hosp. Community Psychiatry **31:**693-696, Oct., 1980.

Bayer, Mary: Easing mental patients' return to their communities, Am. J. Nurs. **76:**406-608, 1976.

Bellak, Leopold, and Barten, Harvey H., editors: Progress in community mental health, vol. 3, New York, 1975, Brunner/Mazel, Inc.

Carter, A.B.: Rural emergency psychiatric services, Am. J. Nurs. **73:**868-869, 1973.

Carter, James: Treating black patients: the risk of ignoring critical social issues, Hosp. Community Psychiatry **32:**281-282, April, 1981.

Caton, Carol, Goldstein, Jill, Serrano, Oscar, and Bender, Rose: The impact of discharge planning on chronic schizophrenic patients, Hosp. Community Psychiatry **35:**255-262, March, 1984.

Collins, James, Mathura, Clyde, and Rosher, Debra: Training psychiatric staff to treat a multicultural patient population, Hosp. Community Psychiatry **35:**372-376, April, 1984.

Davies, M.: Continuity care unit: a model of services for chronic psychiatric patients, J. Psychosol. Nurs. Ment. Health Serv. **19:**42-45, Feb., 1981.

Donaldson, Ken: Looking back, Ment. Hyg. **60:**5-9, Spring, 1976.

Geller, Joseph J.: The relationship between psychoanalysis and the Community Mental Health Program, Perspect. Psychiatr. Care **13:**113-118, July-Sept., 1975.

Gorman, Mike: Community absorption of the mentally ill: the new challenge, Community Ment. Health J. **12:**119-127, Summer, 1976.

Hitchcock, Janice E.: Community mental health nursing: an innovative use of the nurse's evolving role, Community Ment. Health J. **7:**3-12, March, 1971.

Huey, Karen: Conference report—patient re-entry into the community, Hosp. Community Psychiatry **31:**52-56, Jan., 1980.

Johns, Marion Meaux: What has been done about the mental health of minorities? Ment. Hyg. **60:**21-30, Spring, 1976.

Jones, Robert: Street people and psychiatry: an introduction, Hosp. Community Psychiatry **34:**807-812, Sept., 1983.

Kaplan, Howard M., and Bohr, Ronald H.: Change in the mental health field, Community Ment. Health J. **12:**244-251, Fall, 1976.

Krauss, Judith B.: The chronic psychiatric patient in the community—a model of care, Nurs. Outlook **28:**308-314, May, 1980.

Lamb, H. Richard: Deinstitutionalization and the homeless mentally ill, Hosp. Community Psychiatry **35:**910-913, Sept., 1984.

Lamb, H. Richard: Young adult chronic patients: the new drifters, Hosp. Community Psychiatry **33:**465-468, June, 1982.

Lamb, H. Richard, and Peile, Roger: The need for continuing asylum and sanctuary, Hosp. Community Psychiatry **35:**798-802, Aug., 1984.

Langsley, Donald, and Barter, James: Psychiatric roles in the community mental health center, Hosp. Community Psychiatry **34:**729-733, Aug., 1983.

Lego, Suzanne: The community mental health system: is it an improvement over the old system? Perspect. Psychiatr. Care **13:**105-112, July-Sept., 1975.

Levy, Rona L.: Behavior therapy techniques as a fulfillment of community mental health ideology, Community Ment. Health J. **12:**415-421, Winter, 1976.

Lewis, Nolan D.C.: American psychiatry from its beginning to World War II. In Arieti, Silvano, editor: The American handbook of psychiatry, vol. 1, ed. 2, New York, 1974, Basic Books, Inc., Publishers, pp. 28-42.

Lowery, Barbara J., and Janulis, Diane: Community mental health and the unanswered questions, Perspect. Psychiatr. Care **11:**26-28, Jan., 1973.

Lyon, Glee G., and Hitchins Emily A.: Ways of intervening with the psychotic individual in the community, Am. J. Nurs. **79:**490-493, March, 1979.

Mark, Barbara: From "lunatic" to "client": 300 years of psychiatric patienthood, J. Psychosoc. Nurs. Ment. Health Serv. **18:**31-36, March, 1980.

Miles, James: A psychiatric outreach project to a rural community, Hosp. Community Psychiatry **31:**822-825, Dec., 1980.

Mirelowitz, Seymour: Alienation and bureaucratization of mental health organizations, Ment. Hyg. **56:**6-21, Winter, 1972.

Morrissey, Joseph, and Goldman, Howard: Cycles of reform in the care of the chronically mentally ill, Hosp. Community Psychiatry **35:**785-792, Aug., 1984.

Murray, Jacquelyn E.: Failure of the community mental health movement, Am. J. Nurs. **75:**2034-2036, 1975.

President's Commission on Mental Health: Report to the President, vol. 1, Washington, D.C., 1978.

Rosenblatt, Aaron: Concepts of the asylum in the care of the mentally ill, Hosp. Community Psychiatry **35:**244-250, March, 1984.

Rosen, Arnold, Olarte, Silvia, and Masnik, Ruth: Utilization patterns in an urban ghetto area, Hosp. Community Psychiatry **31:**702-704, Oct., 1980.

Ruiz, Pedro, and Langrod, John: The role of folk healers in community mental health services, Community Ment. Health J. **12:**392-398, Winter, 1976.

Schlesinger, Roxy: Cross-cultural psychiatry: the applicability of Western anglo psychiatry to Asian-Americans of Chinese and Japanese ethnicity, J. Psychosoc. Nurs. Ment. Health Serv. **19:**26-30, Sept. 1981.

Silverman, Wade H., and Val, Eduardo: Day hospital in the context of a community mental health program, Community Ment. Health J. **11:**82-90, Spring, 1975.

Stein, Edna, and Sorenson, Karl Dan: A cooperative apartment for transitional patients, Ment. Hygiene **56:**68-74, Winter, 1972.

Test, Mary Ann, and Stein, Leonard I.: Practical guidelines for the community treatment of markedly impaired patients, Community Ment. Health J. **12:**72-82, Spring, 1976.

Thompson, James, Bass, Rosalyn, and Witkin, Michael: Fifty years of psychiatric services: 1940-1990, Hosp. Community Psychiatry **33:**711-717, Sept., 1982.

Tripp-Reimer, Toni, Brink, Pamela, and Saunders, Judith: Cultural assessment: content and process, Nurs. Outlook **32:**78-82, March/April, 1984.

Two hundred years of mental health care in America: Hosp. Community Psychiatry (entire issue), July, 1976.

Weinstein, Abbot, and Cohen, Morris: Young chronic patients and changes in the state hospital population, Hosp. Community Psychiatry **35:**595-600, June, 1984.

Wilson, Lawrence, Ries, Richard, and Bokan, John: The community mental health center: does it treat patients? Hosp. Community Psychiatry **31:**815-819, Dec., 1980.

Of particular interest

Jansson, D.P.: Return to society: problematic features of the re-entry process, Perspect. Psychiatr. Care **13:**136, 1975.
Some of the realities of the reentry process are discussed here with recommendations for interventions to accomplish this process effectively.

Pardes, H., and Pincus, H.: Treatment in the seventies: a decade of refinement, Hosp. Community Psychiatry **31:**535-542, Aug., 1980.
This article is a review of the changes in the treatment of mental disorders over the decade of the seventies.

Scholberg, H., Becker, A., and McGrath, M.: Planning the phasedown of mental hospitals, Community Ment. Health J. **12:,** Spring, 1976.
This article addresses some of the challenges to the accomplishment of continuity of care in the community mental health model.

chapter two

the mental health team

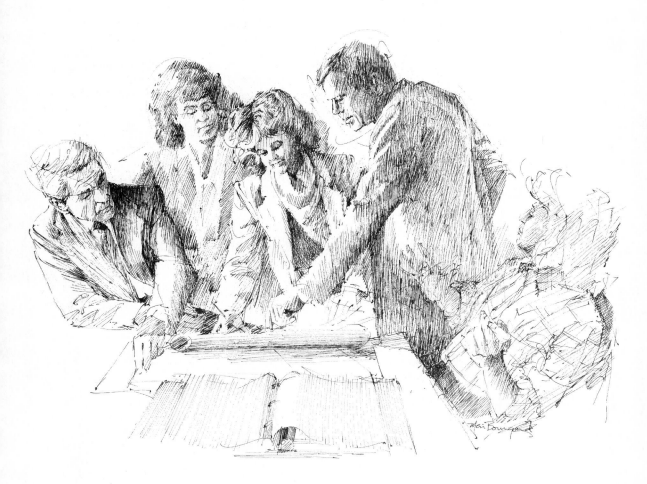

Which one of us is best prepared to be the primary therapist for Mrs. Jackson?

LEARNING OBJECTIVES

After studying this chapter the student will be able to:

1   State the origins of the health care specialties of psychiatric nursing, psychiatry, psychology, psychiatric social work, and activity therapies.

2   Differentiate among the roles and functions of the psychiatrist, psychologist, psychiatric social worker, and activity therapist.

3   Describe the roles and functions of the nurse who works in a mental health setting.

Four health care professions constitute the core mental health disciplines: psychiatric nursing, psychiatry, clinical psychology, and psychiatric social work. They all emerged as specialties within their repsective professions during the last half of the nineteenth century at the time when behaviorally disturbed persons were generally viewed as being ill rather than as being possessed by demons or morally corrupt.

HISTORICAL PERSPECTIVE

The first school of nursing in a psychiatric setting was established at McLean Hospital in 1882, 9 years after the first schools of nursing in the United States had been founded. Up to this time poorly trained, nonprofessional workers had dominated the care of patients in psychiatric institutions and the purpose of this school was to improve the care of the mentally ill by upgrading the skills of attendants. The first class of 15 women graduated in 1886. By 1917 41 mental institutions were operating training schools for nurses. Unfortunately, the standards for admission and graduation established by most of these schools were much lower than those of schools of nursing in general hospitals. Beginning in 1906 nurse educators began to work toward establishing affiliations in psychiatric situations for students enrolled in schools of nursing in general hospitals but it was not until 1955 that all schools of nursing offered an experience in psychiatric nursing as a required part of the curriculum. Schools of nursing in psychiatric hospitals no longer exist.

Although the superintendents of the asylums were physicians, the specialty of psychiatry was not known until 1846 when the practice of hospitalizing the mentally ill made possible the systematic observation and study of mental disorders. It was not until after World War I that the specialty was given any significant attention in the curriculums of medical schools.

Unlike psychiatry, which had its origin in the practice setting, psychology began within the university as an academic, research-oriented discipline, devoted to the scholarly study of human behavior. The first psychological clinic was established in 1896 at the University of Pennsylvania, followed shortly by the establishment of psychological laboratories in such hospitals for the mentally disturbed as McLean Hospital in Massachusetts, St. Elizabeth's Hospital in Washington, D.C., and Boston Psychopathic Hospital.

Social work began as an organized profession in the 1870s but the specialty of psychiatric social work did not emerge until 1906 as a result of the aftercare movement, which was designed to provide adequate financial, medical, and moral assistance to patients released from mental hospitals. Mary C. Jarrett, believed to be the first psychiatric social worker, directed the first formal training course for psychiatric social workers at Smith College in 1918.

Emphasis on prevention and recognition of early stages of mental illness began in the early part of the twentieth century, largely due to the efforts of Clifford Beers. Having spent several years in various mental institutions as a patient, he emerged in 1907 to write his famous book *A Mind That Found Itself*. This book about his experience as a mentally ill patient provided the impetus for the beginning of the mental health movement in the United States.

Child guidance clinics developed and flourished in this country from the early 1920s through the 1930s. The staffing pattern of the traditional clinic team, which included a psychiatrist, a psychologist, and a social worker is a heritage from this era. The nurse was omitted from this pattern. This oversight was undoubtedly related to the prevailing view of the role of women at that time as well as to the belief that the nurse's expertise lay solely in caring for the physically ill. Because most children who required help from child guidance clinics were not physically ill, the usefulness of the nurse in such clinics was thought to be limited or nonexistent.

The number of mental health professionals remained relatively small for the first half of the twentieth century because there was little to attract persons to the field. However, at the conclusion of World War II, the nation was shocked to learn that there had been more psychiatric casualties than injuries caused by combat. This realization led to the passage of the National Mental Health Act in 1946 and the establishment of the National Institute of Mental Health in 1949. In 1950 training grants were provided for the preparation of psychiatrists, psychologists, psychiatric social workers, and psychiatric nurses. These federal funds dramatically increased the number of health care professionals prepared to care for the mentally ill. The provision of training funds for nurses along with the other three disciplines firmly established the nurse as an integral part of the mental health team.

Although not considered a core mental health discipline, no discussion of the mental health team would be complete without mention of the activity therapies. The disciplines that make up the activity therapies include occupational therapy, recreational therapy, music therapy, rehabilitation counseling, educational therapy, and patient library services (bibliotherapy). Within these specialties other services may be provided, such as dance therapy, drama therapy, art therapy, horticulture therapy, and manual arts therapy. The history of occupational therapy, the oldest of the activity therapies, is cited here because of its intimate connection with nursing.

The first book written on the subject of occupational therapy was written by a nurse, Susan E. Tracy. This book, *Studies in Invalid Occupation*, was published in 1910. Miss Tracy also gave the first course of instruction on the subject in 1906 at the Adams Nervine in Boston. As such, nurses were the first occupational therapists, although that term was not used until 1921.

Some physicians also saw the potential therapeutic benefit of a planned activities program. As early as 1892 Dr. E.N. Brush wrote that even the most simple and routine tasks keep the mind occupied, awaken new trains of thought and interest, and divert the client from the delusions or hallucinations that harass and annoy him. Dr. Brush particularly advocated the use of outdoor activities in the belief that physical exertion had a beneficial effect on the emotional health of the client. Since the nursing staff was responsible for initiating and supervising all client activities, a book titled *Occupation Therapy, a Manual for Nurses* was published in 1915. The author was Dr. William Rush Dunton, one of the earliest leaders in the field of occupational therapy. Dr. Dunton advised that the nurse "provide herself with an armamentarium which should consist at least of the following: playing cards, dominoes or card dominoes, cribbage board, scrap book with puzzles and catches, and one or more picture puzzles. . . . She is also urged to cultivate a particular craft in order that she may herself have a hobby and also that she may have special ability in instructing her client."*

ROLES AND FUNCTIONS OF MENTAL HEALTH PROFESSIONALS

Nurses are professionals whose initial educational preparation is through an associate degree, baccalaureate degree, or diploma program. After this preparation the nurse becomes licensed as a registered nurse through successful completion of state board examinations. Without additional educational or experiential preparation this nurse can function as a generalist in any setting. An increasing number of nurses with baccalaureate degrees have continued their education to attain master's degrees in a particular clinical specialty. Nurses prepared at the graduate level in psychiatric-mental health nursing have advanced preparation in promoting the mental health of individuals, groups, families, and communities, as well as in assisting these persons in increasing the effectiveness of their adaptations. The nursing profession administers an examination process whereby these expert nurses can be certified, although there is no legal mandate requiring this. It is becoming increasingly common to refer to the nurse with a master's degree in psychiatric-mental health nursing as a *psychiatric nurse* and to the nurse without a master's degree who works with the mentally ill as *a nurse who works in a mental health setting*. This distinction is more than a semantic one, indicating the fact that psychiatric nursing is a specialty in nursing. The specific roles and functions of the nurse who works in a mental health setting are discussed in detail later in this chapter.

Psychiatrists are physicians who have had several years of supervised residency training in the medical specialty of psychiatry. The law does not require licensing beyond that necessary for any physician, but the medical profession makes available a vol-

*Dunton, William Rush: Occupation therapy, a manual for nurses, Philadelphia, 1915, W.B. Saunders Co., p.8.

untary examination in this clinical specialty. Physicians who successfully complete this examination are "Board Certified" and identify themselves as such. This designation helps to ensure the lay public of the services of a physician with advanced knowledge and experience in psychiatry. Psychiatrists function in private practice as well as treating hospitalized clients. In the latter instance the psychiatrist may be the leader of the treatment team, although there is a trend toward the treatment team leader being the person who is most knowledgeable about the client, regardless of professional discipline. The psychiatrist's unique function is the prescribing of medications and the administration of other somatic treatments such as electroconvulsive therapy. In addition the psychiatrist is the only professional equipped to make a medical diagnosis and is particularly skilled in identifying and treating persons whose problems have highly interrelated emotional and physiological components.

Psychologists are professionals who have advanced education in the study of mental processes and the treatment of mental disorders. They are not physicians but hold doctoral degrees. As is true in the field of medicine and nursing, psychology has become such a broad discipline that most psychologists specialize. Those who are most directly involved in the diagnosis of mental illness and in the treatment of the emotionally ill are called *clinical psychologists*. Those clinical psychologists concerned with the diagnosis of mental illness have developed expertise in the use of inferential tools that are designed to assist in the diagnostic process and assessment of treatment effects. Such tools are projective techniques best exemplified by the Rorschach test, personality inventories such as the Minnesota Multiphasic Personality Inventory, and intelligence tests. Only clinical psychologists are trained in the use and interpretation of these highly complex instruments. Other clinical psychologists have chosen to develop expertise in the treatment of the emotionally ill. Since the entire education of these psychologists has been geared to the study of human behavior, they are particularly effective when the problems of the individual or the family are clearly psychogenic in origin and manifestation. Most clinical psychologists work in close collaboration with a psychiatrist who assists in the treatment program if somatic therapies seem indicated. Some states make legal certification mandatory for practice as a clinical psychologist.

Social workers are health professionals many of whom have educational preparation at the master's degree level. Although social workers are prepared to work with individuals and families who have a wide variety of physical, emotional, and social problems, some specialize in psychiatric social work. *Psychiatric social workers* are particularly skilled in assessing familial, environmental, and social factors that contribute to the dysfunctional behavior of the individual and the family. They also are major contributors to the planning and implementation of follow-up care.

All *activity therapists* are required to hold a minimum of a bachelor's degree in their field and many have advanced degrees. A master's degree is required for entry into art therapy. Although each form of activity therapy has a specific focus, they share the principle that it is helpful to the emotionally disturbed person to be engaged in an activity that focuses on objects outside himself. The concept of *object relations* is a fundamental one in activity therapies. This concept includes not only the materials used in the therapy but also the setting, the therapist, and the other participants. These objects all have symbolic value, and through their use the individual expresses feelings, needs, and impulses. In this sense, all activity therapies are creative and therefore can be used in varying ways and for varied purposes. They are developed into a program based on psychodynamic insights but are highly individualized to meet the needs of the person for whom they are designed.

The following four goals are common to all activity therapies in a mental health setting:

1. To provide opportunities for structured normal activities of daily living. Activities are designed to help the clients deal with their basic problems. In addition, the activities permit the maintenance as well as reinforcement of the healthy aspects of the client's personality.
2. To assist in diagnostic and personality evaluation. As trained members of the health care team, activity therapists can assist with diagnostic and personality evaluations through their observations of clients as they participate in

the activities. In addition, the process of participation, such as the type of activity chosen and the interaction that takes place between the client and the therapist and between the client and other participants, gives the therapist much valuable information about the personality structure of the client.

3. To enhance psychotherapy and other psychotherapeutic measures. The activity prescribed for the client often provides a nonverbal means for the client to express and resolve the feelings that are being discussed verbally in other settings. In addition, the interpersonal relationship established between the client and the therapist provides another vehicle for the provision of corrective emotional experiences.

4. To assist the client in making the transition from the sick role to becoming a contributing member of society. Some activities provide opportunity for work experience, often with the use of community resources. Through these activities the client is able to learn a skill that may be marketable. Other activities in this category focus on the development of the client's talents and interests so that he might learn to use his time in ways that are satisfying to him.

All activity therapies have in common the fact that they are designed to achieve a specified goal, and the role of the therapist is to observe, direct, and guide the client in the activity. The therapist continuously assesses the client's reactions to the activity both as a means of providing information to other members of the treatment team and as a basis on which to alter the activity as the needs of the client change.

It should be noted that anyone may legally call himself or herself a psychotherapist or psychoanalyst, and these designations do not guarantee a level of expertise. All reputable therapists and analysts, however, have years of advanced education and supervised clinical training in their particular discipline.

ROLES AND FUNCTIONS OF THE NURSE

The nurse's role shifts frequently as she strives to make her contacts with clients therapeutic. She is the creator of a therapeutic environment when she provides opportunities for clients to experience acceptance in the milieu. Frequently she fills the role of socializing agent when she helps individuals or groups to plan and participate in social events. The nurse finds that she must assume the role of counselor when clients need someone to listen with understanding and empathy while they talk about troublesome problems. The nurse is sometimes a teacher, especially when she helps clients learn to function in more socially acceptable ways. Frequently she fills the role of mother surrogate when she gives emotional support and understanding or when she performs a nurturing activity such as feeding a client. Sometimes she functions in the familiar technical role of nurse as she performs such nursing duties as administering medications or treatments. Some nurses who have advanced educational preparation function in the therapist role by meeting with individuals, families, or groups at specified times and engaging them in a process designed to help them make fundamental system changes.

The nurse probably never functions in any single role at any given time; usually she fulfills all or several of them at once. For the sake of clarity, however, these roles will be discussed separately.

The nurse as creator of a therapeutic environment

One of the major therapeutic contributions the nurse can make is to develop a warm, accepting atmosphere. Although this atmosphere is related superficially to the furnishings and decor of the environment, these attributes are no substitute for genuine human warmth, which springs solely from other human beings. If the situation is to be therapeutic for clients, it is essential that the nursing staff who are in close daily contact with the clients be honest, sincere, friendly people who really care about others. If the nurse is able to establish a warm, accepting atmosphere, the way will have been prepared so that the contributions of all members of the mental health treatment team can be of maximum effectiveness.

A feeling of security is an essential element in developing a therapeutic climate. When clients are provided with an emotionally secure climate, feelings of acceptance, friendliness, warmth, safety, and relaxation are present. Many emotionally ill people enter a treatment setting because they are fearful, anxiety-ridden, and insecure in their relationships with other people. A therapeutic climate should make it possible for such individuals to behave as they need to behave because of their illness, secure in the knowledge that they will not be rejected and that they do not need to fear retaliation.

Another essential element in creating a therapeutic climate is an attitude that anticipates positive change and growth. If the climate is to be therapeutic everyone working with clients must project an attitude that encourages improvement and positive change in behavior.

The nurse as socializing agent

Another important role is that of socializing agent. In fulfilling this role the nurse helps clients participate successfully in group activities. Physical facilities in many mental health settings are ideal for organizing and directing group activities. In a residential setting, group activities are particularly needed during that period in the day which comes after the evening meal. Many scheduled activities stop before supper, and clients are frequently faced with long, unoccupied evenings. The nurse who cares for clients during the evening hours has a significant opportunity to contribute to the mental health of these persons. Such a simple activity as an evening snack period can be the focus for group singing, group games, or group conversation. Activities organized by the clients themselves uncover and use hidden talent. In this way the group has an opportunity to recognize and encourage its own members and to contribute to developing the strengths of individuals. A dining room situation may lend itself to group activity. In such a situation the nurse has an opportunity to create an experience from which a feeling of belonging can develop. Mealtime is too often viewed solely from the standpoint of nutrition. Sometimes clients are hurried so that the staff can get on to some other activity. Conversation is sometimes discouraged because it slows up eating. The nurse who is with clients during mealtime may view her task solely from the standpoint of getting the clients fed as efficiently and quickly as possible. When the nurse ascribes to these views, she misses a valuable opportunity to facilitate positive learning experiences for clients.

In a nonresidential treatment setting, the nurse can assist clients to improve their social skills by introducing them to each other and then encouraging conversation by bringing up a neutral topic such as the weather. The community-based nurse who sits in an office waiting for the client to keep his appointment misses an important opportunity to assist clients to develop social skills in the common social setting of the waiting room.

The nurse makes a contribution to improving the social skills of clients by encouraging and developing the healthy aspects of their personalities. Many mentally ill persons have used withdrawal because of their extreme sensitivity and anxiety in relation to other people. The treatment setting provides opportunities for these individuals to learn to achieve success in social situations by creating opportunities through which they develop feelings of security with other people.

The nurse as counselor

Empathic listening is another important aspect of psychiatric nursing. There is probably no more important task than listening to a client in a positive, dynamic, empathic way without at the same time giving advice, stating opinions, or making suggestions. This type of active listening encourages the client to think through his problems and to arrive at a decision that is helpful to him. It helps the client to discharge anxiety and tension. It tells the client that the nurse really cares.

Empathic listening demands a great deal from the nurse both in time and emotional energy. It demands that she be skillful in reflecting the client's comments to him in such a manner that he will realize she is interested in the discussion and wants to hear as much as he needs to tell. Some nurses may not understand the vital importance of this kind of listening and may feel that they should stop the client's outpouring of problems. Unfortunately this is easily done by a comment such as, "You can tell all that to your therapist tomorrow. He's the one who needs to know these things." The nurse may respond with the even less helpful comment, "Things will be better tomorrow. Just keep a stiff upper lip." Clients often share their problems more freely with the nurse than with anyone else. The nurse and the other members of the mental health team need to determine their mutually therapeutic roles with the client so the nurse and client can assess which concerns may appropriately be channeled to which team member.

The role of the nurse is to help the client with problems of reality that deal with the here and now. There are scores of times when clients discuss problems with the nurse that do deal with the areas that are her special concern, and it is in these situations that her role as a counselor is most frequently helpful.

Among the nurse's therapeutic responsibilities as a counselor is the giving of reassurance. Many situations in the life of a client require that someone give some reassurance. Sometimes the nurse may suggest that reassurance should more logically be provided by the psychiatrist, religious counselor, or social worker. The nurse needs to learn what services are available and how she can help to procure the assistance the client needs. However, more often than not it is up to the nurse to provide the needed reassurance. Such needs appear in every area of the client's life. There is the client who cannot sleep because he fears the treatment scheduled for the morning; the client who is upset because her husband did not visit as he had promised and she is now sure that he does not love her; the client who believes he is doomed forever because he has committed an unpardonable sin; and the client who is afraid of everything. The list is endless, and the needs for reassurance frequently appear at 11 PM or at 3 AM when no help may be readily available. It is for this reason that many day-care centers provide staff members who are available by phone during the entire 24-hour period. Often the staff members are nurses or trained mental health aides whose prompt intervention can prevent the need for hospitalization.

Obviously no set of rules or suggestions will serve as a solution in each of these many situations. Probably the most effective reassurance for fearful, upset clients is a nursing staff that does not change frequently and whose members are consistently kind and accepting. Sitting beside a client may in itself be reassuring to him. This may help him feel that someone on whom he can depend is there, ready to help in whatever way possible. Listening is one of the better ways of offering reassurance. Although logical, reasonable answers are frequently not helpful, they may be reassuring for some clients. Effective reassurance is dependent on the situation, the nurse, her relationship with the client, and his personality. Obviously a suspicious client will require a different kind of help than will a depressed one.

Another aspect of the nurse's counseling role is in helping clients find acceptable outlets for anxiety. The client who is found sobbing hopelessly may be helped by a simple suggestion that she walk up and down the hallway with the nurse. Another client who is tense or excited may respond to the nurse's suggestion that she take a warm tub bath before going to bed. Some other ways in which the nurse may help clients find outlets for anxieties include assisting clients to participate in simple tasks, to become involved in some group activity, or to talk about their feelings.

**The nurse as
teacher**

If purposeful therapeutic interventions can provide the individual with opportunities to learn to live more happily and more successfully with other people, they will make a significant contribution to the client's emotional growth. If the client is merely treated for the purpose of safeguarding his family, the community, or himself, and if he relies entirely on the judgment of professional personnel, it is questionable how worthwhile the experience can be. It is in helping the client to learn to cope in a more mature way with interpersonal relationships that the nurse has a role as a teacher.

Problems of behavior manifested by mentally ill persons are as varied as life itself and encompass every aspect of living. Some clients, like children, must learn many simple tasks involved in living. They need help in learning to dress appropriately for the occasion; to assume responsibility for tasks assigned; to care for physical needs so that they can be acceptable to others; to eat in socially prescribed ways; to accept a reasonably flexible schedule for eating, sleeping, and bathing; and to cope with many other aspects of group living.

The nurse may fill the role of teacher as she helps a client learn a new game, dance step, or song so that he may participate more actively in recreation. She may actually take the role of dance partner or may participate in a game to help a shy, frightened client become integrated into a group. The nurse may participate in an activity requiring only two persons to help a hostile, suspicious client learn that some people can be trusted. She may continue to participate with this client over a period of time until he is able to participate in a group activity without her supporting presence.

In her role as a teacher the nurse helps clients learn to participate in more socially acceptable and satisfying living activities.

**The nurse as
mother surrogate**

Traditionally in this culture the nurse has been a trusted person who performs personal services for sick people. Many of these services are similar to those a mother performs for children. Nurses who consistently function in mental health settings almost invariably become mother surrogates for some of the clients with whom they are closely associated. The role of mother surrogate is part of the traditional role of the nurse, and, although it does not imply becoming the client's mother, it includes many mothering activities that may be required for some persons who are mentally ill. Although most mentally ill persons are able to bathe, dress, and feed themselves, there are a few who are too emotionally ill to carry out these simple tasks. For some of these persons the nurse may need to assume the traditional protective, supportive, mothering role when she gives physical care.

The nurse, like an effective mother, realizes that is is important for clients to assume responsibility for their own physical care as soon as possible. Thus she gives physical care to emotionally ill persons in an empathic and understanding way but looks for and seizes every opportunity to encourage them to assume responsibility for their own care as soon as possible. The effective nurse withdraws from the task of feeding or bathing a client just as rapidly as he is able to take over the responsibility for himself. In this way the nurse supports the client's increasing autonomy.

The nurse not only carries out the mothering role in relation to the physical needs of clients, but she is also like a mother in relation to managing the treatment setting. It is she who develops many of the policies concerning the environment, that profoundly affect the clients' lives. She is indirectly responsible for almost every aspect of the time the client spends in the treatment setting, from housekeeping to securing emergency medical care. The nurse sets the tone of the treatment situation, much as a mother sets the tone of the family.

One of the most therapeutic aspects of the nurse's traditional role as mother surrogate is in assisting individuals and groups of clients to set limits for their own behavior. This aspect of the nurse's role probably overlaps the teacher role.

Clients who interact with each other over time may react toward each other as if they were members of the same family. These reactions are usually unconscious but are nonetheless real and may serve as a basis for much emotional and social unlearning and relearning. Therefore the nurse's role as mother surrogate offers her an opportunity to provide clients with healthy experiences in the area of emotional relationships.

While serving as the object of many of the angry, hostile feelings that some clients cannot otherwise admit or express, the nurse may be able to supply the warm, accepting, nurturing relationship that some persons require to move toward more mature behavior. In conjunction with other members of the mental health team, the nurse is able to provide experiences that may prove to be corrective of the client's earlier unsatisfactory interpersonal experiences.

The technical nursing role

The traditional role of the nurse includes those technical aspects involved in pouring and administering medications, monitoring vital signs, carrying out medical and surgical treatments, and observing and recording client behavior. Recently numerous nurses have become skilled in performing routine physical examinations. This activity, once limited to physicians, is becoming increasingly important for nurses to master as the inextricable relationship between the mind and body is recognized. Occasionally a mentally ill person can accept a nurse as a helpful counselor or teacher only after her ability to carry out the technical aspects of the role has been demonstrated. Therefore the nurse needs to be alert to the fact that such procedures as administering medications and taking vital signs provide her with an opportunity to enhance the therapeutic relationship with the client as well as to achieve the primary goal of the procedure.

One of the nurse's most significant responsibilities is the accurate and perceptive observation and recording of the client's behavior. In carrying out this function skillfully and meaningfully the nurse contributes to the understanding that all members of the mental health team bring to bear on the client's problems. Nurses are the professional persons who are with clients for the longest period of time; as such they have a unique opportunity to help other professional workers understand clients' needs through effective recording of samples of conversation, sleep patterns, interpersonal relationships, socialization activities, and descriptions of personal habits.

It is suggested that the client's behavior be described rather than labeled. Not only do labels have stereotypical meanings, they may also convey different messages to different readers. Instead of recording that a client is hallucinating, it is more meaningful to record exactly what was observed. The following is an example of this type of recording: "Stood near the ventilator for 10 minutes with hand cupped around ear as if trying to hear better. Carried on an animated conversation. Although no other person was present, the client could be heard saying, 'How dare you call me those names! You are a liar!' "

Instead of recording that the client is disoriented and misidentifies people, it would be more meaningful to record the following: "Mr. J. greeted the nurse by saying, 'Good morning, Mary. Have you cooked breakfast yet?' In the afternoon he asked, 'When are we going to have breakfast?' Client believes that this nurse is his wife, and he is not able to differentiate between morning and afternoon."

By recording her observations in this manner, the nurse permits the reader to make his own assessment of the meaning of the client's behavior.

The nurse as therapist

For a number of years some nurses who have had the benefit of an appropriate educational experience in psychiatric nursing have been developing the role of the nurse therapist. When the nurse functions in the role of nurse therapist, she uses the principles developed through the practice of psychotherapy.

Nursing therapy has developed differently in each situation, but basically it follows the same general guidelines. The role of the nurse therapist is carefully explained to all levels of the professional staff and to all clients in the clinical situation. Every attempt is made to be sure that the role is understood before any therapeutic activity is initiated. The nurse collaborates with other mental health professionals in the situation and confers regularly with those responsible for developing the treatment plans for the clients with whom she is working. The nurse's intervention becomes a part of the total treatment plan for the client.

As is the case with all therapists, it is essential that the nurse identify a skilled professional therapist to function on a regular basis as her perceptor or her supervisor while she is working as a nurse therapist. By doing so the nurse therapist enhances the effectiveness of her interactions with the client as well as increases her own knowledge and skill.

The nurse therapist should record each therapy session so that it can be used to (1) review the dynamics of the relationship, (2) analyze the problems that have been presented, and (3) evaluate client progress against the established treatment goals.

CONCLUDING STATEMENTS

1. The four health care professions of psychiatric nursing, psychiatry, clinical psychology, and psychiatric social work constitute the core mental health disciplines.
2. In recognition of the need for improving the care of the mentally ill, the first school of nursing in a psychiatric setting was established at McLean Hospital in 1882. It was not until 1955

that all schools of nursing offered an experience in psychiatric nursing as a required part of the curriculum.

3. Psychiatry emerged as a specialty in 1846 as a result of the availability of hospitalized mentally ill persons whose mental disorders could be observed and studied.

4. Psychology began as an academic, research-oriented discipline devoted to the scholarly study of human behavior.

5. Psychiatric social work emerged in 1906 as a result of the aftercare movement.

6. The number of mental health professionals increased rapidly as a result of training grants made possible through provisions in the National Mental Health Act of 1946.

7. Although not considered a core mental health discipline, activity therapy was viewed as therapeutic as early as 1892.

8. The psychiatrist is the only professional equipped to make a medical diagnosis and to prescribe somatic treatments.

9. The psychologist is uniquely skilled in the administration and interpretation of inferential tools designed to assist in the diagnostic process and assessment of the treatment effects.

10. Psychiatric social workers are major contributors to the planning and implementation of follow-up care of the mentally ill.

11. All activity therapies are based on the principle that it is helpful to the mentally ill person to engage in activities focusing on objects outside himself.

12. The nurse's role shifts frequently as she strives to make each contact with the client therapeutic.
    a. In the role of creator of a therapeutic environment the nurse develops an accepting atmosphere.
    b. In the role of socializing agent the nurse can provide opportunities for clients to achieve greater success in social situations by helping them to develop feelings of security with other people.
    c. In the role of counselor the nurse performs the critical task of listening to a client in a positive, dynamic, empathic way without at the same time giving advice, stating opinions, or making suggestions. The nurse is concerned with the client's reality problems that deal with the here and now.
    d. The nurse has a role as a teacher in helping the client

learn to participate in socially acceptable and satisfying living activities.

e. The nurse's role as a mother surrogate offers her an opportunity to provide experiences that may correct earlier unsatisfactory interpersonal experiences.

f. The technical aspects of the nurse's role are of great value in themselves and also as a means of enhancing the therapeutic relationship.

g. Providing therapy through the nurse-client relationship is one of the most challenging roles being accepted by psychiatric nurses today.

SUGGESTED SOURCES OF ADDITIONAL INFORMATION

Classical

Dunton, William Rush, and Licht, Sidney: Occupational therapy, principles and practice, ed. 2, Springfield, Ill., 1957, Blackwell Scientific Publications.

Gregg, Dorothy E.: The psychiatric nurse's role, Am. J. Nurs. **54:**848-851, 1954.

Gregg, Dorothy E.: The therapeutic roles of the nurse, Perspect. Psychiatr. Care **1:**18-28, Jan.-Feb., 1963.

Hays, Joyce Samhammer: The psychiatric nurse as a social therapist, Am. J. Nurs. **62:**64-67, June, 1962.

Irwin, B.: Play therapy for a regressed schizophrenic patient, J. Psychiatr. Nurs. **9:**30-32, Sept.-Oct., 1971.

Leininger, Madeleine M.: Trends, issues and problems, Perspect. Psychiatr. Care **10:**11-20, Jan.-Feb., 1969.

Meldman, M.J., McGowan, Marjorie, Higgins, Joan, and Schaller, Donna: Nurse psychoterapists in a private practice, Am. J. Nurs. **69:**2412-2415, 1969.

Mereness, Dorothy: Problems and issues in contemporary psychiatric nursing, Perspect. Psychiatr. Care **2**(1):14-16, 1964.

Peplau, Hildegarde E.: Historical development of statement of some facts and trends, presented at the Working Conference on Graduate Education in Psychiatric Nursing, Williamsburg, Va., 1956 (mimeographed).

Rosenblum, Gershen, and Hassol, Leonard: Training for new mental health roles, Ment. Hyg. **52:**81-85, 1968.

Contemporary

Adelson, Gerald, and Leader, Marcia: The social worker's role: a study of private and voluntary hospitals, Hosp. Community Psychiatry **31:**776-780, Nov., 1980.

Ames, Beatrice: Art and a dying patient, Am. J. Nurs. **80:**1094, 1980.

Burch, J.W., and Meredith, J.L.: Nurses as the core of the psychiatric team, Am. J. Nurs. **74:**2037-2038, 1974.

Chamberlain, Jeanettte: The role of the federal government in the development of psychiatric nursing, J. Psychosoc. Nurs. Ment. Health Serv. **21:**11-18, April, 1983.

Davis, Ellen D., and Pattison, E. Mansell: The psychiatric nurse's role identity, Am. J. Nurs. **79:**298-299, Feb., 1979.

Flaskerud, Jacquelyn: Community mental health nursing: its unique role in the delivery of services to ethnic minorities, Perspect. Psychiatr. Care **20:**37-43, Jan.-March, 1982.

Gaston, Edward: Developing a motivating organizational climate for effective team functioning, Hosp. Community Psychiatry **31:**407-412, June, 1980.

Gerace, Laina, and Rosenberg, Lisa: The use of art prints in group therapy with aftercare patients, Perspect. Psychiatr. Care **17**(2):83-86, March-April, 1979.

Gregg, Dorothy E.: Hildegard Peplau: her contributions, Perspect. Psychiatr. Care **16:**118-121, May-June, 1978.

Hediger, Karen H: The place of the dream in therapy, Perspect. Psychiatr. Care **17:**223-227, Sept.-Oct., 1979.

Hyde, Naida: Psychotherapy as mothering, Perspect. Psychiatr. Care **8:**73-78, March-April, 1970.

Kasiman, C.M.: Issues between professional and paraprofessional nursing staff in community mental health, J. Psychiatr. Nurs. **12**(5):31-35, 1974.

Krispin, A. Laurence: Nursing—a role in multidisciplinary treatment planning, J. Psychosoc. Nurs. Ment. Health Serv. **18:**14-16, April, 1980.

Labarca, Judith R.: Communication through art therapy, Perspect. Psychiatr. Care **17:**118-124, May-June, 1979.

McDonagh, M.J., Tribles, V., and Crum, A.: Nurse-therapists in a state psychiatric hospital, Am. J. Nurs. **80:**103-104, 1980.

Moffie, H. Steven, Patterson, Guy, Lavol, Ramon, and Adams, George: Paraprofessionals and psychiatric teams: an updated review, Hosp. Community Psychiatry **35:**61-67, Jan., 1984.

Nelson, Priscilla: Involvement with Betty: an experience in reality therapy, Am. J. Nurs. **74:**1440-1441, 1974.

Romoff, V., and Kane, I.: Primary nursing in psychiatry: an effective and functional model, Perspect. Psychiatr. Care **20:**73-78, April-June, 1982.

Sills, Grayce M.: Hildegard Peplau: leader, practitioner, academician, scholar and theorist, Perspect. Psychiatr. Care **16:**122-128, May-June, 1978.

Of particular interest

Ethrenwald, J.: The history of psychotherapy, New York, 1976, Jason Aronson, Inc.
This book is an excellent resource for the various models of psychotherapy.

Leinenger, Madeleine M., editor: Contemporary issues in psychiatric nursing, Boston, 1973, Little, Brown & Co.

This excellent book is a compilation of articles from nursing leaders on the topics of psychiatric nursing as it relates to various social sciences.

Peplau, Hildegard: Some reflections on earlier days in psychiatric nursing, J. Psychiatr. Nurs. Ment. Health Serv. **20:**17-24, Aug., 1982.
The reflections of a renowned leader in psychiatric nursing are found in this article.

Ujhely, G.: The nurse as psychotherapist: what are the issues? Perspect. Psychiatr. Care **11:**155-160, July-Aug., 1973.
In this article the author focuses on several important aspects of the role of the nurse as psychotherapist.

section II

concepts basic
to psychiatric
nursing

chapter three

general systems theory
and stress
and adaptation

a conceptual
framework

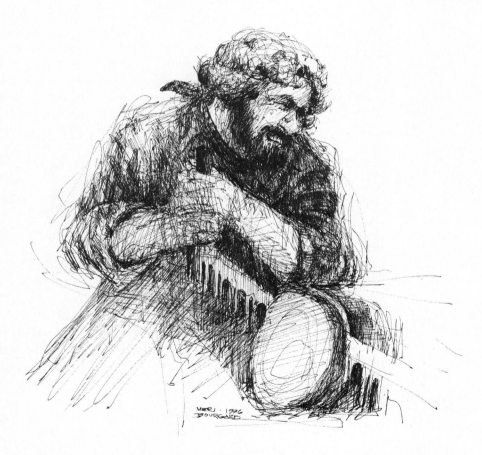

It's amazing how good I feel emotionally when I work hard physically.

LEARNING OBJECTIVES
After studying this chapter the student will be able to:

1 State the purpose of a conceptual framework.

2 Discuss the concepts of general systems theory as applied to human systems.

3 Discuss the concept of stress and adaptation as a process used by human systems.

4 State an example of a nursing intervention utilizing the conceptual framework of systems theory and stress and adaptation.

For nurses to practice efficiently and effectively, they must do so within the context of a conceptual framework. The purpose of a conceptual framework is to organize information in a manner that enables the practitioner to plan, implement, and evaluate nursing care. A conceptual framework also provides consistent and meaningful terminology. Numerous conceptual frameworks could be used effectively to direct nursing care of the mentally ill. In other words, there is no right or wrong conceptual framework. Rather, a conceptual framework is more or less appropriate; its appropriateness is determined by its applicability and utility. An appropriate conceptual framework must help explain the phenomena of concern and thus provide direction for nursing assessment, intervention, and evaluation. It must also be broad enough to be applicable to most, if not all, clinical situations, but not so broad as to be meaningless.

The conceptual framework chosen for this text utilizes general systems theory and the theory of stress and adaptation.

HISTORICAL PERSPECTIVE

General systems theory, as discussed in this chapter, was first discussed by Ludwig von Bertalanffy in 1968. However, other theorists, notably Kurt Lewin, had used its principles decades earlier to formulate their theories. General systems theory has been enthusiastically embraced by the helping professions because it is so useful in explaining relationships among apparently disparate entities. Nevertheless, some critics of this theory believe it is too mechanistic to apply to human systems.

In the 1930s Walter Cannon was the first theorist to mention the role of stress as a factor in causing disease. However, the foremost authority on the theory of stress and adaptation is probably Hans Selye whose pioneering work on the subject was limited to a biochemical model of stress and adaptation. Since that time much research has demonstrated the same processes in the emotional and social realms. Perhaps the most widely publicized results of research in these areas has been the Social Readjustment Rating Scale developed by Holmes and Rahe and published in 1970. This scale ranks various developmental and situational life events according to the amount of change, and therefore stress, each event is likely to evoke in an individual. It has been demonstrated that there is a positive relationship between the number and type of life events experienced by an individual within a year and the probability of his becoming ill, particularly with a stress-related disease. It is a comment on the rapidly changing nature of the society in which we live that some life events on the original scale are no longer considered as stress provoking as they were in 1970, and that other contemporary stressful life events are not included.

GENERAL SYSTEMS THEORY

A *system* is commonly defined as a complex of elements in interaction wherein a relationship between these elements and their properties can be theoretically demonstrated. Since all elements can be theorized to ultimately have a direct or indirect interactional relationship, the only true system is the universe. For example, it is often said that the emotional problems of an individual are due in large part to problems within his family. The family's problems in turn are attributed to problems within the community whose problems in turn result from state, regional, and national concerns. These concerns in turn are closely related to international problems.

Obviously the study of the universe as the true system is not possible or desirable because of the enormous amount of data that would have to be considered. Consequently, it is necessary to delineate a subsystem and define it as "the system" for the purposes of study.

Systems are delineated by the establishment of *boundaries,* which enclose those elements determined to have the greatest interactional qualities in terms of energy, matter, or both. The aggregate of elements that fall within the boundary is referred to as the "system"; each element becomes a component or a *subsystem* of the newly defined system. For example, mental health workers often define the family as the system of concern and the individuals who comprise the family as components or subsystems of the family system.

Each subsystem has its own elements, which are components or subsystems of that system. For example, the individual as a system is made up of a variety of subsystems such as the physiological, psychological, and social subsystems. These subsystems, when viewed as systems themselves, consist of their own subsystems. For example the physiological system consists of the cardiovascular and gastrointestinal subsystems, among others.

Elements that lie outside the boundary serve as the system's *environment*, which is in reality composed of other systems. Therefore the community system serves as an environment for the family system; the family system serves as an environment for the individual system; the physiological system serves as an environment for the psychological system; and so on.

It cannot be overemphasized that boundary delineation is an artificial demarcation of one aspect of the whole—artificial, but necessary, to limit the focus of concern to that which is relevant and thereby increase the probability of comprehending the system. Because boundary delineation is artificial and is intended to enable the nurse to understand the system, boundaries can be enlarged or reduced as experience with the system dictates. For example when the family is the system of concern an initial assessment might indicate that the system should be limited to those members living under the same roof. After working with this system, however, the nurse may discover that the grandparents who live in another state are integral components of this family system. The nurse would then enlarge the original system to include this subsystem, rather than viewing it as part of the environment.

The boundaries of a system have the necessary characteristic of permeability. This permeability may be greater or lesser when systems are compared; the degree of boundary permeability may also change at various times and places within any given system. The permeability of the system boundary regulates the exchange of matter and energy between the system and its environment. Matter and energy that move from the environment through the boundary into the system are referred to as *input*. Matter and energy that move from the system through the boundary into the environment are referred to as *output*.

In a system, matter and energy are an integral part of both the system and the system's environment. *Matter* is defined as anything that has mass and occupies space. *Energy* is defined as the ability to do work. There are two types of energy: potential and kinetic. *Potential energy* is that energy not currently engaged in work, but is available for use. It is stored energy. In contrast, *kinetic energy* is that which is being currently utlized and is therefore unavailable for additional work.

Energy can neither be created nor destroyed; it can only be converted from one form into another or transported from one place to another. When energy is used it does not disappear but merely goes elsewhere or is changed to another form. The principle that energy can neither be created nor destroyed is the first law of thermodynamics; it is reminiscent of Freud's concept of psychic or libidinal energy as explained in Chapter 4.

Systems are in a constant state of dynamic movement as they exchange matter and energy within themselves and between themselves and their environments. Any attempt to study a system is to artificially suspend this motion and therefore run the risk of an inaccurate assessment. Nevertheless, it is necessary to take this risk if systems are to be studied, but any conclusions should take this factor into account.

Systems are characterized by the concept of *non-summativity*, which states that the whole of the system is greater than the sum of its parts. The parts of a system are that system's subsystems, and the system in its totality cannot be understood or appreciated by a mere summation of its subsystems. Perhaps the most familiar example of this concept is the Indian folk tale of the six blind men who each felt a part of an elephant's body. Each then described that part to the others, and as a group, they attempted unsuccessfully to describe the whole. The primary reason that the whole is greater than the sum of its parts is that each subsystem interacts directly or indirectly with all other subsystems by exchanging matter and energy, a concept called *wholeness*. The uniqueness of the system results from the transformations of matter and energy that take place in this exchange, a process known as *throughput*.

Because of the interactional quality of the system's components, changes in any one component will automatically effect compensatory changes in all other components. These changes are compensatory because a system continuously strives to maintain itself as it is. In other words, the system continuously regulates itself to attain a steady state. When referring to living organisms, this process is known as *homeokinesis*.

Human beings are complex systems of interrelated and interdependent subsystems in constant interaction with each other and with their environments. Therefore alterations in any aspect of the system require responsive alterations in other aspects of the system. For example, a person who is physically ill, for whatever reason and to whatever degree, has concomitant emotional reactions to this lack of physical wellbeing. Conversely, there are physical side effects of emotional reactions, such as the stomach upsets, the lightheadedness, and the heart palpitations that accompany severe anxiety or fear.

This holistic view of human beings also provides direction for assessing the individual as an integral part of his social system, simultaneously affecting that system and being affected by it. This view implies that an individual cannot be assessed accurately in isolation from his family, his community, and the reference groups to which he belongs. Nurses new to working with the mentally ill have had the experience of assisting an individual to achieve a higher level of emotional wellness only to be surprised by the observation that the behavior of another member of his family becomes increasingly disturbed. This common phenomenon reflects the fact that the family operates as a system and change in one member requires a compensatory reaction by the family system, often manifested by altered behavior in other family members.

Those human systems that are most successful in achieving their goal of maintaining themselves as close to their original state as possible, ironically are systems whose very existence is in jeopardy. These systems are *relatively closed systems*. The boundaries of relatively closed systems have little permeability, and there is relatively little exchange of matter or energy with the environment. However, boundaries cannot be totally closed in a living system. Some permeability is necessary to exchange matter and energy, a process necessary for life. The bulk of energy in a relatively closed system is used in maintaining a steady state, leaving little potential energy available to respond to input. Because input into the system is minimal, there is ultimate energy loss into the system's environment, leading to increased system disorganization. This situation is termed *entropy*.

The student is probably familiar with a family that does not respond to notes from school about the children's poor academic performance, initially resulting in the family system being undisturbed by this news and thereby maintaining a steady state. Ultimately, however, this system's inability to recognize and process relevant input may lead to the children being left back and perhaps eventually dropping out of school. This in turn means that the children are poorly prepared to leave home and to function as financially independent adults, resulting in the family's financial resources becoming increasingly depleted. In the long run this fictional family does not change and grow but rather becomes increasingly ineffective in fulfilling its functions. This example, although oversimplified, illustrates the counterproductivity of a system attempting to achieve a steady state by maintaining relatively closed boundaries.

In contrast, a system that survives, grows, and develops is characterized by a semipermeable boundary that allows for exchange of matter and energy with its environment and by the availability of a sufficient amount of potential energy to utlize input in the service of system growth. This type of system is known as a *relatively open system* and is characterized by movement toward integration and growth, a situation referred to as *negentropy*.

Finally, an understanding of systems theory must take into account the concept of *feedback*, a unique form of input derived from previous output. The input, throughput, output, and feedback cycle is often referred to as the *feedback loop*. Feedback is the message that the system receives about the degree to which it is successful in attaining a steady state. In other words, feedback is essential to enable the system to adjust or regulate itself. Feedback may emanate from within the system itself or from the system's environment, but in either instance there is a time lag between the system's perception of the feedback and its ability to utilize it in the service of self regulation.

Positive feedback reinforces the system, thereby encouraging the maintenance of a steady state and leading to entropy. *Nega-*

tive feedback is information that indicates change is necessary within the system for the system to grow. These concepts are often difficult for students to understand because of the belief that positive feedback is desirable and negative feedback is to be avoided. It is true that positive feedback reinforces behavior, encouraging people to continue those behaviors which are rewarded. However, inadvertently perhaps, positive feedback discourages growth if altered behavior is necessary for growth. Negative feedback, on the other hand, is growth-producing only if the system has the energy available to utilize the feedback and alter itself. For example, a very intelligent student is not motivated to achieve his potential if his minimal efforts are rewarded with high grades. On the other hand, a student who is not as intellectually capable and who is working to capacity but receiving low grades will not be helped to do better merely through criticism of his work. He does not have the energy available to utilize the negative feedback, whereas his highly intelligent counterpart does.

This brief discussion of general systems theory demonstrates its applicability to nursing practice in regard to describing the structure of human systems. However, its language and concepts only hint at explaining the process. For example, we know that energy is exchanged between systems, but systems theory alone does not allow us to describe the nature of that energy. Therefore to better understand the nature of the processes in which systems engage, we need to turn to another theory, that of stress and adaptation.

STRESS AND ADAPTATION THEORY

Human beings are continuously exposed to a wide variety and large number of stimuli. These stimuli may be physical, emotional, physiological, social, or spiritual and may take the form of matter or energy. These stimuli are input to the system and may emanate from within the system through the feedback loop or from external sources. The system's boundary screens and sorts input to protect the system from becoming overwhelmed while at the same time allowing sufficient input to transcend the boundary and ensure the system's viability.

In the terminology of stress and adaptation theory, system input is called a *stressor*. A stressor, in and of itself, is neither positive nor negative but rather has a positive or negative effect, depending on the way the system processes it. This concept helps to explain why different people respond differently to the same stressor. For example, the death of a spouse is considered to be a negative event in our society. However, after the initial grieving period the surviving spouse may respond with more vigor and interest in life than before the spouse's death. Conversely, the birth of a baby is generally considered to be a positive event, but for some families an additional child to raise may strain emotional and financial resources unbearably.

Stressors may be classified as developmental or situational. The significance of this classification is that developmental stressors can be anticipated but situational stressors cannot. Rather, situational stressors are untoward events. For example, the adolescent is assaulted with physiological, emotional, and social stressors. Because these are a normal expected part of the maturation process, anticipatory guidance of the adolescent and his family can greatly strengthen the resources this system has available for dealing with these stressors. In contrast, the situational stressor of a middle-aged executive with two children in college who loses his job must be dealt with after it happens.

Regardless of whether a stressor is developmental or situational, the variables that determine a system's response to a stressor are multiple but always reflect the amount of potential energy available to deal with the stressor and the meaning of the stressor to the system. For example, a mild laryngitis would not greatly disrupt the system of a dock worker but would be a major stressor to the opera singer.

When a stressor transcends the system's boundary it disturbs the system's steady state, automatically thrusting the system into a condition of stress. Therefore *stress* is defined as a condition in which the human system responds to input that has disturbed its steady state. As such stress is necessary to life and is neither positive nor negative, although it is capable of causing either positive or negative effects. This technical view of stress differs markedly from the way the term is used in everyday language. One often hears the term "stress" used only in a negative sense and often as descriptive of an event rather than the condition of being.

Stress in human beings is a subjective phenomenon that cannot be observed directly, but rather must be inferred from the person's response to the stressor. This response is called an *ad-aptation*. Integral to the theory of stress is the concept that the human system adapts holistically to stress. Regardless of the nature of the stressor, the human being responds in all spheres. A physiological stressor elicits not only a physiological adaptation, but also psychological and social adaptations. In like manner a social stressor elicits social, physiological, and psychological adaptations. In other words, the human system is not able to selectively respond to stressors. This generalized nonspecific response to stress is called the *general adaptation syndrome* and is consistent with the systems theory concept of wholism. For example an adolescent experiencing the stress of her first date responds with fear about the appropriateness of her appearance and behavior. However, this response is not limited to the emotion of fear, but also affects her physiological subsystem by raising her blood pressure and decreasing the blood supply to the digestive subsystem, rendering her unable to eat. This response is actually preparing her for "fight or flight" as if the stressor were life-threatening. It is this fight or flight response that, if prolonged with no outlet, results in the stress-related diseases that constitute major health problems in today's society.

In addition to the general adaptation syndrome, there may be a specific adaptation to the stressor. While the general adaptation syndrome is involuntary and unconscious, adaptations specific to a stressor may be either voluntary or involuntary and conscious or unconscious. When adaptations are voluntary and conscious they are called *coping mechanisms;* when they are involuntary and unconscious, they are called *defense mechanisms.* For example, a student in a state of stress because of an impending examination might adapt by voluntarily and consciously planning time to study and then adhering to the plan. Another student might respond to the same stressor by involuntarily utilizing the unconscious defense mechanism of rationalization by believing the exam is less important than attending social events, and therefore plan not to study. On the surface it would seem that the second student was more successful than the first in returning to the desirable state of homeokinesis in that this second student unlike the first is no longer under stress. It should be remembered however that the second student must use some of his available energy to remain unaware of the reality of the situation; he then has less energy available to deal with subsequent stressors. In either event this example is not complete until the outcome of each adaptation is examined. When the time of the examination arrives, it can be conjectured that the first student who studied would be prepared and therefore would do well on the test. The feedback he would receive is positive, thereby reinforcing the behavior of studying prior to an exam. The second student, however, would be unlikely to do well, and the feedback would be negative, thereby disrupting the system further and causing additional stress with less available energy to deal with it. If sufficient energy were available, however, the student could benefit from this negative feedback by utilizing it to alter his behavior and plan to study for exams in the future.

Once again, this example is overly simplistic in that it implies a linear cause-and-effect relationship between the stressor and the adaptation. In reality, the human system is always being affected by multiple stressors and its adaptations reflect the system's ability to test reality, its previous adaptations, and its amount of potential energy. Human systems that cannot regain homeokinesis because of an inability to test reality, or that have had no previous experience with the stressor, or that lack sufficient energy to adapt to the number and potency of the stressors encountered are in a state of crisis. This condition is discussed fully in Chapter 22.

The student of psychiatric nursing should be aware of the fact that Axis IV of the third edition of the *Diagnostic and Statistical Manual of Mental Disorders* (DSM-III) (see Appendix) requires an assessment of the severity of psychosocial stressors. The fact that this parameter is included for the first time in this manual of psychiatric diagnoses reflects a growing recognition of the role that psychosocial stressors play in mental illness. On examination of this Axis, the student will note that suggested examples of stressors range from those likely to have minimal effect, such as a minor violation of the law, to those anticipated to have a catastrophic effect, such as imprisonment in a concentration camp. It should also be noted that the list of examples includes not only negative events but also those usually considered to be positive, such as pregnancy or job promotions.

Implications for nursing

The conceptual framework of systems theory and stress and adaptation provides nurses with organizing theories within which to understand human behavior and to intervene based on this understanding. Simply stated, the goal of all nursing interventions is to protect the system from noxious stressors or to increase the system's potential energy, thereby enhancing its ability to adapt to the stressor or to diminish the potency of the stressor. The following case history exemplifies how these goals can be achieved.

Mary Smith, a 16-year-old unmarried high school student, informed her parents that she was 2 months pregnant. Although this news was extremely upsetting to all, Mary's parents rallied around her and after many family discussions, often late into the night, the family made several decisions. Mary would not marry the child's father because they had little in common other than a strong sexual attraction. She would carry the baby to term and after its birth she would give it up for adoption so that she would be able to continue her education by going to college and perhaps fulfill her life-long dream of becoming a lawyer. It was also decided that Mary would continue to attend the local high school. Mary's parents met with the school administrators who agreed to this plan. They also contacted an adoption agency to initiate plans for the adoption of the unborn child. These decisions were congruent with the values of the family, were agreeable to all, and seemed feasible to implement. Having adapted to the stressor of Mary's pregnancy, the Smith family regained its homeokinesis by devoting themselves to accomplishing the many household and business tasks left undone while its energy was focused on coping with this system change.

Things went well for the Smith family until the fifth month, at which time Mary was visibly pregnant. Her fellow classmates began openly taunting her, her best friends no longer telephoned her or invited her to their homes, and the school board received a petition from irate parents demanding that Mary be suspended from school until the baby was born. Although the school board did not take this action and Mary's parents remained empathic and supportive Mary became increasingly depressed, unable to eat or sleep. Mr. and Mrs. Smith became alarmed and made an appointment at the mental health clinic. After several sessions at the clinic, it was decided that it would be best for Mary if she were to move to her grandparents' home in a different school district for the duration of her pregnancy (protecting the system from noxious stressors). While she was there she would continue to receive counseling focused on helping her to cope with the birth and subsequent adoption of her child, as well as exploring responses she might use when she was questioned about her pregnancy (increasing the system's potential energy). Finally, the mental health counselors in Mary's home town were concerned about the larger issue of the attitudes of the townspeople, not only for Mary's sake, but also because of what this attitude of intolerance meant to the mental health of her classmates. Because part of the mission of the mental health clinic was community education, the personnel organized evening seminars under the auspices of the school. These seminars were designed to assist interested students and parents to explore their interpersonal relationships and human values.

This case history depicts a family system thrust into a state of disequilibrium by changes in one of its subsystems (Mary's pregnancy). The fact that the family system did not go into a state of massive disequilibrium on experiencing this change shows that it had potential energy available to bring to bear on the situation. It appears that the family utilized a problem-solving approach as the members engaged in many family discussions. The fact that this system's boundaries were relatively open is attested to by the parents' meeting with the school administrators and sharing their plans with them. They also were able to seek help from the mental health clinic when Mary's behavior alarmed them. A system with relatively closed boundaries would be unlikely to be able to exchange information effectively with other systems in its environment.

The decision for Mary to move out of the school district to her grandparents' home is an example of an intervention that utilized available resources to protect Mary from the noxious stressor of peer rejection with which she was apparently unable to cope. Increasing her potential energy, thereby enhancing her ability to adapt to future criticism, was accomplished by the reality-oriented counseling she continued to receive while at her grandparents' home. Finally, the action of the mental health clinic in conducting human relations seminars for the townspeople is an example of an intervention designed to diminish the potency of the stressor.

Although this situation does not specifically refer to the nurse as the mental health professional involved, the interventions employed are well within the scope of the nurse functioning in a community mental health clinic.

CONCLUDING STATEMENTS

1. The purpose of a conceptual framework is to organize information in a manner that enables the practitioner to plan, implement, and evaluate nursing care.

2. A *system* is a complex of elements in interaction wherein a relationship between these elements and their properties can be theoretically demonstrated.
3. Systems are delineated by the establishment of *boundaries* that enclose elements that have the greatest interactional qualities.
4. Each element within a system is a *subsystem.*
5. Elements outside the system's boundary form the system's *environment.*
6. Because boundary delineation is an artificial process boundaries can be enlarged or reduced as experience with the system dictates.
7. System boundaries have the characteristic of being permeable, allowing the exchange of energy and matter between the system and its environment. Matter and energy that move from the environment through the boundary into the system are called *input.* Matter and energy that move from the system through the boundary into the environment are called *output.*
8. *Matter* is defined as anything that has mass and occupies space.
9. *Energy* is the ability to do work and is of two types, *potential* or stored energy and *kinetic* energy.
10. Systems are characterized by the concept of *nonsummativity* of the system; that is, the whole is greater than the sum of its parts.
11. The uniqueness of each system results from the transformations of matter and energy between and among subsystems, a process known as *throughput.*
12. Systems constantly regulate themselves to attain a steady state, a process known as *homeokinesis.* Therefore changes in one component of the system automatically effect compensatory changes in all other components.
13. Human beings are complex systems of interrelated and interdependent subsystems in constant interaction with each other and with their environments.
14. The boundaries of *relatively closed systems* have little permeability and the bulk of the system's energy is bound in maintaining a steady state, leading to energy loss and increased system disorganization. This situation is called *entropy.*

15. The boundaries of *relatively open systems* allow for adequate exchange of matter and energy, and a sufficient amount of potential energy to utilize input in the service of system growth and integration is available. This situation is called *negentropy*.
16. *Feedback* is a unique form of input that sends a message to the system about the degree to which it is successful in attaining a steady state. Feedback may emanate from within the system or from the system's environment.
17. *Positive feedback* reinforces the system and encourages a steady state, therefore discouraging growth and change and leading to entropy. *Negative feedback* disrupts the system, encouraging change and growth if the system has potential energy available to utilize the input, and leads to negentropy.
18. In the terminology of stress and adaptation theory system input is called a *stressor*. A stressor is neither positive or negative but has a positive or negative effect on the system.
19. Stressors may be developmental or situational. Developmental stressors result from the normal maturational process and thus can be anticipated and dealt with through anticipatory guidance. Situational stressors are untoward events that cannot be anticipated and therefore must be dealt with after the occurrence.
20. The variables that determine a system's response to a stressor are many but always reflect the amount of potential energy available and the meaning of the stressor to the system.
21. *Stress* in human beings is defined as a condition of being wherein the human system responds to input that has disturbed its steady state. It is neither positive nor negative but is necessary to life. It is a subjective phenomenon that must be inferred from the person's response.
22. The human system's response to stress is called an *adaptation*.
23. Human systems respond holistically to stress. This generalized nonspecific response to stress is termed the *general adaptation syndrome*.
24. There may also be a specific adaptation to a stressor, which may be voluntary or involuntary and conscious or unconscious.
25. When specific adaptations are voluntary and conscious they

are called *coping mechanisms;* when they are involuntary and unconscious they are called *defense mechanisms.*

26. The adaptations of a human system reflect the system's ability to test reality, its previous adaptations, and its amount of potential energy.
27. The goal of all nursing interventions is to protect the system from noxious stressors, increase the system's potential energy, or diminish the stressor's potency.
28. Axis IV of the DSM III requires an assessment of the severity of psychosocial stressors. This recognizes the role that psychosocial stressors play in mental illness.

SUGGESTED SOURCES OF ADDITIONAL INFORMATION

Classical

Bertalanffy, Ludwig von: General systems theory: foundations, development, and applications, New York, 1968, George Braziller, Inc.
Cannon, William B.: Bodily changes in pain, hunger, fear and death, ed. 2, New York, 1929, Appleton-Century-Crofts.
Caplan, Gerald: Principles of preventive psychiatry, New York, 1964, Basic Books, Inc., Publishers.
Lewin, Kurt: A dynamic theory of personality, New York, 1935, McGraw-Hill Book Co.
Lewin, Kurt: Field theory in social science; selected theoretical papers (edited by D. Cartwright), New York, 1951, Harper & Row, Publishers.
Lewin, Kurt: Principles of topological psychology, New York, 1936, McGraw-Hill Book Co.
Selye, Hans: Stress without distress, New York, 1974, J.B. Lippincott Co.
Selye, Hans: The stress of life, New York, 1956, McGraw-Hill Book Co.
Wolff, Harold: Stress and disease, Springfield, Ill., 1953, Charles C Thomas, Publishers.

Contemporary

Blattner, Barbara: Holistic nursing, Englewood Cliffs, N.J., 1981, Prentice-Hall, Inc.
Bloom, Bernard: The logic and urgency of primary prevention, Hosp. Community Psychiatry **32:**838-843, Dec., 1981.
Brown, Martha, and Fowler, Grace: Psychodynamic nursing: a biosocial orientation, ed. 4, Philadelphia, 1972, W.B. Saunders Co.
Burnside, Irene Mortenson, Ebersole, P., and Monea, H.E.: Psychosocial caring throughout the life span, New York, 1979, McGraw-Hill Book Co.
Carter, Frances M.: Psychosocial nursing, ed. 2, New York, 1976, Macmillan Publishing Co.
Fife, Betsy: Childhood cancer is a family crisis, J. Psychosoc. Nurs. Ment. Health Serv. **18:**29-34, Oct., 1980.

Finesilver, Cynthia: Reducing stress in patients having cardiac catheterization, Am. J. Nurs. **80:**1805-1807, 1980.

Flynn, Patricia A.-R.: Holistic health: the art and science of care, Bowie, Md., 1980, Brady Communications Co., Inc.

Hagen, Diane: The relationship between job loss and physical and mental illness, Hosp. Community Psychiatry **34:**438-441, May, 1983.

Hall, J.E., and Weaver, B.R.: Distributive nursing practice: a systems approach to community health, New York, 1979, J.B. Lippincott Co.

Hill, Martha: When the patient is the family, Am. J. Nurs. **81:**536-538, 1981.

Lazarus, Richard: Psychological stress and the coping process, New York, 1966, McGraw-Hill Book Co.

Luft, Joseph: The johari window model. In Cathart, R.S., and Samover, L.A. editors: Small group communication, a reader, ed. 2, Iowa, 1974, Wm. C. Brown Group.

Murray, Ruth Beckman, and Zentner, J.P.: Nursing assessment and health promotion through the life span, Englewood Cliffs, N.J., 1979.

Murphy, Shirley: After Mt. St. Helen's: disaster stress research, J. Psychosoc. Nurs. Ment. Health Serv. **22:**8-18, July, 1984.

Norman, Elizabeth: PTSD: the victims who survived, Am. J. Nurs. **82:**1696-1698, 1982.

Oleck, L., and Yoder, S.: Holism or hypocrisy? Perspect. Psychiatr. Care **19:**65-67, March-April, 1981.

Spiegel, John: Transactions: the interplay between individual, family, and society, New York, 1971, Science House.

Tierney, M.J., and Strom, Lane: Stress type A behavior in the nurse, Am. J. Nurs. **80:**915-918, 1980.

Trusley, Martha: The use of family therapy in terminal illness and death, J. Psychosoc. Nurs. Ment. Health Serv. **20:**17-22, Jan., 1982.

Of particular interest

Gray, William, Duhl, F.J., and Rizzo, N.D., editors: General systems theory and psychiatry, Boston, 1969, Little, Brown & Co.
This excellent resource is a collection of articles by 28 authors, focusing on the history of general systems theory and its relevance to psychiatry.

Hazzard, Mary E., editor: A systems approach to nursing, Nurs. Clin North Am. **6:** entire issue, Sept. 1971.
This issue is a collection of articles by nurse professionals describing concepts of systems theory and exploring their use in nursing care.

Holmes, T.H., and Rahe, R.H.: The social readjustment rating scale, J. Psychosoc. Res. **11**(1): 213-218, 1967.
This is the widely publicized Social Readjustment Scale, which ranks various stressful life events.

personality:
its structure
and development

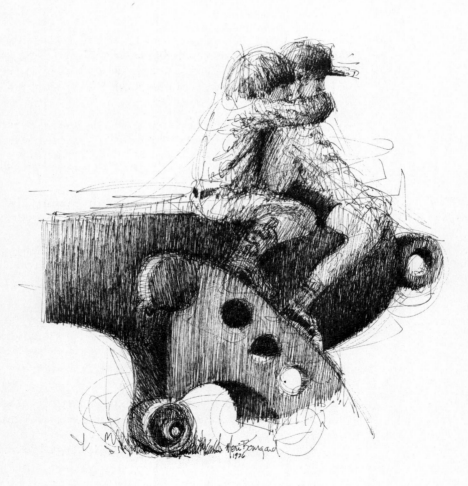

*Being friends with you
makes me feel good about myself.*

1 Describe briefly the history of the study of personality development.

2 Define the term *personality*.

3 Discuss the major concepts underlying the Freudian, Eriksonian, and Sullivanian theories of personality development.

4 Discuss each stage of personality development in terms of its process and outcomes.

Understanding human behavior and the many adjustment problems that arise in the lives of people depends to a large extent on understanding the process through which the personality develops. While the understanding of personality development is integral to the practice of psychiatric nursing it is also essential to the general practice of nursing because nursing interventions must be geared to the developmental level of the recipient if they are to be effective.

HISTORICAL PERSPECTIVE

Before the beginning of the twentieth century the physical and emotional development of human beings was poorly understood. Children were viewed as miniature embodiments of adults and, as such, were treated with little or no understanding of their developmentally related needs. Furthermore, the attainment of physical maturity was equated with the achievement of emotional maturity. If growth was complete, so was development. Throughout history wise and loving mothers of large families certainly must have noticed similarities in their children's behavior at the same periods of their lives. However, it was not until the early twentieth century that the study of personality development of children began in earnest. Interest in the personality development of adults took longer to emerge, but now it is the subject of much study because the number of persons of middle and older age is rapidly increasing.

Much of our current knowledge about the evolution of personality is based on theories proposed by Sigmund Freud (1856-1939). He did much of his important work in Vienna around the turn of the century and is given most of the credit for developing the foundational theories of personality development. It was

Freud's writing that first stressed the crucial importance of early childhood experiences in the development of human personality and the relationship between some of the emotional problems in adult life and the negative influences that sometimes occur during the early years. Freud's theory of personality development is called the *psychosexual theory* of development.

During and after Freud's pioneering work, many other theorists addressed themselves to the study of personality development to better understand human behavior. Investigators such as Erik Erikson and Harry Stack Sullivan have adapted, modified, and enlarged on Freud's basic theories; their work has resulted in theories that are seen as significantly different from those of Freud.

Erik Erikson was born in Frankfurt, Germany, in 1902 of Danish parents. His mother and father had separated before he was born and when he was about 3 years old, his mother married a pediatrician who was a German Jew. With this mixed cultural heritage Erikson had difficulty establishing his own sense of identity. In fact, he made up the name Erik Erikson, which reflects the concept that the child (Erik) is the father (son of Erik) of the man (Erik Erikson). It is likely that his own personal quest for identity was a major factor in the development of his theory of personality development, referred to as the *Eight Ages of Man*. At age 25 Erikson left Germany to go to Vienna where he studied the new discipline of psychoanalysis. He immigrated to Boston, Massachusetts in 1933, fleeing fascism, and has spent the remainder of his life in the United States.

Harry Stack Sullivan was born in Norwich, New York, in 1892 and died in 1949. Sullivan became a psychiatrist during the early years of Freud's profound influence on American psychiatry. However, unlike many of his colleagues, he studied only in the United States, working closely with a group of psychoanalysts and social psychologists who were pulling away from the classical psychoanalytical model established by Freud. Sullivan's theories postulate that the most critical factor in personality development is the individual's relationship with other significant people. His theories emphasize the nature and the quality of these relationships. This fact is best illustrated by his reference to the *mothering one* to distinguish between the roles of the biological mother and the person (male or female) who provides nurturing experiences for the infant. Although Sullivan viewed the relationship between the infant and the mothering one as fundamental to personality development, he also placed great emphasis on the importance of relationships with significant others such as peers, spouse, and offspring as the person progresses throughout life. Therefore Sullivan's theory is called the *interpersonal theory of psychiatry*. In view of the fact that the nurse's role with mentally ill persons is almost totally focused on the relationship that is developed with them, Sullivan's theory seems to be particularly applicable to nursing practice.

DEFINITION OF PERSONALITY

Before a discussion of personality development can become meaningful, it is essential to understand the definition of the term *personality* used by students of human behavior. Unfortunately this word has been used to convey many different meanings and ideas. In ordinary conversation it usually refers to the personal response that the individual evokes from others. It is not unusual for someone to comment that an individual has a pleasing personality or that a certain person has a poor personality. When used technically, the word personality refers to *the aggregate of the physical and mental qualities of the individual as these interact in characteristic fashion with his environment.* Thus it can be seen that personality is expressed through behavior. The characteristic combinations of behavior distinguish one individual from another and endow individuals with their own unique identity.

This definition of personality includes the individual's biological and intellectual endowment, the attributes he has acquired through experience, and his conscious and unconscious reactions and feelings. Personality development is a complex and dynamic process. As such, the personality is constantly evolving from what it was to something different, yet always retains a certain identifiable consistency. It is important to remember that from birth to death personality is ever changing and ever developing. This fact makes it possible for individuals of all ages to profit from corrective experiences and to modify behavior in a positive direction. This is the rationale underlying all psychotherapeutic endeavors on the behalf of clients.

**BASIC
CONCEPTS OF
PERSONALITY
DEVELOPMENT
Freudian
concepts**

Although some psychiatrists feel that is is important to adhere strictly and consistently to the tenets of one school of thought, psychiatric theories currently in use in the United States are becoming increasingly eclectic. That is, concepts from various schools of thought are being used in combination to develop a usable theory of personality development. The necessity of an eclectic approach is particularly apparent in nursing practice; the role of the nurse in interaction with patients is probably more varied than in any other discipline. Consequently the following discussion will outline the basic concepts of Freud, Erikson, and Sullivan with a subsequent discussion of each stage of personality development as described by these theorists. It is hoped that this approach will enable the student to compare and contrast these theories and use that which is applicable as she plans, implements, and evaluates nursing care.

Freud's theories are often referred to as *intrapsychic*, because they emphasize the internal emotional life of the individual as the most significant factor in the development of the personality. Even though Freud deviated widely from the accepted medical theories and practices of his day, his theories are largely based on a biological model. For example, Freud believed that each individual is born with a genetically determined amount of *libidinal energy*, a form of psychic energy that seeks pleasure in an attempt to avoid tension or pain. In this sense libidinal energy is viewed as sexual energy. This energy cannot increase or decrease in amount but must be shared among the various parts of the personality. Freud developed his conception of the stages of personality development largely around the concept of libidinal energy, and delineated each stage of development according to the area of the body on which he believed the energy was focused. For example, the first stage of development is characterized by the libidinal energy being concentrated on the mouth. It is through the mouth that the infant expresses tension and pain, and through the mouth that pleasure is perceived. As the child matures physiologically, the libidinal energy shifts from the mouth to other parts of the body until adulthood when the libidinal energy is focused on the genital area, enabling the individual to establish a mature heterosexual relationship, which Freud saw as the hallmark of the normal development of personality. Therefore Freud delineated only five stages of personality development, seeing this process as being complete at adulthood with major personality alterations unlikely thereafter under usual circumstances. It is because of the libidinal energy theory and its relationship to the development of the personality, that Freud's theory of personality development is called the *psycho- sexual theory.*

Freud's topographical descriptions of the psyche are impor- tant for the student to understand, since these concepts are used almost universally in the United States and contribute much to understanding human behavior.

Levels of consciousness. One way in which Freud described the mind topographically was from the standpoint of levels of consciousness. These levels are referred to as the conscious, the preconscious or subconscious, and the unconscious parts of the mind.

The *conscious* part of the mind is aware of the here and now as it relates to the individual and his environment. It functions only when the individual is awake. The conscious mind is con- cerned with thoughts, feelings, and sensations. It directs the in- dividual as he behaves in a rational, thoughtful way.

The *preconscious* or *subconscious* is that part of the mind in which ideas and reactions are stored and partially forgotten—it is not economical for human beings to burden the conscious mind with a multitude of facts that are infrequently used and currently not in demand. The preconscious also acts as a watch- man; it prevents certain unacceptable, disturbing unconscious memories from reaching the conscious mind. These two functions make the preconscious an extremely valuable device. Material relegated to this handy storehouse can usually be brought into conscious awareness if the individual concentrates on recall.

The *unconscious* is by far the largest part of the mind and is sometimes compared to the large hidden part of an iceberg that floats under the water. In this comparison the small part of the iceberg that appears above the water represents the conscious mind. The unconscious is the storehouse for all the memories, feelings, and responses experienced by the individual during his entire life. The unconscious is one of Freud's most important con- cepts. Freudian theorists believe that the human mind never ac- tually forgets any experience but stores in the unconscious all knowledge, information, and feeling about all experiences. These memories cannot be recalled at will. The individual is rarely aware of the unconscious mind, except as it demonstrates its presence through such means as dreams, slips of the tongue, unexplained behavioral responses, jokes, and lapses of memory. Psychotic symptoms are expressions of unconscious thoughts or feelings. Material stored in the unconscious has a powerful influence on behavior because the accompanying feelings continue to act as motivating, dynamic forces. The individual is unaware of the ideas themselves, but he may continue to experience an emotional reaction as if the material were in the conscious mind. This theory underlies the belief that all behavior has meaning. In other words, no behavior occurs by accident or chance; rather, all behavior is an expression of feelings or needs of which the individual frequently is not aware.

Structure of the personality. The second topographical description developed by Freud is frequently referred to as the structure of the personality. This structure includes the concepts of the id, the ego, and the superego.

The *id* is part of and derived from the unconscious. It is unlearned, primitive, selfish, and the source of all libidinal energy. It contains the instinctual drives, included in which are the drive for self-preservation, the drive to reproduce, and the drive for group association. The id is without a sense of right and wrong and ruthlessly insists on immediate satisfaction of its impulses and desires.

When the new individual is born, he is said to be a bundle of id, seeking only to satisfy his needs and to find release for physiological tensions. By crying, the infant insists on receiving attention when tensions build up. He disregards all other factors in his environment as he demands that his needs be met.

During the individual's entire life the id persists in pushing the organism toward the achievement of its primitive, instinctual goals. It is described as operating on the basis of the *pleasure principle*. That is to say, the id presses for avoidance of pain at all costs and seeks to maintain pleasure. *Pleasure* in this sense refers to release of tension and the establishment of emotional and physiological equilibrium. *Pain* refers to tensions that are present when the infant is cold, hungry, frightened, or anxious. As the child matures, the concept of pain encompasses additional aspects of body equilibrium, including sexual tension, tensions that result from cultural pressures, and tension from physiological needs. Throughout the individual's entire life the id insists that the individual seek release of tension, regardless of the social outcome. It is the duty of other parts of the personality to censor the id and to keep it under control.

The development of the *ego* is a result of the individual's interaction with the environment. It is initiated when the infant recognizes the breast or the bottle as part of the environment rather than as part of his own body. The ego promotes the individual's satisfactory adjustment in relation to his environment. Its main function is to effect an acceptable compromise between the crude pleasure-seeking strivings of the id and the inhibitions of the superego. The means through which the ego achieves this goal is reality testing. The ego deals with the demands of reality as it strives to control and derive satisfaction from the environment. Thus as the individual matures the ego becomes the rational, reasonable, conscious part of the personality and strives to integrate the total personality into a smoothly functioning, unified, coherent whole. In the mature adult it is the ego that represents the self to others and individualizes him from other human beings.

Chronologically, the *superego* develops last. Its development is partially a result of the socialization process that the child undergoes. The superego incorporates the taboos, prohibitions, ideals, and standards of the parents and the other significant adults with whom the child associates. It operates mostly at the unconscious level and at this level is an inhibitor of the id. The superego is blindly rigid, strictly moralistic, and as unrelenting and ruthless as the id. There are two aspects of the superego. One is called the *conscience*. The conscience is the part of the superego that punishes the individual through guilt and anxiety when his behavior deviates from the strict standards of the superego. The other aspect is called the *ego ideal*. The ego ideal rewards the individual through feelings of euphoria and well-being when his behavior emulates those standards believed by the superego to be desirable. It is important to understand that neither the punishing nor the rewarding functions of the superego are based on the reality of the situation. Rather, they are based on the individual's internalized standards of right and wrong, good and bad, which were learned at an early age and which are stored for the most part in the unconscious mind.

Eriksonian concepts

If the individual does not develop an ego strong enough to arbitrate effectively between the id and the superego he will surely develop intrapersonal and interpersonal conflicts. When the id is not controlled effectively, the individual functions in antisocial, lawless ways because his primitive impulses are expressed freely. If the superego is so strong that the individual's life is dominated by its restrictions on behavior, he is likely to be inhibited, repressed, unhappy, and guilt-ridden. Thus a mature, effective, stable adult life depends on the development of an ego powerful enough to adequately test reality and then to mediate successfully between the demands of the id and the superego.

Erikson's theories build on and include Freudian concepts. However, their emphasis is not on Freud's intrapsychic theories but rather on the ability of the ego to develop in a healthy, adaptive manner given a facilitative environment. Therefore Erikson's theories are variously referred to as neo-Freudian, ego psychology, and cultural. Erikson has also extended the stages of personality development to include the totality of the life span, introducing the very important idea that personality development does not cease at the achievement of adulthood. This belief helps to explain the fundamental changes in an individual's feelings and behavior that characteristically occur during his adult life.

A major contribution Erikson has made to the understanding of personality development is his identification of *developmental tasks* for each developmental period. These developmental tasks are age-specific achievements that are largely culturally determined. Achievement of each task increases the ego strength of the individual and enhances the probability of satisfactory achievement of subsequent tasks. Erikson sees the individual's ability to complete each developmental task satisfactorily as dependent not only on his genetic endowment and intrapsychic development, but also primarily on the quality of his interaction with the environment. It is important to understand that the developmental tasks identified by Erikson include both positive and negative outcomes. This means that the individual who has not satisfactorily achieved the developmental task for a specific stage of development will develop, as a result, a nondesirable and less healthy attribute in its stead. The most obvious example is the developmental task of the first developmental period—basic trust versus basic mistrust. The infant who is not successful, for whatever reason, in developing a sense of basic trust will not be left with an ego structure that demonstrates a mere lack of trust. The alternative is the development of an even more negative characteristic—a sense of basic mistrust. The significance of this paradigm is illustrated simply by the difference between the feelings of "I'm not sure that I can trust you," and "I'm sure that I cannot trust you." Therefore to understand Erikson's theory of personality development fully, the student must understand the negative as well as the positive outcomes of each developmental period.

Sullivanian concepts

Sullivan's theories are firmly based on the belief that human beings are more basically different from, than similar to all other animals. The uniqueness of human beings, according to Sullivan, lies in their interdependence; it is as a result of their interactions with others, not their physiological endowment, that the human personality is developed. As previously stated, Sullivan's theories are referred to as *interpersonal*, because of their emphasis on human interaction. Sullivan believed that all human behavior is goal directed toward the fulfillment of two needs: the need for satisfaction and the need for security. The need for satisfaction represents the biological needs of the person for such things as air, food, and sex. The need for security represents the emotional needs of the individual for such feelings states as interpersonal intimacy, status, and self-esteem. When these needs are perceived, internal tension results, and the individual employs a variety of methods to meet them and thereby reduce the tension. Sullivan called these methods *dynamisms*, and it is partially around the dynamisms characteristic of each age group that he built his theory of personality development. For example, during the first stage of development the oral cavity is used almost exclusively by the infant as the method to meet his needs for satisfaction (by crying to be fed) and his needs for security (by crying to be held). Therefore the stage of infancy is characterized by the oral dynamism, and the oral cavity becomes important because it is the means through which the individual establishes interpersonal contact, which in turn is the means through which his needs are met and tension is reduced. In fact the individual not only gets his needs met through interpersonal contact but also through this contact he establishes the fact of his own existence. Sullivan believed that an individual's self-concept is developed as a result of the quality of his interpersonal relationships with significant others in his infancy and childhood. In fact Sullivan defined the self-concept as the result of the reflected appraisals of significant others.

The concept of anxiety is central to Sullivan's theory of personality development. He postulated that anxiety is a response to feelings of disapproval from a significant adult. It is important to understand that these feelings may or may not be based in reality, and that the adult whose disapproval is feared may be real or a symbolic representation. According to Sullivan, then, the development of the personality consists of a series of interpersonally based learnings in which dynamisms are used as the individual attempts to gain approval and avoid the anxiety associated with disapproval.

DEVELOPMENT OF THE PERSONALITY

It has been said that the first 6 years in a child's life contribute the most to personality development. When one considers that these years provide the foundation for future patterns of behavior, this statement appears to be true. However the student must understand the influence of all stages of development on the personality to accurately assess the behavior of the adults for whom she provides nursing care. The following is a description and discussion of each of the developmental stages according to the theories of Freud, Erikson, and Sullivan.

Infancy

The period of infancy roughly extends over the first year and a half of life. Freud referred to this period as the *oral stage* because the child's libidinal energy is focused on his mouth and its functions to the exclusion of all other considerations. This singular focus on self is technically referred to as *primary narcissism*, which means self-love.

In the first months of life the infant is unable to differentiate between himself and his environment. He therefore feels that all that happens to him is caused by him. This feeling of being all powerful is termed *omnipotence*. The infant's awareness of himself is in terms of comfort or discomfort, and his total being is focused on fulfilling the demands of the id, which insists on relief from hunger and cold, which are perceived as a diffused tension. He seeks relief from this tension by using his mouth, lips, and tongue to cry, suck, and swallow. These activities provide him with the greatest pleasures, since they reduce discomfort. In the earliest months the infant is dependent on a nurturing adult to supply the nipple that meets his need for sucking and through which he obtains milk to swallow, appeasing the tension caused by hunger. Accidentally the infant soon finds his thumb and discovers that he can meet his own needs for sucking. Although sucking his own thumb provides pleasure it is experienced as being different from sucking the nipple. Through this simple realization the infant begins the complex, lengthy process of differentiating himself from the environment. In this way the ego or the recognition of the self or the "me" begins to develop.

When weaning is initiated the infant begins to receive fewer oral satisfactions from his environment. When the cup and solid food are substituted for the breast or bottle the infant feels frustrated. With the adoption of more rigid schedules the infant is denied the complete attention of the mother. He may react to these frustrations orally in an aggressive, sometimes destructive way and may begin to bite and may seek symbolic oral gratification by sucking other objects.

Because food and love are given simultaneously during the oral period, oral needs become synonymous with protective love and security. These needs are universal and continue throughout life in one form or another. In adult life release of tension through oral gratification is achieved through chewing gum, smoking, eating, and drinking. Freud believed that these activities are residuals of the oral stage of personality development.

Erikson's view of infancy is very similar to the Freudian view just described, although he terms it the *oral-sensory stage*. Unlike Freud, however, Erikson emphasizes the significance of the mother-child relationship in the achievement of the developmental task of the oral stage: *basic trust versus basic mistrust*. Erikson theorizes that if the infant's great need for love and attention is met consistently and unconditionally by a giving, loving mother, he will learn to trust her. Since the infant cannot help but view his mother as representative of the world at large, this attitude of basic trust in her will strongly influence his perceptions of other people and the environment. Therefore a healthy resolution of this stage of personality development, according to Erikson, results in the development of a basic sense of trust in the mother, which serves as the basis for the development of future trusting relationships. On the other hand, if the infant's experiences with his mother are characterized by inconsistencies and anxiety, he will learn to mistrust her and subsequently generalize this attitude to the world at large. It does not take much imagination to appreciate the many great differences between the feelings and behaviors of adults who have achieved a sense of basic trust and those who have achieved a sense of basic mistrust.

Sullivan referred to the first year and a half of life as the stage of infancy, rather than the oral stage, because he believed that the oral cavity has significance only in that it is the vehicle through which the infant establishes interpersonal contact. Sullivan introduced several very important concepts regarding the first stage of development. He coined the term *mothering one* to reflect the belief that the most important person in the infant's life is the individual who consistently nurtures him, and that this person does not necessarily have to be the biological mother. In fact, whether the mothering one is the biological mother or not, Sullivan believed that this person and the infant have to establish an interpersonal relationship, wherein they become highly significant to each other. This relationship is unique to the stage of infancy and is characterized by the *empathic linkage*, a symbolic emotional umbilical cord that makes the infant and the nurturing adult highly sensitive to each other's feeling states. Other theorists refer to this process as bonding. It is through the empathic linkage that both positive feelings of love and acceptance and negative feelings of anxiety and rejection are conveyed. Sullivan also believed that the development of the *self-concept* begins in the stage of infancy and is closely related to the quality of the infant's feeding experiences. Since the self-concept develops as the result of the reflected appraisals of significant others, if the infant frequently experiences satisfaction and security from the mothering one during the feeding process, he begins to see himself as being a worthwhile individual; that is, he will begin to develop a "good me" self-concept. Conversely, if the infant's experience with the mothering one is frequently fraught with tension and inconsistency, the foundation is laid for the development of a "bad me" self-concept, wherein the individual begins to see himself as being not worthwhile. If the infant is severely deprived during this stage, he will respond with massive amounts of anxiety that threaten his very life. To preserve his life the infant defends himself by disassociating the anxiety-generating experiences. As a result, he cannot develop a sense of self from reflected appraisals, so he develops a "not me" self-concept. This situation lays the foundation for the subsequent development of severe emotional problems.

Once the foundation is laid for its development, the self-concept tends to perpetuate itself. For example the child whose earlier reflected appraisals of significant others have led to the development of a "good-me" self-concept feels he is a worthwhile, valued person and tends to behave as such. This behavior, in turn, evokes further positive feedback from significant others and thereby reinforces the existing "good-me" self-concept. However, as the child grows he inevitably encounters people who do not respond to him in the accustomed manner. This unfamiliar experience evokes anxiety and is dealt with by the use of what Sullivan terms *security operations*, enabling the child to ignore this differing input. This process is just as applicable to people who have developed "bad-me" and "not-me" self-concepts and helps to explain why some persons succeed against all odds and others fail despite all advantages.

All three theorists agreed that the successful resolution of the first stage of personality development greatly enhances the probability of a successful resolution of subsequent stages.

Early childhood

The period of early childhood is a phase of personality development that occurs roughly between the ages of 18 months and 3 years. Freud termed this period of time the *anal stage*, because the libidinal energy shifts from the oral cavity to the anus and the urethra.

In the early part of this period the child freely gratifies his love of self with the pleasurable sensations involved in evacuating the bladder and bowels naturally and without restriction. Although the mouth remains an important zone of pleasure, the child derives his greatest pleasure from the anus and the urethra during these early years.

Ego development continues in this period as the child continuously develops a better defined concept of self. Superego development is initiated as the mother begins to insist that the child accept certain restrictions and controls regarding toileting. It is at this point that the child experiences the first major frustration of his id drives. He is forced to come to terms with the reality of the situation. To retain the love of the mother the child must learn to postpone the immediate pleasure of urinating or evacuating until the appropriate time and place are available. The necessity for adapting to the wishes of the mother regarding toileting places the child and the mother in conflict. As the mother makes demands on the child in an attempt to force him to accept her standards in relation to toileting, the child develops ambivalent feelings toward her, that is, he simultaneously loves and hates her.

Freud believed that if great stress is placed on the child in relation to remaining clean during this period, he may grow up to be compulsively clean and meticulous. On the other hand, he may unconsciously deal with his anxiety by the use of reaction formation as a defense mechanism and become very untidy and unconcerned about cleanliness in his adult life. Other adult attitudes thought to be traceable to rigid toilet training include stubbornness, hoarding and collecting, excessive concern with bowel function, and sadistic or masochistic tendencies.

Erikson refers to this stage of development as the *muscular-anal stage* and identifies *autonomy versus shame and doubt* as the developmental task to be addressed. Of great significance, according to Erikson, is the mother's response to the child's interest in assuming control over himself by controlling his urine and feces. If she treats the child with respect as an individual who is separate from her, he will begin to develop a sense of autonomy, or self-sufficiency. On the other hand, if his efforts to do for himself are ridiculed or interfered with, he will develop a sense of shame and doubt of his capabilities.

Sullivan used the term *early childhood* to refer to this period of life. He acknowledged the shift in the child's interest from his mouth to his anus but emphasized the sense of power the child feels as he attempts to control himself and others, particularly the mothering one. This feeling of power often puts the child and the mothering one in conflict as the mothering one attempts to toilet train the child. The process and outcome of this power struggle are believed to serve as the prototypical experience for similar interpersonal conflicts in later life. Of equal importance during this stage of development is Sullivan's belief that the child sees his feces as an extension of himself, and therefore the mothering one's response to the child's pleasure in his feces is seen by the child as a reflection of her view of him. In that way

Later childhood

the self-concept established in the stage of infancy is reinforced or altered.

The period of later childhood is a phase of development that includes the ages from 3 to 6. Freud called this period the *phallic stage*. This descriptive term refers to the fact that the focus of pleasurable sensations has shifted from the mouth and the excretory organs to the genitalia and that the child begins to identify with the parent of the same sex and unconsciously wishes to replace that parent in the family situation. Thus it is not uncommon to hear a girl in this age-group speak of "marrying Daddy" or a little boy say, "Go away, Daddy, I will take care of Mommy."

Between the ages of 3 and 6 years children begin to examine purposefully their own bodies and the bodies of their playmates. They discover that pleasurable sensations can be aroused from manipulation of the penis or the clitoris. The difference between the sexual structure of men and women is of great interest to them, and they wonder about the girl's lack of an obvious sexual organ. Children of this age may conclude that the penis can be lost in some way, since some people whose bodies they have observed have apparently lost this organ. Anxiety about the loss of the sex organ may develop among children in this age-group. Fears may be expressed by a little boy concerning the loss of his penis through punishment or an accident. These fears are referred to as *castration fears*. Unfortunately some parents reinforce these fears by threatening to cut off the penis if the child is observed fondling it. A little girl notices that she has no penis and may conclude that she lost it or that it has been taken away. She naturally wants what she observes some other children possess. This attitude on the part of a little girl is called *penis envy*. It is sometimes basic to the problem of *sibling rivalry*.

It should be noted that some theorists believe that any evidence of castration anxiety or penis envy in children of this age is a result of cultural conditioning and not an inherent element in personality development. This view is particularly popular among feminists, and a serious student of human behavior would be wise to keep an open mind, observing for behavioral changes in children as cultural changes take place.

During this period the little boy who has always had a great deal of attention and love from his mother begins to feel very possessive toward her. He wants her for himself, and he resents the close tie that he feels exists between his mother and father. He develops competitive feelings toward his father and tries to become a rival with him for his mother's love. The father is such a large and formidable opponent that the little boy develops a good deal of resentment and fear of him. This situation is referred to as the *Oedipus complex*. It may precipitate castration fears, because the little boy may begin to fear that the father will punish him for his resentment toward him and his attempt to replace him in his mother's life. Eventually the little boy concludes that being like his father is a more effective way of achieving his mother's love and attention. Thus he begins to take on the masculine behavior of his father. This is referred to as *identification*. In this way the little boy begins to learn the role of the male in the culture.

Similarly, during this period the little girl begins to identify with the feminine role. The process through which the girl passes in identifying with the parent of the same sex is not as clearly understood as is the process for little boys. The girl feels that somehow her mother is responsible for the fact that she does not have a penis. She also notices that she does not have breasts as her mother does. She may blame her mother for not having provided her with a complete body and may display a good deal of hostility and antagonism toward her. The little girl turns to her father for love and affection and frequently competes openly with the mother for his attention. She begins to imitate her mother because she feels that in this way she may be able to please her father. This is a difficult period for the little girl who must keep her mother's love and approval because she is still dependent on her. It is essential that the child maintain a positive relationship with her mother if she is to accomplish the task of identifying with the feminine role.

The birth of a baby in the family at this time presents both boys and girls of this age with a particularly difficult adjustment problem. The 3- to 6-year-old uses almost all of his energy in controlling his incestuous desires toward the parent of the opposite sex and his rage toward the parent of the same sex. The necessity to compete with a helpless infant for the attention of the parents often results in a great deal of overt sibling rivalry.

Superego development is also at its height at this time, since in most societies the issues being addressed are seen as moralistic ones. Therefore unless this stage is successfully resolved the potential exists for the child to develop long-lasting feelings of guilt because of his incestuous wishes for the parent of the opposite sex and his rage against the parent of the same sex.

Erikson refers to this stage of development as the *locomotor-genital stage* and describes it as having the developmental outcomes of *initiative versus guilt.* He agrees with Freud that children of this age desire to exclusively possess the parent of the opposite sex. To achieve this goal the child makes the first move, that is, he takes the initiative. In a healthy family environment the child inevitably fails to achieve his goal, but he learns a great deal about being assertive and is able to turn his failure into the process of learning how to become a spouse and parent in the future. If, on the other hand, he experiences a great deal of punitiveness and withdrawal of basic approval, his feelings of guilt that are already present will be reinforced and remain in subsequent stages.

Sullivan designated this period of life as *later childhood.* Sullivan believed that the major significance of this stage of personality development is that the child becomes capable of giving up his personal and private language and substitutes language that has universal meaning. The importance of the acquisition of the tool of language cannot be overemphasized, since it allows the child to begin to check out his perceptions and feelings with others. The term that describes this process is *consensual validation.* The ability to consensually validate experiences with others is a major factor in enabling the child to develop relationships with peers in the neighborhood or in the nursery school.

Latency

The stage of personality development that occurs roughly between the ages of 6 and 12 was called *latency* by Freud. This term was chosen because Freud believed that the child's libidinal energy was not focused on any one area of the body as it had been in the previous three stages. He believed that this energy was lying dormant, and therefore nothing of psychosexual significance occurred during this stage. The relatively stable behavior and even-tempered nature of most children of this stage attest to the temporary intrapsychic equilibrium established by the id, ego, and superego.

Erikson recognizes the very important role that school experiences play in the personality development of the child during this period. Although he agrees with Freud that no specific area of the body is of particular interest to children during this stage, he believes that psychic energy is being actively used in pursuit of knowledge and skills. In other words, the child is purposefully involved in acquiring tools through which he can deal with his environment both in the present and in the future. According to Erikson, if the child is successful in this endeavor, he will have achieved the developmental task of *industry*. If the child is unsuccessful, he will feel inadequate and develop a sense of *inferiority*.

Sullivan saw this period of time as being very critical to the development of a healthy adult personality. He divided Freud's and Erikson's 6-year span into two periods: the *juvenile era*, lasting roughly from ages 6 to 10; and *preadolescence*, lasting roughly from ages 11 to 12, or the onset of puberty. During the juvenile era the child turns away from his parents as being the most significant people in his life and looks to peers of the same sex to fill the functions of providing him with a sense of security and companionship. This is the period of gang formation and fierce gang loyalties. The gang requires strict adherence to the rules of the group, and the child slavishly complies with them. During this period the child tries to find his place among his peers. In so doing he acquires two very important interpersonal tools: the ability to compete and the ability to compromise. As the child tests out these modes of behavior with his peers their responses help him to learn to use both appropriately.

Another very important function of the peer group is the reinforcement or alteration of the self-concept. A child who enters this stage of development with a positive or "good me" self-concept is very likely to behave in a manner that elicits responses from his peers that confirm and reinforce his view of self. In instances when the child enters this period with a negative or "bad me" self-concept, positive reflected appraisals from his peer group can do much to alter his view of self. This fact indicates what a very significant role the peer group plays in the life of the child during this period.

During preadolescence the child maintains great interest in the group but simultaneously develops an intense love relationship with a particular person of the same sex who the child perceives to be very similar to himself. Sullivan called this special relationship a *chum relationship*. Up until this time the child's love has been self-centered, but in the chum relationship the child experiences for the first time the capacity to put the needs of someone else ahead of his own. Sullivan saw this experience as a necessary prerequisite to the establishment of a satisfactory heterosexual relationship in subsequent stages of development. The emotional intimacy that the chums experience also helps them to explore and clarify their feelings in a way that builds self-esteem.

Sullivan also stressed the importance of the school experience in the development of the child's personality. It is at school that children meet significant adults who greatly influence the development of their self-concepts. In this culture success at school is rewarded with much approval whereas lack of success often begins a series of defeats that carry over into adult life. The self-concept of children who do poorly in school may be irreparably damaged by the reactions of teachers, the significant adults in that important environment. On the other hand, understanding, helpful teachers may provide the child with a positive basis for self-evaluation and in some instances may constitute an opportunity for corrective interpersonal experiences with adults. Teachers are of tremendous importance in the lives of children and need to be aware of their potential for providing therapeutic experiences in their day-to-day contacts with children.

Puberty and adolescence

The stage of puberty and adolescence covers the years from age 12 to approximately age 18. Because all theorists agree that this stage of development is initiated by the active functioning of the sexual glands and because individuals mature physiologically at different rates, it is difficult to make a definite statement concerning the span of years included in adolescence.

Freud saw adolescence as the final stage of personality development characterized by a reactivation of libidinal energy and the focusing of this energy on the genital area. As such he designated this period as the *genital stage*. Although Freud believed that this final stage lasted for the rest of the person's life, he emphasized that the intense work of this period was completed when the individual achieved a satisfactory heterosexual relationship with a mate and began the life cycle anew by establishing a family.

Adolescence may be the most problematic stage of personality development. As the adolescent matures physiologically he is faced with the necessity of handling powerful sexual urges that threaten to put the influence of the id out of balance with the influences of the ego and superego. Because of this imbalance of psychic forces, unresolved conflicts and unsolved problems of earlier developmental periods often reemerge at this time. This is particularly true of the Oedipal conflict because of the similarity of the sexual urges experienced at both stages. Therefore the adolescent is simultaneously drawn toward his parents and driven away from them. This ambivalence is manifested by much conflict between the adolescent and his parents as the adolescent vacillates between behaving in a dependent, immature, childlike way and in an independent, mature, adult manner.

Erikson builds on Freud's theory by elaborating on the conflictual nature of the parent-child relationship. Erikson sees the developmental task of puberty and adolescence as the development of a sense of *identity versus role diffusion*. It is during this time that the individual must emancipate himself from his parents, not only physically but also emotionally by establishing for himself his own sense of identity. He must answer the most fundamental questions of "Who am I?" and "What am I?" This requires many decisions regarding familial, occupational, and social roles. To be sure, the adolescent is strongly influenced by his family's norms and values as he struggles to make these decisions. However, if he is to successfully master this developmental stage, he must accept these norms and values as his own, or reject them and establish new guidelines for himself. In other words, the adolescent's primary task is to develop an ego that has integrated previous learnings and experiences so that he develops a sense of continuity and sameness in his life. Unsuccessful mastery of this stage results in a diffuse, fragmented sense of self, the most problematic aspect of which is often the shifting between an adult and a child orientation.

Sullivan designated the period between 12 and 17 or 18 years of age as *early adolescence*. As the person experiences sexual urges (termed *lust* by Sullivan), he turns from the chum relationship to the task of establishing a relationship with a peer of the opposite sex. The peer group remains an important aspect of the adolescent's life during this stage because it serves the important function of providing security and consensual validation of the adolescent's feelings and behaviors. The influence of the peer group in regulating the adolescent's behavior is very strong.

Successful resolution of the stage of adolescence is greatly impeded when the child is seen as unacceptable by his peer group, perhaps because of physical handicaps or major cultural differences. The consequence of this nonacceptance may be a prolonged clinging to parents or parent figures to feel a sense of security and belongingness. Another pitfall of this stage occurs when the adolescent's peer group is composed of individuals who are antisocial in nature and engage in delinquent behavior. Although the adolescent will avoid the anxiety of isolation by identifying with this group, it is also likely that he will develop behaviors that are antagonistic to the society at large and that will impede him in the successful achievement of subsequent developmental tasks.

Young adulthood

The period of young adulthood has its onset at the end of adolescence and continues until adulthood. It is almost impossible to state a chronological age range for this period with any degree of accuracy, although many authorities state that it usually begins sometime in the person's twenties and is concluded in the late thirties or early forties. As the life span increases and the entry into the adult work world is delayed by the need for increasingly advanced education, it is obvious that the age ranges of the later developmental periods will have to be reevaluated.

As previously stated Freud believed that the healthy young adult will have achieved psychosexual maturity. By this he meant that the individual will have integrated his libidinal drives in a manner that enables him to love a member of the opposite sex with whom he hopes to establish a home and nurture a family. At the same time the healthy young adult retains enough self-love to seek satisfaction for his own needs without being destructive to others. In addition he is able to direct positive feelings toward other people in his environment, to work effectively, to achieve creatively, and to fully use the capacities with which he has been endowed without being hampered by crippling anxieties. The ability to achieve these mature capabilities depends to a large extent on the person's heredity and constitutional endowment. However, psychosexual development is powerfully influenced by the experiences that the person has during his early formative years.

Although Freud's theory of psychosexual development does not preclude the potential influence of events on personality in the individual's adult life, Freud postulated that the early developmental stages were critical and that the final stage begins in the late teens and lasts for the remainder of the person's life, with major personality development alterations being unlikely during this time under usual circumstances.

Erikson, on the other hand, sees the personality as continuing to develop dynamically throughout the remainder of the life span. During young adulthood Erikson sees the necessity for the individual to continue making decisions about significant aspects of life, such as choosing a mate with whom the individual can experience both physical and emotional intimacy. Erikson expresses this by stating that the task to be mastered during this period is the development of *intimacy versus isolation*. The ability to develop an intimate relationship with an adult of the opposite sex is highly dependent on satisfactory mastery of previous developmental tasks and leads to the establishment of a safe and congenial family environment in which children can be raised. Accepting the role of parent and the responsibility for nurturing, safeguarding, and rearing children is essential if the culture is to be perpetuated. Obviously the individual's ability to be successful in these activities is determined to a large extent by his experiences as a child within a family—hence the expression that the child is the father of the man. Erikson also emphasizes the significance of successfully building one's lifework during this stage. Children cannot be effectively nurtured unless the family has a reasonable degree of social and financial security. Thus acceptance of family responsibilities requires that the young adult be reasonably effective in performing some aspect of work.

If the developmental task of intimacy and its concomitant responsibilities are not achieved, the young adult is likely to develop a sense of emotional isolation having the sense that he "does not fit." Although the young adult who retreats into isolation often does so to avoid the emotional pain risked by the vulnerability associated with intimacy, he ironically discovers that the price of self-protection is not having his needs met, which increases the need to protect himself.

Sullivan referred to young adulthood as the stage of *late adolescence*. He believed that the major task of this period is the incorporation of intimacy (which developed during preadolescence with a chum) with lust (which became the mode of relating during early adolescence) so that these are not experienced in isolation from each other. Sullivan viewed this mode of relating as the hallmark of adult maturity, and therefore did not identify any subsequent stages of development.

Adulthood

As previously stated neither Freud nor Sullivan identified developmental dynamics beyond the achievement of adolescence or early adulthood. However, both these theorists implied that it may take the remainder of the individual's life for him to develop the maturity that theoretically should have been achieved by those periods. Erikson, however, continued to elaborate on developmental tasks specific to later life.

According to Erikson, the developmental task of adulthood is the development of *generativity versus stagnation.* Erikson believed that as the emotionally healthy individual grows older it becomes increasingly important to him that he transmit his values to the next generation, thereby helping to ensure his own immortality through the perpetuation of his culture. Therefore it is not unusual to see the adult become very involved in activities that are concerned with his community and the society at large. On the other hand, the individual who developed a sense of isolation during the previous period becomes increasingly self-absorbed and is often acutely aware of "marking time." This person gets little fulfillment from interpersonal relationships or work and has few if any meaningful goals. Hence Erikson's descriptive term, *stagnation.*

Current literature about the stage of adulthood makes it clear that this period is one about which we still need to learn more. Several authorities believe that the adult, because of physiological alterations, aging parents, an increasing awareness of community and societal needs, and grown children who lead lives independent of him, confronts his own mortality for the first time. It is believed that this confrontation results in much uneasiness about the status quo and a subsequent reevaluation of one's goals and purposes in life. Persons who have previously led relatively unexamined lives often find themselves in a state of crisis, which they may attempt to hide from others, since to them their concerns do not seem to be reality based. Societal manifestations of this turmoil are a marked increase in the divorce rate and major shifts in career patterns. For example the woman who has been relatively satisfied as a homemaker for the past 15 or 20 years feels as if she has been left out of the mainstream of life and suddenly develops a need to become involved in a career outside the home. Likewise, it is not uncommon for a husband and father at this stage of life to feel that the occupation in which he has been involved for the previous 20 years is unsatisfying, regardless of his monetary or social success.

It is understandable that this reaction on the part of either wife, husband, or both, causes much disequilibrium in the family system. As a result, it is believed, many middle-aged persons decide they have made a mistake, not only in choice of vocation, but also in marriage partner, geographical location, and hobbies. It is unfortunate that many decisions are made precipitously on the basis of these feelings and that these feelings are not recognized as being valid within the developmental context in which they occur.

Margaret Mead, world famous anthropologist, eloquently pointed out that the needs and requirements of marital partners, like those of their children, change as the relationship matures. Thus the maintenance of a happy and successful marriage relationship requires that the partners continuously seek to relate to each other as individuals whose needs are in a process of dynamic evolution.

Maturity

The role of aged individuals who have retired from an active social and economic life is unique in this culture. Unfortunately the wisdom they have accumulated through the years is not considered to be of value as it is in some cultures. Aging persons find it necessary to adjust to a reduced income, waning physical strength, and deteriorating health. This may be an anxiety-producing experience, since it represents a loss of power and independence. Loneliness is another experience with which elderly people must cope. Frequently their friends and marital partners die, leaving them in social isolation. Such lonely individuals who are no longer able to cope efficiently with their own physical requirements need to adjust to the establishment of living arrangements that are acceptable, while at the same time being faced with the need to accept a dependent role. Older persons need to establish social relationships with a group of interested, sympathetic peers. This need leads many older individuals to seek an affiliation with a "golden age" club or a similar organization.

The preceding statements about the stage of maturity are pessimistic in tone because of the current nature of the society in which we live and the ways in which elderly people are viewed. It should be clear that the older person must inevitably make many adjustments to altered physiological, social, and financial states. If his previous developmental tasks have been satisfactorily achieved, however, it is quite possible for him to make the necessary adjustments with grace, dignity, and a minimum of undue anxiety.

The major dynamic of the stage of maturity is the acceptance of the inevitability of death. To develop this acceptance the individual engages in a life review. If on the whole the aged person is able to feel satisfied with the uniqueness and achievements of his past life, Erikson believes the person will develop a sense of *ego integrity*, which in turn enables him to view death as the ultimate conclusion of life. If, on the other hand, the individual's life review finds him lacking, he will develop a sense of *despair*, because time is too short for him to undo and redo his life to achieve the sense of fulfillment he lacks.

As with adulthood, maturity is a stage of life about which much more can be learned. Interest in and concern about this stage of development are increasing as the number of older persons in our society increases.

Table 4-1 outlines the age-related interpersonal experiences and behavioral outcomes experienced by human beings as they traverse the eight ages of man identified by Erikson. They are outlined here because of their comprehensiveness and applicability to nursing practice.

CONCLUDING STATEMENTS

1. The understanding of personality development is integral to the practice of psychiatric nursing but it is also essential to the general practice of nursing.
2. Before the beginning of the twentieth century the physical and emotional development of human beings was poorly understood. It was not until the early twentieth century that the study of personality development of children began in earnest. Interest in the personality development of adults took longer to emerge.

Table 4-1   interpersonal age-related experiences and behavioral outcomes based on Erikson's theory of personality development

ages of man	interpersonal age-related experiences	age-related behavioral outcomes	ego qualities
ORAL-SENSORY			
Positive	Infant is held lovingly and tenderly by mother; needs met with sensitivity and consistency.	Infant sleeps and feeds easily; is usually relaxed and snuggles closely when held.	Basic trust
Negative	Infant continuously experiences anxiety in contact with mother; needs met inconsistently.	Infant generally tense and crying; not comforted by holding; rages when left by mother.	Basic mistrust
MUSCULAR-ANAL			
Positive	Toddler's efforts to stand on own feet are respected and encouraged; relaxed, unhurried toilet training.	Toddler takes pride in self-expression, whether making bowel movements or playing.	Autonomy
Negative	Toddler experiences rejection as efforts at self-sufficiency are ridiculed; cleanliness overemphasized	Toddler is self-conscious, hiding face or self from others; is stubborn and has temper tantrums.	Shame and doubt
LOCOMOTOR-GENITAL			
Positive	Child's need to explore body is accepted matter-of-factly; sexual curiosity handled without anxiety.	Child begins to imitate parent of the same sex; approaches tasks with enthusiasm.	Initiative
Negative	Child's masturbatory activities are condemned and punished; sexual curiosity ignored or rebuked.	Child experiences nightmares, often symbolic of castration; hides masturbatory activities.	Guilt
LATENCY			
Positive	Child's efforts at learning are supported; new interests and friendships encouraged.	Child is obedient, prefers order and limits; works on projects to completion with peers.	Industry
Negative	Child is ridiculed in front of peers; friends and interests criticized.	Child fears failure and gives up; does not try to do or to learn.	Inferiority
PUBERTY AND ADOLESCENCE			
Positive	Youth's beginning emancipation from family is accepted; vocational choices supported.	Youth turns from parents to peer groups, joining cliques and clubs; develops crushes on other figures.	Identity
Negative	Youth's rapidly changing body, awkwardness, and interest in opposite sex are ridiculed; parents try to dominate.	Youth is unable to separate from parents; is embarrassed over physical changes; is unable to make job choice.	Role diffusion

Adapted from Lofstedt. *Mereness' Essentials of Psychiatric Nursing Learning and Activity Guide,* St. Louis, 1982, The C. V. Mosby Company.

Table 4-1 interpersonal age-related experiences and behavioral outcomes based on Erikson's theory of personality development—cont'd

ages of man	interpersonal age-related experiences	age-related behavioral outcomes	ego qualities
YOUNG ADULTHOOD			
Positive	Young adult experiences support, interest, approval, and tenderness in love relationship; has job satisfaction.	Young adult is well-rounded; has varied interests in family, job, friends, and hobbies.	Intimacy
Negative	Young adult's choice of partner is rejected by parents; parents try to hold and control offspring.	Young adult sacrifices relatedness for work and drive to succeed; is unable to give emotionally to others.	Isolation
ADULTHOOD			
Positive	Adult experiences orgasm with loved, trusted, and respected partner; experiences love and respect from offspring.	Adult is productive and creative; bears and nurtures children; teaches and gives to others.	Generativity
Negative	Adult experiences rejection and hostility in adult relationships; takes no pleasure in community affairs.	Adult experiences impotence/frigidity; becomes bored and resentful with job.	Stagnation
MATURITY			
Positive	Individual experiences love and respect from maturing offspring; has satisfying past recollections.	Individual looks forward to retirement as opportunity to try new things; recalls past with pleasure.	Ego integrity
Negative	Individual experiences alienation from family; loneliness occurs as friends, spouse, and others die.	Individual faces death with fear, preoccupied with reliving life because of dissatisfaction with the past.	Despair

3. Much of our current knowledge concerning personality development is based on the theories proposed by Sigmund Freud (1856-1939). Freud's theory of personality development is called the *psychosexual theory* of development.
4. Erik Erikson, born in 1902, built on Freud's theories by identifying eight developmental stages that encompass the entire life span, referred to as the *Eight Ages of Man*.
5. Harry Stack Sullivan, an American psychiatrist (1892-1949), developed a theory of personality development that emphasizes the uniqueness of human interdependence. Sullivan's

theory is called the *interpersonal theory* of psychiatry.

6. The term *personality* refers to the aggregate of physical and mental qualities of the individual as these interact in characteristic fashion with his environment.

7. A theoretically eclectic approach to the understanding of personality development is particularly applicable to the practice of nursing.

8. The levels of consciousness were described by Freud as the conscious, the preconscious, and the unconscious.

9. According to Freud, the structure of the personality includes the id, the ego, and the superego.

10. Erikson's theory of personality development emphasizes the ability of the ego to develop in a healthy, adaptive manner given a facilitative environment. Therefore it is variously referred to as neo-Freudian, ego psychology, or cultural.

11. Sullivan theorized that personality development consists of a series of interpersonally based learnings in which dynamisms are used as the individual attempts to gain approval and avoid the anxiety associated with disapproval.

12. Freud identified five stages of personality development: the oral stage, the anal stage, the phallic stage, the stage of latency, and the genital stage. These descriptive terms represent the area of the body on which the libidinal energy is focused.

13. Erikson identifies developmental tasks specific to eight stages of development. These are basic trust versus basic mistrust, autonomy versus shame and doubt, initiative versus guilt, industry versus inferiority, identity versus role diffusion, intimacy versus isolation, generativity versus stagnation, and ego integrity versus despair.

14. Sullivan identified significant interpersonal learnings that take place during each of seven stages of development. During the stage of infancy, the self-concept is learned; during early childhood, the use of power; during later childhood, the use of language that can be consensually validated; during the juvenile era, the ability to compete and to compromise; during preadolescence, the ability to experience intimacy; during early adolescence, the development of a heterosexual orientation; and during late adolescence, the integration of intimacy and lust in a heterosexual relationship.

SUGGESTED SOURCES OF ADDITIONAL INFORMATION

Classical

Berlien, Ivan C.: Growth as related to mental health, Am. J. Nurs. **56:**1142-1145, 1956.

Bowlby, John: Maternal care and mental health, Series No. 2, Geneva, 1952, World Health Organization.

Brill, A.A.: Freud's contribution to psychiatry, New York, 1944, W.W. Norton & Co., Inc.

Caplan, Gerald: Prevention of mental disorders in children, New York, 1961, Basic Books, Inc., Publishers.

Committee on Psychiatric Nursing, National League for Nursing Education: Psychological concepts of personality development, Am. J. Nurs. **50:**122-125, 182-184, 242-243, 1950.

English, O. Spurgeon, and Pearson, G.H.J.: Emotional problems of living; avoiding the neurotic pattern, ed. 3, New York, 1963, W.W. Norton & Co., Inc.

Munroe, Ruth L.: Schools of psychoanalytic thought, New York, 1955, The Dryden Press, Inc.

Sullivan, Harry Stack: The interpersonal theory of psychiatry, New York, 1968, W.W. Norton & Co., Inc.

Thompson, Clare: The different schools of psychoanalysis, Am. J. Nurs. **57:**1304-1307, 1957.

Contemporary

Arnold, Helen M.: Snowwhite and the seven dwarfs: a symbolic account of human development, Perspect. Psychiatr. Care **117**(5):218-222, Sept.-Oct., 1979.

Bowlby, John: Attachment, New York, 1980, Basic Books, Inc., Publishers.

Bowlby, John: Separation, New York, 1980, Basic Books, Inc., Publishers.

Cumming, Elaine, and Henry, William E.: Growing old; the process of disengagement, New York, 1979, Arno Press, Inc.

Dilman, I: Freud and human nature, Oxford, England, 1983, Basil Blackwell, Ltd.

Dresen, Sheila E.: Staying well while growing old: autonomy, a continuing developmental task. V. Am. J. Nurs. **78:**1344-1346, Aug., 1978.

Ehmann, Virginia E.: Empathy: its origin, characteristics, and process, Perspect. Psychiatr. Care **9:**72-80, March-April, 1971.

Geller, Joseph: Developmental symbiosis, Perspect. Psychiatr. Care **13:**10-12, Jan.-March, 1975.

Gibney, Helen A.: Masturbation: an invitation for an interpersonal relationship, Perspect. Psychiatr. Care **10:**128-134, July-Sept., 1972.

Graves, Joy Dan: Psychoanalytic theory—a critique, Perspect. Psychiatr. Care **11**(3):114-120, 1973.

Howell, Elizabeth, and Bayes, Marjorie, editors: Women and mental health, New York, 1981, Basic Books, Inc., Publishers.

Lanza, Marilyn: Originals of aggression, J. Psychosoc. Nurs. Ment. Health Serv. **21:**11-16, June, 1983.

Lidz, Theodore: The person, his and her development throughout the life cycle, New York, 1976, Basic Books, Inc., Publishers.

May, Robert: Sex and fantasy: patterns of male and female development, New York, 1980, W.W. Norton & Co., Inc.

Pinch, Winifred: Feminine attributes in a masculine world, Nurs. Outlook **29:**596-599, Oct., 1981.

Powers, Mary Ellen: Universal utility of psychoanalytic theory for nursing practice models, J. Psychosoc. Nurs. Ment. Health Serv. **18:**28-30, April, 1980.

Rouslin, Sheila: Developmental aggression and its consequences, Perspect. Psychiatr. Care **13:**170-175, Oct.-Dec., 1975.

Schutzenhofer, Karen K.: The development of autonomy in adult women, J. Psychosoc. Nurs. Ment. Health Serv. **21:**25-30, April, 1983.

Sheehy, Gail: Passages—predictable crises of adult life, New York, 1976, E.P. Dutton, Inc.

Woods, Nancy Fugate: Human sexuality in health and illness, ed. 2, St. Louis, 1979, The C.V. Mosby Co.

Woosley, Debra Gooden: A working concept of intellectualization, J. Psychosoc. Nurs. Ment. Health Serv. **18:**36-39, Jan., 1980.

Of Particular Interest

Erikson, Erik H.: Childhood and society, ed. 2, New York, 1964, W.W. Norton & Co., Inc.
This classic text presents the author's psychosocial theory of personality development in a sensitive, insightful manner.

Rogers, C.: On becoming a person, Boston, 1961, Houghton Mifflin Co.
Personal growth is discussed in this text both from the individual's point of view and as it affects the therapeutic process.

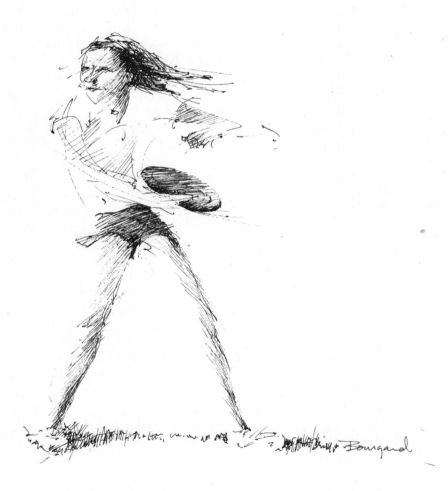

Gotta keep moving, gotta keep busy.

LEARNING OBJECTIVES
After studying this chapter the student will be able to:

1 Define the concept of anxiety and list its characteristics.

2 Discuss the process through which anxiety originates as theorized by Freud and by Sullivan.

3 Discuss how ego defense mechanisms, security operations, and coping mechanisms serve as adaptations to anxiety.

Anxiety is the most universal of human emotions and is experienced by all persons throughout their entire life span. Despite its all-pervasive nature, however, anxiety cannot be observed directly. Rather, its presence can be inferred only from behavior.

Anxiety is simultaneously an adaptation and a stressor. It functions as an adaptation in that it is a response to system disequilibrium and initially reduces the level of stress by obscuring the nature of the stressor. In the long run anxiety is a nonproductive adaptation because it prevents the system from focusing on and directly dealing with the source of the stress. Nevertheless, its existence is a signal that the system is having difficulty maintaining homeokinesis and in that sense it serves a valuable function.

Anxiety also serves as a stressor in that it, unlike any other emotion, is always perceived as negative. Thus its presence thrusts the system into a state of stress, sometimes compounding rather than relieving the original stress. Because anxiety is always perceived as being negative, the system employs a variety of mechanisms to deal with it that are themselves adaptations.

Because anxiety is a basic factor in the development and manifestation of human behavior, it is necessary for the nurse to acquire an in-depth understanding of its characteristics, origin, and the usual adaptations to it.

HISTORICAL PERSPECTIVE

It is reasonable to assume that people have experienced anxiety since the dawn of humanity. Until recently, however, human beings have had to struggle merely to survive. Consequently it is likely they more frequently experienced the emotion of fear than that of anxiety.

The emotions of fear and anxiety are indistinguishable to the person experiencing them. Fear is a response to a real stressor that threatens the very existence of the system. Because the stressor can be identified, it becomes possible to deal with it directly by fighting it or fleeing it. These adaptations provide a direct outlet for the physiological and psychological tension resulting from the emotion of fear.

Such is not the case when the adaptation to a stressor is anxiety. In this instance the feeling perceived is the same as that known when fear is present but the stressor is unknown to the person. Consequently there is no direct outlet for the built-up tension; the anxiety becomes a stressor itself.

Sigmund Freud was the first theorist to emphasize the importance of anxiety in the development of human behavior. He first demonstrated the use of ego defense mechanisms as an adaptation to anxiety and believed that the necessity for their use indicated a greater or lesser degree of psychopathology. In contrast, contemporary theorists believe that psychopathology exists when the individual utilizes defense mechanisms as the predominant mode of dealing with anxiety, thereby obscuring reality, or when the individual utilizes only one or two such mechanisms to the exclusion of all others. In other words, it is acknowledged that a sparing use of a wide variety of mental mechanisms is within the range of healthy behavior. It should be noted, however, that as the society becomes more complex and therefore more stressful, anxiety and its adaptations become more frequent causes and effects of mental disorders. Mental disorders specific to anxiety to its adaptations are discussed more fully in Chapter 15.

DEFINITION AND CHARACTERISTICS OF ANXIETY

Anxiety is defined as a vague sense of impending doom, an apprehension or sense of dread, which seemingly has no basis in reality. Lay persons refer to anxiety as "being nervous."

As observed earlier anxiety is the only emotion that is always perceived as being negative. In contrast to anxiety, emotions that are usually considered to be painful sometimes bring pleasure. For example, most people do not enjoy being angry. On occasion, however, it is satisfying to experience anger when one feels it is justified and shares it in common with others. Another characteristic of anxiety is its extreme communicability. Almost like a living organism, anxiety is transferred with amazing rapidity from one individual to another, often below a level of awareness.

When the individual experiences anxiety he cannot distinguish it from fear, a feeling state that occurs in response to a specific identifiable environmental threat. Because anxiety cannot be distinguished from fear the physiological response is the same in that the autonomic nervous system is activated and the body becomes ready for "fight or flight." Since an identifiable environmental threat is not present the individual cannot discharge the tension of anxiety by fighting or fleeing and consequently may experience such symptoms as a pounding heart and a dry mouth, the perception of which serves to increase anxiety. Furthermore, when an individual becomes aware of being anxious he often frantically searches for a reason to explain this feeling in the hope of abolishing it. He is rarely successful, and his explanation often describes the result of his anxiety, not its cause. For example, a young woman who believes she is anxious because of the responsibilities she must assume in the care of her young infant may really be experiencing a conflict between a desire to be dependent and the need to be independent, which in turn creates anxiety, making her increasingly less able to care for the infant. Therefore her explanation of her anxiety is not its cause but rather its manifestation.

Anxiety occurs in degrees. Although it is never seen as desirable, mild anxiety serves the function of motivating the person and making him more physically and mentally alert. When the level of anxiety is extremely high the individual may be incapable of action or may react with unusual behavior or what appears to be irrational behavior. This irrational behavior is referred to as a panic state.

ORIGIN OF ANXIETY

Most authorities believe that anxiety occurs most often as an adaptation to a threat to biological integrity, an unconscious symbolic conflict, or a threat to the self-concept.

Freud believed that anxiety is a response to the emergence of id impulses that are unacceptable to the superego. In other words the ego detects a real or potential conflict between the id and the superego, which results in anxiety, thereby alerting the ego to the necessity for intervention. He believed that all persons experience anxiety initially during the birth process when the respiratory and cardiovascular systems must undergo rapid, extensive changes to support extrauterine life. He also viewed the birth process as the prototypical separation. These two factors—the threat to life and separation—are associatively linked to each other and to the experience of anxiety. In subsequent developmental stages, he theorized, unconscious conflicts are perceived as life threatening, are associated with separation, and result in anxiety.

Sullivan viewed anxiety as always occurring in an interpersonal context. That is, anxiety is generated when the individual anticipates or actually receives cues that signal disapproval from one or more significant others. This presents an individual with an approach-avoidance dilemma in that there is a desire to approach or please the other person because he is seen as being significant, but to do so incurs the risk of disapproval of self—a threat to the very existence of the individual as he knows himself. According to Sullivan the human being first experiences anxiety as an infant when either his need for satisfaction, which is physiologically based, or his need for security, which is interpersonally based, is not met by the mothering one. The student will remember that Sullivan's theory of personality development also emphasized the empathic linkage between infant and mothering one through which anxiety is readily communicated. The empathic linkage makes the infant and mothering one uncommonly sensitive to discomfort in each other. Because of his inability to solve problems, the infant has no alternative but to believe that the mothering one's anxiety, which is communicated to him via the empathic linkage, is caused by him, even though the source of this discomfort may be external to him. This phenomenon, which all adults have experienced, by definition, during their infancy, is the basis for Sullivan's belief that anxiety is interpersonally based.

Some authorities distinguish between normal anxiety and pathological anxiety. In reality this distinction refers to the nature of the stressor that precipitates the response of anxiety rather than to the nature of the anxiety itself. *Normal anxiety* arises from a realistic apprehension of a previously unencountered situation that has symbolic meaning to the individual. For example, the anxiety a bridegroom experiences before his wedding very likely arises in response to his unconscious concern about his ability to assume the role of husband and therefore his view of the wedding as a symbolic threat to his identity as an adequate male.

In contrast, *pathological anxiety* is often a response to thoughts, feelings, wishes, or desires that, if conscious, would be unacceptable to the individual himself or that, if known, would cause the loss of approval or love from significant others. Therefore situations that evoke such unacceptable thoughts, feelings, wishes, or desires are associated with anxiety against which the individual must defend in order to maintain his self-concept. For example, a young man who has unconscious homosexual desires that if known to him would be repugnant might react with massive amounts of anxiety when circumstances such as college force him to live in close physical proximity with other young men.

ADAPTATIONS TO ANXIETY

Because moderate to high levels of prolonged anxiety can prove lethal to the human system, some method of relieving anxiety is essential if the system is to regain homeokinesis. The human being usually is able to relieve anxiety through a form of adaptation referred to as mental mechanisms. *Mental mechanisms* are patterns of thinking and behaving that are used to protect the individual from threatening aspects of his environment or from his own feelings of anxiety. Mental mechanisms are learned as being effective adaptations to anxiety during one of the phases of personality development. They are further developed and elaborated upon as the individual grows and struggles with problems. Thus the use of these mechanisms is a matter of resorting to earlier patterns of thinking and behaving that have already proved helpful in relieving anxiety. Many of these methods of thinking and behaving are wholly unconscious, whereas others are partly conscious and partly unconscious. All, however, are a means of protecting the individual from situations he perceives as dangerous. In this regard they serve a very important function by helping the person to maintain biological integrity and self-esteem.

Ego defense mechanisms are one type of commonly used mental mechanism. These are utilized when the individual unconsciously experiences a basic conflict between id impulses and the demands of the superego. The ego unconsciously uses some of its energy to initiate a defense mechanism that effects a compromise between the demands of the id and the superego, thereby relieving anxiety.

Another form of mental mechanism is called *security opera-*

tions. These were identified by Sullivan and are called into play when anxiety is a response to a threat to the self-concept. Security operations, like ego defense mechanisms, operate without the awareness of the individual employing them.

Although the sparing use of mental mechanisms is considered healthy and serves the function of lowering anxiety, thereby enabling the system to regain homeokinesis, this use does exact a toll. The price of this adaptation is the use of system energy, resulting in less potential energy available for growth. Furthermore the stressor, whether it be a conflict or threat, is not directly addressed or resolved.

Another adaptation to anxiety is that of *coping mechanisms.* A coping mechanism, unlike an ego defense mechanism or a security operation, is based on a conscious acknowledgment that a problem exists. As a result the individual engages in reality-oriented problem-solving activities designed to reduce tension. It is for this reason that coping mechanisms are considered to be more healthy adaptations than ego defense mechanisms or security operations. For example, when a student unexpectedly fails an examination he would be using the ego defense mechanisms of projection if he believed that he failed bcause the teacher was inadequate. Although this would reduce his anxiety it would not be helpful in enabling him to pass the course. On the other hand, if this student were able to acknowledge his failure to himself he would then be able to use the coping mechanism of going to the instructor for help. If he understands his errors not only is his anxiety reduced but he is also able to learn what is necessary to pass the course.

Ego defense mechanisms

The following is a discussion of commonly used ego defense mechanisms as identified by Freud. The student should remember that these defenses emanate from the unconscious and use psychic energy derived from the ego as they protect it from anxiety. Furthermore it should not be forgotten that an ego defense mechanism may originate in more than one stage of personality development, or it may originate in one stage and be reinforced in others. Ego defense mechanisms are not clear-cut and almost never appear as isolated phenomenon.

Compensation. Compensation is a pattern of adaptive behavior by which anxiety resulting from feelings of inadequacy or weakness is relieved as the individual emphasizes some personal or social attribute that overshadows the perceived inadequacy or weakness and gains social approval.

The origins of this adaptation can be seen in the young infant who substitutes his thumb or toy for the nipple or bottle to relieve tension and compensate for some of the pleasurable sensations of sucking that may be lacking in quantity.

Obviously compensation is far more complicated in adults than in infants and is usually prompted by feelings of guilt or inferiority. It may explain much of the behavior observed in adults who work zealously to promote philanthropic enterprises. Compensation may be operating in the behavior of a man who is very small in physical stature but who is extremely successful in the business world through his aggressive practices. It may also be one of the mechanisms operating when a young person who is paralyzed as a result of a car accident is able to achieve many honors for outstanding scholarship in college.

Displacement. Displacement is a defense mechanism used when an individual unconsciously believes he would be in great danger if his feelings about another person were known to that person. The adaptation to the resultant anxiety is the discharge of feelings onto a person or object entirely different from the one to which they actually belong. Displacement may be used by a teacher who is angry with an immediate supervisor and does not show these feelings in his presence but reacts with unreasonable anger when a pupil accidentally breaks a windowpane on that same day. The teacher may be displacing angry feelings by expressing them toward the student rather than toward the supervisor. Actually the teacher has unconsciously substituted the student for the supervisor and has displaced the feelings accordingly.

Denial. Denial is the adaptation often employed to defend the system against the stress of the sudden onset of massive amounts of anxiety. It is a process whereby the individual truly does not recognize the existence of an event or feeling. Although denial is a commonly used defense in severe emotional illnesses such as schizophrenia, it is often seen as a reaction of the healthy individual when he is unexpectedly confronted by a disastrous situation. For example, the wife of a policeman who has just been killed in the line of duty may calmly respond to the informant, "You must have made a mistake! I just had breakfast with him no more than

2 hours ago. I'm getting ready to shop now, so you'll have to excuse me.''

It is important to understand that the mechanism of denial operates on a totally unconscious basis in response to the sudden onset of massive amounts of anxiety. Denial should not be confused with lying, which is a conscious effort to avoid responsibility in a situation.

Fixation. Fixation refers to the point in the individual's development at which certain aspects of the emotional development cease to advance. For reasons that are usually obscure, further development seems to be blocked. This blocking appears to arise from the inability of the individual to solve problems that occurred during the specific phase of development at which progress ceased. Thus the individual is unable to achieve the developmental tasks of that phase, and since it is not possible to entirely bypass a stage, he is always handicapped in proceeding to the stages that follow. For example, individuals who have not experienced the love and security required for the satisfactory resolution of the first stage of development may spend the remainder of their lives attempting to achieve gratification through the oral cavity. Some individuals fixated at this stage of personality development may drink huge quantities of alcohol or compulsively overeat, because food and liquid intake are so closely allied to love and security in the unconscious emotional life.

Sublimation. In the mechanism of sublimation the energy involved in anxiety-producing primitive impulses and cravings is unconsciously redirected into constructive and socially acceptable channels. This is one of the chief mechanisms operating when a child learns to redirect the pleasurable sensations involved in expelling excrement at will into the more socially acceptable patterns of toilet training.

Sublimation is one of the more positive adaptations to anxiety and is at least partially responsible for much of the artistic and cultural achievement of civilized people. It is operating when a woman redirects her sexual drives, which might be expected to result in a home and children, into a successful career as a nursery school teacher. It is probably operating when a young man who has lost his lover turns to writing poetry about love.

Reaction formation. Reaction formation can occur when an individual experiences anxiety resulting from unconscious feelings or wishes that are unacceptable to him and relieves the anxiety by expressing an attitude or acting in a way that is directly opposite to that which he really feels. Thus the individual is denying, in a sense of the word, his true feelings or desires. People who are extremely friendly, overly polite, and very socially correct frequently have unconscious feelings of anger and hatred toward many people. These true feelings may be evident in slips of the tongue or in biting humor.

Reaction formation sometimes develops out of rigid toilet-training experiences. One evidence of reaction formation may be observed in adults who are untidy about their homes and their personal hygiene but whose mothers required meticulous conformity to rules of cleanliness and tidiness.

Identification. Identification is a much used and extremely useful mechanism because it plays a large part in the development of a child's personality and in the process of acculturation. Through the process of identification the individual defends against anxiety resulting from feelings of inadequacy by unconsciously taking on desirable attributes found in people for whom he has admiration and affection. He integrates these attributes into his own personality. Thus the little boy takes on masculine attributes that he admires in his father. The student integrates into his personality makeup the attributes he admires in his professor. Another form of identification is observed when an individual develops an unreasoning sympathy for a criminal because of an unconscious sense of guilt.

Introjection. The mechanism of introjection is closely related to identification. However, whereas the mechanism of identification adds to the individual's personality, introjection tends to replace all or part of the personality. This defense is based on the psychoanalytic concept of oral receptivity and refers to the unconscious symbolic swallowing of an aspect of a significant person in response to anxiety precipitated by the real or perceived loss of this person. Introjection is operating when the child develops the superego by incorporating the ideals and standards of the parents. When introjection is operating in adults it suggests that the entire personality of a second person has been incorporated and has replaced the original personality. A psychotic patient who claimed to be Moses wore a beard, let his hair grow long, talked in biblical phrases, and acted as Moses might have acted. What he believed to be the personality of Moses had been incorporated by the patient, and he had given up his own personality. Introjection may operate in a less constructive way than identification, especially when it is observed in adults. For instance, a depressed person may have unconsciously incorporated another person and attempt to commit suicide to kill the introjected person whom he unconsciously hates.

Undoing. In the mechanism of undoing the individual engages in certain behaviors as a means of symbolically canceling out unconscious thoughts or feelings that are unacceptable and therefore associated with anxiety. Although the individual is aware of his behavior he is not aware of its purpose, and his behavior often seems irrational even to him. Undoing is seen as the basis of compulsive behavior. Undoing behavior is frequently highly repetitive, because it does not achieve its aim of actually canceling out the anxiety-producing thought or feeling. A famous example of this defense mechanism is found in Shakespeare's play *Macbeth*. Lady Macbeth, the wife of the main character, compulsively washes her hands exclaiming, "Out, out damned spot!" after having goaded her husband into murdering the king.

Isolation. Isolation is a phenomenon where the feeling is detached from the event in the individual's memory, enabling the person to recall the event without its attendant anxiety. This mechanism is evident in situations when an individual relays a harrowing experience without any evidence of emotion.

Rationalization. Rationalization is a mental mechanism that is almost universally employed. It is an attempt to make one's behavior appear to be the result of logical thinking rather than the result of unconscious desires or cravings that are anxiety producing. It is used when the individual has a sense of guilt about something he does or believes or when he is uncertain about his behavior. It is a face-saving device that may or may not deal with the actual truth. Rationalization should not be confused with falsehoods or alibis, since the latter are conscious avoidance maneuvers. Rationalization is almost totally unconscious, and although it is used to put the individual in the best possible light, it does not have the deliberate aspect of other conscious avoidance maneuvers.

The person who does not want to keep an appointment because to do so would create anxiety and says that the appointment slipped his mind is not telling a falsehood, but rather is using rationalization as a defense mechanism. Although rationalization relieves anxiety temporarily, it is not an effective mechanism of adjustment because it assists the individual to avoid facing the reality factors in the situation.

Repression. Repression is a widely used and completely unconscious mechanism. Painful experiences, unacceptable thoughts and impulses, and disagreeable memories are forcibly dismissed from consciousness to relieve the anxiety associated with them. The psychic energy with which they were invested becomes an active free-floating source of anxiety in the unconscious mind. Many painful experiences are repressed during early childhood and become unconscious sources of emotional conflict in later life. Selfish, hostile feelings and sexual impulses are frequently repressed. Such repression always causes internal conflict. This repressed material may find escape through conversion into physical symptoms, or into obsessions or pathological anxiety that arises without apparent reason.

Regression. Regression occurs when an individual is faced with anxiety stemming from a conflict or problem that cannot be solved by using the adaptive mechanisms with which he customarily solves problems. In such a situation he may unconsciously resort to behavior that was successful at an earlier stage in his development but which he had presumably outgrown. Thus regression is a return to patterns of behavior appropriate to an earlier developmental stage. Any retreat into a state of dependency on others to avoid facing acute problems can be called a regressive trait. "Crying on someone's shoulder" is symbolic of the infant's seeking comfort on the maternal bosom. Although some seeking for a dependency relationship is a benign form of regression, this mechanism may become the main element in the development of a serious psychosis.

Projection. Projection is a frequently used unconscious mechanism that relieves anxiety by transferring the responsibility for unacceptable ideas, impulses, wishes, or thoughts to another person. The mechanism is used when the individual's own hostile, aggressive thoughts are unacceptable to him and thus cause anxiety. Although all people use this mechanism to some extent it is not a healthy method of adaptation and is more frequently used by mentally ill persons than by more healthy individuals. It is operative in such psychotic symptoms as delusions and hallucinations. In the latter, the individual hears voices saying things about him that he unconsciously fears are true. The paranoid person may project his own inner hate of others by saying that a group of people is plotting to kill him. Less pathological use of projection is evident when a worker blames the boss for his difficulties on the job or when a student blames the teacher for his failure on an examination. Paranoid persons frequently project their feelings of sexual inadequacy on others. Thus a common delusion concerns the unfaithful spouse when the actual lack of fidelity is in the mind of the accuser.

Symbolization and condensation. A symbol is an idea or object used by the conscious mind in lieu of the actual idea or object, which if consciously perceived would be anxiety producing. Instinctual desires may appear through symbols, the meanings of which are not clear to the conscious mind. For example, a man who unconsciously harbors feelings of inadequacy about his masculinity may defend against this anxiety by owning only large automobiles despite the fact he cannot afford to purchase or operate them. The phallic symbolism of large automobiles serves to reassure this individual about his adequacy as a male.

Symbols are the language of the unconscious. Such symbols appear in dreams or in fantasies and may emerge through various rituals or obsessive behavior. Symbols may become further merged by condensation to represent a wide range of anxiety-producing ideas that become lumped together so as to lose their painful significance. When they rise to the conscious level they take the form of an apparently incoherent jumble of words, the real meaning of which is hidden in the unconscious. Such condensations of thinking are frequently noted in the apparently irrational language of the schizophrenic individual. However these condensations have meaning and significance for him.

Conversion. Conversion refers to the expression of emotional conflicts through a physical symptom for which there is no demonstrable organic basis. The use of this mechanism is preceded by the use of repression whereby the anxiety resulting from the emotional conflict was previously adapted to by repressing the conflict into the unconscious. When the conflict reappears as a physical symptom the individual is unaware of any connection between the two phenomena. Thus a child who is highly anxious because of chronic friction between her parents, both of whom she loves, may find herself suddenly blind. This symptom literally relieves her of the necessity of seeing such incompatibility. In like manner, a young soldier who simultaneously loves his country but abhors killing may suddenly develop a paralysis of his right hand rendering him unable to pull the trigger of a gun.

Although the physical symptom is symbolically related to the nature of the conflict, conversion is not always expressed in a direct and easily recognized manner. Frequently it is difficult to determine just what repressed conflicts in the unconscious produce a certain physical symptom. The symptom always serves to distract attention from the individual's real problems. This mechanism is entirely unconscious and is not used by mature, well-adjusted individuals.

The following is a discussion of the security operations identified by Sullivan as protective measures against anxiety. It should be remembered that Sullivan stressed that anxiety emanates from an interpersonal context and is highly communicable.

Apathy. The security operation of apathy is similar to the ego defense of isolation wherein the individual defends against anxiety by not allowing himself to feel the emotion associated with an anxiety-producing event. Thus the individual utilizing apathy manifests an extreme indifference to an event that would usually elicit a high degree of emotion. This security operation protected a young wife against massive amounts of anxiety when her husband was convicted of involvement in organized crime and sentenced to 15 years in prison. Although she had no previous knowledge of his business she was able to recount to her parents the events which transpired after his arrest without any emotion, leading them to conclude that she didn't care.

Somnolent detachment. The security operation of somnolent detachment manifests itself by the individual falling asleep when confronted by a highly threatening, anxiety-producing experience. It has its origin in the developmental stage of infancy where the baby can be observed to fall asleep after his crying fails to bring the mothering one to feed him. Although somnolent detachment is a primitive defense it can be observed in adults who are in a state of great stress. For example, a young woman sitting for the licensure examination in nursing falls asleep less than a half hour after the exam begins and fails the exam.

Security operations

Selective inattention. Selective inattention is the mechanism whereby anxiety-producing aspects of a situation are not allowed into awareness, thereby enabling the individual to maintain an adequate level of system homeokinesis. For example the security of a woman whose husband is having an affair is threatened so she selectively inattends the many clues to his behavior and is genuinely surprised when he asks for a divorce to marry his lover.

Preoccupation. The security operation of preoccupation is manifested by a consuming interest in a person, thought, or event to the exclusion of the anxiety-producing reality. Preoccupation was used as a protective measure by a devout Christian woman who routinely made home visits in her community to invite others to worship at her church. One Saturday she was severely bitten on her left leg by a large dog in the yard of the home she was approaching. The dog's attack caused her to fall on her right knee and she became preoccupied with the bruise on this knee to the exclusion of concern about her mangled left leg. The anxiety she was experiencing was due not only to the suddenness of the dog's attack but more fundamentally to a threat to her security that was based in part on the belief that God would always protect her when she was doing His work.

Coping mechanisms

The variety and number of coping mechanisms are as great as the creativity and resources of human beings. They cannot all be listed and defined but they can be categorized into short- and long-term adaptations. This categorization is based not only on a time factor but also on the object and effect of the adaptation. It should be remembered that all coping mechanisms are conscious, learned adaptations to anxiety based on problem solving and result in altered behavior.

Short-term coping mechanisms. Short-term coping mechanisms are conscious maneuvers focused on the anxiety itself rather than on its source and are designed to effect a relatively immediate relief from anxiety. Consequently, short-term coping mechanisms represent avoidance or escape behaviors. A commonly used short-term coping mechanism is *suppression*. Although historically considered an ego defense mechanism, it does not emanate from the unconscious. Rather, suppression is the conscious and intentional dismissal to the preconscious mind of impulses, feelings, and thoughts that are unpleasant or unacceptable to the individual. Suppressed material is easily recalled and is thus available to the conscious mind. Perhaps the most famous example of suppression is that used by Scarlett O'Hara in *Gone With The Wind*. When Scarlett's sense of security was repeatedly threatened, she would exclaim, "I'll think about that tomorrow." Other examples of short-term coping mechanisms are the decisions to drink or eat when anxious, or to avoid conflictual situations by pleading illness. Although these maneuvers are successful in relieving anxiety they do not help the individual to adapt better to similar anxiety-producing situations in the future. Furthermore, the result of a frequently used short-term coping mechanism can become a stressor itself. For example, consistent overeating can lead to obesity.

Long-term coping mechanisms. Long-term coping mechanisms are characterized by efforts to address the source of anxiety. Therefore, the anxiety is not relieved immediately but rather continues while its source is being sought. Long-term mechanisms tend to represent confrontational behaviors in that the source of the anxiety is dealt with rather than avoided. An example of a long-term coping mechanism is the housewife's decision to attend college to prepare herself to become financially independent, thereby coping with the anxiety caused by being financially dependent upon her husband.

Long-term coping mechanisms are more productive than short-term mechanisms since they provide the individual with patterns of behavior that increase self-esteem and can be built upon in future anxiety-producing situations. However, they can be used only in instances in which the individual is able to experience anxiety without too much system disequilibrium.

CONCLUDING STATEMENTS

1. Anxiety is the most universal of all emotions. It cannot be observed directly but must be inferred from behavior.
2. Anxiety is simultaneously an adaptation to system disequilibrium and a stressor to which the system must adapt.
3. Anxiety if defined as a vague sense of impending doom, an apprehension, or a sense of dread.
4. Anxiety has the following characteristics:
   a. It is always perceived as a negative feeling.
   b. It is extremely communicable.

    c. It cannot be distinguished from fear by the individual experiencing it.

    d. It occurs in degrees.

5. Anxiety occurs most often as a result of a threat to biological integrity, an unconscious symbolic conflict, or a threat to the self-concept.
6. Freud believed that anxiety results from the emergence of id impulses that are unacceptable to the superego.
7. Sullivan viewed anxiety as occurring when the individual anticipates or actually receives cues that signal disapproval from one or more significant others.
8. Ego defense mechanisms were identified by Freud. They use psychic energy derived from the ego and serve to protect the ego from anxiety.
9. Most ego defense mechanisms are initiated early during the development of the personality. They are not clear-cut and almost never appear as isolated phenomena.
10. Sullivan identified protective measures against anxiety, which he called security operations.
11. Coping mechanisms are conscious, reality-oriented problem-solving activities designed to relieve anxiety. They can be categorized into short-term and long-term adaptations.

SUGGESTED SOURCES OF ADDITIONAL INFORMATION

Classical

Freud, Anna: The ego and mechanisms of defense, New York, 1967, International Universities Press.

Horvath, Kathy: Incorporation: what is the nurse's role? Am. J. Nurs. **72:**1096-1100, 1972.

Nehren, Jeanette, and Gilliam, Naomi R.: Separation anxiety, Am. J. Nurs. **65:**109-112, Jan., 1965.

Peterson, Margaret H.: Understanding defense mechanisms, Am. J. Nurs. **72:**1651-1674, 1972.

Contemporary

Bloom, Michael: Adolescent-parental separation, New York, 1980, Gardner Press, Inc.

Elliot, Susan M.: Denial as an effective mechanism to allay anxiety during a stressful event, J. Psychosoc. Nurs. Ment. Health Serv. **18:**11-15, Oct., 1980.

Kerr, Norine: Anxiety: theoretical considerations. Perspect. Psychiatr. Care **16**(1):36-40, Jan.-Feb., 1978.

King, Joan M.: Denial, Am. J. Nurs. **66:**1010-1013, May, 1966.

Knowles, Ruth: Dealing with feelings: managing anxiety, Am. J. Nurs. **81:**110-111, Jan. 1981.

Laughlin, H.: The ego and its defenses, New York, 1979, Jason Aronson Press.

Lidz, Theodore: The person: his and her development throughout the life cycle. New York, 1976, Basic Books, Inc., Publishers.

Snyder, Joyce C., and Wilson, Margo F.: Elements of a psychological assessment, Am. J. Nurs. **77:**253-239, Feb., 1977.

chapter six

the determinants of mental health and mental illness

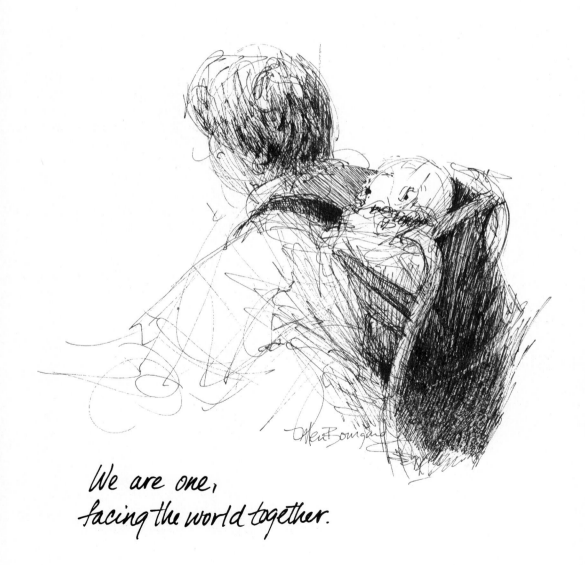

We are one,
facing the world together.

LEARNING OBJECTIVES

After studying this chapter the student will be able to:

1. Discuss the personality attributes believed to serve as determinants of mental health in adults.

2. Discuss the genetic, physiological, intrapersonal, interpersonal, and cultural factors believed to serve as determinants of mental illness in adults.

3. Discuss the genetic, physiological, interpersonal, and cultural factors believed to contribute to the prevention of mental illness in adults.

On few topics is there as little exact information available as there is on mental health and the cause and prevention of mental illness. Completely satisfactory definitions of mental health and mental illness have yet to be developed. To a large extent these concepts are culturally determined and are defined differently in various parts of the world. Behavior that might be characterized as abnormal or mentally sick in one culture may be accepted and encouraged in another. For example, men who sit most of the day staring at the sun might be considered mentally ill in the United States, but in India they are considered holy and are provided for through the benevolence of the community.

Nevertheless, it is necessary for the nurse to understand current theories about the determinants of mental health and mental illness to effectively plan, implement, and evaluate nursing care.

HISTORICAL PERSPECTIVE

Because behaviors indicative of mental health or mental illness are defined by the society in which the individual lives, it seems reasonable to assume that the prevailing view of the determinants of mental health and mental illness is also culturally defined. For example, a society that explains other phenomena on the basis of supernatural powers would be likely to attribute aberrant behavior to the same cause. This was certainly the case in Biblical times when demented individuals were considered to be possessed by satanic forces. This belief continued more or less unabated until the nineteenth century. In like manner a society that possesses and values highly developed scientific knowledge and technology is likely to view all manifestations of mental illness as resulting from scientifically based phenomena, often to the exclusion of other factors. In other words, beliefs about the determinants of mental illness have changed as the knowledge, skills, and values of the society have shifted.

Such has not been the case in regard to the determinants of mental health. In fact little attention was paid to the description and determinants of mental health until the mid-twentieth century. Until that time mental health, like physical health, was assumed to be present when illness was absent. In the case of mental health this often meant the absence of socially unacceptable behavior. It cannot be overemphasized that behavior considered socially unacceptable differs from society to society and over time within any given society. Thus mental health like mental illness has never been an absolute concept, but rather is relative to time and place.

The first attempts to describe the characteristics of the mentally healthy individual were based on inferences drawn from what was known about the mentally ill, often leading to erroneous conclusions. Consequently, mental health was described in negative terms, such as the absence of incapacitating anxiety. It was not until the late 1950s that psychologist Marie Johoda identified criteria of positive mental health. This work was done under the auspices of the Joint Commission on Mental Health Illness and Health, whose report was published in 1961.

It can be concluded therefore that human beings have been concerned about aberrant behavior since the beginning of time, although the definition of aberrance and the delineation of its causes have differed markedly over the centuries. In contrast, interest in and understanding of the manifestations and determinants of mental health are very recent.

PERSONALITY ATTRIBUTES OF THE MENTALLY HEALTHY ADULT

Although it is impossible to provide a definition of mental health that would be universally acceptable to all authorities in all cultures, it is possible to discuss the attributes usually identified as being present in the personality structures of those adults who appear to successfully adapt to stress. The ability to adapt to the recurrent stresses of living and to achieve a relatively effective adjustment is referred to as mental maturity by many authorities, emotional maturity by others, and mental health by some.

Mental health is closely related to physical health because the human being is a unified, integrated whole. The dichotomy of body and mind has persisted much too long among some groups because the cause and effect relationship between the two is not always precisely demonstrable.

Presently, different standards exist for evaluating mental health and physical health. Those applied to mental health are stated in terms of personality attributes, adaptations to stress, interpersonal capacities, and the ability to cope with reality. Evaluations in these terms are of necessity complex and imprecise. In contrast, much evaluation of physical health can be done in terms of precise measurement in such areas as weight, blood pressure, biochemical content of the blood, and urinalysis.

Few people can be said to have achieved complete mental health or emotional maturity. Thus it is probably more helpful to assess the individual in terms of relative strengths or limitations in relation to the social norms and values existing in the community in which the individual lives. Because the behavior of mentally ill people reflects some strengths as well as limitations, the line of demarcation between mental health and mental illness is sometimes difficult to describe and is sharply defined in only a limited number of individuals.

Margaret Mead wrote that mental health is actually determined by a set of ratios involving the emotional, social, and psychological strengths with which an individual is fortified, the events he has experienced throughout life, the stress he is currently experiencing, and the expectations society has established for him. Thus a young lawyer who loses his wife and two children in an automobile accident will be able to maintain emotional equilibrium and continue to carry on his law practice and his personal life after a reasonable period of grieving if the ratios stated above are favorable. His ability to carry on will depend on the strengths within his personality, the supports his family and friends provide, the number of crises he has experienced in the past, and the expectations of significant people in his life. If he has had other traumatic personal losses in the past, if his family and friends are not able to be with him or do not provide him with emotional support, if he is disappointed by not receiving the political appointment he was promised shortly before his wife was killed, and if he perceives that significant people in his life subtly believe that his burdens are overwhelming and he will not be able to carry on, he may unconsciously seek refuge in mental illness.

Mental health is always relative. It is relative to time, place, and situation. It has been demonstrated that the ability of individuals to maintain emotional equilibrium in the face of a devastating situation differs, depending on whether the problem is being faced alone or as a member of a group. Group membership is emotionally supportive and is usually a positive factor. This fact has been exemplified by the prisoners who were returned to the United States at the end of the Vietnam War. Although many of them had suffered tremendous deprivation for several years and had often undergone torture, most of these men were in much better mental health than psychiatrists had anticipated. Another example of the same phenomenon is the mental health of the 52 Americans after being held hostage in Iran for 444 days. The explanation for these unexpected outcomes was the group relationship that was maintained throughout both ordeals. Individually these persons felt they were not alone in their misery. Their membership in the group was reassuring and supportive. In addition, as a group they were actively engaged in trying to do something about the situation, although this activity often had to be in the form of organized passive resistance.

Most authorities agree that one of the major attributes of the mentally healthy or emotionally mature individual is the capacity to love and to be loved in return. This capacity is usually thought to embrace the ability to establish a satisfying heterosexual love relationship and the ability to carry through this relationship to its usual eventual conclusion of marriage and the establishment of a safe home environment for the nurturing of children. It follows that the establishment of a home and the nurturing of children require the capacity to effectively cope with a work situation.

The ability to love and be loved also includes the many appropriate levels of love shared by the individual with parents, siblings, friends, and other individuals with whom he is involved. This ability is described by some authorities such as Marie Jahoda as adequacy in interpersonal relations.

The individual's level of self-acceptance and the way he perceives reality are usually mentioned as two other capacities significant in the development of emotional maturity. These capacities involve how effectively the individual has learned to accept his own limitations and abilities. In other words, the capacity to live comfortably with oneself is considered to be an important attribute. The way the individual perceives the world around him is equally important, since he copes with it in terms of his perceptions. Thus if the individual's view of his environment leads him to perceive it as dangerous, hostile and threatening, he will probably display attacking, suspicious, cautious behavior. On the other hand, if the individual perceives his environment as friendly, interesting, and rewarding his method of coping with reality will be more acceptable, at least in this culture. Self-acceptance and the individual's perception of reality greatly influence another capacity, environmental mastery, which is almost always mentioned by authorities when writing about the emotionally mature, mentally healthy individual. Environmental mastery suggests that the individual feels in control of himself and his environment and has made an investment in living that has necessitated the high-level development of his inherent abilities.

In addition, the mentally healthy or emotionally mature individual will have developed the capacity for independent thinking and action. This capacity is described by some as efficiency in problem solving and by others as autonomy or self-determination.

A final capacity usually included in such a discussion is the ability of the individual to effect a balance or synthesis of all psychological functions and personal attributes, which provides a unifying, integrated outlook on life and a sense of direction to the individual in relation to his role in it.

Thus it can be seen that mental health or emotional maturity is a highly individual attribute; that it cannot be defined in terms of the absence of disease; that it cannot be understood in terms of isolated symptoms; and that it is intimately related to the norms of the society in which the individual finds himself.

FACTORS THAT MAY SERVE AS DETERMINANTS OF MENTAL ILLNESS

It is impossible to be definitive about the causes of a behavioral response that may be diagnosed as mental illness or to be specific about how this illness might have been prevented. The individual must be viewed as a totality in constant interaction with his environment. No single set of facts can be considered separately when seeking the determinants of mental illness. All the facts must be studied together if the behavior of any individual is to be understood. The only reasonable approach to the study of the determinants of mental illness is a consideration of an individual's total life experience, with emphasis on genetic, physiological, intrapersonal, interpersonal, and cultural factors, each of which may have contributed to the problem. The following discussion presents the possible role each of these factors may assume in producing mental illness.

Genetic factors

Current knowledge concerning human heredity has not developed to a state in which definitive statements can be made about the influence of heredity on the development of mental illness. Around the turn of this century it was a generally accepted belief that mental illness was inherited and that the tendency to develop certain psychotic reactions was transmitted with regularity from one generation to another. These ideas seemed to have validity when it was observed that manic-depressive and schizophrenic syndromes did appear frequently in more than one generation of the same family. More recently it was thought that the tendency to develop similar psychotic reactions among members of the same family might be a response to the environmental factors within the family rather than a result of heredity. It is reasonable to believe that children learn to behave in unusual ways when they are reared by parents who habitually respond in unusual ways to other people, to social situations, to work responsibilities, and to parenthood. Today most well-read people take the rational view that both environmental and genetic factors significantly influence the way in which the individual reacts to life experiences.

One of the most significant studies to demonstrate the influence of genetic factors in the development of specific forms of mental illness was conducted by Franz Kallmann between 1930 and 1950. Kallmann carried out longitudinal studies of identical twins who were raised in widely different environments. He found that if one twin developed schizophrenia the other became ill with schizophrenia in 86% of the cases, even though these children were not reared in the same families and were not subjected to the same environmental influences. In the same study he found that if one twin developed bipolar manic-depressive psychosis the other twin developed the same illness in 96% of the cases.

**Physiological
factors**

The biological heredity of an individual may be an indirect genetic determinant of mental illness because the genetically determined qualities of body type, sex, intelligence, temperament, and energy endowment all influence the nature and quality of the individual's adaptations to stressors throughout his life. In a sense the individual also inherits the family milieu into which he is born and the cultural forces to which he will be required to adapt. These factors surely influence an individual's total response to life and play a large part in his ability to maintain an emotional equilibrium throughout life.

As knowledge about human behavior evolves scientists recognize the urgent need for more research and study of human genetics as it relates to the causation of mental illness.

A large number of persons suffer from symptoms of mental illness in conjunction with a physical illness but because of the temporary character of most of these mental reactions they are not recognized as being psychiatric conditions. It is interesting to note that the same organic problem may produce a wide variety of mental reactions in different persons. This suggests that personality plays an important role in behavioral response even when brain tissue is involved.

Traumatic brain damage is one of the common organic problems to which the human organism reacts with abnormal mental symptoms. Such an injury may result in a variety of mental symptoms, depending on the location and severity of the injury and the age and personality of the individual. The aftereffects of brain injury are frequently serious because of the progressive intellectual and emotional degeneration that may occur and the possibility that this degeneration may be accompanied by convulsive seizures.

Brain tumor is an organic condition that may be accompanied by a variety of mental and physical symptoms. The symptoms depend on the location of the tumor, its size, and, to some extent, on the type of tumor. Surgery is frequently helpful but may result in the same sequelae that follow brain injury.

Delirium resulting from toxins in the blood or from a high blood level of certain drugs is a temporary condition that requires consideration and treatment of both the mental and physical symptoms. Bromides, barbituric acid derivatives, sulfa drugs, morphine, cocaine, marijuana, thiocyanates, and lead are examples of agents that produce such problems.

Withdrawal from a heavy and consistent intake of alcohol over a short period of time without adequate food intake can produce an acute condition called delirium tremens. A prolonged, excessive alcoholic intake can produce a chronic irreversible dementia that is accompanied by a gradual personality deterioration.

Cortisone and adrenocorticotropic hormone (ACTH) may produce psychotic reactions in selected individuals. The symptoms usually disappear when the drugs are withdrawn. Thyroid and pituitary diseases may result in overactivity, emotional lability, anxiety, and overt fear or confusion and depression. These symptoms usually disappear when the physical condition is corrected.

Encephalitis, or inflammation of the brain, may cause specific abnormalities and may lead to psychic and physical disorders, depending on the organism that caused the condition, the age and personality of the individual, and the treatment provided. The acute form of encephalitis is characterized by lethargy, delirium, confusion, and stupor. In its chronic form it is recognized clinically as paralysis agitans and is characterized by shaking palsy associated with increasing irritability, insomnia, and neurotic behavior.

Increasing numbers of researchers are engaged in studies that point to a neurochemical correlate of mental illness, especially the schizophrenic and manic-depressive psychoses. Some hypotheses are (1) schizophrenics produce more or fewer corticoids than do normal individuals, (2) schizophrenia might result from faulty transmethylation of catecholamines, yielding a mescaline-like compound found more frequently in the urine of schizophrenic subjects than in the urine of normal persons, and (3) a disturbance in catecholamine metabolism is a major factor in manic-depressive psychosis. Although these and other research findings have promise in enlarging our understanding of factors that contribute to mental illness, it is unlikely that a singular, definitive causative factor will be identified in the near future. This pessimism is warranted because of the methodological problems encountered when studying human subjects and the large number of diverse behaviors labeled as indicative of mental ill-

Intrapersonal factors

ness in our society. Nevertheless, research in this area should continue to receive both cooperation and financial support.

Intrapersonal factors are those conscious and unconscious thoughts and feelings that the individual brings to bear on all situations he encounters. When the situation is unfamiliar or otherwise threatening to his sense of self, the individual's anxiety level rises. Because high levels of anxiety or prolonged anxiety cannot be tolerated for long the anxious person adapts by utilizing ego defense mechanisms, security operations, or coping mechanisms. For example, an individual may relieve guilt feelings about a sexual transgression by blaming his partner and claiming that it was not his fault but the fault of the woman whose behavior was seductive. A student may unconsciously defend himself against feelings of inadequacy by rationalizing and stating that although he failed a college entrance examination he can play football better than anyone on his team. These are simple examples of normal ego defense mechanisms used to help an individual relieve anxiety when intrapersonal feelings are involved, thereby enabling him to regain homeokinesis.

If intrapersonal feelings continue to cause increased anxiety it may become necessary for the individual to use more elaborate mental mechanisms. As time goes on the elaborate defenses may prove inadequate and he may begin to use bizarre ways of defending himself. When this kind of defense becomes necessary the individual is said to be mentally ill.

Situations that precipitate intrapersonal difficulties are as varied as the people involved because they are perceived in the context of each person's unique personality organization. However, situations likely to require adaptations beyond the capacity of some people are those that symbolize a threat to the person's identity or to his security. Such a situation is often referred to as a *precipitating factor* rather than as a cause of mental illness, since it is the situation in interaction with the individual's mental mechanisms that results in behavior indicative of mental illness.

There are some periods in life when the individual is more vulnerable emotionally than others. During these critical periods psychotic episodes are more likely to occur than during other times throughout the life cycle. At these times individual defenses may not be adequate to adapt successfully to the stress usually associated with the developmental stage. These critical periods occur during the development of adolescence, middle age, and old age. They are stressful periods from both physiological and psychological standpoints.

During adolescence the young person is attempting to integrate rapid physical growth and genital maturity into his personality pattern. The individual is struggling to sever close family ties while at the same time seeking to be loved and accepted both at home and by the peer group. The adolescent's desperate need to belong to his peer group causes him to be influenced greatly by the social standards of his peers, which may be at variance with his own values. Many of life's most significant decisions such as the choice of employment and a lifetime marital partner are made during this period. These stressors may create overwhelming stress to which the adolescent may have difficulty adapting. Some actually become mentally ill. Young people seem to be most vulnerable between the ages of 17 and 25, years during which some adolescents or young adults develop schizophrenia.

Some women and men become mentally ill during late middle age. This critical period occurs during the late forties for women and during the late fifties for men. It is a critical period in life for several reasons, one of which is the declining activity of the reproductive function, which many men and women consider to be the factor that determines their masculine or feminine identity. Equally as important in the causation of mental illness during this period is the recognition that if their most cherished lifetime goals have not been achieved, there is little chance that they will be. Some women with successful, busy husbands and children who are almost grown suddenly begin to feel that their life's work has been completed and that they are no longer useful or needed. Some men anticipate retirement with dread, for much the same reason. This period is often perceived as the midpoint of life. If the future is viewed as being entirely downhill, a midlife depression can result.

After the age of 60, emotional disorders increase. This is an extremely critical period in the lives of many individuals because feelings of insecurity are brought on by the changes in life-style caused by retirement, the threat of financial dependency resulting from the loss of income, and the fear of the loss of physical

Interpersonal factors

competence. In addition, degenerative conditions of the brain and nervous system may occur after age 60, rendering some older individuals totally incapable of functioning independently.

Interpersonal factors refer to the relationships that individuals develop with significant persons in their environment. Actually the development of positive feelings about the self and others depends to a great extent on the kind of interpersonal relations developed between the individual and the significant people in his environment during his very early life. Feelings of security, well-being, personal value, and self-esteem in the adult originate and are powerfully influenced by the relationship developed with the mothering persons in the earliest months of the individual's life. Likewise experiences with other significant persons during childhood influence the feelings the child will have toward himself and others in later life. It is possible to relate many of the anxiety-producing situations in an individual's adult life to faulty relationships that existed with significant adults during his early life.

Early family relationships, especially with mother and father, influence the individual's ability to successfully adapt to the stress of adult life. If faulty relationships in some aspect of the individual's early life have never been corrected, he may not be able to adapt successfully to the stressors of adult life.

Faulty relationships that may influence the individual's future adjustment are referred to as *predisposing factors*. This suggests that they are dormant in the individual's unconscious life and may cause difficulty in the future, provided that a certain amount of intrapsychic stress occurs at a time when the individual is more vulnerable than usual. For example, a young man may be able to complete college, accept a responsible position, and carry on what appears to be a well-adjusted life until he becomes engaged to be married. The stress of assuming this additional financial and social responsibility combined with the self-doubt that may develop concerning his ability to assume the masculine role in a marriage relationship may produce more anxiety than he is able to tolerate. At such a time his unconscious need for a defense against anxiety may become so great that he may resort to unusual or bizarre ways of behaving.

Cultural factors

The culture into which an individual is born superimposes on him many values and ideas with which he must deal for the remainder of his life. It presents the individual with many conflicts between bodily drives and acceptable ways of directing these drives. For example, young people are physically ready for marriage long before our culture sanctions marriage.

In the past, the roles of men and women have been clearly defined, but within the last 30 years these have been changing rapidly. The effect that sex-related role blurring or role changes will have on the mental health of future generations is yet to be determined. Some authorities believe that the effect will be to increase the incidence of mental illness, because children will find it difficult to identify with appropriate sex roles that are based on distinct functions for each sex. Conversely, other experts believe that the incidence of mental illness will decrease because children will be encouraged by the society to engage in functions most suitable to them as persons, regardless of their gender. As with any other major cultural change it will require several generations of alterations in child-rearing practices before any of these theories can be confirmed.

Minority groups face problems superimposed on them by the culture. Members of a group that is different because of race or religion may face many situations that cause them as individuals to feel unsure, inadequate, and unwanted and to fear the loss of personal security.

High cultural value has been placed on marriage and a certain amount of disapproval is meted out to individuals who fail to marry after they have reached early adulthood. Single people eventually become members of a minority group and suffer some of the same discriminations with which minority groups must cope.

These examples should be sufficient to suggest that cultural conflict can lead to adjustment problems that may result in such a high level of anxiety that the individual is forced to use abnormal defenses.

FACTORS THAT MAY CONTRIBUTE TO THE PREVENTION OF MENTAL ILLNESS

There are few if any facts on which to base definitive comments concerning the prevention of mental illness. Until there is a clear definition of mental illness it will be difficult to know exactly what preventive measures are required. Furthermore, since mental illness takes so many forms it is unlikely that any single measure will prove to be effective in preventing all mental illness.

Genetic factors

Following is a brief discussion of preventive measures that could be taken in regard to some of the factors previously identified as contributing to mental illness.

Although there is little or no evidence that most forms of mental illness are genetically transmitted, continuing research is promising in regard to the major psychoses of schizophrenia and bipolar affective disorder. Genetic counseling could be helpful to individuals who have a history of these illnesses in their families.

Procedures such as amniocentesis make available information about the likelihood of an unborn child being physically or mentally impaired. This information gives parents the option to terminate the pregnancy so as to prevent unmanageable stress on themselves or on the child who may be biologically ill equipped to adapt to the usual stressors of life. However, it should be emphasized that for most people a decision to abort a fetus is a major stressor in and of itself. Furthermore, it must be acknowledged that forced family planning either through genetic counseling or abortion is an unacceptable practice in a free society. Finally, any role that genetic engineering will play in the future to prevent mental illness is yet to be determined.

Physiological factors

Many forms of acute and chronic mental illnesses that are secondary to physical illnesses could be prevented by enhancing physical health, preventing physical illness, and continuing to develop early, effective treatment for physical illness. For example, syphilitic meningoencephalitis, which in the past accounted for approximately 10% of all admissions to psychiatric hospitals, has been essentially eradicated due to the discovery of antibiotics that effectively treat syphilis in its early stages.

Although the antipsychotic drugs have been widely used since 1956, they have had no effect on curing or preventing mental illness, except to the degree that they make persons amenable to other forms of treatment by decreasing the distressing symptoms of the major psychoses. Recently, however, lithium carbonate has become increasingly prominent as a drug that prevents the recurrence of bipolar manic depression when the optimum serum lithium level is established and maintained. This breakthrough supports the belief that biochemical deficiencies ultimately may be identified as causing some forms of mental illness. If this proves to be the case chemical substitutes could be taken throughout life, thereby preventing the onset of mental illness.

Interpersonal factors

It appears at this point in our understanding of human behavior that a stable, secure, loving family life, especially during the earliest years, is essential to the development of attitudes about self and others that make it possible for individuals to satisfactorily adapt to the stresses of adult life and to live in a satisfying and productive way. It is the responsibility of the home and the school, both of which deal with children during their early and formative years, to help children develop the capacity to live mentally healthy adult lives and to provide corrective experiences for children who have had negative relationships with individuals whose parenting behaviors were inadequate. However, merely saying this is not sufficient. Private and publicly supported programs designed to teach young people effective parenting behaviors and to support them in their efforts are essential. In addition, more emphasis should be placed on child guidance theories in teacher education programs.

Cultural factors

Many authorities believe that prevention of mental illness will not be achieved on a widespread scale until efforts are directed at improving the quality of life for all persons in our society. These authorities conclude that many of our social problems such as poor housing, racial, religious, and sexual discrimination, and unavailability of quality health care to all are major elements in the cause of mental illness. Therefore these persons support broad social reform programs designed to alter the basis of these social ills. Although great strides have been made over the past few decades in alleviating some of these social problems, effective and economical means of eliminating them are yet to be determined.

CONCLUDING STATEMENTS

1. Human beings have been concerned about aberrant behavior since the beginning of time, although the definition of abberance and the delineation of its causes have differed markedly over the centuries. In contrast, interest in and understanding of the manifestations and determinants of mental health are very recent.
2. Mental health or emotional maturity is thought to be the ability to adapt successfully to recurrent stresses of living and to achieve a relatively effective adjustment to life.
3. Because few people can be said to have achieved complete mental or emotional maturity, it is more helpful to assess the

individual's relative strengths or limitations in relation to social norms and values.

4. Mental health is always relative and is determined by a set of ratios involving the emotional, social, and psychological strengths with which an individual is fortified, the events he has experienced throughout life, the stress he is currently experiencing, and the expectations society has established for him.

5. Mental health or emotional maturity is assessed in terms of personality capacities that involve interpersonal relations, self-acceptance, perceptions of reality, environmental mastery, self-determination, and resistance to stress.

6. The only reasonable approach to the study of the determinants of mental illness is a consideration of an individual's total life experience with emphasis on genetic, physiological, intrapersonal, interpersonal, and cultural factors.

7. Present knowledge concerning human heredity has not developed to a level at which definitive statements can be made about the influence of heredity on the development of mental illness.

8. Scientists recognize the urgent need for more research and study of human genetics as it relates to the cause of mental illness.

9. The same organic problem may produce a wide variety of mental reactions in different persons, which suggests that personality plays an important role even in individual responses to involvement of brain tissue.

10. Present research indicates that alterations in a person's neurochemistry may be a contributing factor in the development of the schizophrenic and manic-depressive psychoses.

11. There are some periods in life when the individual is more vulnerable emotionally than others. These critical periods are adolescence, middle age, and old age.

12. Interpersonal factors refer to the relationships that an individual develops with significant persons in his environment which, in turn, exert a powerful influence on his mental health.

13. Cultural conflict can lead to adjustment problems that may result in such a high level of anxiety that the individual is forced to use abnormal defenses.

14. Until there is a clear definition of mental illness it will be difficult to know exactly what preventive measures are required, although it is unlikely that any single measure will be effective in preventing all mental illness.
15. The availability of genetic counseling and procedures such as amniocentesis give adults who have a familial history of mental illness options in regard to bearing children.
16. Lithium carbonate prevents recurrences of bipolar manic-depressive episodes when a recommended serum level is established and maintained.
17. A stable, secure, loving family life assists individuals to develop attitudes about self and others that make it possible to adapt to the stresses of adulthood and to live a satisfying and productive life.
18. Eradication of major social problems such as poor housing and discrimination may be a major factor in preventing mental illness on a widespread scale.

SUGGESTED SOURCES OF ADDITIONAL INFORMATION

Classical

Caplan, Gerald: Principles of preventive psychiatry, New York, 1964, Basic Books, Inc., Publishers.

Galdston, Iago: The American family in crisis, Ment. Hyg. **42:**229-236, 1958.

Hollingshead, August B., and Redlich, Frederick C.: Social class and mental illness, New York, 1958, John Wiley & Sons, Inc.

Jackson, Don D., editor: The etiology of schizophrenia, New York, 1960, Basic Books, Inc., Publishers.

Kallmann, Franz J.: Heredity in health and mental disorder, New York, 1953, W.W. Norton & Co., Inc.

Mead, Margaret: Mental health in our changing culture, Ment. Hyg. **56:**6-8, 1972.

Myers, Jerome K., and Bean, Lee L.: Family and class dynamics in mental illness, New York, 1964, John Wiley & Sons, Inc.

Norris, Catherine N.: Psychiatric crises: practical considerations, Perspect. Psychiatr. Care **5:**20-28, Jan.-Feb., 1967.

Opler, Marvin K., editor: Culture and mental health, New York, 1959, Macmillan Publishing Co., Inc.

Robischon, Paulette: The challenge of crisis theory for nursing, Nurs. Outlook **15:**28-32, July, 1967.

Contemporary

Aguilera, Donna C., and Messick, Janice M.: Crisis intervention: theory and methodology, ed. 4, St. Louis, 1981, The C.V. Mosby Co.

Ahr, P., and Gorodezky, M. and Won Cho D.: Measuring the relationship of public psychiatric admissions to rising unemployment, Hosp. Community Psychiatry **32**(6):398-401, 1981.

Akiskal, H., and Tashjian, R.: Affective disorders: II. Recent advances in laboratory and pathogenic approaches, Hosp. Community Psychiatry **34**(9):822-830, 1983.

Bloom, Bernard: The logic and urgency of primary prevention, Hosp. Community Psychiatry **32**(12):838-843, 1981.

Burton, Arthur: Operational theories of personality, New York, 1974, Brunner/Mazel, Inc.

Chesler, Phyliss: Women and madness, Garden City, N.Y., 1973, Arno Press, Inc.

DeCourcy, Peter, and DeCourcy, Judith: A silent tragedy: child abuse in the community, Port Washington, N.Y., 1973, Alfred Publishing Co.

Deutsch, Stephen, and Davis, Kenneth: Schizophrenia: a review of diagnostic and biological issues, I., Hosp. Community Psychiatry **34**(4):313-321, 1983.

Deutsch, Stephen, and Davis, Kenneth: Schizophrenia: a review of diagnostic and biological issues, II., Hosp. Community Psychiatry **34**(5):423-437, 1983.

DeYoung, Carol D.: Nursing's contribution in family crisis treatment, Nurs. Outlook **16**:60-62, Feb., 1968.

Eichenbaum, L., and Orbach, S.: Understanding women: a feminist psychoanalytic approach, New York, 1983, Basic Books, Inc., Publishers.

Fishel, Anne H., and Jefferson, Carolyn B.: Assertiveness training for emotionally disturbed women, J. Psychosoc. Nurs. Ment. Health Serv. **21**:22-28, Nov., 1983.

Gershon, E.: The impact of biology on modern psychiatry, New York, 1977, Plenum Press.

Hagen, Diane: The relationship between job loss and physical and mental illness, Hosp. Community Psychiatry **34**(5):438-441, 1983.

Hickey, Brian: Transitional relatedness and engaging the regressed borderline client, J. Psychosoc. Nurs. Ment. Health Serv. **21**:26-30, Jan., 1983.

Howell, Elizabeth, and Bayes, Marjorie, editors: Women and mental health, New York, 1981, Basic Books, Inc., Publishers.

Insel, T., and Goodwin, F.: The dexamethasone suppression test: promises and problems of diagnostic laboratory tests in psychiatry, Hosp. Community Psychiatry **34**(12):1131-1138, 1983.

Jacobson, Ann: Melancholy in the 20th century: causes and prevention, J. Psychosoc. Nurs. Ment. Health Serv. **18**:11-21, July 1980.

Kerr, Norine J.: The tyranny of the shoulds, Perspect. Psychiatr. Care **22**:16-19, Jan.-March, 1984.

Kolb, Lawrence C.: Modern clinical psychiatry, ed., Philadelphia, 1977, W.B. Saunders Co.

Landsberg, Gerald: The state of prevention in mental health, Perspect. Psychaitr. Care **15**(1):15-17, 1977.

Luchins, Daniel: Developments in biological psychiatry: clinical applications to the major psychoses, Hosp. Community Psychiatry **33**(5):355-361, 1982.

May, Rollo: Power and innocence: a search for the sources of violence, New York, 1972, W.W. Norton & Co., Inc.

Myers, Jerome K., and Bean, L.L.: A decade later: a follow-up of social class and mental illness; in collaboration with Max P. Pepper, New York, 1968, John Wiley & Sons, Inc.

Plunkett, Richard J., and Gordon, John E.: Epidemiology and mental illness, New York, 1979, Arno Press, Inc.

Resing, Marcia: Mental health problems of vietnam veterans, J. Psychosoc. Nurs. Ment. Health Serv. **20**:40-43, Sept., 1982.

Rosenthal, David: The genetics of schizophrenia. In Arieti, Silvano, and Brody, Eugene B., editors: American handbook of psychiatry, ed. 2, vol. 3, New York, 1974, Basic Books, Inc., Publishers, pp. 588-600.

Schlesser, Michael, and Altshuler, Kenneth: The genetics of affective disorder: data, theory, and clinical application, Hosp. Community Psychiatry **34**(5):415-422, 1983.

Singer, Ann: Mothering practices and heroine addiction, Am. J. Nurs. **74**:77-82, 1974.

Stone, Michael: The borderline syndromes: constitution, personality and adaptation, New York, 1980, McGraw-Hill Book Co.

Stuart, Gail Wiscartz: Role strain and depression: a causal inquiry, J. Psychosoc. Nurs. Ment. Health Serv. **19**:20-28, Dec., 1981.

Usden, Earl: Biochemistry of mental disorders: new vistas, New York, 1978, Marcel Dekker, Inc.

Of particular interest

Jahoda, Marie: Current concepts of positive mental health, New York, 1979, Arno Press, Inc. (Edited by Gerald Grob.)

This text is a classic presentation defining positive mental health and describing criteria of positive mental health.

Rosenhan, D.L.: On being sane in insane places, Science **179**:250-258, 1973.

This article provokes consideration of the definition of mental illness through description of an experiment testing mental hospitals' response to psychiatrically "sane" people.

section III

the tools of psychiatric nursing

chapter seven

the self-awareness of the nurse

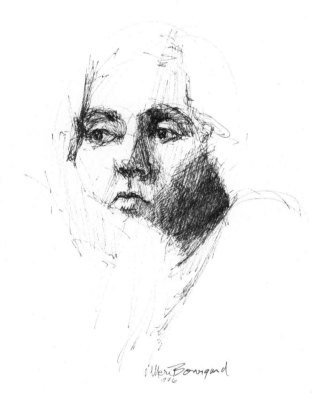

*I never knew
I affected people that way!*

1 State the importance of self-awareness to the effective practice of psychiatric nursing.

2 Discuss the relationship between the nurse's beliefs and feelings and the quality of nursing care she provides.

3 Identify seven principles of psychiatric nursing, discussing the beliefs and feelings on which each principle is based.

4 Define psychiatric nursing.

In many ways mentally ill persons are the most challenging group of individuals with whom the nurse has an opportunity to work. In a very real sense the relationship the nurse and the client develop can be one of the most important factors in the client's therapeutic experience. Whether the nurse can be a force for developing a truly therapeutic situation for the client depends on her ability to provide him with new and more positive experiences in living with other people. To accomplish this the nurse continuously strives to understand the client's behavior and the emotional needs expressed by that behavior. However, since it is the relationship between the nurse and the client that has the potential for becoming a therapeutic experience for the client, it is not sufficient for the nurse to understand only the client. In addition she must develop self-awareness.

To practice psychiatric nursing effectively the nurse must constantly adjust and readjust her approaches, attitudes, and feelings. To do so she gives much thought and consideration to her own behavior as it influences the behavior of others. In other words the nurse needs to be prepared to make positive use of her own personality, her primary tool, as she works therapeutically with clients. Many nurses successfully make therapeutic use of their personality without actually recognizing it or being able to analyze how they succeed. However nurses who work with the mentally ill cannot trust to luck in the hope of developing the self-awareness fundamental to being therapeutically effective. Although the effective practice of psychiatric nursing probably does not require unique personality attributes or attitudes, it does require a consistent, thoughtful effort directed toward developing awareness of self and others.

HISTORICAL PERSPECTIVE

The importance of self-awareness when working with emotionally ill persons was not recognized until Freud's revolutionary discovery of the unconscious mind and its role in influencing behavior. Freud demonstrated by his treatment of patients how the origins of present behavior often lay in repressed emotions and experiences of early childhood. He logically concluded that what was true of his patients was also true of all human beings, namely, that much behavior is determined by beliefs and feelings that are beyond awareness. He also believed that if one is to help others one must have an in-depth understanding of one's own beliefs and feelings so as not to inadvertently interfere with the progress of the patient. Psychoanalysis, the treatment procedure developed by Freud, therefore required the analyst to undergo much the same rigorous process of self-examination prior to being qualified to treat others.

While Freud emphasized the importance of self-understanding, it soon became apparent that most mental health professionals could not or would not avail themselves of such a lengthy, costly, and emotionally disruptive process. In the 1960s and 1970s it became evident that increasing one's self-awareness had value to all persons, not just those involved in providing human services. It was during this era that sensitivity training and encounter groups became popular and a plethora of groups designed to enhance self-awareness abounded. The Johari window, described in this chapter, is a tool that became popular at that time. It was named for its developers, Joseph Luft and Harry Lipton.

Although the popularity of these self-awareness groups has diminished somewhat it is now well accepted that increased self-awareness is desirable for all persons but is mandatory for those who, like nurses, work to assist others in achieving emotional growth.

THE NATURE AND IMPORTANCE OF SELF-AWARENESS

The major therapeutic tool of the nurse who works with the mentally ill is her use of self in the interpersonal context. Since behavior is largely determined by one's beliefs and feelings, the nurse's ability to use herself as a therapeutic tool depends on her adopting beliefs and feelings conducive to the effective practice of psychiatric nursing. Many nurses already hold these attitudes, but unless they are brought to a level of awareness they cannot be used purposefully. Furthermore, nurses whose beliefs and feelings are not conducive to the effective practice of psychiatric nursing cannot hope to alter them unless they can become aware of them. While it is desirable for all nurses to learn to examine their beliefs and feelings, it is imperative for the nurse who works with the mentally ill to do so.

The reader will note that the desired goal is self-awareness, not self-understanding. Self-understanding implies a knowledge of why one believes and feels as one does and this often requires a lengthy, in-depth process of self-examination guided by a qualified professional. Not many nurses have the opportunity to engage in this process, nor is it necessary for most. However, all nurses can become aware of what they believe and feel without necessarily having to understand why they believe and feel as they do. Self-awareness is within the grasp of all persons if they are willing to work at achieving it. They can consider their own responses, and they can develop the habit of studying responses they evoke from others. Nurses can develop the practice of recognizing and acknowledging their beliefs and feelings and examining them in group discussions with other professional people who are also striving to develop and improve awareness of self. They can learn a great deal by studying their own behavior and the behavior of others and by asking themselves such questions as, "What beliefs and feelings underlie what I did?" "How can I use these beliefs and feelings to elicit a desirable response from others?"

A helpful model for understanding the concept of self-awareness is the Johari window (Fig. 7-1). The upper left quadrant of the window represents a person's beliefs and feelings that are known to him and to others. This quadrant is termed "open." For example, a nurse may believe that acutely psychotic persons are very amenable to therapeutic intervention. Furthermore, she may be aware that she is the type of person who is gratified by relatively rapid changes in a client's behavior. Consequently, she often volunteers to assume the nursing care of acutely psychotic clients, allowing others to infer this particular belief and feeling from her behavior.

The upper right quadrant, the "blind" quadrant, represents those beliefs and feelings hidden from a person's awareness, usually because of their anxiety-producing nature. The person defends against awareness of such beliefs and feelings by using ego

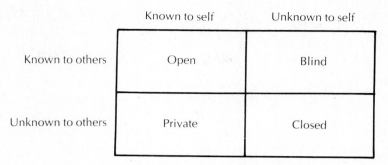

Fig. 7-1. Johari window.

defense mechanisms or security operations. However, his behavior reveals these beliefs and feelings to others. For example, the nurse may believe that clients who abuse alcohol are morally degenerate and any contact with them makes her angry. This belief and feeling may be unacceptable to her and so not exist at a level of awareness. However, her comments about these clients and her behavior when around them reveal her negative feelings to others, including the clients.

The lower left quadrant of the Johari window represents beliefs and feelings known to the person but purposefully and consciously concealed from others. This quadrant is termed "private" and usually exists because the individual fears rejection if his beliefs and feelings were known. For example, the nurse may believe that clients who seek readmission to the hospital at the end of the month when they have run out of money are really malingerers and therefore she feels they are undeserving of care. Being aware of this belief and consequent feeling but fearing she would be criticized by her peers if they were known, she extends herself to provide care for these clients in an effort to conceal her attitude toward them.

Finally, the lower right quadrant (the "closed" quadrant) represents beliefs and feelings so deeply buried in the person's unconscious mind that they are unknown both to him and to others. This does not imply that these beliefs and feelings do not affect the persons' behavior but rather that behavioral manifestations are likely to be indirect and therefore not easily understood by either the person or others.

Using the Johari window as a model the goal of self-awareness can be understood to be the decrease of the size of the blind and private quadrants, thereby enlarging the size of the open quadrant. In this way a greater number of beliefs and feelings will become known to the person and to others. Working toward this goal has two major advantages. First, it requires energy to conceal beliefs and feelings from oneself or from others. Therefore an increase in self-awareness and self-disclosure can free energy that can then be used more profitably. Second, an increase in self-awareness and self-disclosure gives the person more control over his own behavior as well as a better understanding of others' response to him.

Under usual circumstances it is unlikely that the size of the closed quadrant will be reduced, but as is true of self-understanding, the effective practice of psychiatric nursing does not require complete self-awareness.

BELIEFS AND FEELINGS

For the nurse to expand her self-awareness, she must examine her beliefs and her feelings about the mentally ill and about psychiatric nursing. These combined beliefs and feelings constitute the nurse's philosophy of psychiatric nursing and provide the bases for the principles that direct her nursing care.

In contrast to facts, *beliefs* are thoughts held to be true but not proven to be so. Some beliefs ultimately will be tested and proven to be either facts or falsehoods. Others are not amenable to testing because of their very nature. For example, a belief that stems from a value, such as the belief that human beings are basically good, does not lend itself to known methods of research.

The current state of knowledge about human behavior is at best imprecise. It consists mostly of beliefs, and many of these beliefs are incompatible. For example, the medical model of health care holds the belief that aberrant behavior is a reflection of an individual illness that is hypothetically amenable to treatment by somatic means. In contrast, a sociological model of health care dictates the belief that aberrant behavior is a sign of deviance rather than illness and must be assessed and treated within the larger context of the society. This contrast illustrates the diversity of currently held beliefs about human behavior and the necessity for all health professionals to develop an awareness of the beliefs that guide their professional practice.

Becoming aware of one's beliefs is necessary but not sufficient to the expansion of self-awareness. In addition, the nurse must examine her feelings about the mentally ill and about psychiatric nursing. *Feelings* are the affective states the nurse brings with her from past experiences and applies to the current situation.

As previously stated, the combination of beliefs and feelings constitutes the nurse's philosophy and provides direction for the development of principles that will guide her nursing care. *Principles* are rules or laws that have proved to be applicable in most if not all, situations. The identification of principles of psychiatric nursing allows the nurse to operationalize her beliefs and feelings in nursing care.

To aid the student in expanding her self-awareness the remainder of this chapter discusses my beliefs, feelings conducive to the effective practice of psychiatric nursing, and the resultant principles of psychiatric nursing to which I adhere.

A PHILOSOPHY OF PSYCHIATRIC NURSING

Human beings are viewed as complex systems of interrelated parts, the whole of which is greater than the sum of the parts. This belief represents a holistic perspective, a stance that acknowledges the interdependence and interrelatedness of the parts to each other, to the person, and to the environment. Therefore alterations in any aspect of the system require responsive alterations in other aspects of the system.

Nurses new to the care of the mentally ill sometimes believe that the slightest change in the environment of a mentally ill person will precipitate an untoward emotional response. It is also not unusual for such a nurse to believe that the mentally ill individual is so emotionally fragile that he can be traumatized by an inexpertly phrased statement. These beliefs may cause some nurses to fear that they may injure clients emotionally, and as a result they may avoid contact with them.

This fear and its resultant behavior are particularly unfortunate and unwarranted if the nurse views the client as a system. It is important to remember that emotionally ill persons are not defenseless and that they withstand the inappropriate approach of new workers remarkably well. It may be helpful to note that if clients were in fact defenseless it would be a relatively easy matter to interact with them in a manner that would result in emotionally corrective experiences. Rather, clients, like all human beings, are complex organisms who are usually able to sense the innate friendliness behind the nurse's approach even if it is not skillfully executed. Furthermore, the nurse who is new to the mental health setting has developed expertise in many other areas of nursing practice that can be brought to bear on the interaction. Consequently, the nurse can develop the *feeling that she has the potential to be helpful to the client,* even though she may not yet have developed expertise in the care specific to the emotionally ill.

A major principle of psychiatric nursing that stems from this belief and feeling is that *the nurse views the client as a holistic being with a multiplicity of interrelated and interdependent needs.* The implications of this principle are numerous. First, the nurse caring for the mentally ill individual must be skilled in understanding the interrelatedness of all the client's subsystems. For example, mental illness does not provide immunity to physical illness and mentally ill persons are as prone to the development of physical illness as are other members of the population. Therefore the nurse needs to be constantly alert to the possibility that a mentally ill client may develop a physical illness, and thereby avoid the pitfall of assuming that all symptoms are simply manifestations of emotional stress. The individual must also be viewed as an integral part of his social system, simultaneously affecting the system and being affected by it. Therefore he canot be assessed accurately in isolation from his family, his community, and the reference groups to which he belongs. As a result the well-prepared nurse who works in a mental health setting must not only have effective interpersonal skills but also current knowledge about pathophysiology and about the norms and practices of various subcultures and religions. This principle is often cited as the rationale for employing a nurse whose educational background includes preparation in the biophysical and psychosocial realms, instead of a nursing assistant whose on-the-job training focuses only on the psychosocial realm.

A second belief is that *each individual has some strengths and a potential for growth,* that is, a potential for developing increasingly effective adaptations to stress. I do not mean to suggest that all individuals have an equal number or the same type of strengths, or the same potential for growth, but rather that each individual has some strengths and some potential for growth, no matter how small or great.

Sometimes nurses who are new to working with the mentally ill feel despair at the slow progress some clients are able to make. In fact, some nurses feel hopeless about effecting any improvement in the mentally ill. This feeling often emanates from inexperience in working with persons who have a chronic illness and for whom there may be no specific treatment. However, as the nurse gains experience and adopts the belief that each individual has potential for growth, despair will be replaced by hope. Interestingly, *the feeling of hope is therapeutic* in and of itself, since it conveys to the client the feeling that change is possible.

The principle of psychiatric nursing that is derived from this belief and from the feeling of hope is that *the nurse focuses on the client's strengths and assets, not on his weaknesses and liabilities.* All clients have some strengths, no matter how few or insignificant they may seem. These strengths should be built on to encourage the emotional growth of the individual. For example the client who dresses himself without undue difficulty can build on his behavior by being encouraged to choose clothing appropriate to the occasion and weather. As the client learns to make these choices he may very well develop an increasing sense of autonomy, which in turn may carry over to other areas of his daily living. This example may seem overly simplistic, but it is given to illustrate how this principle can be used in frequently encountered situations.

When mental health care was limited to institutional care an illness orientation was all-pervasive. A client who was cooperative was all too often seen as being overly submissive; if the same client becomes assertive he ran the risk of being labeled rebellious. The focus on illness not only tended to reinforce the condition and therefore stifle the client's growth, it also may have contributed to the development of illness. A positive outcome of the community mental health movement has been the necessity to focus on the healthy aspects of the client in an effort to enable him to maintain himself in the community and outside the institution. In many instances this orientation has been even more successful than had been originally anticipated. Some authorities believe this may be due to the fact that when an individual is helped to identify and accept his strengths, he is less threatened and therefore more open to exploring and altering his dysfunctional behaviors. It should be noted, however, that a focus on the individual's strengths and growth potential does not mean that his limitations should not be taken into account when assessing his behavior. Failure to do so and subsequent misjudgments have accounted for many of the failures that have also accompanied the community mental health movement.

I endorse the belief that *each individual, although sharing much in common with other persons, is unique and has inherent value*. This belief is consistent with the view of human beings as complex systems that transform energy and matter in a unique way. The belief that each individual has inherent value is a product of the Judeo-Christian heritage of our society and is manifested in numerous ways through societal practices.

In contrast, American culture also places great value on an individual's capacity to contribute to the society and thus covertly devalues those persons who are unable or who choose not to do so. Certainly many mentally ill persons are not able to make an identifiable contribution to the welfare of the society and therefore some nurses have the feeling that the mentally ill have less inherent value than do other more productive members of the population. It is important for the nurse to recognize this feeling if it exists and attempt to overcome it by focusing on the humanness of the client, regardless of his level of productivity. Valuing the client may also be difficult because of his appearance or his behavior. Once the nurse is able to view these factors as indicators of the client's ineffective adaptations, she is more likely to be able to *appreciate his uniqueness and inherent value*.

The principle of psychiatric nursing that stems from the belief in and feeling about the uniqueness and inherent value of each human being is that *the nurse accepts the client as a unique human being who has value and worth exactly as he is*. In fact, most authorities agree that this principle is the most basic to the effective practice of psychiatric nursing.

The conviction that each individual is unique implies that the nurse has a responsibility to observe and listen carefully to each person as if he were the only one to whom care has ever been given. The nurse must not "tune him out," even though his story has been told 100 times before. Psychological experiments have demonstrated that each person's perceptions of and reactions to the same situation are always different, depending on many variables such as previous experience and present state of being.

This principle guides the nurse in respecting the worth and dignity of persons at all times, without regard to the acceptability of their behavior. Thus the effective nurse treats clients with respect even though their behavior may be unacceptable. Inherent in this principle is the attitude that information about clients is treated with appropriate professional confidentiality and that client problems must not become topics for social chatter. This principle also implies that the treatment methods in which health professionals engage must not in themselves be dehumanizing, even though such methods may have desirable outcomes. In other words, if all human beings have inherent worth and value, treatment modalities that are dehumanizing do not justify even desirable ends.

Although the nurse needs to convey to the client a belief in his potential to change and grow, acceptance of him must not depend on his reaching these goals. That would be conditional acceptance and may convey, "I value you only because of what you could become." Most clients have a long history of being rejected in social relationships because their behavior did not measure up to usual societal expectations. Therefore such individuals enter treatment situations fully expecting the responses with which they are so familiar. If they do in fact receive these negative responses, they might just as well not have sought treatment, because they will be receiving very little constructive help. Since the nurse spends more time with the client than any other professional person, she has the greatest opportunity to convey a feeling of acceptance to him. Calling the client by his surname, such as Mr. Smith, until the client requests otherwise is an example of how acceptance can be conveyed.

In apparent contradiction to the belief that each individual is unique is the belief that *all human beings are sufficiently similar that there is a basis, no matter how small, for understanding and communicating with one another.* Harry Stack Sullivan has said that we are all more human than otherwise. I ascribe to this belief of similarity among human beings and further believe that differences in feelings and behavior are more likely to be differences in quantity rather than in quality. For example, all persons have experienced anxiety although most individuals have not been forced to adapt to anxiety by withdrawing from reality. Almost everyone knows what it means to feel sad, or happy, or ex-

cited. Those who are mentally ill experience these same emotions, but to an exaggerated or diminished degree.

The very nature of this belief may elicit in the nurse a fear
that she herself may become mentally ill. Not too many decades
ago it was commonly believed by lay people that if a person
worked with the mentally ill for too long a period, he too would
become mentally ill. This belief had its origins in the lack of understanding of the causes of mental illness and in the observation
that many who did work with the mentally ill were in fact emotionally disturbed themselves. This latter phenomenon was a result of the fact that the care of the mentally ill was seen as such
an undesirable job that only socially deviant persons who could
not find employment elsewhere were willing to work in the asylums.

The nurse of today brings into the mental health setting all
the biases and prejudices of the society at large. When the nurse
realizes that the behavior of most clients is not as bizarre as she
had expected, another fear may be elicited—the fear that she has
more problems than the clients appear to have. Consequently,
some nurses initially believe that they require psychiatric treatment or hospitalization. Although this may be true in a very few
instances, the nurse will learn that most persons enter a treatment situation because of an increasing inability to perform the
usual activities of daily living in regard to both work and family
life. In contrast, the nurse who is functioning despite the emotional problems she may have learns that the ability to function
productively is an important criterion of mental health.

Beginning students of psychiatric nursing frequently experience anxiety about their state of mental health as they learn
more about the dynamics underlying mental illness. This probably results from the fact that the student can more easily identify
with the mentally ill person than with the physically ill person.
All human beings have experienced emotional trauma, anxiety,
guilt, anger, and other emotions, but not all have experienced
appendicitis, myocardial infarcts, or other forms of major physical illnesses.

Once again, it is important for the nurse to remember that
none of the feelings and few of the experiences of mentally ill
persons are different in kind from those she has personally
known. In fact, the nurse will learn to *use her familiarity with the*

various emotions as a tool through which to develop empathy with the client's feelings.

The principle of psychiatric nursing that is based on belief in the similarity of all human beings and the nurse's empathy with the client's feelings is that *the nurse has the potential for establishing a relationship with most if not all clients.* This principle implies that nurses who interact with the mentally ill must continuously strive to discover the area of similarity between the person and themselves that can serve as a means of establishing communication. Nurses cannot hide behind the belief that it is useless to try to help an individual because his background, experience, and behavior are different from anything with which they are familiar. This does not suggest that a common cultural or experiential background between a client and a nurse may not be helpful in establishing communication, but rather that nurses must continue to strive to communicate with clients even if their frame of reference is not immediatey understood. Furthermore, in some situations when the nurse and the client share a great deal in common the nurse may fail to recognize the client's uniqueness and inappropriately attribute to him her own feelings and reactions. This principle does not mean, however, that any one nurse should or could have a relationship with all clients. The student will learn that to engage effectively in a therapeutic relationship with a client is very time consuming and an emotionally and intellectually draining activity. Therefore such interventions should be undertaken with clients who are most likely to benefit from the nurse's personality and style of interaction. However, the nurse can interact with every client in a helpful way if she continuously looks for areas of similarities between them to use as a basis for increasing her understanding of the client.

A belief central to the effective practice of psychiatric nursing is that *all behavior is purposeful and designed to meet a need or to communicate a message.* No behavior is accidental or occurs by chance.

Some nurses fear the clinical practice of psychiatric nursing not only because it is a new experience but also because of many preconceived ideas about the behavior of mentally ill persons. Nurses may have heard discussions about unusual and frightening behavior of such individuals. These discussions often exaggerate the behavior being described and tend to arouse fear on the part of the listener.

The nurse with these feelings can cope more readily with the situation by acknowledging any concerns about personal safety, by facing the fact frankly, and by examining these fears to discover what they involve. It is usually helpful to discuss such attitudes in situations in which students and teacher can help each other in examining, understanding, and coping with these feelings. This method is particularly effective when the discussion focuses on a specific individual whose behavior is causing concern.

Much of the fear of mentally ill persons grows out of cultural attitudes and beliefs handed down from one generation to another. In spite of attempts to educate the public about mental illness, there are still many persons who believe that all mentally ill individuals are dangerous and require drastic measures to control their behavior. Nurses being introduced to a mental health setting will be surprised at the large number of clients whose behavior is socially acceptable. They will be surprised to find that many mentally ill persons seem content to be inactive. Instead of requiring controls, many clients require stimulation and need to be helped to develop an interest in the available activities. Once the nurse has become familiar with the clients in the mental health setting and has gained more knowledge about human behavior, it will be possible for her to replace her fear of client behavior with a *feeling of curiosity about its meaning.*

The principle of psychiatric nursing that stems from the belief that all behavior is purposeful and the accompanying curiosity about its meaning is that *the nurse explores the client's behavior for the need it is designed to meet or the message it is communicating.* This principle does not imply that all behavior must be accepted or condoned as it is expressed. On the contrary, tolerance of all behavior, no matter how antisocial it may be, can convey to the client the idea that he is not important enough for the nurse to explore his behavior with him. The helpful nurse will make an effort to convey to the client her understanding that his behavior has meaning and her willingness to help him meet the need or communicate the message in a socially acceptable way. Some clients have never become aware that there are socially acceptable means through which their needs can be met. When the nurse helps the client to evaluate the consequences of his present behavior and test new patterns of behavior she will do a great deal in furthering his feeling of being a worthwhile human being. By treating the client's socially unacceptable behavior in this manner the nurse communicates that she is not being punitive or judgmental, but is primarily concerned about the client's welfare.

Another belief regarding the nature of human behavior is that *it was learned as an adaptation to earlier stressors,* especially those experienced during the influential years of infancy and childhood when the foundation of the personality is laid. Therefore *the individual's present behavior is believed to represent the best possible adaptation he is capable of making at the time.* It should be noted that all behavioral adaptations were effective in maintaining homeokinesis at the time they were learned. If, however, the interpersonal environment in which the behavioral adaptation was learned was unique or unhealthy, the behavior that was effective in the original situation becomes ineffective and dysfunctional when the person moves to a subsequent developmental stage or into the larger social system that functions in a more usual or healthy manner.

Even when they are seeking help mentally ill persons may be shy, suspicious, withdrawn, and preoccupied with their own thoughts and problems. The nurse may interpret these behaviors as a dislike of her and react with the socially familiar response of disliking the client. As the nurse develops an understanding of mental illness she will realize that some clients behave in this manner even when they want very much to become acquainted with the nurse because they fear that they will not be accepted by her. The nurse cannot expect to thoroughly like all clients nor can she expect all clients to genuinely like her. However, it is realistic to expect that she will develop some understanding and acceptance of all clients and learn not to view all their behavior as a reflection of their feelings toward her. She will also be able to develop *the ability to care about clients even though they may not reciprocate this feeling* if she works at developing a support group among her peers rather than looking to clients for approval and gratitude.

The principle of psychiatric nursing based on the above beliefs and feelings is that *the nurse views the client's behavior nonjudg-*

mentally while assisting him to learn more effective adaptations. This principle is central to the effective practice of psychiatric nursing because it implies that it is possible for the client to un-learn old adaptations and relearn new, more effective adaptations if provided with an environment that facilitates and supports this goal. Further, this principle also implies that the nurse is likely to accept the client's behavior, withholding judgment. For example, adherence to this principle makes it inappropriate for the nurse to say that the client refuses to participate in group therapy; rather, the nurse is more likely to understand that at this time the client is not able to participate. In addition, this principle helps to dispel the aura of hopelessness that often surrounds the care of the mentally ill. Although it is important to be realistic about the changes any one individual can make it is inappropriate to believe that a person's behavior cannot change or that his overall adaptation to the stresses of life cannot become more effective.

A final belief integral to the effective practice of psychiatric nursing is the understanding that *an individual learns behavioral adaptations primarily in interaction with significant people in his environment.* Human beings do not exist in a vacuum; their survival depends on interaction with other human beings. However, an individual cannot be expected to learn new behavioral adaptations if he is not given an opportunity to interact with others who provide experiences that are more positive than those he has known previously.

Nurses beginning an experience in psychiatric nursing sometimes find they have a strong desire to be helpful but simultaneously feel they are not skillful enough to assume a significant role in the treatment of the mentally ill person. These feelings present nurses with an uncomfortable personal dilemma from which they may seek to escape by becoming indifferent. To allow this feeling to develop would be unfortunate, because indifference is one of the reactions that most mentally ill persons have already experienced much too often in their relations with family and friends. In contrast, nurses are encouraged to become emotionally involved with their clients. In fact, without such involvement the nurse can be of little real therapeutic help. However, it is essential to understand the meaning of involvement. *Involvement* implies that the nurse is genuinely and sincerely interested in the client, that she gives of her time and of herself without expecting anything in return, and that she interacts in a way that meets the need of the client instead of her own. Although initially the nurse may feel that her interpersonal skills are not developed to a level that makes her feel adequate in the situation, with guidance, practice, and persistent study of self, the early feelings of inadequacy will be replaced with *feelings of competency in her ability to interact therapeutically* with the mentally ill.

The principle of psychiatric nursing derived from the belief and feeling just discussed is that *the quality of the interaction in which the nurse engages with the client is a major determinant of the degree to which the client will be able to alter his behavioral adaptations in the direction of more satisfying, satisfactory interpersonal relationships.* When the individual seeks help from a treatment setting he has little impetus to alter his adaptive mechanisms if his characteristic behavior is met with the same negative, judgmental attitudes he has experienced from society. On the other hand, if in spite of his behavior the individual becomes involved with an interested, concerned nurse who values his worth and dignity, positive satisfactory behavioral adaptations are likely to be elicited. This principle is particularly germane to the practice of psychiatric nursing because the nurse is the professional person who is likely to spend the greatest amount of time with the client and therefore is the person who has the greatest opportunity to create the environment in which the client can unlearn previous ineffective adaptations and learn new more effective adaptations.

DEFINITION OF PSYCHIATRIC NURSING

The nurse's philosophy of psychiatric nursing provides direction for stating a definition of psychiatric nursing. The philosophy just discussed leads me to define psychiatric nursing as a process whereby the nurse assists persons, as individuals or in groups, to develop a more positive self-concept, a more satisfying pattern of interpersonal relationships, and a more satisfactory role in society. The achievement of these goals results from assisting clients to increase and utilize their potential energy to enlarge their effective adaptations to the stresses of life, thereby enabling them to increase system openness and maintain homeokinesis.

The student is encouraged to examine her own beliefs and feelings about the mentally ill and about psychiatric nursing so

TABLE 7-1 beliefs, feelings, and principles conducive to the effective practice of psychiatric nursing

belief	feeling	principle
Human beings are complex systems of interrelated parts, the whole of which is greater than the sum of the parts	The nurse feels she can be helpful to the client, since she has expertise in many areas of nursing	The nurse views the client as a holistic being with a multiplicity of interrelated and interdependent needs
Each individual has some strengths and a potential for growth	The nurse is hopeful about the client's ability to grow	The nurse focuses on the client's strengths and assets, not on his weaknesses and liabilities
Each individual is unique and has inherent value	The nurse appreciates the uniqueness and inherent value of the client	The nurse accepts the client as a unique human being who has value and worth exactly as he is
All human beings are sufficiently similar that there is a basis for understanding and communicating with one another	The nurse feels empathy with the client's feelings	The nurse has the potential for establishing a relationship with most if not all clients
All behavior is purposeful and is designed to meet a need or to communicate a message	The nurse feels curious about the meaning of the client's behavior	The nurse explores the client's behavior for the need it is designed to meet or the message it is communicating
Behavior is learned as an adaptation to an earlier stressor and is the best possible adaptation the individual is capable of making at the time	The nurse cares about clients even though they may not reciprocate her feeling	The nurse views the client's behavior nonjudgmentally while assisting him to learn more effective adaptations
An individual learns behavioral adaptations primarily in interaction with significant people in his environment	The nurse feels competent in her ability to interact therapeutically with the mentally ill	The quality of the interaction in which the nurse engages with the client is a major determinant of the degree to which the client will be able to alter his behavioral adaptations in the direction of more satisfying, satisfactory interpersonal relationships

that she might state a philosophy and definition of psychiatric nursing to guide her nursing care.

CONCLUDING STATEMENTS

1. The major therapeutic tool of the psychiatric nurse is her use of self in the interpersonal context.
2. The nurse's ability to use herself as a therapeutic tool is de-

pendent on her adopting beliefs and feelings conducive to the effective practice of psychiatric nursing.

3. All nurses can become aware of that which they believe and feel without having to understand why they believe and feel as they do.

4. Self-awareness and self-disclosure free energy that can be used more profitably and give the person an increasing degree of control over his behavior.

5. For the nurse to expand her self-awareness she must examine her beliefs and feelings that, combined, constitute her philosophy of psychiatric nursing and provide the bases for those principles that direct her nursing care.

6. The belief that human beings are complex systems of interrelated parts, the whole of which is greater than the sum of its parts, combined with the nurse's feeling of being potentially helpful to the client, are the bases of the principle that the nurse views the client as a holistic being with a multiplicity of interrelated and interdependent needs.

7. The belief that each individual has strengths and a potential for growth, combined with the nurse's feeling of hope about the client's ability to grow, are the bases of the principle that the nurse focuses on the client's strengths and assets and not on his weaknesses and liabilities.

8. The belief that each individual is unique and has inherent value, combined with the nurse's appreciation of the client's uniqueness and inherent value, are the bases of the principle that the nurse accepts the client as a unique human being who has value and worth exactly as he is.

9. The belief that all human beings are sufficiently similar that there is ground for understanding and communicating with each other, combined with the nurse's feeling of empathy with the client's feelings, are the bases of the principle that the nurse has the potential for establishing a relationship with most if not all clients.

10. The belief that all behavior is purposeful and designed to meet a need or to communicate a message, combined with the nurse's feeling of curiosity about the meaning of the client's behavior, are the bases of the principle that the nurse explores the client's behavior for the need it is designed to meet or the message it is communicating.

11. The belief that behavior is learned and is the best possible adaptation the individual is capable of making at the time, combined with the nurse's caring about the client, are the bases of the principle that the nurse views the client's behavior nonjudgmentally while assisting him to learn more effective adaptations.

12. The belief that an individual learns behavioral adaptations in interaction with significant others, combined with the nurse's feeling of competency in her ability to interact therapeutically, are the bases of the principle that the quality of the nurse-client interaction is a major determinant of the degree to which the client will be able to alter his behavioral adaptations.

13. Psychiatric nursing is defined as a process whereby the nurse assists persons, as individuals or in groups, to develop a more positive self-concept, a more satisfying pattern of interpersonal relationships, and a more satisfactory role in society.

SUGGESTED SOURCES OF ADDITIONAL INFORMATION

Classical

Black, Sister Kathleen M.: An existential model for psychiatric nursing, Perspect. Psychiatr. Care 6:178-184, July-Aug., 1968.

Brill, Norman Q.: The importance of understanding yourself, Am. J. Nurs. 57:1325-1326, 1957.

Frances, Gloria M.: How do I feel about myself? Am. J. Nurs. 67:1244-1245, 1967.

Goldsborough, Judith D.: On becoming nonjudgmental Am. J. Nurs. 70:2340-2343, 1970.

Goldstein, Joan: Exploring attitudes that affect nursing care, Nurs. Outlook 16:50-51, June, 1968.

Holmes, Marguerite J.: What's wrong with getting involved? Nurs. Outlook 8:250-251, May, 1960.

Hyde, R.M., and Coggan, C.M.: When nurses have guilt feelings, Am. J. Nurs. 58:233-236, 1958.

Jacobs, Linda M.: Beginning practitioner's adjustment to a psychiatric unit, Nurs. Outlook 18:28-31, Oct., 1970.

Johnson, Betty Sue, and Miller, Lynne C.: The interpersonal reflex in psychiatric nursing, Nurs. Outlook 15:60-63, May, 1967.

Lewis, Garland K., and Holmes, Marguerite J.: Meddling with emotions, Nurs. Outlook 9:405-407, 1961.

Lewis, John A.: Reflections on self, Am. J. Nurs. 60:828-830, 1960.

Luft, J.: Of human interaction, Palo Alto, California, 1969, National Press Books.

Peplau, Hildegard E.: Professional closeness—as a special kind of involvement with a patient, client, or family group, Nurs. Forum **8:**342-359, 1969.

Rogers, C.R.: On becoming a person, Boston, 1970, Houghton Mifflin Co.

Schwartz, Morris S., and Shockley, Emmy Lanning: The nurse and the mental patient, New York, 1956, John Wiley & Sons, Inc.

Stevens, Leonard F.: Understanding ourselves, Am. J. Nurs. **57:**1022-1023, 1957.

Sullivan, Harry Stack: The interpersonal theory of psychiatry, New York, 1953, W.W. Norton & Co., Inc.

Tuteur, Werner: As you enter psychiatric nursing, Am. J. Nurs. **56:**72-74, 1956.

Contemporary

Aiken, L., and Aiken J.L.: A systematic approach to the evaluation of interpersonal relationships, Am. J. Nurs. **73:**863-866, 1973.

Benfer, Beverly A.: Clinical supervision as a support system for the caregiver, Perspect. Psychiatr. Care **171:**13-17, Jan.-Feb., 1979.

Chapman, Nadine: An essay on the art of nursing, Perspect. Psychiatr. Care **21:**66-69, April/June 1983.

Clark, Carolyn C.: Inner dialogue: a self-healing approach for nurses and clients, Am. J. Nurs. **81:**1191-1193, June 1981.

Dormer, Aline: The miracle of caring, J. Psychosoc. Nurs. Ment. Health Serv. **18:**21-24, Aug., 1980.

Duldty, Bonnie: Helping nurses to cope with the anger-dismay syndrome, Nurs. Outlook **30:**168-174, March 1982.

Fagin, Claire: Accountability, Nurs. Outlook **19:**249-251, 1971.

Flynn, Patricia Ann Randolph: Holistic health: the art and science of care, Bowie, Md., 1980, Robert J. Brady Co.

Gedan, Sharon: This I believe . . . about psychiatric nursing practice, Nurs. Outlook **19:**534-536, 1971.

Gunderson, Kathleen, et al.: How to control professional frustration, Am. J. Nurs. **77:**1180-1183, July 1977.

Johnson, R., Richardson, H., Von Endt, L., and Lindgren, K.: The professional support group: model for psychiatric clinical nurse specialists, J. Psychosoc. Nurs. Ment. Health Serv. **20:**9-13, Feb., 1982.

Kalisch, Beatrice J.: An experiment in the development of empathy in nursing students, Nurs. Res. **20:**202-211, 1971.

Knowles, Ruth: Dealing with feelings: coping with lethargy, Am. J. Nurs. **81:**1465, Aug., 1981.

Knowles, Ruth: Dealing with feelings: handling anger: responding vs reacting, Am. J. Nurs. **81:**2196, Dec., 1981.

Knowles, Ruth: Dealing with feelings: managing guilt, Am. J. Nurs. **81:**1850, Oct., 1981.

Knowles, Ruth: Dealing with feelings: overcoming guilt and worry, Am. J. Nurs. **81:**1663, Sept., 1981.

Krikovian, Diana, and Paulanka, B.: Self awareness—the key to a successful nurse-patient relationship, J. Psychosoc. Nurs. Ment. Health Serv. **20:**19-21, June, 1982.

Lenarz, Dorothea M.: Care is the essence of practice, Am. J. Nurs. **71:**704-707, 1971.

Levinson, Richard: Sexism in medicine, Am. J. Nurs. **76:**426-431, 1976.

McGoran, Saralee: On developing empathy: teaching students self-awarness, Part 1, Am. J. Nurs. **78:**859-861, May, 1978.

Oiler, Carolyn: Nursing reality as reflected in nurse's poetry, Perspect. Psychiatr. Care **21:**81-89, July/Sept., 1983.

Pilette, Patricia: Caution: Objectivity and specialization may be hazardous to your health, Am. J. Nurs. **80:**1588-1599, Sept., 1980.

Rawnsley, Marilyn M.: Toward a conceptual base for affective nursing, Nurs. Outlook **28:**244-247, April, 1980.

Reich, Stephen, and Geller, Andrew: The self-image of nurses employed in a psychiatric hospital, Perspect. Psychiatr. Care **153:**126-128, 1977.

Robinson, Lisa: Psychiatric nursing as a human experience, Philadelphia, 1977, W.B. Saunders Co.

Schoffstall, Carole: Concerns of student nurses prior to psychiatric nursing experience. An assessment and intervention, J. Psychosoc. Nurs. Ment. Health Serv. **19:**11-14, Nov., 1981.

Sinkler, Gail H.: Identity and role, Nurs. Outlook **18:**22-24, Oct., 1970.

Slimmer, Lynda Walton: Helping students to resolve conflicts between their religious beliefs and psychiatric-mental health treatment approaches, J. Psychosoc. Nurs. Ment. Health Serv. **18:**37-39, July 1980.

Ujhely, Gertrud B.: Am I my brother's keeper? Perspect. Psychiatr. Care **17:**204-211, Sept.-Oct., 1979.

Van Devort, Dolores Walters: Both hands clapping, Am. J. Nurs. **73:**999-1000, 1973.

Zimmerman, Beverly: Human questions vs human hurry, Am. J. Nurs. **80:**719, April, 1980.

Of particular interest

Albiez, Sr. A.: Reflecting on the development of a relationship, J. Psychiatr. Nurs., pp. 25-27, Nov.-Dec., 1970.
This article is especially relevant for the beginning student. The author describes her feelings during her first student psychiatric nursing experience.

American Nurses' Association, Division of Psychiatric and Mental Health Nursing Practice: Standards of psychiatric-mental health nursing practice, Kansas City, Mo., 1982.
This is important reading for students of psychiatric nursing. The American Nurses' Association (ANA) describes each of the standards of psychiatric nursing, the rationale for each, and the assessment factors for each.

Coad-Denton, A.: Therapeutic superficiality and intimacy. In Longo, D., and Williams, R., editors: Psychosocial nursing: assessment and intervention, New York, 1978, Appleton-Century-Crofts.

The differences between an intimate social relationship and an intimate therapeutic relationship are discussed by the author. Included are nursing interventions designed to promote therapeutic intimacy.

Peplau, H.: Interpersonal relations in nursing, New York, 1952, G.P. Putnam's Sons.

This classic book provides the reader with a description of psychiatric nursing. Included are discussions of the roles of psychiatric nursing, its functions, and its impact on various settings, all within an interpersonal conceptual framework.

effective communication

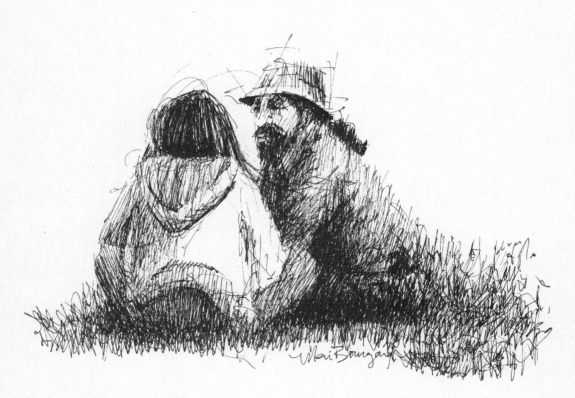

I'm listening.

LEARNING OBJECTIVES
After studying this chapter the student will be able to:

1   Define the communication process.

2   Discuss the three modes of communication.

3   Give examples of effective verbal and nonverbal communication.

4   Identify special problems and their solutions in communicating with the mentally ill.

Communication refers to the reciprocal exchange of information, ideas, beliefs, feelings, and attitudes between two persons or among a group of persons. As such it is a dynamic process requiring continual adaptations by those involved. Communication is effective when it accurately and clearly conveys the intended messages.

The communication process is basic to all nursing practice and when effective greatly contributes to the development of all therapeutic relationships. Knowledge of and skill in effective communication are essential for the nurse who works with the mentally ill because her ability to be therapeutic is highly related to the effectiveness of her communication skills.

HISTORICAL PERSPECTIVE

Communication is not unique to human beings. Other species of animals communicate with each other. Only humans, however, have the ability to engage in the complex interaction evidenced by the use of language. In fact, the ability to use language is seen by many as an essential characteristic of being human. Effective communication is a major means by which people express many of their needs and subsequently have them met, thereby experiencing satisfying, satisfactory relationships with others.

The needs of primitive human beings most certainly centered around issues of physical survival. Therefore their ability to listen for and respond appropriately to sounds that warned of danger or assured safety was essential. Effective communication was achieved when verbal and nonverbal forms of communication were accurately transmitted and interpreted. Feedback about the effectiveness of the communication was likely to be immediate. During this period of human development communication was limited to face-to-face interaction between individuals and among small groups.

Although the alphabet was developed around 2000 BC major changes in the communication process did not occur until the invention of the printing press in the fifteenth century. This invention made possible the mass production of the written word and essentially changed the culture of communication from a speaking-listening orientation to a visual orientation.

This change in orientation coincided with and contributed to a change in the standard of living wherein the peoples of the Western world could afford to be less concerned about survival issues and more concerned about higher level needs related to interpersonal relationships. Paradoxically, as concern with these needs intensified there was an increased dependence on the written word, which by definition is devoid of human contact. Some authorities believe that this dependence on the written word and consequently on a visual orientation to communication has diminished the ability of many contemporary human beings to engage in the effective verbal and nonverbal communication that characterizes satisfying interpersonal relationships. In fact, some believe that continuous ineffective communication between parent and child is a major contributing factor to the subsequent development of mental illness in the child. Whether this is the case or not, it is well documented that ineffective communication patterns are a predominant symptom of many forms of mental illness and that engaging in effective communication with clients can have therapeutic results.

Because of the complexity of the communication process and its pivotal role in interpersonal relationships, effective and disturbed communication patterns have been the subject of much study by contemporary theorists. One of the best known, psychiatrist Jurgen Ruesch, has written that communication is therapeutic when it is helpful. The following discussion of communication is designed to provide the nurse with guidelnes for the development of helpful and therefore therapeutic communication patterns.

MODES OF COMMUNICA-TION

Everyone is familiar with communication through the written word. When written material is read, the reciprocal aspects of communication are limited to the reader's ability to understand and react to the ideas and concepts that the author is attempting to convey. If the reader does not receive the intended message effective communication has not been achieved.

Another mode of communication with which everyone is familiar is the spoken word or *verbal communicaton*. If persons who are speaking together understand the same language, a major reciprocal element is present as they exchange, question, challenge, clarify, and enlarge on statements.

A mode of communication of which people are not always aware is *nonverbal communication*, which is closely related to verbal communication and is usually an integral part of it. Nonverbal communication refers to the messages sent and received through such means as facial expression, voice quality, physical posture, and gestures. Thus a person's behavior conveys a great deal to the astute observer. Nonverbal communication is often referred to as *body language*. Because nonverbal communication, or body language, is always present, it has been said that a person cannot *not* communicate.

Inner feelings are expressed by the manner in which an individual conducts himself in even such simple activities as walking down the hall, opening and closing doors, reclining in an easy chair, speaking to other people, and asking questions. The nonverbal aspects of communication sometimes convey general attitudes, feelings, and reactions more clearly and more accurately than do spoken words. An understanding of the implications of nonverbal communication is important for all nurses, especially those who work with the mentally ill. Not only is it important for therapeutic reasons that the nurse be aware of the client's nonverbal communication, she must also be aware of her own nonverbal communication. Mentally ill persons are more aware of the nurse's nonverbal behavior than many nurses realize. The nurse who works rapidly, walks down the hall briskly, closes doors emphatically, and answers questions sharply is likely to be seen as an angry, unapproachable person. The nurse who smiles, speaks in a warm, friendly manner, and approaches her work calmly conveys an acceptance that may prompt the client to turn to her for help.

Another mode of communication, rarely recognized on a conscious level, is *metacommunication*. Metacommunication refers to the role expectation individuals have of each other in the context in which verbal and nonverbal communication take place. These role expectations strongly influence the nature of the verbal and nonverbal communication. For example, when a salesperson says to a customer, "May I help you?" it is understood by both indi-

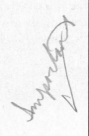

viduals that she is asking whether she can be of assistance in helping the customer to make a purchase. On the other hand, when the nurse in a treatment setting asks the same question of a client it is understood by both that she is asking if there is something she might do, such as listening or helping the client with activities basic to his needs. Metacommunication and nonverbal communication are present in all situations in which there are two or more persons, although verbal communication may be absent at times.

Communication is most effective when the three previously mentioned modes of communication—verbal, nonverbal, and metacommunication—are congruent. Imagine the reaction of the previously mentioned salesperson if the customer responded: "Yes, you can help me. My child is ill and I am very worried about her." In this situation the customer's reply indicates that she is responding only to the verbal communication of the salesperson and is ignoring the metacommunication. Therefore the customer's reply illustrates incongruency between her verbal communication and her metacommunication, which is likely to result in an increase in the anxiety levels of both persons involved.

DEVELOPING EFFECTIVE MODES OF COMMUNICATION

Developing modes of communication that are effective within the family, the culture, and the society in which one lives is an exceedingly complex learning process that begins at birth and comprises a large part of subsequent developmental stages. Although some of this learning takes place in a formal way through such societal agencies as the school, the foundation of the communication process is laid within the family long before the child is ready to attend school. In this respect the family acts as the representative of the society at large.

Much of the teaching and learning about communication within the family structure is achieved indirectly. For example, the child learns certain words by hearing them used in the home and without anyone actually teaching him to associate the word with the object. This is illustrated by the 4-year-old child of two college professors who was asked by his nursery school teacher to identify pictures of objects. His classmates identified one as a *suitcase* or *bag*, but he identified the same object as an *attaché case*. Furthermore, he was unable to identify the object called *apron* by the rest of his classmates. The strong academic influ-

cultural
input
input

ence and lack of domestic interest in this child's home were clearly demonstrated by the nature of his vocabulary.

In the same way the meaning of nonverbal communication is learned. In some cultures a loud tone of voice signifies anger. In other cultures the opposite is true—that is, silence signifies anger, whereas loud, animated talking is indicative of nothing more than enthusiasm. To survive, children must learn to attach meaning to both the verbal and nonverbal communications of their family members, since they are highly dependent on these persons for having their needs met. It is a comment on the great intellectual potential of human beings to note how quickly the child does learn the meaning of highly complex messages.

It is not sufficient, however, for the child merely to learn the meaning of the messages he receives. He must also learn ways of responding that are acceptable within the family structure, and this is no simple task. Witness for example the child who lives within a family in which the verbal response to situations that are frustrating or anger-producing is to swear. Not infrequently the first time the child repeats a swear word in response to his anger or frustration, he is told by the adults that he is using a bad word that is forbidden and if he continues to use it, he will be punished.

Despite the complexity of learning the communication process, the majority of children are capable of doing so in a relatively short period of time and quickly become able to adapt that which they have learned in the home to the demands of the larger society. The previously mentioned 4-year-old quickly learned what an apron was and how it was used and that an attaché case is only one type of bag. In some instances, however, effective adaptation is not possible or becomes possible only after experiencing much stress. The stress of adapting to the communication in a different culture can be observed when adults travel rapidly between countries by jet airplane. Many travel agencies give their customers brochures describing the customs and frequently used words of the countries to be visited to lessen the communication shock experienced by the traveler.

The preceding examples illustrate communication problems that are normal from the standpoint of mental health. There are instances, however, when the learning of the communication process is fraught with such a high level of stress that it produces a

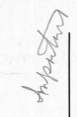

pattern of communication that is ineffective within either the family itself or society at large. *For our purposes, we can consider any communication to be ineffective if it does not accurately and clearly convey the message intended.* All persons occasionally experience ineffective communication. However, when this becomes a pattern (the rule rather than the exception), it frequently is a manifestation of mental illness and, in addition, is a factor in perpetuating the illness.

USING EFFECTIVE COMMUNICATION IN THE CARE OF THE MENTALLY ILL

Mentally ill individuals need the opportunity to communicate with others who are sincerely interested in their problems and who care about them as people. It is important for the nurse to learn to communicate in such a way that her conversation will become a part of the total therapeutic environment. The ability to communicate therapeutically with clients requires that the nurse have an attitude of acceptance and genuine interest in them.

A climate of mutual trust and respect must be developed before mentally ill persons can feel safe enough to communicate with a nurse. This is not an easy climate to establish; it requires time, patience, knowledge, and skill. However, the nurse is rewarded for her efforts by the knowledge that when a client is helped to converse effectively with a professional person, an emotionally supportive experience often results.

Initiating a conversation

When the nurse joins the professional staff of a treatment facility, she and the clients are strangers to one another. They must become acquainted before therapeutic communication can take place. Most clients approach the nurse cautiously at first, as they approach other strangers. Some individuals may not approach the nurse at all. A few may insist on monopolizing her total attention. The wise nurse will use some of the same skills in building a relationship with a mentally ill person that she has used successfully to build relationships with other strangers.

If the nurse has not already been introduced to the clients she will begin by introducing herself. It will be helpful if she explains her status at the same time. This can be done by saying, "I am Miss Jones, a student nurse, and I will be here for 4 weeks." Or she might say, "I am Miss Smith, a graduate nurse, and I have come to work here for a while." If the nurse does not know the name of the person to whom she has introduced herself, she might say, "Will you please help me learn your name? I am sorry that I do not know it." With this invitation most persons will introduce themselves. Having learned the name of the client she uses it when speaking to him. This simple but important technique helps to individualize the conversation and encourages the client to focus his attention.

After the nurse and the client have been introduced, it is appropriate for the nurse to initiate a conversation. A conversation is one of the most common of the shared activities in which people engage. It is the logical beginning for any relationship. Just as the nurse initiates the conversational topics with other strangers, she may find it helpful with clients to introduce a neutral conversational topic appropriate for the time and place. If the time of year is right, baseball may be an appropriate topic. If the client seems interested in baseball, the nurse may choose to initiate a conversation with a question about a recent game. For example, she may begin by saying, "I did not have a chance to follow the game yesterday. What was the final score?" Othe neutral topics that may be used include the headlines in the newspaper, the weather, or an approaching event. If the nurse notices that one person is holding a newspaper, she may begin a conversation by inquiring, "What interesting happenings are in the headlines today?"

Having introduced a topic, the sensitive nurse will wait for a response and will not feel compelled to avoid silences by immediately adding her own comments or opinions. After ample opportunity has been given for a response, it is suggested that she introduce a second conversational idea that logically follows the first.

Clients often ask new nurses personal questions such as, "Are you married?" or "What nursing school are you from?" or "Where do you live?" The natural curiosity of clients about the personal life of the professional staff is understandable. However, if the conversation is allowed to be focused on the personal life of the nurse, it quickly loses its original goal—to achieve communication that is therapeutic for the client. If the nurse wishes to do so it would seem logical for her to respond to factual questions such as, "Are you married?" with a simple "Yes" or "No." If the client continues to ask personal questions she might state "It seems you are very interested in me," or ask, "I wonder if we could not find

**Developing
effective verbal
communication**

a topic other than my personal life to discuss?" Frequent personal questions directed to the nurse alert her to the need for focusing future conversation more carefully. It may suggest that the individual in question hopes to direct attention away from his own problems.

To be effective, the nurse's verbal communication must be guided by goals. The nurse's therapeutic potential will be greatly increased if a conscious effort is made to establish a goal for each interaction before initiating a conversation. The identified purpose for the interaction will provide a guide as to the appropriate approach and attitude to be used, the approximate length of the conversation, and the manner in which it will be terminated.

Certainly the nurse should avoid approaching anyone with a barrage of words. In their desire to communicate effectively, nurses sometimes resort to asking a series of questions. Unfortunately this is too often the type of conversation that is reported when nurses are asked to tell about a recent conversation with a client. "How are you today?" is one of the usual questions with which many nurses begin a conversation. Such an opening sentence usually does little to develop a conversation.

Frequently the nurse interacts with the client for the purpose of giving or getting specific information. Although the attitude toward the client should be friendly, the nurse should initiate the conversation by explaining the purpose of the questions she will ask. In this instance it is appropriate that the questions be more direct than those usually employed. Such a conversation would be brief and terminated with an expression of thanks for the client's cooperation.

Direct questions may be perceived by a mentally ill person as threatening to personal security, "Why did you come to the hospital?" or "How do you feel about your job?" may touch on sensitive feelings. Thus direct questions are usually helpful only when specific information must be obtained or when the person is confused. When a client is responding to intrapsychic stimulation, it may be necesary to use direct questions to communicate with him.

A second goal for initiating an interaction may be to establish a beginning rapport that can serve as a basis for developing a meaningful future relationship. With such a goal, attention would be focused on the client in a friendly, relaxed way to convey a willingness to listen. In such a situation, emphasis is on getting acquainted and establishing a feeling of mutual trust.

If the purpose of the interaction is to encourage the person to express his thoughts and feelings, a nondirective approach would undoubtedly achieve the most positive results. In such a situation the client would be encouraged to initiate the conversation. Responding to his comments by reflecting his thoughts back to him might be helpful in encouraging him to continue expressing his feelings without introducing new or unrelated ideas. For example, if the client speaks of his unhappy home life, the nurse might respond by saying, "It sounds to me as if you are saying that your home life is unhappy." In addition, this type of response gives the client an opportunity to either accept or reject the nurse's impression of his communication.

Once having encouraged the client to express his thoughts and feelings, the nurse may not be prepared to hear what he has to say and may respond judgmentally. Such an attitude is reflected in statements such as, "Don't be silly!" or "How could you possibly think that?" Responses such as these discourage the client from further divulging his thoughts and feelings. To be helpful, it is important that the nurse withhold her personal opinion about what the client is saying and avoid the use of words that connote a judgment.

A general rule to follow when talking with clients is to encourage them to take the conversational lead. Although the nurse may initiate communication and may keep the conversation alive, the conversation must focus on the interests and concerns of the client if it is to be of value.

Some nurses attempt to communicate with clients by doing most of the talking while the client sits or stands passively nearby. If the client responds at all in a situation like this, it is usually to give a one-word answer. When the nurse communicates in such a way, her comments usually fall into the category of giving advice or persuading the client to do something that someone believes will benefit him. Neither advice or persuasion is of much help if the goal is to assist the client to become a self-directing adult. Giving advice suggests that one person is attempting to impose his values and personal choices on a second person who is not capable of making such choices. The giver of advice often begins the conversation by saying, "If I were you."

The nurse is not the client and cannot know the choices that are best for him to make in most situations. She does not know all the past experiences that influence his present thinking and feeling and therefore is not qualified to make suggestions about his many problems and concerns. Advice may result in a temporary and positive response because it may relieve the client from the responsibility of making an immediate decision. In the long run it is likely to encourage the client to remain dependent on some other person for decisions.

Furthermore giving advice is not always a safe practice. If the advice is accepted and the situation remains unimproved or worsens, the giver of the advice is likely to be blamed. Instead of offering advice, it is more helpful to explore mutually the positive and negative aspects of the possible decisions that are available. Ultimately the goal of the professional person is to help the client identify the decision he can feel most comfortable about making.

Nurses make many comments that they hope will give reassurance but actually fall short of this goal. Even though the nurse intends to be helpful, it is rarely helpful to make comments such as the following: "Don't worry," "Your doctor says this medicine will help you." "There are a great many people who are worse off than you are," and "Don't cry, you don't want people to see you crying." Such comments are meaningless and are likely to convince the client that the nurse is not able to understand his problems. Reassurance is never achieved by use of meaningless clichés. Instead, reassurance is more likely to be achieved by the nurse's spending time with the client and by listening to his expressions of feelings as long as he seems to need to talk. It is reassuring to the client if the nurse considers the problem thoughtfully and asks intelligent, reality-oriented questions about the situation. It is reassuring to the client when the nurse accepts his tears without comment or assures him that crying is a reasonable thing to do under the circumtances, provided, of course, the circumstances do warrant such expression. It is reassuring to the client when the nurse listens to his personal problems without showing surprise or disapproval when he talks about past social behavior that is unusual or below the nurse's standards. It is reassuring when the nurse agrees that the client has a problem and works with him in trying to problem-solve. It is reassuring when the nurse reflects to the client the tone of the feeling she hears him expressing. For the nurse to say, "It sounds to me as if you are really upset," conveys to the client that his feelings as well as the content of what he is saying is being understood. Once again, it should be noted that the nurse is not imposing a feeling on the client by a statement such as this but rather expressing her own response. It may be reassuring to the client if the nurse sits with him even when he does not feel like talking, thereby conveying a genuine interest in his problem and acceptance of him.

Persuasion suggests that some pressure is being placed on the client to accept a prescribed course of action. This, like advice, does not encourage self-reliance.

Suggestion is an aspect of communication that may be helpful to some individuals. Much can be done to stimulate interest in activities and to help individuals alter social attitudes by using skillfully phrased suggestions. For instance, encouraging a client to participate in the activities offered by the occupational therapist may be accomplished by telling him about the activities available and by using suggestions such as, "You might enjoy the finger-painting class." At another time a second comment about this activity might be, "Many clients seem to have an interesting time when they go to occupational therapy; I think you might too." The client who refused to wash his hair for several weeks may do so if several people with whom he is acquainted comment about his attractive appearance when his hair was clean a few weeks before. One suggestion is usually not sufficient to alter an attitude or help a person accept a new idea. Suggestion must be used frequently and skillfully by persons whose opinion the client respects.

Developing effective nonverbal communication

One of the first steps the nurse can take in developing effective nonverbal communication is to examine her own feelings toward clients and, if possible, to focus her activities on those for whom she has genuine feelings of interest and acceptance. If the nurse attempts to work closely with clients with whom she has many negative feelings, she will surely communicate these feelings nonverbally. The nurse needs to recognize the importance of her personal feelings in developing a reciprocal relationship with a client. It is also essential to recognize the role of nonverbal communication and to understand that it is impossible for every nurse to develop a therapeutic relationship with every mentally ill person. Equipped with this knowledge and understanding, the nurse can feel comfortable in admitting that she is not the appropriate person to provide care to a specific individual with whom she has not been able to establish a positive relationship.

After examining her own feelings toward clients the nurse can take a number of specific steps to engage in effective nonverbal communication. One of the most important of these steps is to sit near a client when talking to him. Some nurses hesitate to sit beside clients even when they are trying to converse with them. This hesitancy probably comes from experience in previous nursing situations in which the nurse was expected to administer physical comfort measures or therapeutic treatment procedures.

When the nurse stands during a conversation she conveys the idea that she is in a hurry, that she expects the conversation to be a short one, and that she is prepared to remain for only a few minutes. In such a hurried atmosphere no one can expect a client to feel that there is interest or time enough for him to talk about anything important. Conversely, when sitting with a mentally ill person, it is important not to sit in such a way that the person feels trapped or in danger of attack. Astute observation of the client's nonverbal behavior will quickly reveal if the nurse is sitting in a position that produces the best climate for conversation. Examples of behaviors likely to indicate that the client feels uncomfortable are the movement of his body or chair away from the nurse, his focusing his eyes elsewhere, and physical signs of anxiety such as restlessness and agitation. The nurse should not hesitate to alter her position if this seems appropriate from her observations of the client's behavior. When the nurse conveys her sincere interest in the client through her position and through the warmth of her voice and facial expression, the first step has been taken toward the establishment of a therapeutic nurse-client relationship.

Another important step the nurse can take in developing effective nonverbal communication is to develop her listening skills. Listening implies silence, but it does not imply passivity. The listener can and should be an active, alert, and interested participant, even though she may make very few verbal contributions. The nurse gives evidence of interest by being genuinely interested in the client and in what he is saying. This interest cannot be feigned. Evidence of genuine, sincere interest is shown by the expression on the listener's face, by the way the listener looks at the speaker, and by the verbal encouragement that is given to the speaker. Nodding the head to suggest that one understands or agrees is one way of giving encouragement. Comments such as, "That must have been difficult for you" or "I see, go on" are encouraging when said at an appropriate time with a friendly, interested tone. If the listener cannot follow the logic of the speaker or the sequence of the related incidents, it is best to ask the speaker to review that part of the story again. The nurse might say, "Could you explain that last statement again for me? I do not believe I understood it clearly." Or she might say, "I'm sorry, I didn't understand what you said a minute ago. Could you go over the last point again?" If the nurse fails to ask for clarification when it is needed, the client will soon discover that she has lost the sequence and meaning of the conversation and is trying to act as if she understands when she does not. This is one way of losing the client's confidence.

Effectively concluding a conversation

The conclusion of a conversation is as important as is the initiation of a conversation. The conclusion of a conversation will often set the tone for subsequent conversations between the nurse and the client. When the nurse needs to leave, she should break off the conversation so that it can be resumed at another time. Thus she might say, "I have been interested in what you have been telling me, and I hope we can continue this discussion later on." Of course, such a statement must be true. If she has promised to talk with the client at another time, she must find time for resuming the conversation. She might begin by saying, "I have been thinking about our conversation of yesterday and I am wondering if we could talk some more about the last point that you were making." The nurse would use this statement only if it were true. If such a statement were not true, she would choose another that would be appropriate for the conversation.

SPECIAL PROBLEMS IN COMMUNICATING WITH THE MENTALLY ILL

Congruent communication is necessary when one is attempting to relate therapeutically with mentally ill persons. They have had much previous experience in interaction with significant others who have communicated incongruent messages, particularly in regard to simultaneous verbal and nonverbal modes of communication wherein the nonverbal message contradicted the verbal message. The consequence of this communication is that the receiver must decide which message he will respond to, aware that whichever choice he makes he will be incorrect. When this type of communication is usual rather than the exception it may result in the receiver becoming unable to respond at all because he becomes immobilized by anxiety. Some theorists believe that this pattern of communication is characteristic of dysfunctional families in which one or more members become schizophrenic as an adaptation to the stress of this form of disturbed communication. The technical term for this type of disturbed interaction is *double bind communication*.

As the professional person spending the most time with the client in the treatment setting, the nurse has the greatest opportunity to create an environment in which the client can experience congruent communication. She can help the client to learn modes of adaptation that are more reality oriented and therefore more useful than his previous adaptation of retreating from reality into a psychosis.

For the nurse to express congruent messages she must be aware of herself and her own feelings, a concept discussed in Chapter 7. A helpful suggestion is for the nurse to make clear to the client what she is feeling, that is, to bring into verbal communication her nonverbal messages rather than letting the client guess their meaning. An example of this might be the nurse who says after being purposely tripped, "The feeling your behavior evokes in me is irritation." It is important to note that this statement conveys a very different message than if the nurse were to say, "You irritate me." In the former statement the nurse is expressing and owning her own feelings and not rejecting the client, whereas in the latter statement she is blaming and rejecting the client, which is likely to end the possibility of any further communication.

Since nonverbal aspects of communication usually convey the intended message most clearly, mentally ill persons, like all others, usually accurately sense the sincerity and kindness of the staff. Thus it has been observed that a staff member who is gruff and outspoken with clients may be respected and loved by them because he communicates nonverbally a basic attitude of kindness and a sincere interest in their welfare. A nurse who has adopted an unusually saccharine approach may be deeply resented by clients because nonverbally she conveys a feeling of rejection.

Many mentally ill persons struggle with the problem of not being able to trust other people. One of the ways a nurse can help such a person is to demonstrate that she can be trusted. If a client can begin to trust one person, it is possible that trust can eventually be extended to other people. When trying to help a client learn to trust her, the nurse sometimes finds herself in a dilemma. A client with whom the nurse is establishing a relationship may confide information that places her in an untenable position. On the one hand, she wishes to respect his confidences, while at the same time she hopes to carry out her responsibilities as a member of the professional staff. The following situation precipitated such a dilemma.

A client confided that he was planning to leave the city during the next weekend, ostensibly to visit his family. He told the nurse that he had stolen enough money from his friends to purchase a train ticket to a distant city where he was unknown and where he hoped to make a fresh start. The client cautioned the nurse not to tell anyone about these plans until after he was gone. The nurse had reason to be concerned about the client's safety, and now was in conflict about keeping the confidence, while still fulfilling her role as a member of the professional staff. She was understandably distressed about the situation.

It is important for the nurse to inform the client at the beginning of their relationship that she will share information essential to his treatment or safety with other members of the treatment team. When the client begins to confide information to the nurse that should be shared with other members of the professional staff, she has a responsibility to remind him that she must report the conversation to the appropriate people. The nurse might say to the client, "You know it will be necessary for me to share what you are telling me with the treatment team." Given this reminder, the client must then decide whether he will continue the discussion. A reasonable guide to follow is that the nurse has a responsibility to tell the client's therapist and the nurse in charge if the client tells her of plans that are dangerous to him or others or that interfere with the treatment plan.

When the nurse has established a relationship with the client that makes it possible for him to express his thoughts and feelings freely to her, she has a responsibility to listen with acceptance and understanding. The fact that the client confides in the

TABLE 8-1   behavioral examples of effective verbal and nonverbal approaches

verbal approach	nonverbal approach
Introduces self and explains status	Conveys acceptance and genuine interest
Uses client's name when speaking to him	Waits patiently for responses
Introduces a neutral topic appropriate to time and place	Focuses attention on client
Asks questions for the purpose of obtaining specific information	Listens to client's expression of feelings
Encourages client to take conversational lead	Sits quietly with client if he does not wish to talk
Reflects client's comments back to him	Focuses efforts on clients for whom she has positive feelings
Avoids a barrage of words	Sits near client but not so that he feels trapped or in danger of attack
Avoids personal opinions and words that connote judgment	Actively listens by nodding head appropriately and looking at client
Focuses conversation on interests and concerns of client	
Avoids giving advice or persuasion	
Withholds false reassurance	
Asks intelligent, reality-oriented questions about the situation	
Suggests activities and behaviors that may be helpful to client	

nurse indicates that an atmosphere of trust has been established. However, at times a client confides feelings and thoughts to the nurse that may be more appropriately discussed with his therapist. The nurse may not be in a position to be most helpful to the client in the particular situation. In this instance the nurse can suggest that this information be shared with the client's therapist and that she could assist the client in doing so, if he desires. It is also necessary that the nurse and the therapist have an opportunity to discuss the client's behavior and his problems.

Behavioral examples of verbal and nonverbal communication approaches that may prove to be effective are summarized in Table 8-1.

CONCLUDING STATEMENTS

1. Communication refers to the reciprocal exchange of information, ideas, beliefs, feelings, and attitudes between two persons or among a group of persons. It is a dynamic process requiring continual adaptations by those involved.

2. Communication is effective when it accurately and clearly conveys the intended messages.
3. Knowledge of and skill in effective communication is essential for the nurse who works with the mentally ill because her ability to be therapeutic is highly related to the effectiveness of her communication skills.
4. Verbal communication, nonverbal communication, and metacommunication are three modes of communication. Nonverbal communication and metacommunication are present in all situations in which two or more persons are interacting; verbal communication may be absent at times.
5. Communication is most effective when the three modes of communication are congruent.
6. A climate of mutual trust and respect must be developed before mentally ill persons can feel safe enough to communicate with the nurse.
7. The therapeutic potential of the nurse's verbal interaction with the client will be greatly increased if it is guided by goals established before the conversation is initiated.
8. When the goal of the conversation is to give or to get specific information, the nurse may appropriately ask questions that are more direct than those usually employed.
9. When the goal of the interaction is to establish a beginning rapport with the client, attention should be focused on the client in an attempt to convey a willingness to listen.
10. If the purpose of the interaction is to encourage the client to express his thoughts and feelings, a nondirective approach is most appropriate.
11. Clients should be encouraged to take the conversational lead.
12. Neither advice nor persuasion is helpful when the therapeutic goal is to help the client become a self-directing adult.
13. Reassurance can be helpful to clients if the method used is appropriate for the client and his problem, but statements that represent meaningless clichés are rarely reassuring.
14. Skillfully phrased suggestions are useful in altering social attitudes, in changing ideas, and in stimulating interest in therapeutic activities.
15. One of the first steps the nurse can take in developing effective nonverbal communication is to examine her own feelings toward clients and, if possible, to focus her activities on those for whom she has genuine feelings of interest and acceptance.

16. The need for congruent communication is great when one is attempting to relate therapeutically with mentally ill persons.
17. Clients must be helped to understand that the nurse has a responsibility to share confidences with the treatment team when clients confide behavior that may be dangerous to themselves or others or may interfere with the treatment goals.

SUGGESTED SOURCES OF ADDITIONAL INFORMATION

Classical

Davis, Anne J.: The skills of communication, Am. J. Nurs. **63:**66-70, Jan., 1963.

Ehmann, Virginia E.: Empathy: its origin, characteristics, and process, Perspect. Psychiatr. Care **9:**72-80, March-April, 1971.

Gerber, Claudia B., and Snyder, Deanne, F.: Language and thought, Perspect. Psychiatr. Care **8:**230-233, 237, 1970.

Goldin, Phyllis, and Russell, Barbara: Therapeutic communication, Am. J. Nurs. **69:**1928-1930, 1969.

Goldsborough, Judith D.: On becoming nonjudgmental, Am. J. Nurs. **70:**2340-2343, 1970.

Hewitt, Helon E., and Pesznecker, Betty L.: Blocks to communicating with patients, Am. J. Nurs. **64:**101-103, July, 1964.

Lewis, Garland K.: Communication; a factor in meeting emotional crises, Nurs. Outlook **13:**36-39, Aug., 1965.

Lewis, Garland K.: Nurse-patient communication, Dubuque, Iowa, 1978, William C. Brown Co., Publishers.

Peplau, Hildegard E.: Talking with patients, Am. J. Nurs. **60:**964-966, 1960.

Peplau, Hildegard E.: Interpersonal techniques; the crux of psychiatric nursing, Am. J. Nurs. **62:**50-54, June, 1962.

Robinson, Alice M.: Communication with schizophrenic patients, Am. J. Nurs. **60:**1120-1123, 1960.

Schwartz, Morris S., and Shockley, Emmy Lanning: The nurse and the mental patient, New York, 1965, John Wiley & Sons, Inc.

Travelbee, Joyce: What do we mean by rapport? Am. J. Nurs. **63:**70-72, Feb., 1963.

Contemporary

Amacher, Nancy Jean: Touch is a way of caring, Am. J. Nurs. **73:**852-855, 1973.

Bolzoni, N.J., and Geach, Barbara: Premature reassurance: a distancing maneuver, Nurs. Outlook **23:**49-51, 1975.

Burgess, Ann Wolbert, and Lazare, Aaron: Interviewing techniques. In Psychiatric nursing in the hospital and the community, ed. 2, Englewood Cliffs, N.J., 1976, Prentice-Hall, Inc., pp. 155-174.

Burkett, Alice D.: A way to communicate, Am. J. Nurs. **74:**2185-2187, 1974.

Dethomaso, Marita Tribou: "Touch power" and the screen of loneliness, Perspect. Psychiatr. Care **9:**133-118, May-June, 1971.

Field, William E.: Watch your message, Am. J. Nurs. **72:**1278-1280, 1972.

Gluck, Miriam: Learning a therapeutic verbal response to anger, J. Psychosoc. Nurs. Ment. Health Serv. **19:**9-12, March, 1981.

Gruber, Louis N.: The no-demand, third person interview of the nonverbal patient, Perspect. Psychiatr. Care **15**(1):38-39, 1977.

Haggerty, Virginia C.: Listening, Nurs. Forum **10**(4):382-387, 1971.

Harden S., and Halaris, A.: Nonverbal communication of patients and high and low empathy nurses, J. Psychosoc. Nurs. Ment. Health Serv. **21:**14-20, Jan., 1983.

Impey, Lorraine: Art media: a means to therapeutic communication with families, Perspect. Psychiatr. Care **19:**70-77, March/April, 1981.

Kalisch, Beatrice J.: What is empathy? Am. J. Nurs. **73:**1548-1552, 1973.

Karns, P., and Schwab, T.: Therapeutic communication and clinical instruction, Nurs. Outlook **30:**39-43, Jan., 1982.

Kerr, Norine J.: Discussion of "common errors in communication made by students in psychiatric nursing," Perspect. Psychiatr. Care **16:**184-187, July-Aug., 1978.

Knowles, Ruth D.: Building rapport through neurolinguistic programming, Am. J. Nurs. **83:**1010-1013, July, 1983.

Laughlin, Sister Noel: Symbolism as a memory tool in learning therapeutic communication techniques, Perspect. Psychiatr. Care **21:**9-17, Jan.-March, 1983.

Loesch, Larry C., and Loesch, Nancy A.: What do you say after you say mm-mm? Am. J. Nurs. **75:**807-809, 1975.

Mitchell, Ann C.: Barriers to therapeutic communication with black clients, Nurs. Outlook **26:**109-112, Feb., 1978.

Platt-Koch, Lois: Soap opera: catalyst to communication, Am. J. Nurs. **84:**1244-1246, Oct., 1984.

Ruffin, Janice E.: The relevance of racism to the goals of psychotherapy, Perspect. Psychiatr. Care **14:**160-164, 1976.

Sayre, Joan: Common errors in communication made by students in psychiatric nursing, Perspect. Psychiatr. Care **16:**175-183, July-Aug., 1978.

Tobiason, Sara J.B.: Touching is for everyone, Am. J. Nurs. **81:**728-730, April, 1980.

Underwood, Patricia R.: Communication through role playing, Am. J. Nurs. **71:**1184-1186, 1971.

Veninga, Robert: Communications: a patient's eye view, Am. J. Nurs. **15**(2):66-71, 1973.

Yoder, Susan A.: Alienation as a way of life, Perspect. Psychiatr. Care **15**(2):66-71, 1977.

Of particular interest

Reusch, J., and Bateson, G.: Communication: the social matrix of psychiatry, New York, 1968, W.W. Norton & Co., Inc.

These renowned authors discuss basic communication theory as it relates to psychiatric theory. It is highly recommended for the beginning student.
Snyder, J.C., and Wilson, M.F.: Elements of a psychological assessment, Am. J. Nurs. **77:**235, 1977.
In a concise, carefully organized format the authors present a model for psychological evaluation. Throughout is an emphasis on self-understanding and communication between nurse and client.

interpersonal interventions

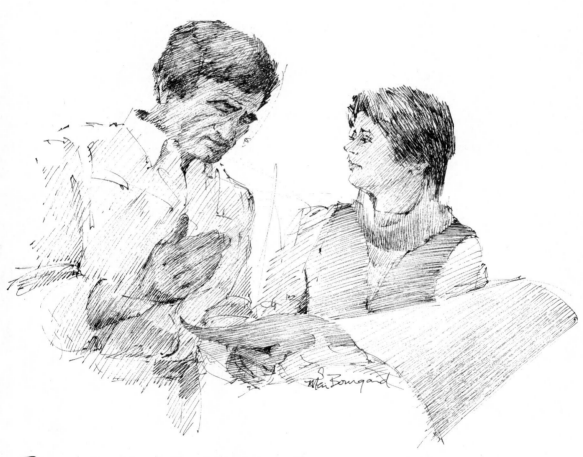

Showing me what he's written is like giving me a gift.

LEARNING OBJECTIVES

After studying this chapter the student will be able to:

1 State common patterns of nontherapeutic interpersonal interventions.

2 Discuss the concepts of acceptance and consistency as they relate to all interpersonally based therapeutic interventions.

3 Discuss three types of interpersonal interventions in terms of their goals and degree of nurse-client involvement.

4 Discuss the developmental phases of the nurse-client relationship.

5 Differentiate between a social and a therapeutic relationship.

All interpersonally based interventions take place within the context of human interaction. Although interventions that are therapeutic possess common elements, they are developed differently by each person, depending on the characteristics of the individuals involved. If an intervention is to become therapeutic, it is necessary to recognize the client as a unique, important human being who experiences hopes, fears, joys, and sorrows as do all other people. It is necessary to understand that the client has his own special set of problems and reactions to life. It is important for the nurse to interact with him so that she develops and reflects an understanding of his emotional responses and the probable meaning of his behavior. Through her sensitivity the nurse can develop a recognition of some of the client's emotional needs and an appreciation for some of the ways in which she can be helpful to him. In many instances the nurse will be most helpful to the client by interacting with him in a way that is different from the previous social interactions he has experienced. Many mentally ill persons have a long history of having failed at establishing and maintaining satisfying interpersonal relationships. To the degree that the nurse's interactions with the client reflect acceptance of him and consistency in response to him, they will be therapeutic by providing experiences that are corrective of earlier, less helpful interpersonal experiences.

HISTORICAL PERSPECTIVE

In 1947 McGraw-Hill Book Company published *Nurse Patient Relationships in Psychiatry* by Helena Willis Render. She was the first author to introduce the idea that the relationship the nurse establishes with the client has a significant therapeutic potential. This book stimulated much attention on the part of nurses concerning the potential therapeutic possibilities inherent in their work role in psychiatric settings. In 1952 G.P. Putnam's Sons published the book *Interpersonal Relations in Nursing* by Dr. Hildegard E. Peplau, an active nurse clinician and educator. This book in many ways revolutionized the teaching and practice of psychiatric nursing in this country. Peplau's text focused on the therapeutic potential of the one-to-one relationship. It was not, however, until the widespread use of the psychotropic drugs rendered clients amenable to interpersonally based treatment modalities that psychiatric nursing began to take the form it has today, making use of the concepts originally proposed by Render and Peplau.

Currently it is acknowledged that the use the nurse makes of her own personality can be a great therapeutic influence in the experience of the client if she uses understanding and skill. It is the only tool that is uniquely hers and that she alone directs. Although the nurse may give dozens of daily medications and may assist with other somatic therapies, the major way in which she directly influences the care of the client is through the use she makes of herself as she deals with the client in face-to-face interactions.

COMMON PATTERNS OF NONTHERAPEUTIC INTERPERSONAL INTERVENTIONS

Some of the characteristic ways in which nurses intervene nontherapeutically with clients are discussed here in the hope of assisting readers to examine the quality of their own professional behavior.

Some nurses prefer to view their work role as a series of tasks to be performed. Such a nurse is probably seen by clients as a person who is busily engaged in performing tasks as a means of avoiding contact with them. She may interact with clients only when she is involved in performing a specific technical nursing task. Such a nurse should ask herself why she finds it necessary to remain aloof from clients. An evaluation of her professional behavior may reveal fears or an attitude toward mentally ill persons that can be altered.

Some nurses interact with clients solely through socialization. This approach might be called the role of the social technician. A nurse who uses this approach may spend much time initiating social activities and encouraging clients to participate. She may focus all conversation with clients on social activities. This approach makes it possible for her to avoid involving herself with clients except superficially, and it discourages clients from sharing emotionally upsetting problems with her. Clients often do need help in participating in social activities, but this is only one of their many needs. The nurse who focuses only on the social needs of clients limits her effectiveness.

Inexperienced nurses sometimes relate to clients of the opposite sex in a seductive way. This often appears to be the only approach that some nurses are able to make to clients of the opposite sex. Nurses who use this method of relating to mentally ill persons confuse their professional and social roles. They probably give little thought to the meaning their behavior has for the client. Such an approach suggests that the nurse is not fully aware of the client's emotional problems and does not realize that seductive behavior may add to already disturbing feelings with which the client is trying to cope. Nurses who use seductive behavior in relating to mentally ill persons should seek the guidance of a mature counselor. They may need help in finding more appropriate channels through which they can express their own emotional needs.

Some nurses attempt to control all situations, usually as an adaptation to their own anxiety. However, the nurse who rigidly controls the environment will not be able to create a climate in which the client can achieve maximum emotional and social growth because these achievements depend on the client's being able to make his own decisions and to direct his own behavior.

The quality of the interaction between the nurse and the client is closely related to the motivation that underlies the nurse's attitude toward nursing and her perception of her role as a nurse. Because motivations are partially if not wholly unconscious, it is difficult to examine one's own motivations. Therefore the nurse will need guidance in evaluating her characteristic approaches to clients. It is suggested that this can be accomplished best through a series of conferences with an expert in psychiatric nursing, during which nurse-client interactions are discussed in depth. As a result of these discussions and of the increased knowledge and experience gained, the nurse can often develop other more therapeutic approaches to clients.

DEVELOPING THERAPEUTIC INTERPERSONAL INTERVENTIONS

The foundation of all interpersonally based therapeutic interventions is *acceptance*. This is a commonly used word among nurses, although it is not universally understood or operationalized by them. Other behaviors that are equally important in psychiatric nursing are those expressed by the adjectives *nonjudgmental* and *consistent*. All these concepts are basic in developing therapeutic interventions with any client. They are discussed here in the hope of helping the nurse to make effective use of them in caring for mentally ill persons.

Acceptance implies that the nurse treats the client as an important individual who has inherent worth and not as a diagnostic entity or a set of psychiatric symptoms. Actually, the use of diagnostic terms may encourage the nurse to adopt an impersonal attitude toward the client. The nurse implies that she is accepting the client by calling him by name and by recognizing that he has the same basic personal rights she herself possesses. Acceptance implies that the nurse tries to understand the meaning the client is conveying through his behavior. An accepting nurse recognizes that the client handles his behavior as well as he is able at a given time. She encourages the client to express his feelings to her, realizing that in this way he is able to relieve emotional tensions. She does not censor him for statements and feelings that may not be conventionally acceptable, realizing that his behavior is an expression of his illness. She recognizes that his comments may not be directed toward her personally.

The word *nonjudgmental* is usually used in conjunction with the word *attitude* and is closely related to the concept of acceptance. One cannot be achieved without the other. A nonjudgmental attitude is neither condemning nor approving. Through tone of voice and manner the nurse conveys to the client a helpful attitude without morally judging his behavior. A nonjudgmental attitude toward the behavior of a mentally ill person implies that the nurse recognizes that behavior, like physical symptoms displayed by physically ill persons, is neither good or bad nor right or wrong but rather a learned adaptation to stress. As such she also realizes that the client has the potential to change his behavior by learning new adaptations to stress.

Acceptance of mentally ill persons and their behavior is often difficult to achieve and almost everyone occasionally falls short of the ideal. The behavior of some mentally ill persons is offensive at times. This is true for example of the behavior of clients who are so confused that they soil themselves. It may be impossible for the nurse to avoid feeling repelled by the sight of a person grossly soiled, but it is possible for her to avoid making him feel that he is an offensive person. Joking in front of a client about his behavior or describing his shortcomings to others within his hearing is neither respecting nor accepting him.

Consistency is another important characteristic of therapeutic interventions. The consistent nurse maintains the same basic attitude toward the client so that he derives security from being able to predict her behavior. Not only should the client be able to expect the same positive attitudes and approaches from an individual nurse, but also the entire nursing staff should interact with consistency from the standpoint of basic attitudes and overall policies. Consistency helps lessen the client's anxiety by simplifying decision making and by avoiding uncertainties.

All mentally ill persons experience some loss of self-esteem and self-confidence. If an intervention is to be helpful to a client it must assist him in reestablishing his self-confidence and restoring his self-esteem. This is a slow process that requires consistent work over a period of time. Recognizing the client as being an important human being, expressing genuine interest in him, spending time with him, conversing with him, and listening with understanding to his expressions of feeling are all ways of helping him feel worthwhile, important, and wanted. On the other hand indifference, insincerity, and an impersonal attitude toward the client reinforce his sense of unimportance and further convince him of what he may already believe—that he is lacking in value as a person.

It is not possible for a nurse to intervene in a way that has the same therapeutic potential and the same meaning for each individual client. It is possible, however, for the nurse to learn to know the names and something of the needs of all clients with whom she comes in close contact. With many of these persons the nurse can expect to develop a positive relationship. With a limited number she will be able to interact in a way which will lay the foundation for the development of a therapeutic relationship. It is with these individuals she will be able to carry on discussions that have therapeutic potential, because she will know them well and will have developed a genuine interest in them as people.

TYPES OF THERAPEUTIC INTERPERSONAL INTERVENTIONS

The nurse is often involved in at least three types of one-to-one situations. These situations are differentiated on the basis of the degree of nurse-client involvement and whether the goal of the intervention is immediate, short-range, or long-range. As the nurse engages in each of these situations with clients she variously assumes the roles of creator of a therapeutic environment, socializing agent, counselor, teacher, mother surrogate, and technical nurse. Therapeutic use of these roles is discussed at length in Chapter 2.

The first situation in which the nurse and client are likely to engage is one in which the nurse and the client do not know each other and the client is in immediate, severe difficulty that requires the nurse to intervene. In other words, an emergency exists. The nature of the emergency can range from a life-threatening situation, such as a suicidal attempt, to the client's being overwhelmed by a particular emotion, such as grief, and expressing this behaviorally. Ideally the person who intervenes in such situations should be one who knows the client and understands the plan of treatment for him. This however is not always possible because of the necessity for immediate action or the unavailability of the appropriate staff member or because the client is new to the treatment setting. When such situations arise, the nurse must not avoid intervening merely because she does not know the client. Rather, she must bring to bear on the situation her knowledge of the dynamics of human behavior and her skill in psychiatric nursing. In these emergency situations the nurse will do well to employ the principles of psychiatric nursing and good common sense. The client has a right to be protected from harming himself, either physically or emotionally, and from harming others.

Needless to say once the emergency situation is resolved immediate efforts should be made to contact those mental health personnel who are involved with the client's treatment or to establish a long-range treatment plan and begin its implementation if one has not already been developed.

The second situation is one in which the nurse and client

know each other but the nurse does not have major responsibility for this particular client's treatment. Unfortunately, some nurses believe that if they are not assigned to the care of a particular client they have little or no responsibility to behave in a thoughtful, goal-directed manner when interacting with him. This is not the case and in fact, the value of the therapeutic interventions of other staff can be lessened by the thoughtless, offhand behavior of a particular nurse. Although it is not possible for the nurse to have in-depth knowledge of all the clients in any treatment setting, it is possible and important for her to be aware of the treatment goals for all clients with whom she is likely to come in contact, no matter how superficially. With this awareness the nurse's on-the-spot interactions with the client can be designed to support and enhance the treatment that is being implemented by other nurses and mental health personnel.

This situation is particularly common in psychiatric nursing, since, unlike many physically ill persons, emotionally ill persons usually have physical mobility and are not dependent on the nurse to approach them at the bedside. It is not uncommon for an emotionally ill person to seek out a nurse other than the one to whom he is assigned to validate statements made to him by his assigned nurse or to otherwise engage the two nurses in a power struggle. The client's motivation may or may not be conscious and may be a manifestation of the stage of the relationship in which the client and his nurse are engaged. In any event, the manner in which the nurse responds is frequently an important factor in enhancing or impeding the therapeutic endeavors of others. These on-the-spot, seemingly casual interactions should have as their goal support of the overall treatment of the client.

The third one-to-one situation the nurse encounters is one in which she seeks to develop a therapeutic relationship with a client in an effort to provide corrective interpersonal experiences. Because such a relationship requires an in-depth knowledge of the client and much of the nurse's time and energy, it is possible for the nurse to have only a few such relationships in progress at any point in time. An understanding of the process of these relationships will make clear that it is inappropriate to use the term *nurse-client relationship* to describe all interactions between the nurse and all clients with whom she comes in contact. This is not to say that all nurse-client interactions should not be therapeutic, but rather that in only a few will the nurse be intensely involved in an ongoing relationship with the client that is designed to provide corrective interpersonal experiences. Since the nurse can be involved in only a few nurse-client relationships at any one time it is important that she make the best use of her time, energy, and skills by devoting them to those clients whose nursing diagnosis indicates a potential for benefiting from this type of nursing intervention. Not all nurses work equally effectively with all clients, since the nurse's own personality is the major tool she has for intervention. Therefore when the nursing care plan indicates that a nurse-client relationship is desirable, the nurse who develops such a relationship should be one whose self-awareness indicates that she would be likely to be effective with the particular client. Since both nurses and emotionally ill persons are more human than otherwise and have the same wide variety of personality structures, it is unlikely that there ever would be a client for whom a suitable nurse were not available.

TABLE 9-1   types and characteristics of interpersonal interventions

type of intervention	degree of nurse-client involvement	goal of intervention
Emergency	None	Immediate—resolution of a severe difficulty
Interaction	Nurse and client know each other; nurse does not have major responsibility for client's treatment	Short range—support and enhance treatment efforts of others
Relationship	High degree	Long range—provide corrective interpersonal experiences for client

DEVELOPMENTAL PHASES OF THE NURSE-CLIENT RELATIONSHIP

Every therapeutic relationship that a nurse develops between herself and a client has an initial phase, referred to as the *orientation phase* or the *getting acquainted period*. It is during this phase that the nurse and client agree on a mutually acceptable contract that serves to establish the parameters of the relationship. The goals of this phase are the development of trust and the establishment of the nurse as a significant other to the client.

Although in some instances the client initiates the relationship, more frequently it is the nurse who first approaches the client. She does so by introducing herself by name and position and suggesting that she would like to work with him on his problems by meeting with him for a specific period of time and at a specified time and place. It is also important for the nurse to ask the client how he would like to be addressed. Most clients respond positively to this approach, ironically because the nurse is not yet an important part of their life and the idea of developing a relationship with her is not threatening. Once the time and place of their conversations is agreed on it is imperative that the nurse adhere strictly to this schedule. The nurse should also suggest a duration for each conversation, for example 45 minutes. This period of time must be adhered to, despite the fact that the client may at various times attempt to entice the nurse to stay longer with him by bringing up highly charged emotional issues 5 minutes prior to the end of the session. The nurse can handle this by acknowledging that the issues at hand sound important and by suggesting that the client reintroduce them at the beginning of their next meeting. This approach is therapeutic because it demonstrates that the nurse will follow through on what she had promised—in this instance, sessions of a 45-minute length—and therefore can be trusted to do what she says. It is important to understand that clients sometimes unconsciously introduce highly significant issues shortly before the end of planned sessions as a means of letting the nurse know what is disturbing them without running the risk of having to discuss these issues at length because they know that the session will soon be over. If the nurse succumbs to the temptation to continue the discussion beyond the agreed time the client will learn that he has to be more guarded with her in the future.

Some clients, rather than attempting to lengthen the sessions, try to shorten them by overt means such as walking away or covert means such as falling asleep. The nurse can effectively deal with such situations by remembering that this period of time is set aside solely for interaction with this client and by stating this to him. If the client then still walks away or falls asleep the nurse should remain in the designated meeting place for the remainder of the decided time. This behavior of the nurse also indicates to the client that she can be trusted to do what she has promised, despite his behavior.

As the nurse becomes more meaningful to the client his behavior toward her often appears increasingly negative. He may not appear for the scheduled sessions or his language may become profane or he may resist talking about himself and state a preference for discussing the nurse's personal life. At this point many nurses become discouraged and disappointed, since the earlier sessions had seemed to proceed smoothly. In contrast, the nurse has reason to feel encouraged since at this point in the relationship, the client's behavior most likely indicates that the nurse is becoming a significant other to him. Mentally ill persons have had much previous experience in familial and social relationships with persons who have initially accepted them but subsequently rejected them when their behavior became inappropriate. Therefore the client has a need to test the nurse's reliability before finally allowing himself to trust her. If the nurse does not view this change in the client's behavior as a test to determine just how much he can rely on her to be accepting and nonjudgmental of him, she might feel discouraged and decide to end the relationship. To act on this feeling would be a mistake, since it would confirm the client's view of the nurse as being no different than others who have disappointed him. More importantly, it would also confirm his view of himself as being unworthy and unacceptable. Rather than discontinuing the relationship the nurse must respond to the client's behavior with meticulous consistency. For example, if she has agreed to meet with him at a specified time and place she must be there even if he does not appear. If she continues in this manner the client will soon have less need to test her, and the first phase of the relationship will be over.

The second phase in a therapeutic relationship between a nurse and a client is called the *maintenance* or *working phase.* The goal of this phase is the identification and resolution of the client's problem. Therefore the characteristics of this phase are highly individualized to the nature of the client's problems. Because each individual is unique and because the working phase of a relationship is so highly individualized to the particular client and nurse, few specific parameters can be given to guide the progress of this phase. An exception, however, is the necessity for limit setting, which often arises during this phase.

Limit setting is required when the client is threatening physical harm to himself or others, when he is destroying property or threatening to do so, and when his verbal hostility is upsetting and causing other clients or personnel to become tense and upset. If the client who requires limit setting is willing to discuss his behavior, it may be sufficient for the nurse to point out that he is causing a dangerous and disturbing situation and to request that he stop. For some persons such a request will be sufficient. However, others will require a more direct approach. In such an instance the nurse must speak firmly and explain that unless his disruptive behavior stops, he will have to be segregated from the group and placed in a room alone or will be given a medication to assist him to gain control of his behavior.

If the nurse initiates and enforces limit setting in an empathic and nonpunitive manner, the client will often feel a sense of relief from anxiety because another person has assumed the responsibility for identifying and enforcing the boundaries of his behavior. Rather than damaging the relationship, limit setting often serves to further convince the client that the nurse cares about him as a worthwhile individual.

In summary, the maintenance or working phase of the nurse-client relationship is the time to identify and address the client's problems. Unless both the nurse and the client are actively involved in this process the relationship cannot be effective. In maintaining a therapeutic relationship with a client, the nurse encourages him to express his concerns, fears, hopes, and problems. Sometimes she will be able to achieve this by asking direct and specific leading questions. The nurse needs to recognize when she is able to intervene in the client's expressed concerns and when it is necessary to refer the client to other members of the clinical team who are prepared to cope with the specific problem. Therefore it is important for the nurse to understand how she and the other members of the clinical team share responsibility for the client's therapy.

The third phase of the therapeutic relationship is referred to as the *termination* or *concluding phase*. It is unrealistic to expect a relationship to continue indefinitely. This fact should be recognized and planned for in the orientation phase of the nurse-client relationship.

When the nurse learns that it will be necessary for her to leave the client, she should discuss this fact with him as soon as possible. If the nurse knows at the outset of the relationship that it will be terminated at a specific time, the plans for the work of the nurse and the client should always include this fact. Terminating a relationship can be a traumatic experience for both the nurse and the client because they have shared much that is personal and important. At such a time many clients express the feeling that the nurse is forsaking them. The loss of a trusted nurse is an especially difficult problem for a client who has been unable to trust other people. It is not unusual for clients to act out their frustration at the news of the impending loss of a trusted nurse.

In view of the possible traumatic difficulties that the departure of the nurse presents to the client, the nurse must seek to understand the client's sense of loss and to help him express his feelings and cope with them. The goal of this phase of the relationship is to help the client to review what he has learned through the process of the relationship and to transfer these learnings to his interactions with other persons.

Although the client with whom the nurse has established an ongoing therapeutic relationship will require special help in accepting her departure, the entire group of clients with whom the nurse has been working will respond in a variety of ways to her expected loss. Ideally, clients in a psychiatric setting should experience a relatively constant professional staff with whom they can establish meaningful relationships and work out emotional problems. Clients, like all people, will react to an anticipated loss in a variety of ways, depending on the characteristic way in which they respond to loss, their unique emotional needs, and the relationship they have developed with the departing staff member. Some clients may become depressed and unconsciously believe that they have been personally responsible for the loss of the nurse. Other clients may not be able to accept the loss of this valued person and may repress the knowledge. They may report that no one told them that she was leaving. Other clients may respond with anger and may insist that the administrator take steps to see that the nurse does not leave.

When the nursing staff members are prepared for a variety of responses on the part of clients, they can understand, accept, and cope with their behavior. This means that they will need to spend time talking with and listening to clients. They will need to make

themselves more available than usual to deal with the clients'
many feelings about the situation and to reassure clients that
they are not being abandoned. Sometimes it is helpful to encourage the clients to channel their feelings into some constructive
activity. One way to redirect clients' concerns is to help them organize and carry out a party to honor the departing nurse.

It is unfortunate when clients are not given an opportunity to
express their feelings about such a situation or helped to handle
their feelings. When this happens, as it does when a valued staff
member simply disappears without any explanation, the feelings
are not avoided but appear in many unusual behavioral reactions. A group of clients who have suffered such an unexplained
loss may suddenly rebel against the entire nursing staff, or the
physician may find that many former symptoms that clients had
previously experienced have been reactivated.

The client is not the only person who must cope with feelings
of loss when the nurse-client relationship is terminated. By virtue

**TABLE 9-2   goals of and nurse behaviors in each phase
of the nurse-client relationship**

phase of nurse-client relationship	goal	nurse behaviors
Orientation	Development of trust Establishment of nurse as a significant other to client	Establishes mutually accept-able contract Responds to testing behavior of client by adhering strictly to terms of contract
Maintenance	Identification and res-olution of client's problems	Highly individualized to the nature of the client's prob-lems Empathic nonpunitive limit setting
Termination	Assist client to review what he has learned and to transfer this learning to interac-tion with others	Understands client's sense of loss Helps client express his feel-ings and cope with them Encourages client to channel feelings into constructive activity such as a farewell party Recognizes own feelings of loss

of having established and maintained a relationship with the client the nurse has invested a great deal of time, energy, thought, and emotion in the client. As a result she also will experience a sense of loss when the relationship is terminated. If she does not allow herself to recognize these feelings she might express them indirectly by showing undue concern for the client's future welfare, by encouraging him to stay for a few more sessions, or by otherwise encouraging his dependence on her. As is true of the client, the nurse's previous experiences with and responses to loss are major determinants of her ability to effectively cope with the sense of loss she feels when a nurse-client relationship is terminated. Most nurses find it helpful at this time to seek the guidance of the professional who is supervising the relationship. The nurse must remember that if the termination phase is not handled skillfully by encouraging the client to assume the independence he is ready for, the nurse can negate the value of the work that has been done in the preceding phase. Table 9-2 summarizes the goals of and nurse behaviors in the nurse-client relationship.

DIFFERENTIATING BETWEEN SOCIAL AND THERAPEUTIC RELATIONSHIPS

Sometimes it is difficult for nurses to differentiate between social and therapeutic relationships when dealing with mentally ill persons. The problem is even more complicated because mentally ill individuals usually are not physically ill and therefore are not bedridden. They frequently give the superficial impression of being socially and emotionally healthy. Nurses who have not developed an understanding of emotional illness may find it difficult to accept the fact that they are interacting with people who are ill. Thus their role confusion is understandable.

In a social relationship the needs of both the involved individuals are considered. The needs of both must be met in a satisfying way if the relationship is to continue. A social relationship usually develops spontaneously without a conscious plan. The goal of such a relationship is usually shared by the participants and is frequently limited to personal pleasure. The participants in a social relationship share mutual concern regarding reciprocal approval. This may develop more or less satisfactorily without conscious awareness of the emotional significance of the relationship.

In contrast, the therapeutic relationship focuses on the personal and emotional needs of the client. Such a relationship is therapeutically oriented and is planned after consideration has been given to the needs of the client and the therapeutic ability of the nurse. There is always a therapeutic goal toward which the nurse directs her interventions, but it is not always shared by the client. When the nurse has accepted this role, she must strive to be consciously aware of the developing relationship and its meaning. She should seek help in reflecting objectively on the meaning of the interaction between herself and the client so that she will be prepared to guide the client in developing more appropriate behavior. In a therapeutic relationship the nurse does not necessarily seek the client's approval. She reevaluates the situation constantly so that she can distinguish between the client's actual needs and his demands. When it is time for the relationship to be terminated the nurse releases the patient emotionally and strives to help him move forward to more appropriate relationships.

Following are examples of the development of both a social and a therapeutic relationship between a nurse and a client.

A young student of nursing, Miss S., was assigned to a unit where she was to have an initial experience in psychiatric nursing. The unit was populated by young men and women in their late teens or early twenties. The living quarters for the two groups were divided by a large living room. The clients gathered in the living room for group meetings, social activities, and conversations. Clients came and went freely in this unlocked unit. Some of the clients were employed during the day and returned to the hospital in the evening. Other clients were continuing their schoolwork in a nearby high school.

Miss S. participated enthusiastically in the social activities of the group. She frequently sought permission to participate in some of the activities planned for the evening hours. Permission was granted because it was the only possible way for her to become acquainted with several of the clients. When it was learned that Miss S. did not know how to dance, some of the young men volunteered to teach her. She learned quickly and was particularly successful in dancing with one young man, Jim L. They were approximately the same age and had a few friends in common, since they had grown up in the same general area in the city. The student nurse began to focus a good deal of attention on Jim. At client parties she insisted that he dance with her most of the time. Because Jim was popular with the female clients, they became annoyed with the student nurse and complained about her to the physician in charge. When Miss S. was asked to stop attending ward parties, she arranged to meet Jim in the afternoon away from the hospital. She began writing Jim daily notes that were delivered by fellow students.

When the instructor became aware of this problem, she asked Miss S. to come to her office for a talk. Miss S. discussed the situation freely. She said that she enjoyed having the opportunity to associate with Jim and could see no reason why questions were being raised. She admitted that she planned to drop the relationship as soon as the psychiatric nursing experience was completed. Miss S. said her friendship with Jim was an interesting interlude for both of them while it lasted. She was surprised to learn that Jim had requested a transfer from the unlocked unit to a unit where he would not be allowed so many privileges. She did not realize that Jim was desperately afraid of falling in love with a girl and that her relationship with him had reactivated many of his old fears and self-doubts.

In this situation the nursing student focused on her own social needs and on what she believed were Jim's social needs. Her stated goal for the relationship was immediate personal pleasure. Miss S. had given little thought to the meaning this relationship had for Jim or what effect her behavior would have on her professional role with other patients. She did not seek guidance in evaluating the relationship. As a result of Miss S.'s failure to differentiate between a social and a professional relationship, her experience with Jim was not helpful to him or satisfying for her.

On this same unit another nurse was able to develop an effective therapeutic relationship. Miss L., a young graduate nurse, came to work on the unit shortly after Miss S. left.

Miss L. became interested in Bill A., a young man approximately the same age as Jim. He was painfully shy and avoided social contact with other people. He did not know how to dance and felt so inadequate that his only role in social situations was that of an observer. He did not take advantage of the privileges available to clients in this unlocked unit. He was intellectually capable but had quit high school because of his shyness and fear of people.

Miss L. was sorry that Bill had not completed high school; as a result of discussions with the clinical team, it was decided that her goal would be to help him free himself of his fear of people to the extent that he would be able to return to school. She realized that this was a long-term goal and that it would be necessary for Bill to take many small steps forward before he could make such a move. She began her work immediately by sitting beside him for a few minutes each day. Getting acquainted with him was difficult because he was always deeply involved in reading. At first he was almost rude when she asked if she might sit down for a few minutes to talk. After many days Bill seemed to look forward to their daily meetings. Finally she noticed that he closed the book when she approached.

After several weeks Miss L. suggested that they take a walk together to the occupational therapy department to see what was going on there. He reluctantly accompanied her. On their tour of this department she talked about the many interesting available activities. She discovered that Bill had once done oil painting but feared criticism so much that he destroyed each painting before it was completed. Making use of this knowledge, Miss L. was able to obtain some oil painting equipment so that Bill could paint in a single room away from inquisitive people. Miss L. stopped to see his work daily and discovered that he had a great deal of talent. Other nurses came to praise his work. Finally he was able to transfer his work to the occupational therapy department and eventually gave his consent to have several of his paintings hung in the lobby of the hospital.

One evening Miss L. gently encouraged Bill to accompany her to one of the social affairs given by the clients. During the first party he began to learn to dance. With encouragement and praise he learned to dance well and attended most of the social activities planned by the clients. He began dancing with other nurses, and finally he felt sure enough of himself to ask young women clients to dance.

After Miss L. had known Bill for over a year, she suggested that they go for a walk together outside the hospital. As usual he was reluctant to comply, but with encouragement he accompanied her. Several months after his first venture outside with Miss L., Bill began going out regularly with other clients to attend movies and football games and to visit art galleries. After working closely with Bill for 2 years, Miss L. suggested that they visit the high school near the hospital. As usual, Bill needed much encouragement, but he finally made the visit with her. Eventually he was able to enroll as a student and completed his high school work.

CONCLUDING STATEMENTS

1. If an interpersonally based intervention is to become therapeutic, it is necessary for the nurse to recognize the client as a unique, important human being who, like all persons, experiences hopes, fears, joys, and sorrows and has his own special set of problems and reactions to life.
2. To the degree that the nurse's interactions with the client re-

flect acceptance of him and consistency in response to him, they will be therapeutic by providing him with encounters that are corrective of earlier, less helpful interpersonal experiences.

3. The use the nurse makes of her personality is the key to her success in face-to-face interactions with clients.

4. The quality of interaction between the nurse and the client is closely related to the motivation that underlies the nurse's attitude toward nursing and her perception of her role as a nurse.

5. The foundation of all interpersonally based therapeutic interventions is acceptance, which implies that the nurse treats the client as an important person who has inherent worth and not as a diagnostic entity or a set of psychiatric symptoms.

6. The nurse who maintains a nonjudgmental attitude realizes that the unusual behavior of the mentally ill person is neither good or bad nor right or wrong but rather a learned adaptation to stress. As such, she also realizes that the client has the potential to change his behavior by learning new adaptations to stress.

7. If the nurse maintains consistency in her approach toward the client, she helps to lessen his anxiety by minimizing uncertainties and by simplifying decision making.

8. If intervening with a client is to be therapeutic, it must assist the client in reestablishing his self-confidence and restoring his self-esteem.

9. There are at least three types of one-to-one situations in which the nurse is usually involved. These situations are differentiated on the basis of the degree of nurse-client involvement and whether the goal of the intervention is immediate, short-range, or long-range.

10. One type of one-to-one situation is called a nurse-client relationship, which has three developmental phases: the orientation or getting-acquainted phase, the maintenance or working phase, and the termination or concluding phase.

11. A therapeutic relationship focuses on the personal and emotional needs of the client, whereas in a social relationship the needs of both the involved individuals are considered.

SUGGESTED SOURCES OF ADDITIONAL INFORMATION

Classical

Bressler, Bernard, and Vause, Mary Ella: The psychotherapeutic nurse, Am. J. Nurs. **62**:87-90, May, 1962.

Burkhardt, Marti: Response to anxiety, Am. J. Nurs. **69**:2153-2154, 1969.

Connolly, Mary Grace: What acceptance means to patients, Am. J. Nurs. **60**:1754-1757, 1960.

Hale, Shirley L., and Richardson, Julia H.: Terminating the nurse-patient relationship, Am. J. Nurs. **63**:116-119, Sept., 1963.

Hays, Joyce Samhammer: Focusing on feelings, Nurs. Outlook **10**:332-333, May, 1962.

Kachelski, M. Audrey: The nurse-patient relationship, Am. J. Nurs. **61**:76-79, May, 1961.

Rogers, Carl R.: A counseling approach to human problems, Am. J. Nurs. **56**:994-997, 1956.

Schwartz, Morris S., and Shockley, Emmy Lanning: The nurse and the mental patient, New York, 1956, John Wiley & Sons, Inc.

Sene, Barbara S.: Termination in the student-patient relationship, Perspect. Psychiatr. Care **7**:39-45, Jan., 1969.

Speroff, B.J.: Empathy is important in nursing, Nurs. Outlook **4**:326-328, June, 1956.

Contemporary

Arnold, Helen M.: Four A's: a guide to one-to-one relationships, Am. J. Nurs. **76**:941-943, 1976.

Bayer, Mary: Saying goodbye through graffiti: it all began when we were about to discharge Hilda, Am. J. Nurs. **80**:271, Feb., 1980.

Bishop, Barbara R.: The psychiatric nurse as a therapist—not a baby sitter, Perspect. Psychiatr. Care **10**:41-43, Jan.-March, 1972.

Burgess, Ann Wolbert, and Lazare, Aaron: Techniques in the therapeutic process. In Psychiatric nursing in the hospital and the community, ed. 2, Englewood Cliffs, N.J., 1976, Prentice-Hall, Inc., pp. 108-128.

Carser, Diane: Primary nursing in the milieu, J. Psychosoc. Nurs. Ment. Health Serv. **19**:35-41, Feb., 1981.

Caudle, Patricia: Found: one person, Am. J. Nurs. **73**:310-313, 1973.

Cloud, Elizabeth D.: The plateau in therapist-patient relationships, Perspect. Psychiatr. Care **6**:112-121, July-Sept., 1972.

Curtin, Leah: Privacy: belonging to oneself, Perspect. Psychiatr. Care **19**:112-115, May-Aug., 1981.

Delgado, Melvin: Therapy Latino style: implications for psychiatric care, Perspect. Psychiatr. Care **17**(3):107-113, May-June, 1979.

Dillon, Kathryn M.: A patient-structured relationship, Perspect. Psychiatr. Care **9**:167-172, July-Aug., 1971.

Eisenman, Elaine P.: Primary care in a mental health facility, Nurs. Outlook **24**:640-645, 1976.

Feather, Roberta, and Bissell, Brenda: Clinical supervision vs. psychotherapy: the psychiatric mental health supervisory process, Perspect. Psychiatr. Care **17**(6):266-272, Nov.-Dec., 1979.

Garant, Carol: Stalls in the therapeutic process, Am. J. Nurs. **80:**2166-2169, 1980.

Gruber, Louis N.: The no-demand, third person interview of the non-verbal patient, **15:**38-39, 1977.

Heineken, Jan: Treating the disconfirmed psychiatric client, J. Psychosoc. Nurs. Ment. Health Serv. **21:**21-26, Jan., 1983.

Johnson, Margie: Self-disclosure: a variable in the nurse-client relationship, J. Psychosoc. Nurs. Ment. Health Serv. **18:**17-20, Jan., 1980.

Karshmer, Judith: Rules of thumb: hints for the psychiatric nursing student, J. Psychosoc. Nurs. Ment. Health Serv. **20:**25-28, March, 1982.

Krikorian, D., and Paulanka, B.: Self-awareness—the key to a successful nurse-patient relationship, J. Psychosoc. Nurs. Ment. Health Serv. **20:**19-21, June, 1982.

Littlefield, Nadine Thompson: Therapeutic relationship: a brief encounter, Am. J. Nurs. **82:**1395-1399, 1982.

Stokes, Gertrude A., and Fitzpatrick, Patricia: Teaching students psychotherapy, Am. J. Nurs. **77:**249-253, 1977.

Thomas, Mary D., Baker, Joan M., and Estes, Nada J.: Anger: a tool for developing self-awareness, Am. J. Nurs. **70:**2586-2590, 1970.

Topf, Margaret, and Dambacher, Betty: Teaching interpersonal skills: a model for facilitating optimal interpersonal relations, J. Psychosoc. Nurs. Ment. Health Serv. **19:**29-33, Dec., 1981.

Vidoni, Clotilde: The development of intense positive counter transference in the therapist toward a patient, Am. J. Nurs. **75:**407-409, 1975.

White, Cheryl L.: Nurse counselling with a depressed patient, Am. J. Nurs. **78:**436-439, March, 1978.

Will, Gwen Tudor: A sociopsychiatric nursing approach to intervention in a problem of mutual withdrawal on a mental hospital ward, Perspect. Psychiatr. Care **8:**11-35, Jan.-Feb., 1970.

Zahourek, Rothlyn P., and Crawford, Carole M.: Forced termination of psychotherapy, Perspect. Psychiatr. Care **16:**193-199, July-Aug., 1978.

Of particular interest

Boettcher, E.: Nurse-client collaboration: dynamic equilibrium in the nursing care system, J. Psychiatr. Nurs. **16:**7, Dec., 1978.
Nurse-client collaboration as it parallels nursing process is the focus of this article. The clinical example used is helpful in planning care, implementing plans, and evaluating outcome.

Lego, Suzanne M.: The one-to-one nurse-patient relationship, Perspect. Psychiatr. Care **18**(2):67-89, March-April, 1980.
In one of the most comprehensive articles of its kind the author discusses the history of the one-to-one therapeutic relationship in psychiatric nursing. She brings together factors such as published research, literature patterns, and related trends that have influenced the emergency of this therapeutic mode.

psychotropic agents

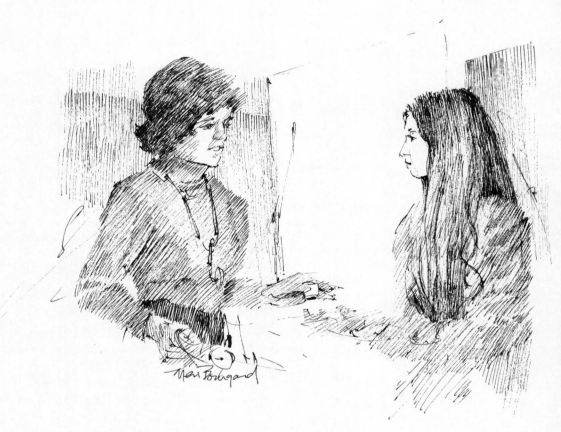

Mary looks more depressed today.
I'd better report that to the charge nurse.

LEARNING OBJECTIVES

After studying this chapter the student will be able to:

1 Name the four categories of psychotropic agents commonly used in the treatment of the mentally ill.

2 State the indications for use of the drugs from each of the four categories of psychotropic agents.

3 Discuss the usual side effects of each category of psychotropic agents.

4 Discuss the adverse effects of each category of psychotropic agents.

5 Discuss the responsibilities of the nurse in the use of psychotropic agents.

The psychotropic drugs have been widely prescribed and remarkably effective in their own right. Because of them, other treatment modalities, such as psychotherapy and the various group therapies, have been made available to large numbers of individuals. Although the psychotropic drugs do not cure mental illness, they do normalize behavior. Thus many people are able, for the first time, to participate therapeutically with others in a variety of group activities. Mental health centers are able to focus more attention on providing therapeutic experiences instead of expending time controlling behavior and keeping individuals fed, clothed, and bathed.

One of the most dramatic results of the use of antipsychotic drugs, one category of psychotropic agents, is the ability of many severely disturbed persons to return to their community after a relatively short period of time. Some are able to reestablish their roles in the family, and others return to their jobs. These drugs have made possible the movement of thousands of individuals out of large public psychiatric hospitals into community treatment centers. Thus the care and treatment of mentally ill people have been dramatically altered by the introduction of the psychotropic drugs.

HISTORICAL PERSPECTIVE

Through the ages the human race has searched for solutions to the problem of mental illness, a problem that has been present among some members of the human family since the beginning of time. Treatment has ranged from trephining the skull, which was used by prehistoric peoples, to soft music and beautiful surroundings, which were used by the ancient Greeks. Floggings, purgings, and starvation were used in more recent times. A variety of primitive shock treatments have been used in past centuries. These have included throwing individuals into a pit filled with snakes and ducking them in ice-cold water. Benjamin Rush, who was America's first psychiatrist, worked at Pennsylvania Hospital in Philadelphia and devised an instrument, the gyrator, for the treatment of mental illness. It employed a system of centrifugal action to whirl the person about to increase the flow of blood to his brain. About 1792 Dr. Rush invented the "tranquilizer," a type of restraint, and the ducking stool.

Many of these strenuous attempts to restore a person's normal behavior were based on the belief that the person had lost his senses as a result of an emotional crisis and that restoration would be achieved when he experienced another equally disturbing event. Tranquility for emotionally disturbed individuals has always been one of the goals of treatment and remains one of the goals today.

In more modern times the cold, wet sheet pack and the continuous tub bath were used in attempts to help individuals achieve more tranquil emotional states. The individual reactions to these measures varied widely.

One of the first drugs to be used for its tranquilizing effect was reserpine, which is the purified alkaloid of *Rauwolfia serpentina*. Although reserpine is somewhat effective in relaxing and quieting overactive individuals, this drug has a delayed action, tends to intensify depression, and is associated with gastrointestinal hemorrhage. It has been largely replaced by the psychopharmacological agents that were first introduced in the United States in 1953 on a research basis. Use of these drugs in the treatment of mental illness has had a dramatic effect on the care of emotionally ill people and on the national attitude toward all aspects of mental illness.

PSYCHOTROPIC DRUGS

The term *psychotropic drugs* refers to any drug that has the effect of altering the mind. Drugs that have an antipsychotic effect such as the phenothiazine derivatives, and drugs that have an antianxiety effect, such as the benzodiazepine derivatives are commonly referred to as major and minor tranquilizers. Many authorities believe that these terms are misnomers in that the main effect of these drugs is not tranquilization, but rather clearing of the sensorium in the case of the antipsychotic drugs, and lowering of anxiety in the case of the antianxiety drugs. To be sure, "tranquilization" often occurs with the administration of these drugs, but it is thought to be a result of the individual's increased ability to test and deal with reality. At the very least the designation of these drugs as major or minor is misleading in that all these drugs are potent chemical agents that have a major effect on the body chemistry. The false belief that the antianxiety drugs are "minor tranquilizers" may have contributed to their being inappropriately prescribed for individuals who are not mentally ill but who are experiencing the anxiety associated with crisis states. In many instances these drugs are abused by individuals who seek relief from anxiety. This practice is dangerous because these drugs not only create a physiological disequilibrium, but may also create a false sense of well-being, decreasing the person's motivation to address and solve those problems from which the anxiety stems.

In addition to the antipsychotic and antianxiety drugs, there are two other categories of commonly used psychotropic drugs: the antidepressants and lithium carbonate. The nurse who works with the mentally ill must be knowledgeable about the actions, side effects, and adverse effects of the drugs in each of these four categories, because their use is so prevalent and because the nurse most often administers them and monitors their effects.

Antipsychotic drugs

In 1956 the most useful of the new drugs, chlorpromazine, was introduced. It was marketed under the name of Thorazine and is only one of several examples of the family of drugs known as the *phenothiazine derivatives*. All the drugs in this group have essentially the same action. They are especially helpful to individuals who demonstrate psychotic symptoms related to schizophrenia. For this reason they are referred to as antipsychotic drugs because they seem to reduce psychotic symptoms. Thus excited, overactive individuals are calmed by these drugs; withdrawn, inactive individuals become normally active; and hallucinatory, delusional people become less symptomatic. Some authorities state that from 65% to 75% of the schizophrenic individuals who receive adequate doses of one of the phenothiazine derivatives become less psychotic.

Because chlorpromazine (Thorazine) proved to be so effective for psychotic individuals, scientists began searching for even more beneficial combinations of the essential chemicals used in the formula. As a result, there are now many phenothiazine derivatives, each with slight variations in its formula. In addition, other antipsychotic drugs with an entirely different chemical formula have been developed. To assist in clarifying the facts about these drugs, Table 10-1 was prepared. The majority of the anti-

TABLE 10-1   antipsychotic psychotropic drugs

generic name	trade name	range of daily oral dosage (mg)	comments
PHENOTHIAZINE DERIVATIVES: DIMETHYLAMINE SUBGROUP			
Chlorpromazine	Thorazine	100-1500	
Triflupromazine	Vesprin	20-200	
Promazine	Sparine	100-2400	
PHENOTHIAZINE DERIVATIVES: PIPERIDINE SUBGROUP			
Thioridazine	Mellaril	100-800	
Piperacetazine	Quide	20-160	
Mesoridazine	Serentil	100-400	Schizophrenia, organic mental disorders, and alcoholism are often treated with Serentil
PHENOTHIAZINE DERIVATIVES: PIPERAZINE SUBGROUP			
Acetophenazine	Tindal	40-120	
Fluphenazine	Prolixin	2-20	Often given intramuscularly at a dosage two to three times *less* than orally
Perphenazine	Trilafon	6-64	
Trifluoperazine	Stelazine	2-40	
BUTYROPHENONE DERIVATIVES			
Haloperidol	Haldol	2-100	Optimum dosage highly variable
THIOXANTHENE DERIVATIVES			
Chlorprothixene	Taractan	100-600	Specific for moderate to severe agitation, anxiety, and tension related to schizophrenia
Thiothixene	Navane	10-60	
DIHYDROINDOLONE DERIVATIVES			
Molindone	Moban	15-225	Specific for use in schizophrenia
DIBENZOXAZEPINE DERIVATIVES			
Loxapine succinate	Loxitane	20-200	

psychotic drugs are listed with their generic name, trade name, and range of daily oral dosage in milligrams.

Antipsychotic drugs are all considered useful in the management of the manifestations of psychotic disorders, although they are usually *not* indicated for psychotic depressions. Drug manufacturers often make claims that a drug is specifically useful in alleviating a particular symptom, implying that there are major differences between drugs within a given chemical group. Clinicians, on the other hand, more commonly report that the effect of the drug seems to be idiosyncratic to the individual and that if a drug in one chemical group is not successful in alleviating the symptomatology without adverse effects, success can often be achieved by the administration of an antipsychotic drug from another chemical group. Because of this observation, Table 10-1 presents the antipsychotic drugs according to chemical group.

Tables 10-2 and 10-3 describe some of the side effects and adverse effects that can be brought on by the use of some of these drugs with selected individuals. The nurse is often the first health care professional to notice the occurrence of adverse effects and therefore must differentiate them from unpleasant but benign side effects and initiate appropriate nursing and medical measures. These measures vary from reassuring the client in instances when side effects occur to withholding the drug and contacting the physician immediately when adverse effects occur.

Antianxiety drugs

In addition to the antipsychotic drugs there is a group of widely used drugs referred to as antianxiety drugs. These drugs were called minor tranquilizers in the past. They do not have an antipsychotic quality and therefore do not help schizophrenics. These drugs are best used to (1) treat individuals suffering from delirium tremens, (2) relieve anxiety in individuals experiencing moderate situational stress (for example, preoperatively), (3) potentiate anticonvulsant drugs, (4) relieve muscle spasm, and (5) reduce high to moderate levels of endogenous anxiety to a moderate or mild level, rendering the client able to benefit from psychotherapy.

Table 10-4 provides the generic name, trade name, range of daily oral dosage in milligrams, and comments about the specific uses for some of the most commonly used antianxiety drugs. It should be noted that the propanediols are less often used than the benzodiazepines because overdoses can be treated success-

TABLE 10-2   side effects of antipsychotic drugs

side effect	comments
Dry mouth, blurred vision, constipation, urinary hesitance, paralytic ileus	These effects result from the drug's interference with acetylcholine. The first three should be treated symptomatically and client reassured. In instances of urinary hesitance and paralytic ileus medication should be withheld until medical evaluation is obtained.
Orthostatic hypotension	Drug used with great caution if cardiovascular disease is present and with the elderly. Individual should be warned about possible occurrences and taught to rise slowly and dangle legs before standing.
Photosensitivity	Protect client from ultraviolet light. Use sunscreen. Occurs most frequently with chlorpromazine. Examine skin frequently.
Endocrine changes	Weight gain, edema, lactation, and menstrual irregularities. Treat symptomatically. Reassure client.
Extrapyramidal reactions	Dose and duration related. Managed by adjusting dose of drug or adding antiparkinsonism drug.
Pseudoparkinsonism	Typical shuffling gait, masklike facies, tremor, muscular ridigity, slowing of movements, and other symptoms mimicking those seen in Parkinson's disease.
Akathisia, dystonia	Continuous restlessness, fidgeting, and pacing occur. Spasm of neck muscles, extensor rigidity of back muscles, carpopedal spasm, eyes rolled back, swallowing difficulties occur. There is acute onset, but condition is reversible with appropriate medication. Reassurance should be provided until symptoms subside.
Akinesia	Lethargy, feelings of fatigue and muscle weakness. Must be differentiated from withdrawal.

fully only with hemodialysis, and intentional overdoses are therefore more likely to result in death.

All antianxiety drugs have the potential for creating physical and emotional dependence. Withdrawal symptoms similar to those experienced following withdrawal from barbiturates and alcohol have occurred following abrupt discontinuance of an-

TABLE 10-3   possible adverse effects of antipsychotic drugs

adverse effect	comments
Skin reactions	Urticarial, maculopapular, edematous, or petechial responses may occur 1 to 5 weeks after initiation of treatment. Withhold drug until after medical evaluation.
Jaundice	Develops in about 4% of the clients and is a dangerous complication; drug should be discontinued.
Agranulocytosis and leukopenia	Chlorpromazine depresses production of leukocytes. Initial symptoms of sore throat, high temperature, and lesions in mouth indicate that drug should be stopped immediately. Outcome may be lethal, but this is rare.
Ocular changes	Corneal and lenticular changes and pigmentary retinopathy may occur with high dosages over long periods of time. Periodic ocular examinations are recommended.
Convulsions	Antipsychotic agents lower seizure threshold, making seizure-prone persons more likely to have seizures. Persons with a history of seizures or organic conditions associated with seizures require an increased dosage of anticonvulsant medication if antipsycotics are used.
Tardive dyskinesia	Insidious onset of fine vermicular movements of tongue occurs, which is reversible if drug is discontinued at this time. Can progress to rhythmical involuntary movements of the tongue, face, mouth, or jaw with protrusion of tongue, puffing of cheeks, and chewing movements. No known treatment; often irreversible. Prevention is imperative. Females over 50 years on prolonged doses are particularly at risk. Do *not* withhold drug until after medical evaluation; symptoms will increase.

tianxiety agents, especially diazepam. Therefore the dosage of the drug should be gradually tapered before its discontinuance, especially with clients who have taken large doses of antianxiety agents over an extended period of time.

Antianxiety drugs have a limited number of side effects. Sedation occurs when large doses are given, and the client needs to be warned not to engage in activities that require complete mental alertness. Ataxia is occasionally observed. Adverse effects are

TABLE 10-4 antianxiety psychotropic drugs

generic name	trade name	range of daily oral dosage (mg)	comments
BENZODIAZEPINE GROUP			
Chlordiazepoxide	Librium	10-100	
Diazepam	Valium	4-40	Useful for relief of skeletal muscle spasm
Oxazepam	Serax	30-120	Particularly useful in older persons
Flurazepam	Dalmane	15-30h.s.	Effective hypnotic agent for temporary use
Clorazepate dipotassium	Tranxene	7.5-60.0	
PROPANEDIOL GROUP			
Meprobamate	Miltown, Equanil	400-1600	Useful as a muscle relaxant

Antidepressant drugs

uncommon; the most serious are those in which a paradoxical reaction in the form of acute excitement, anxiety, hallucinations, increased muscle spasticity, insomina, or rage occurs. The drug should be discontinued if these symptoms appear.

The third major category of psychotropic drugs is made up of the antidepressants, which are extremely useful in the treatment of individuals who are depressed. In fact statistics show that about 70% of the depressed individuals treated with these drugs improve markedly. Unfortunately, when drugs from this category are given, there is a delay of several weeks in the therapeutic effect. This fact suggests that suicidal individuals are best hospitalized during this period, not only for their protection, but also to allow the professional staff to assess the onset of the drug's effect, which clients often do not report because of their depression.

The antidepressants fall into two main chemical structures: the tricyclic antidepressants and the monoamine oxidase (MAO) inhibitors. Table 10-5 gives the generic name, trade name, range of daily oral dosage in milligrams, and comments about the specific uses for some of the most commonly used antidepressant drugs.

Side effects of antidepressant drugs. Dryness of the mouth is experienced by all who take any one of the antidepressants. Other side effects that may be experienced by many who take one of the antidepressants include difficulties in visual accommoda-

TABLE 10-5 antidepressant psychotropic drugs

generic name	trade name	range of daily oral dosage (mg)	comments
TRICYCLIC ANTIDEPRESSANTS			
Imipramine	Tofranil	75-300	More effective when used for retarded depressive reactions of manic-depressive psychosis than for any other condition. Helpful in severe anxiety attacks and enuresis in children.
Amitriptyline	Elavil	75-300	Hypnotic effect useful when depressed individuals have severe sleep disturbance.
Desipramine	Pertofrane, Norpramin	75-200	More quickly effective therapeutically than imipramine or amitriptyline.
Nortriptyline	Aventyl	40-150	
Doxepin	Sinequan	75-300	Has antianxiety effect.
MONOAMINE OXIDASE INHIBITORS			
Isocarboxazid	Marplan	20-60	Monoamine oxidase inhibitors potentiate effects of many other drugs, including sedative, hypnotic actions of alcohol and barbiturates. When cautiously administered with appropriate dietary restrictions and careful observation of blood pressure, their therapeutic effect may outweigh their danger in individuals who have not responded to an adequate trial of tricyclic antidepressants.
Phenelzine sulfate	Nardil	40-60	
Nialamide	Niamid	75-450	
Tranylcypromine	Parnate	20-60	

tion, perspiration about the head and neck, and postural hypotension that often leads to injuries. A mild degree of urinary retention or constipation may also occur. These drugs aggravate glaucoma. In addition, MAO inhibitors may also produce a variety of central nervous system symptoms that may include tremor of the upper extremities, convulsions, twitching, and ataxia. If such symptoms appear, they can be easily controlled by decreasing the dosage.

Adverse effects of antidepressant drugs. Adverse effects of the tricyclic antidepressants include exacerbation of the psychosis and cardiac arrhythmias. The most serious and potentially lethal adverse effect of the MAO inhibitors is a *hypertensive cri-*

sis. Monoamine oxidase is essential in the metabolism of tyramine, a substance contained in many commonly eaten foods that exerts a pressor effect. When a client is taking an MAO inhibitor, particularly tranylcypromine (Parnate), and eats a food containing tyramine, the tyramine cannot be metabolized and this can cause a hypertensive crisis. This syndrome is often referred to as the *Parnate-cheese reaction.* Foods containing tyramine that must be avoided include aged cheese, whiskey, beer, cream, chocolate, canned figs, coffee, licorice, Chianti and sherry wines, live yeast or yeast extracts such as yogurt, fava beans, soy sauce, pickled herring, pickles, chicken liver, sauerkraut, smoked salmon, snails, and raisins. These dietary restrictions should be maintained for at least 2 weeks after the drug is discontinued to allow for the complete resynthesis of the drug.

MAO inhibitors potentiate epinephrine, so clients who are taking these drugs must be warned to avoid other drugs containing ephedrine because this combination may cause extreme hyptertension. Examples of commonly used over-the-counter medications that must not be taken include many cold remedies and antihistamines.

Finally, MAO inhibitors should not be administered with the tricyclic antidepressants. If a client's medication is changed from one category of antidepressant to another, a lag period of at least 2 weeks should elapse to avoid an adverse synergistic effect.

Lithium carbonate

The fourth category of psychotropic drugs is lithium carbonate. This drug is now recognized as effective in the treatment of manic phases and in preventing the recurrence of manic-depressive episodes when given on a maintenance basis. About three fourths of the individuals who have a definite diagnosis of bipolar depression improve remarkably when treatment with lithium is properly carried out. Lithium does not impair intellectual activity, consciousness, or range or quality of emotional life. However, the toxic levels of lithium are close to the therapeutic levels. Adverse effects of lithium, or lithium toxicity, can be monitored by measuring serum lithium levels. Thus facilities for prompt and accurate serum lithium level determinations should be readily available to the client. Clinical symptoms of an adverse reaction to lithium include nausea, abdominal cramps, vomiting, diarrhea, thirst, and polyuria. These symptoms can occur at lithium levels below 2 mEq/L. If the drug dosage is not reduced at the first sign of toxicity, serious central nervous system and cardiovascular system damage may ensue. Recent studies have shown that prolonged use of lithium even without symptoms of adverse reactions may lead to renal tubule damage, cardiac toxicity, and thyroid imbalance. Therefore, despite its effectiveness, lithium is prescribed cautiously and is unlikely to fulfill its promise of curing manic-depressive psychosis.

RESPONSIBILITIES OF THE NURSE

Because of the widespread use of psychotropic agents in the treatment of the mentally ill, it is not unusual for a nurse to spend a large part of her time preparing and administering medications. Unfortunately, some nurses believe that their responsibility has been fulfilled once these tasks are completed. However, such is not the case. The responsibilities of the nurse in regard to clients receiving psychotropic agents are numerous.

Before the client receives any medication, it is essential for a number of assessments to be made. Initially the client's medical history must be obtained, especially in regard to seizure disorder; pregnancy; cardiac, hepatic, or renal disease; and substance abuse. In addition, physiological baseline data about the client should be determined. These include blood pressure, both sitting and standing; pulse, both quality and rate; weight; sleep pattern; gait and movement; and blood chemistry. Many psychotropic agents affect these physiological processes and, except in extreme situations, an accurate assessment of their effect cannot be made unless baseline data are available to which a comparison can be made. In addition, the choice of drug and dosage are influenced by these factors.

As the nurse works with the client before he receives a medication she often is in the best position to ascertain his attitude toward taking medications. Clients vary widely in their response to drug therapy, depending on such variables as their past experiences with psychotropic agents or other mind-altering drugs and their current state of orientation. Some clients are eager to receive medication and see it as the answer to all their problems. Others, particularly those who are suspicious, fear medication because of their feelings of loss of control. In most instances, both of these extreme views are not reality based. The client needs to be helped to develop a realistic picture of what a psychotropic agent can and cannot do.

Once having ascertained the client's medical history, his physiologic baseline, and his attitude toward taking medication, the nurse is in a position to collaborate with the physician in determining the most effective medication, dosage, frequency, and route of administration. Although the physician has the responsibility for prescribing psychotropic medications the assessments of a knowledgeable nurse are often relied on, especially in regard to dosage, frequency, and route of administration. If indicated by the assessment data, the nurse is wise to suggest the medication be ordered by alternate routes, as well as to obtain a *prn* order.

The specific actions of the prescribed drug should address those symptoms of the client's illness which are most distressing to him or to others. These symptoms are called *target symptoms* and the degree to which they are ameliorated increases the likelihood of the client continuing to cooperate with his treatment regimen. For example, a newly admitted schizophrenic client who is distressed by visual hallucinations and for whom an antipsychotic drug is prescribed will often be relieved by the diminution of this disturbing symptom. If he had been previously counseled by the nurse to expect this result his trust in her and in the health care delivery system will be increased. However, it is important that the nurse make clear that if often takes as long as 6 or 8 weeks before improvement in target symptoms is seen.

After a drug has been ordered for the client it is the nurse's responsibility to accurately prepare, administer, and record the medication and its effects. As previously stated, some nurses unfortunately see this phase of the treatment as the only aspect of their role or, if not the only aspect, the most important one. In reality the success the nurse has with this phase of the process depends greatly on the quality of the client assessment she has previously obtained and the degree of physician-nurse collaboration she has been able to establish.

Most nurses have much experience in preparing medications, and doing so in a psychiatric setting does not differ from executing this task in other settings. On the other hand, administering medications to mentally ill persons may be dramatically different than what the nurse is accustomed to. First, most mentally ill clients are ambulatory and the nurse must use caution that the tray of medications intended for a group of clients not be accessible while she is occupied with administering medications to one client. Some clients will try to steal medications for use as barter for items such as cigarettes. In addition, clients may take medications to save until a sufficient amount has been accumulated so they may attempt suicide. Finally, clients may accidentally knock the tray over, resulting in the potential loss of medication and the actual loss of the nurse's very valuable time. Therefore it is a desirable practice for the nurse to keep the tray inaccessible to the client group and to administer medications to one client at a time.

While administering medication the nurse has a valuable opportunity to observe the client for side effects and adverse reactions as well as for changes in behavior. Of equal importance, she has the opportunity to interact with the client in such a way as to gain his acceptance of the medication. In this regard it is most often helpful for the nurse to refer to the drug as "medication" rather than using the word "drug" to prevent confusion with mind-altering street drugs. Nurses sometimes feel so rushed when administering medications that they resent the client's asking questions about his medications or otherwise lengthening the process. As a result it is not unusual for the nurse to be drawn into a power struggle with the client around the issue of whether or not he will take his medication and when he will do so. This common situation is unfortunate not only because it usually takes a great deal of time, but more importantly because it sets a negative tone associated with taking medications. Rather than engaging in a power struggle with the client, the effective nurse takes the time to answer the client's questions and otherwise gives him as much control of the situation as possible. The client has the right and the need to know the name, dosage, actions, side effects, and adverse effects of the medicine he is taking.

Clients who refuse medication present a particular challenge to the nurse. Before the nurse decides to omit the dose or to administer it parenterally she should make an assessment of why the client is refusing. Once again this takes time, but time might be saved in the long run. One chronically ill schizophrenic client was readmitted to the hospital because of an exacerbation of visual and auditory hallucinations probably precipitated by his having stopped his antipsychotic medication a month previously due to lack of money. Even though this client was known to the nursing staff as being cooperative he refused to take his oral medication. Every time the nurse would extend her hand with the medication cup the client would become visibly distressed, perspire profusely, and wrap his arms tightly around himself. Although the staff were agreed that what this client needed most was the prescribed antipsychotic medication, they disagreed about how it should be administered. Some argued that the client should be restrained and given the medication by injection. The nurse who knew him best, however, was struck by his uncharacteristic refusal of the medication and by the consistency of his behavior when offered it. She hypothesized that the client was perceiving the nurse's extended arm as an attack and consequently was experiencing massive amounts of anxiety when efforts were made to give him medication. Based on this assessment she approached the client from the side, laid the medication and water cups on the counter, slowly explained what they were, and gently directed the client to take the medication. Within a very short time the client complied. This thoughtful intervention by the nurse allowed the client to maintain control of the situation, accomplished the nurse's goal, and avoided the difficult and potentially traumatic situation of having to forcibly administer an injection.

It is important that the nurse document and otherwise communicate to other staff members interpersonal interventions that have proven useful in working with clients who resist taking medications. The use of the same approaches will help to ensure consistency in treatment and increase the client's trust in the staff.

Once the client has begun a regimen of psychotropic medications it is the nurse's responsibility to monitor his physiological response to the medication. Obviously, to do so effectively, the nurse must be knowledgeable about the intended effects, side effects, and adverse effects of the drugs the client is receiving. She must observe him carefully and listen to his reports with concern. When side effects appear the nurse can reassure the client that these are anticipated and make suggestions for reducing his discomfort. For example, the dry mouth associated with the pheniothiazines can be diminished by the client chewing sugarless gum or sucking on hard candy. If adverse effects occur the nurse must notify the physician immediately, and in most instances withhold the medication.

The ultimate goal of treatment with psychotropic medications is to enable the client to function at the highest level possible with the least amount of medication. To achieve this goal the nurse is most helpful when she works with the client on developing nonchemical adaptations to his symptoms such as increasing his interpersonal resources and skills. For clients who must remain on maintenance doses of medication, the nurse has the responsibility to help the client learn as much as he is able about the medication he is taking and also to learn how to administer it to himself correctly.

CONCLUDING STATEMENTS

1. The use of psychotropic drugs that help to normalize behavior has had a dramatic effect on the care of mentally ill individuals in this country and on the national attitude toward all aspects of mental illness.
2. Antipsychotic drugs are considered useful in the management of the manifestation of psychotic disorders, particularly schizophrenia.
3. Antipsychotic drugs are found in seven chemical groups. If a drug in one chemical group is not successful in alleviating symptomotology without adverse effects, success can often be achieved by the administration of an antipsychotic drug from another chemical group.
4. Side effects of antipsychotic drugs include dry mouth, blurred vision, constipation, urinary hesitance, paralytic ileus, orthostatic hypotension, photosensitivity, endocrine changes, and extrapyramidal reactions.
5. Adverse effects of antipsychotic drugs include skin reactions, jaundice, agranulocytosis and leukopenia, ocular changes, convulsions, and tardive dyskinesia. When adverse effects occur a physician should be notified and the drug withheld in all instances except tardive dyskinesia.
6. Antianxiety drugs are used to treat individuals suffering from delirium tremens, relieve anxiety in individuals experiencing moderate situational stress, potentiate anticonvulsant drugs, relieve muscle spasm, and reduce high to moderate levels of endogenous anxiety.
7. Antidepressants fall into the chemical groups of the tricyclics and the monoamine oxidase inhibitors.
8. Lithium carbonate is effective in the treatment of manic

phases and in preventing the recurrence of manic-depressive episodes when given a maintenance basis to persons with a diagnosis of bipolar depression.

9. The nurse's responsibility to the client receiving psychotropic medications includes assessing him physiologically and attitudinally prior to and during this treatment.

10. The success the nurse has in administering the prescribed drug is highly dependent on the quality of the client assessment she has previously obtained and the degree of physician-nurse collaboration she has been able to establish.

11. While administering medication to the client the nurse has a valuable opportunity to observe him for side effects and adverse reactions as well as for changes in behavior.

12. The client has the right and the need to know the name, dosage, actions, side effects, and adverse effects of the medicine he is taking.

13. When a client refuses medication the nurse should make an assessment of why he is refusing before she decides to omit the dose or to administer it parenterally.

14. The ultimate goal of treatment with psychotropic medications is to enable the client to function at the highest level possible with the least amount of medication.

SUGGESTED SOURCES OF ADDITIONAL INFORMATION

Classical

Maloney, Elizabeth M., and Johannesen, Lucile: How the tranquilizers affect nursing practice, Am. J. Nurs. **57:**1144-1146, 1957.

Contemporary

Batey, Sharyn, and Ledbetter, James: Medication education for patients in a partial hospitalization program, J. Psychosoc. Nurs. Ment. Health Serv. **20:**7-10, July, 1982.

Battle, E., Halliburton, A., and Wallston, K.: Self medication among psychiatric patients and adherence after discharge, J. Psychosoc. Nurs. Ment. Health Serv. **20:**21-28, May, 1982.

Boettcher, Elaine, and Alderson, Sylvia: Psychotropic medications and the nursing process, J. Psychosoc. Nurs. Ment. Health Serv. **20:**12-16, Nov., 1982.

Cohen, Marcia, and Amdur, Mark: Medication group for psychiatric patients, Am. J. Nurs. **81:**343-345, Feb., 1981.

DeGennaro, M., Hymen, R., Crannell, A., and Mansky, P.: Antidepressant drug therapy, Am. J. Nurs. **81:**1304-1310, July, 1981.

Distasio, Carol, and Nawrot, Marcia: Methaqualone, Am. J. Nurs. **73:**1922-1925, 1973.

Gitlin, Michael, and Jamison, Kay: Lithium clinics: theory and practice, Hosp. Community Psychiatry **35**:363-368, April, 1984.

Halikas, James: Psychotropic medication used in the treatment of alcoholism, Hosp. Community Psychiatry **34**:1035-1039, Nov., 1983.

Harris, Elizabeth: Lithium, Am. J. Nurs. **81**:1310-1315, 1981.

Harris, Elizabeth: Sedative-hypnotic drugs, Am. J. Nurs. **81**:1329-1334, 1981.

Keith, Samuel, Starr, Shirley, and Matthews, Susan: A team approach to pharmacologic treatment of chronic schizophrenia, Hosp. Community Psychiatry **35**:803-805, Aug., 1984.

Kucera-Bozarth, K., and Beck, N., and Lyss, L.: Compliance with lithium regimens, J. Psychosoc. Nurs. Ment. Health Serv. **20**:11-15, July, 1982.

Larken, Anne: What's a medication group?, J. Psychosoc. Nurs. Ment. Health Serv. **20**:35-37, Feb., 1982.

Marder, S., Swann, E., Winslade, W., Van Putten, T., Chien, C., and Wilkins, J.: A study of medication refusal by involuntary psychiatric patients, Hosp. Community Psychiatry **35**:724-726, July, 1984.

Neizo, Barbara, and Murphy, Mary: Medication groups on an acute psychiatric unit, Perspect. Psychiatr. Care **21**:70-73, April-June, 1983.

Pilette, Wilfrid L.: What is an adequate therapeutic trial of psychotropic medication? Perspect. Psychiatr. Care **15**:170-174, Oct.-Dec., 1977.

Rosal-Grief, Victoria: Drug-induced dyskinesias, Am. J. Nurs. **82**:66-69, 1982.

Smith, Janet: Improving drug knowledge in psychiatric patients, J. Psychosoc. Nurs. Ment. Health Serv. **19**:16-18, April, 1981.

Vernon, Amelia Wallace: Classification of psychotropic drugs, J. Psychosoc. Nurs. Ment. Health Serv. **19**:15-17, Nov., 1981.

Wendt, Roselyn L.: Good morning, world. I'm glad to be back, Am. J. Nurs. **79**:949, May, 1979.

Whiteside, Sharon: Patient education: effectiveness of medication programs for psychiatric patients. J. Psychosoc. Nurs. Ment. Health Serv. **21**:16-21, Oct., 1983.

Of particular interest

Harris, Elizabeth: Antipsychotic medications, Am. J. Nurs. **81**:1316-1324, July, 1981.

Harris, Elizabeth: Extrapyramidal side effects and antipsychotic medications, Am. J. Nurs. **81**:1324-1328, 1981.
These articles present a comprehensive discussion of the antipsychotic medications and their extrapyramidal side effects. They are essential reading for all nurses working with psychotic clients.

Hitchens, E.A.: Helping psychiatric outpatients accept drug therapy, Am. J. Nurs. **77**:464-466, 1977.
This is an excellent article on the various issues related to the use of psychotropic medications for discharged psychiatric clients.

chapter eleven

the therapeutic environment

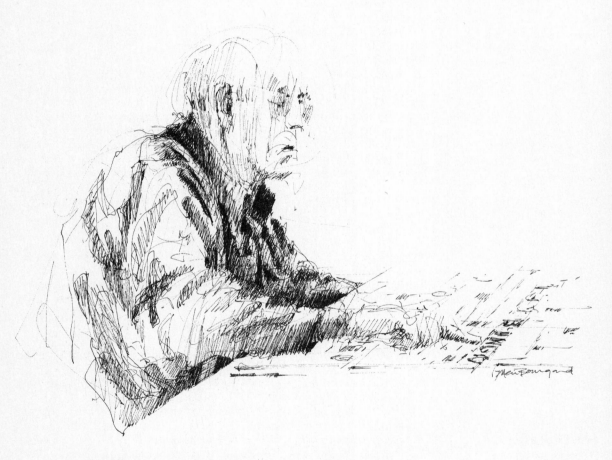

Tomorrow at the unit meeting I'm going to suggest that we play bingo every Friday night.

LEARNING OBJECTIVES
After studying this chapter the student will be able to:

1 State the goals of a therapeutic environment.

2 Discuss the characteristics of a therapeutic environment.

3 Explain the necessity for setting limits in a therapeutic environment.

4 Discuss the influence of the physical environment on the therapeutic environment.

5 State the significant aspects of a therapeutic community.

6 Discuss the implications of the therapeutic environment for the role of the nurse.

The environment in which the mentally ill person is treated is believed to be a major factor in enhancing or impeding the therapeutic effects of other treatment modalities. It is further believed by some that the environment itself has therapeutic potential. These beliefs are consistent with the conceptual framework of systems theory in which the client is seen as a system being affected by and affecting other systems, including the environment with which he interacts. What is questioned, however, is whose responsibility it is to create and maintain a therapeutic environment. For many years the professional staffs of most hospitals encouraged the belief that any planned therapeutic endeavor for hospitalized clients was solely the responsibility of the physician. Today it is believed that a variety of people can provide therapeutic help for mentally ill persons. Because the nurse is with the client for the longest period of time and because both are directly affected by the environment, it seems logical that the nursing staff assume major responsibility for the creation and maintenance of a therapeutic environment.

HISTORICAL PERSPECTIVE

The archives of American psychiatry include records of early successful attempts to develop a homelike atmosphere for mentally ill persons with provision for social and recreational activities. Physicians and their families joined other staff members in initiating and directing some of these activities. Early in the nineteenth century emphasis on a homelike environment, recreational activities, and a sympathetic approach to clients was referred to as *moral treatment*. In 1842 Boston State Hospital was reported to have placed emphasis on moral treatment for mentally ill individuals. The superintendent of one psychiatric hospital in Massachusetts is reported to have invited inmates to his home for Sunday dinner. Intimate discussions of the inmates' personal problems and difficulties were part of the therapy offered in those institutions at that time.

Some authorities believe that the era of moral treatment of the mentally ill ceased to exist because of the large numbers of immigrants who arrived in the United States after the Civil War. Many of these people could not cope with the problems of adjustment presented by the radically different environment they found in this country and were therefore deemed mentally ill. Large numbers of inmates with differing cultural backgrounds and languages swelled the census of mental institutions and made it difficult if not impossible to provide a homelike environment. Thus the era of moral treatment passed.

By 1940 large public hospitals were filled to overflowing. Because of the ever-increasing patient population the task of the hospital personnel was staggering. They were able to do little more than keep the inmates bathed, dressed, and fed.

An unprecedented national concern for the welfare of the mentally ill after World War II and the introduction of the first of the antipsychotic drugs in the early 1950s fostered a resurgence of interest in the therapeutic potential of the hospital environment. It was within this context that *Social Psychiatry*, a small book by Dr. Maxwell Jones, was published in England in 1953.

When published in the United States Dr. Jones' book was titled *The Therapeutic Community*, and it soon became one of the motivating forces in the movement to use the hospital environment therapeutically in the treatment regimen of mentally ill persons. This influential book was a report of efforts at Belmont Hospital in England during and after World War II to rehabilitate neurotic patients through group methods. That experience in group living at Belmont Hospital came to be known as the *therapeutic community*, a specialized form of therapeutic environment. In the therapeutic community, particular attention was paid to the development of the social structure of the hospital and to communication between patients and the hospital staff. Dr. Jones dedicated his book to "The Nursing Staff who have formed a framework around which our therapeutic communities have been built." Although the nurses to whom he referred were not registered nurses, they were intelligent, capable, mature women who used the interpersonal skill and understanding required in psychiatric nursing. The dedication is appropriate. Without a nursing staff with insight, understanding, personal warmth, and skill in directing groups, the concept of a therapeutic community could not have developed into a reality.

GOALS AND CHARACTERISTICS OF A THERAPEUTIC ENVIRONMENT

As with any treatment regimen, a therapeutic environment is most likely to be successful if its implementation is guided by goals. The goals of a therapeutic environment are to help the individual develop a sense of self-esteem and personal worth, to improve his ability to relate to others, to help him learn to trust others, and to return him to the community better prepared to work and live. The probability of these goals being achieved is high in an environment that displays the following characteristics*:

1. The client is familiar with the environment and what is expected of him.
2. The client feels comfortable and unafraid in the environment.
3. The client's immediate physical needs are met.
4. The client has clean surroundings and is cared for with clean equipment.
5. The environment provides the client with optimum safety from injury from his own impulses or from the impulses of others, from anxieties related to his former environment, and from decisions beyond his current level of responsibility.
6. The personnel in the environment respect the client as an individual, recognize his rights, needs, and opinions, and accept his behavior as a learned response to stress.
7. The environment provides for a limited number of restrictions and for opportunities for freedom of choice.

*Adapted from Brown, Martha M., and Fowler, Grace R.: Psychodynamic nursing—a biosocial orientation, ed. 3, Philadelphia, 1972, W.B. Saunders Co.

EMOTIONAL CLIMATE ESSENTIAL TO A THERAPEUTIC ENVIRONMENT

8. The environment provides a testing ground for the establishment of new patterns of behavior.

A quick perusal of these characteristics of a therapeutic environment indicates that they are concerned primarily with its emotional climate.

The most important environmental factor in helping clients achieve the goal of improved emotional health is the interpersonal climate of the unit where the individual is to live during his hospital stay. The establishment and maintenance of this climate should be the responsibility of the nursing staff of the unit. It is interesting to note that of all health care workers only the nursing staff has its "office" on the unit—the nurse's station. Thus the nursing staff is the professional group most affected by and most able to influence the emotional climate of the unit.

Like all people who embark on a new experience, clients need help to become familiar with the hospital situation and to learn what the staff expects of them. Because a new environment may frighten emotionally ill persons, a sensitive nursing staff will strive to develop a climate that encourages clients to see the hospital as a safe place where they are protected from the dangers of the outside world.

Providing safety for a client includes safeguarding him against making significant decisions when he is not well enough to do so. Thus the nursing staff may find it necessary to help him avoid making decisions about such matters as a pending divorce or separation, or the sale of property.

The therapeutic emotional climate in a hospital is established by a nursing staff that is friendly, sensitive, and concerned about clients' welfare. Such staff members are aware of the client's individual rights and needs. They respect him as a worthwhile, important human being, even though his behavior may sometimes be socially unacceptable.

Some clients want and need reassurance that the staff will establish guidelines for both their behavior and the behavior of others. The process of establishing and enforcing such guidelines is referred to as *limit setting*.

Setting limits frequently becomes the responsibility of the nurse, although the psychiatric team usually makes the initial decision concerning the limit to be established. Certainly the nurse would be wise to seek an opportunity to discuss the setting of limits with other professional colleagues when such responsibility is entirely up to her. She will want to be certain that she is not imposing her own personal standards on clients. If a form of client government is operating, much of the limit setting can be established by this group.

An example of a limit frequently established in psychiatric settings is the requirement that all clients attend breakfast fully dressed and ready for the activities of the day. Usually this requirement is made because some mentally ill persons seem to prefer to stay up most of the night and remain in bed most of the day. This habit can help the client avoid participating in most activities of the day and relieve him of the need to relate to people. If the client is required to be up and dressed for breakfast he is then available to participate in group activities. This rule also requires the client to establish some kind of living pattern that involves getting to bed at a reasonable hour in the evening. Some authorities argue that many well persons enjoy sleeping until noon and that they often skip breakfast. It seems reasonable to allow some clients to decide when they will retire and arise and what morning activities they will become involved in, including breakfast. It is apparent that before any rule that regulates client activity is established, all respects of the result of such action should be considered, including the problem of enforcing the rule once it is established. Consideration should be given to how a rule assists or impedes the growth of mature attitudes on the part of clients.

The populations of psychiatric units are likely to include both men and women. This calls for some limit setting concerning the relationship between men and women. Since sexual behavior is often a problem area for many mentally ill persons, they may feel much more comfortable if fairly specific limits are established for their coming and going on the unit where they are to live. The question essentially involves the limits that would be most helpful to men and women who are fearful of each other but who should be helped to establish more mature behavioral patterns in relation to the opposite sex.

The nurse can easily confuse limit setting with control of behavior. She may rationalize that many of the unnecessary controls that may have been imposed are limits placed on the situation for the safety and security of clients. Sometimes unnecessary controls are placed on behavior because of one unfortunate incident. For instance, one psychiatric hospital refused to allow clients to go outdoors for a walk because several years earlier one male client had attacked a nurse with whom he was walking. The responsibility for setting limits should not be assumed by one individual until the proposed action has been discussed with other people and all possible alternatives have been explored.

Although appropriate limit setting is essential to the establishment and maintenance of an emotional climate conducive to a therapeutic environment, the nursing staff also strives to establish as few rules and regulations as possible for client behavior and restricts activity only when necessary. Opportunities for freedom of choice are provided. As the client demonstrates his ability to accept more responsibility for his behavior, opportunities for making choices are increased.

As the client's emotional health improves, he will experiment with new mechanisms of adjustment and develop new ways of responding to others and of coping with stress. Some of these new methods of dealing with problems may not be appropriate. He will require encouragement to continue testing new patterns of behavior until he has achieved a more mature way of relating to other people.

INFLUENCE OF PHYSICAL ENVIRONMENT ON THE THERAPEUTIC ENVIRONMENT

A therapeutic climate for mentally ill persons depends on the attitude of the staff toward mental illness and the needs of the clients and does not develop as the result of any fixed type of hospital architecture. It can be developed in any type of hospital if the staff focuses on meeting the needs of clients. However it is helpful if certain structural features are present. The needs of clients can be met more effectively if facilities for privacy, socialization, and planned activities are available. If such facilities are not already present in the unit where clients live, innovations must be introduced if a therapeutic environment is to be created.

If a person's self-esteem is to be raised it is essential to provide an opportunity for privacy and a place where his personal belongings can be kept. In most settings a substitute has been found for the barrack-like dormitories and public showers with which many large psychiatric hospitals were once equipped. The mass approach to the care of human beings destroys self-esteem and the sense of individual worth. The key to a therapeutic environment is provision for the unique needs of individuals rather than dealing with clients as members of a crowd. In the past the idea that nothing should be arranged for one client unless it could be arranged for the group led many hospital staffs away from treating people as individuals. This attitude sometimes increased the client's difficulties rather than providing opportunities for him to solve problems.

If clients are to receive individualized care, and if the environment is to be therapeutic, living quarters must be attractive and inviting. In most instances no more than two or three persons should share the same room. If possible, single rooms should be provided for individuals who have strong feelings about sharing a room with another person. Clothes closets and dressers or satisfactory substitutes for this equipment must be available. It is important for mentally ill persons to bring personal clothing and other equipment to the hospital so that they can be attractively and appropriately groomed. The use of hospital clothing may be necessary in rare instances, but in the past this dress helped to depersonalize the institution's population and reduced them to a group of human beings with a universal attitude of hopelessness. Because it is therapeutic for clients to assume responsibility for their personal cleanliness, laundry facilities should be available.

Dining room facilities are important in developing a therapeutic environment. Mealtime should be a leisurely experience and a time for sharing ideas and reinforcing friendly relationships. It is not merely a time for the intake of food. Nurses can profitably assume a therapeutic role by serving as hostesses at small tables that seat groups of four to six clients. The role of hostess is more effective if the nurse shares the meal with the clients. This plan has been used successfully in some hospitals. As hostess the nurse can encourage conversation and can help make mealtime a happy, relaxed, and rewarding group experience. Such mealtime experiences cannot be initiated unless there is a dining room attached to the unit itself. Serving meals in large, noisy dining rooms where hundreds of people are fed gets food to clients but makes it impossible to accomplish other therapeutic goals.

Bathrooms should provide privacy. Although locks on doors may not be advisable, it is possible to provide toilet doors that close and shower rooms equipped with screens. The old practice of showering 10 to 15 persons at a time helped to reduce the individual to a member of a crowd and negated other attempts to help him feel like a respected human being. The therapeutic environment can develop most effectively when physical surroundings help clients to feel that they are respected and that their personal preferences are recognized, appreciated, and considered.

THE THERAPEUTIC COMMUNITY— A FORM OF THERAPEUTIC ENVIRONMENT

The therapeutic community is an approach to the care of mentally ill persons through group activity. It is an attempt to introduce democracy into the hospital setting. The therapeutic community strives to involve the client in his own therapy, to restore self-confidence by providing an opportunity for decision making, and to focus his attention and concern away from self and toward the needs of others. It has been organized in various ways in different settings. Sometimes the principles of the therapeutic community are used throughout the hospital and in other situations they may be limited to one or two units where the clients are almost ready to be discharged.

One important aspect of a democratic situation is that the people who are to be influenced by a decision are involved in making the decision. Until recently administrators and professional staffs in hospitals have taken the position that persons who require hospital care are incapable of making wise judgments and therefore must have all decisions made for them. Clients in most hospitals where this philosophy has been implemented have been reduced to a dependent state. Recently there has been a growing realization that forcing an adult person into such a dependent role is not usually necessary and is not therapeutic. Of course, there are some completely dependent persons for whom all decisions must be made. This is obviously true of acutely ill or unconscious patients. However, in spite of the reason for hospitalization a majority of adults are able to make valid decisions about many things involving their welfare. Forcing the dependent role on some mentally ill persons may be particularly unfortunate. Some of them have spent a lifetime struggling against an unconscious desire to accept a dependent role. When hospitalization forces this role on such an individual, he may never be able to relinquish it.

Today there is a growing belief that a therapeutic environment for mentally ill persons should provide an opportunity for them to participate in the formulation of hospital rules and regulations that affect their personal liberties. Following through with such a plan means that clients would be involved in formulating policies that regulate smoking, bedtime, late night privileges, weekend passes, social activities, control of the radio, television, and piano, check-in time when returning to the hospital from a weekend, reporting for meals, and the many other aspects of personal life that are influenced by rules in the usual psychiatric setting. Also, it is thought to be therapeutic to involve clients in making decisions about behavior and relationships among the unit population. Thus clients in a therapeutic community might be given responsibility for rendering a judgment about the infringement of unit rules, settling arguments between clients, judging the appropriateness of granting weekend privileges for certain members of the group, and many other decisions regarding the regulation of life on the unit.

Careful preparation of both the hospital staff and the clients should be assured before a therapeutic community is initiated. The hospital staff may have a good deal of difficulty accepting the activities and responsibilities granted to clients. Before a therapeutic community is initiated a thorough exploration of the implications of such an undertaking should be carried on through group discussions. All levels of hospital workers from physicians to attendants, kitchen helpers, and cleaning people should be involved in these group discussions because all will be affected by this new activity. All members of the staff need to have a thorough understanding of the goals and limitations of the undertaking. Clients in the units where the new philosophy is to be initiated should also have an opportunity to explore its implications through group discussions. These discussions should be directed by the physicians and nurses who will be directly involved in the future activities of the new organization. Both clients and hospital staff need to understand what responsibilities they can and cannot assume.

Active administrative sanction, acceptance, and interest are essential if the therapeutic community is to be successful. Involving clients in decision making represents a drastic change in the entire administrative philosophy of many hospitals. The therapeutic community cannot be expected to function smoothly at all times, and problems will undoubtedly arise. Decisions made by clients will not always be reality based. Unless the entire hospital staff believes that involving clients in decision making is therapeutically valuable and worth the struggle, dissenting forces may destroy the undertaking.

Meetings of the therapeutic community should be held regularly and at specific times if they are to be effective. Meetings should not be allowed to deteriorate into complaint sessions or to focus entirely on what the hospital should do for clients. This can be avoided if the group has some real responsibility for solving problems relating to clients' needs.

In one instance the members of a therapeutic community in a small unit of a large New York psychiatric hospital held a meeting to consider the problem of three suicide attempts made in 1 week by a young woman on the unit. Their decision was to institute a buddy system so that she would be accompanied at all times by one of a group of clients, each of whom would be assigned to spend a specific amount of time with her daily. Several weeks after this decision was made, the system was working well, and the woman had made no further suicide attempts. At this same meeting other problems considered were the problem of a client who did not return on time from a weekend holiday, a fight between two clients, and the request by a new client for a weekend pass.

It is far easier for the hospital staff to make all decisions for clients, but there is little that is therapeutic in this procedure. When clients have the opportunity to make decisions about their own and other people's behavior, they are presented with a realistic learning experience.

Significant aspects of a therapeutic community include the following:

1. The emphasis in a therapeutic community is placed on social and group interaction, with both individual clients and staff as important members of the community.
2. The goal of the therapeutic community is to provide a favorable climate in which clients can gain an awareness of their feelings, thoughts, impulses, and behavior, try new interpersonal skills in a relatively safe environment, increase

personal self-esteem, and realistically appraise the potentially helpful and destructive aspects of their behavior.

3. The work of the therapeutic community and the maintenance of an open network of communication are achieved through a daily meeting attended by all staff members and all clients who work and live on the specific unit.
4. A successful therapeutic community requires that both staff and individual clients become fully aware of their roles, limitations, responsibilities, and authority.
5. Staff members in a therapeutic community make information openly available to clients with whom they share treatment responsibilities.
6. The treatment arena in the therapeutic community includes all relationships among the members of the community, with special attention being given to the network of communication among members.

THE IMPLICATIONS OF THE THERAPEUTIC ENVIRONMENT FOR THE NURSE

It is not possible to develop a therapeutic environment without the strong, intelligent leadership of a nurse. When many of the traditional rules and regulations of the psychiatric unit are discarded and it becomes a place that focuses on meeting the needs of the individual and the group, the nurse is forced to accept a more active therapeutic role with clients. She finds it necessary to assign the clerical work, which formerly kept her confined to the nurse's station, to a secretary to free herself to give leadership to the personnel as they participate with clients in all the planned activities. Mentally ill persons require mature help and guidance in initiating and carrying out social activities.

When clients begin to experiment with new ways of behaving, they will make use of the nurse as an understanding person with whom they can discuss daily problems and emotional stressors. The nurse needs to be more alert than ever to changes in behavior. In a therapeutic environment many of the traditional safeguards are removed, and therefore safety of clients depends more than ever on an alert nursing staff. Thus it becomes the responsibility of the nurse to recognize changes in mood and behavior of clients and to intervene at appropriate times.

Skill in understanding group behavior and in directing groups is essential in the therapeutic environment. The nurse needs to work actively with client government to solve many unit problems. Finally, active, functioning channels of communication are essential. The nurse's ability as a leader will be reflected in the total effectiveness of the psychiatric team and ultimately in the therapeutic climate of the psychiatric unit. To a large extent the effectiveness of the client's total hospital experience will depend on the level of professional leadership provided by the nurse.

CONCLUDING STATEMENTS

1. Because the nurse is with the client for the longest period of time and because both are directly affected by the environment it seems logical that the nursing staff assume major responsibility for the creation and maintenance of a therapeutic environment.
2. The goals of a therapeutic environment are to help the client develop a sense of self-esteem and personal worth, to improve his ability to relate to others, to help him learn to trust others, and to return him to the community better prepared to work and to live.
3. The characteristics of a therapeutic environment are concerned primarily with its emotional climate.
4. Establishing and enforcing limits are necessary to reassure some clients.
5. Limit setting frequently becomes the responsibility of the nurse, although decisions about what limits need to be established are usually made by the entire psychiatric team.
6. The needs of clients can be met more effectively if physical provisions for privacy, socialization, and planned activities are available.
7. The therapeutic community is an approach to the care of the mentally ill through group activity.
8. One important aspect of a therapeutic community is that the people who are to be influenced by a decision are involved in making the decision.
9. The work of a therapeutic community and the maintenance of an open network of communication are achieved in a daily community meeting attended by all staff and all clients who live and work on the specific unit.
10. It is not possible to develop a therapeutic environment without the strong, intelligent leadership of a nurse.
11. In a therapeutic environment the nurse will find it necessary

to be free from clerical work to give leadership to the unit personnel as they participate with clients in planned activities.

Classical

Abrams, G.M.: Defining milieu therapy, Arch. Gen. Psychiatry **21:**553-560, 1969.

Bennet, Leland R.: A therapeutic community, Nurs. Outlook **9:**423-425, 1961.

Berliner, Arthur K.: The two milieus in milieu therapy, Perspect. Psychiatr. Care **5:**266-271, Nov.-Dec., 1967.

Briggs, Dennie Lynn: Social psychiatry in Great Britain, Am. J. Nurs. **59:**215-221, 1959.

Greenblatt, M., York, R.H. and Brown, I.L.: From custodial to therapeutic patient care in mental hospitals, New York, 1979, Arno Press, Inc.

Holmes, Marguerite J., and Werner, Jean A.: Psychiatric nursing in a therapeutic community, New York, 1966, MacMillan Publishing Co., Inc.

Huey, Florence: In a therapeutic community, Am. J. Nurs. **71:**926-933, 1971.

Irvine, LaVerne F., and Deery, S. Joel: An investigation of problem areas relating to the therapeutic community concept, Ment. Hyg. **45:**367-373, 1961.

Jones, Maxwell: Beyond the therapeutic community, New Haven, Conn., 1968, Yale University Press.

Jones, Maxwell: The therapeutic community: a new treatment method in psychiatry, New York, 1953, Basic Books, Inc., Publishers.

Loomis, Maxine E.: Nursing management of acting out behavior, Perspect. Psychiatr. Care **8:**168-173, 1970.

Peplau, Hildegarde E.: Interpersonal relations in nursing, New York, 1952, G.P. Putnam's Sons.

Schwartz, Morris S., and Shockley, Emmy L.: The nurse and the mental patient, New York, 1956, John Wiley & Sons, Inc.

Siegel, Nathaniel H.: What is a therapeutic community? Nurs. Outlook **12:**49-51, May, 1964.

Simpson, George, and Kline, Nathan S.: A new type psychiatric ward, Am. J. Psychiatry **119:**511-514, 1962.

Stainbrook, E.: The hospital as a therapeutic community. In Freedman, A.M., and Kaplan H.I.: Comprehensive textbook of psychiatry, Baltimore, 1975, The Williams & Wilkins Co.

Stanton, A., and Schwartz, M.: The mental hospital. A study of institutional participation in psychiatric illness and treatment, New York, 1954, Basic Books, Inc., Publishers.

Stevens, Leonard F.: What makes a ward climate therapeutic? Am. J. Nurs. **61:**95-96, 1961.

Von Mering, Otto, and King, Stanley H.: Remotivating the mental patient, New York, 1957, Russell Sage Foundation.

Contemporary

Adelson, Pearl Yaruss: The backward dilemma, Am. J. Nurs. **80**:422-426, 1980.

Boettcher, Elaine: Preventing violent behavior: an integrated theoretical model for nursing, Perspect. Psychiatr. Care **21**:54-58, April-June, 1983.

Brooks, Rath E.: Behind the heavy metal door, Am. J. Nurs. **79**:1547-1550, Sept., 1979.

Busteed, Ellen, and Johnstone, Charles: The development of suicide precautions for an inpatient psychiatric unit, J. Psychosoc. Nurs. Ment. Health Serv. **21**:15-19, May, 1983.

Calnen, Terrence: Whose agent? A re-evaluation of the role of the psychiatric nurse in the therapeutic community, Perspect. Psychiatr. Care **10**:210-219, Dec., 1972.

Carser, Diane: Primary nursing in the milieu, J. Psychosoc. Nurs. Ment. Health Serv. **19**:35-41, Feb., 1981.

Carson Verna: Meeting the spiritual needs of hospitalized psychiatric patients, Perspect. Psychiatr. Care **18**:17-20, Jan.-Feb., 1980.

Cavens, Annie, and Williams, Robert L.: The budget plann: (behavior modification of long-term patients), Perspect. Psychiatr. Care **9**:13-16, Jan.-Feb., 1971.

Clark, Carolyn C.: A social systems approach to short-term psychiatric care, Perspect. Psychiatr. Care **10**:178-182, Oct.-Nov., 1972.

Closurdo, Janette S.: Behavior modication and the nursing process, Perspect. Psychiatr. Care **13**:25-36, Jan.-Mar., 1975.

Corton, P., Drake, R., Whitaker, A., and Potter, J.: Dealing with suicide on a psychiatric inpatient unit, Hosp. Community Psychiatry **34**:55-59, 1983.

Craig, Anne E., and Hyatt, Barbara A.: Chronicity in mental illness: a theory on the role of change, Perspect. Psychiatr. Care **16**:139-144, May-June, 1978.

Dall, William: Home is not sweet anymore, Ment. Hyg. **75**:22-24, Winter, 1975.

Devine, Barbara: Therapeutic milieu/milieu therapy: an overview, J. Psychosoc. Nurs. Ment. Health Serv. **19**:20-24, March, 1981.

Fanning, V.: Patient involvement in planning own care: staff and patient attitudes, J. Psychiatr. Nurs. **10**:5-8, Jan.-Feb., 1972.

Fitzgerald, Roy, C., and Long, Imelda: Seclusion and the treatment and management of severely disturbed manic-depressed patients, Perspect. Psychiatr. Care **11**:59-64, 1973.

Gardner, Kathyrn: Patient groups in a therapeutic community, Am. J. Nurs. **71**:528-531, 1971.

Hinds, Pamela: Music: a milieu factor with implications for the nurse-therapist, J. Psychosoc. Nurs. Ment. Health Serv. **18**:28-33, June, 1980.

Islam, A., and Turner, D.: The therapeutic community: a critical reappraisal, Hosp. Community Psychiatry **33**:651-653, Aug., 1982.

Jones, Maxwell: Nurses can change the social systems of hospitals, Am. J. Nurs. **78:**1012-1014, 1978.

Kiev, Ari: The courage to live, New York, 1980, Lippincott & Crowell.

Lacy, Marcia: Creating a safe and supportive treatment environment, Hosp. Community Psychiatry **32:**44-47, Jan., 1981.

Lantz, James: Adlerian community treatment with schizophrenic clients, J. Psychosoc. Nurs. Ment. Health Serv. **20:**25-30, April, 1982.

McCoy, Susan, and Garritson, Susan: Seclusion: the process of intervening, J. Psychosoc. Nurs. Ment. Health Serv. **21:**8-15, Aug., 1983.

McDonagh, Mary Jo, et al.: Nurse-therapists in a state psychiatric hospital, Am. J. Nurs. **80:**102-105, 1980.

Moran, Janet C.: An alternative to constant observation: the behavioral checklist, Perspect. Psychiatr. Care **17:**114-117, May-June, 1979.

Penningrath, Philip E.: Control of violence in a mental health setting, Am. J. Nurs. **75:**606-609, 1975.

Raskinski, Kenneth, Razinsky, Ronald, and Pasulka, Paul: Practical implications of a theory of the "therapeutic milieu" for psychiatric nursing practice, J. Psychosoc. Nurs. Ment. Health Serv. **18:**16-20, May, 1980.

Reuell, Virginia M.: Nurse-managed care for psychiatric patients, Am. J. Nurs. **75:**1156-1157, 1975.

Templin, H. Elaine: The system and the patient, Am. J. Nurs. **82:**108-111, 1982.

Warner, Sandra: Humor and self-disclosure within the milieu, J. Psychosoc. Nurs. Ment. Health Serv. **22:**17-21, April, 1984.

Whaley, Mary, and Ramirez, Luis: The use of seclusion rooms and restraints in the treatment of psychiatric patients, J. Psychosoc. Nurs. Ment. Health Serv. **18:**13-16, Jan., 1980.

Wilmer, Harry: Defining and understanding the therapeutic community, Hosp. Community Psychiatry **32:**95-104, Feb., 1981.

Of particular interest

Jones, J.: Social psychiatry in practice, Harmondsworth, England, 1968, Penguin Books, Ltd.
The author's elaboration on the concept of the therapeutic community is especially relevant for the nurse in considering the impact of institutionally based nursing care.

Wolf, M.S.: A review of literature on milieu therapy, J. Psychiatr. Nurs. **15:**26-33, May, 1977.
This comprehensive overview of milieu therapy is especially relevant for the nurse in considering the ramifications of providing psychiatric nursing care within an institution.

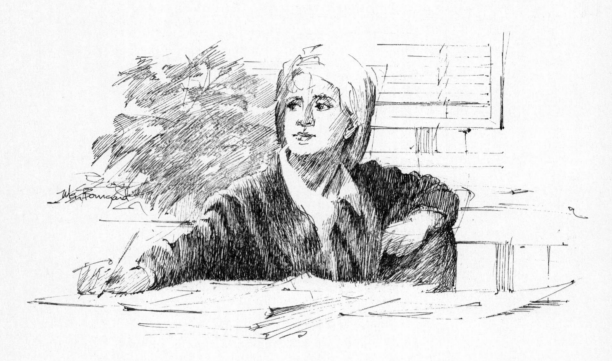

Why hasn't Mr. Smith's behavior changed?

LEARNING OBJECTIVES

After studying this chapter the student will be able to:

1 Describe the five phases of the nursing process.

2 Describe the characteristics of an effective interview.

3 Discuss observation as a means of client assessment.

4 Discuss the role of the conceptual framework of systems theory and stress and adaptation in providing direction for a comprehensive client assessment.

5 State a hypothetical nursing diagnosis in a manner that provides direction for the development of a plan of nursing care.

6 Develop a hypothetical plan of nursing care from a nursing diagnosis.

All too often the same nurse who systematically plans, implements, and evaluates care for the physically ill individual relies on on-the-spot intuitive judgment in administering care to the mentally ill person. This practice is likely to result in therapeutic interactions that occur more by chance than by design, and as a result decrease the probability of the client's attaining a more satisfactory level of emotional well-being. Therefore it is important for the nurse to understand how the *nursing process* can be applied to the care of the mentally ill. Although the terms used to describe the nursing process vary, the process is always an adaptation of the problem-solving technique and involves the phases of assessing, diagnosing, planning, implementing, and evaluating.

HISTORICAL PERSPECTIVE

Nursing began as more an art than a science. Those who cared for the ill had little more to rely on to ease suffering than intuitively administered comfort measures. With the explosion of medical knowledge in the late nineteenth century the nurse depended on the physician to direct her activities. It was not until the mid-twentieth century that a number of factors converged that ultimately led to the development of the nursing process.

The first of these factors was the extreme shortage of nurses during and after World War II. This shortage meant that a few nurses had to care for many patients. In attempting to care for patients in an efficient and effective manner the nursing care plan was developed. The nursing care plan not only standardized care, but also was a major tool in facilitating communication between and among nurses. Much of the nursing care plan, however, consisted of an organization of physician's orders that were carried out by nurses.

At the same time a second factor emerged, namely, the development of psychiatric-mental health nursing as a specialty within the occupation of nursing. Until that time caring for the mentally ill was not a desirable calling. Consequently, those who chose to do so were remarkably free of the strictures imposed by medicine in other areas of health care. It was, therefore these early psychiatric-mental health nurses who were able to design interventions that were within the domain of nursing practice and who documented the effectiveness of these interventions. Thus the independent role of the nurse flourished in the nursing care of the mentally ill.

With an increasing number of independent nursing functions, especially the nurse-client relationship, the need to monitor the quality of nursing care became apparent. In response to this need an adaptation of the problem-solving approach was adopted as a means to systematically plan and evaluate nursing care. This approach became known as the nursing process. The first book describing the nursing process appeared in 1967. Since that time a number of refinements in the process have been made, but its original purpose of defining the problem, designing a plan to address the problem, and evaluating its effectiveness remains.

ASSESSMENT PHASE

The first phase of the nursing process is the assessment phase. The purpose of the assessment phase is to collect data about the client and to organize these data so that they are useful.

The nurse needs to collect data about the client from all appropriate sources. These include the client's chart, other health care workers, relevant texts and journal articles, and the client's family and friends. However, the most important and significant source of information about the client is the client himself. To obtain data from the client the nurse needs to perfect her skills in interviewing and observing.

How to assess

An interview is conducted to obtain specific information. As such, it is not designed to be therapeutic or to convey information, although indirectly it may be helpful or informative to the client. An interview is guided by goals and an effective interview requires that the nurse organize her goals and approaches before meeting with the client. Because an interview is structured it is likely that the nurse will be more directive and ask more questions than she would in an interaction designed to be therapeutic. Thus the nurse is wise to have thought through sample questions, the answers to which will provide the data sought. Questions likely to be most effective in eliciting information are simple, concrete, and direct. For example, "What do you usually eat for breakfast?" is preferable to "Tell me about your usual diet."

On initiating an interview the nurse should tell the client the purpose of the interaction and approximately how long it will last. As with all interactions the nurse should introduce herself to the client if they have not already met and position herself on eye level with the client. Ideally both she and the client should sit in comfortable chairs. However, this is not always possible if the client is too anxious to sit. In that case the nurse may wish to remain standing as well. If the nurse intends to take notes during the interview, she should explain the purpose of her writing at the onset. By orienting the client in this manner the nurse establishes a foundation on which a future trusting relationship with the client can be built, either by her or by another nurse.

One of the most important goals of an initial interview is to ascertain the client's perception of his problems. While it is generally advisable to avoid using "why" questions, they are sometimes desirable when interviewing persons who are psychotic because "why" questions are concrete and direct. For example, a psychotic, hallucinating individual who is asked "What brought you to the hospital?" might very well respond by answering, "A car brought me." In contrast, the same client might respond to "Why did you come to the hospital?" by answering, "To get out of the cold" or "Because I see my grandmother all the time, and I know she is dead." Either of these responses answers the nurse's question, which is not the case when she avoided the use of a "why" question.

Having ascertained the client's perception of his problem, the nurse's next goal is to determine the duration of the problem, what circumstances led up to the problem, who else is involved, and in what way the client expects the hospital or clinic to be of help. A determination of these variables is essential to an accurate, comprehensive assessment and allows the nurse to compare the client's perceptions of the problem with the perceptions of others. Then she can design a plan of care which will be of the greatest help to the client.

Another major goal of the interview is to obtain information about such factual data as the client's daily activities, previous health history, educational level, and occupation. It is important, however, that the client not be bombarded with questions that can be answered by other sources. For example, if the nurse has access to a chart from the client's previous admission she ought not ask for such information as the client's date of birth unless she questions the reliability of the available information or is using the question to assess the client's memory.

The interview should be concluded as close to the time specified as possible. It is helpful to the client for the nurse to repeat what she said earlier about how she will use the information he shared. It is also important that the nurse inform the client what will happen next, such as the fact that she will take him back to the unit, or that he should schedule another appointment with the receptionist.

The other skill that is integral to the assessment phase of the nursing process is that of observation. Observation is a frequently used term for an active goal-directed process that utilizes all appropriate senses. As the nurse talks or otherwise interacts with the client, she looks, hears, feels, and smells. In general, the goal of observation is to determine the appropriateness and congruence of the client's appearance, behavior, and verbalizations with each other and with the situation. This implies, then, that observations are planned. Not meant to be implied, however, is that the nurse should not observe phenomena that she had not anticipated. It is important for the nurse to attend to her own intuitive feelings about a situation. Experience has shown that more often than not these intuitive feelings are manifestations of the nurse's unconscious perceptions that are based on reality. The observer needs to be alert to the client's facial expression, voice quality, neatness and appropriateness of dress and grooming, participation in activities, response to other clients and staff, and many other aspects of his behavior while she is interviewing him and during the time he spends in the treatment setting, whether that be 1, 8, or 24 hours.

To validate the information gained from observations and to determine their significance, observations of the same or similar events need to be made repeatedly. For example, the nurse may observe that on one occasion a client who was unable to purchase his brand of cigarettes swore at the clerk and stalked out of the store. Many people occasionally feel this degree of frustration and sometimes act on it. If the client does not have a similar reaction in future situations, it is likely that this incident is relatively insignificant. On the other hand, if the nurse observes that on subsequent days the same client yells and walks away because he must wait for the elevator, and then later displays the same behavior because his meal contains food he does not like, she would be correct in determining that she had identified a theme or pattern in this client's behavior likely to be most indicative of his problems. In some instances, however, behavior that is strikingly uncharacteristic of the client may be highly significant and should be recorded and communicated to other members of the professional team. As the nurse learns to understand more about the meaning of human behavior and learns to know the client as an individual, she will become more skillful in recognizing significant behavior.

What to assess

To assess the client comprehensively, the nurse needs to adopt a conceptual framework that will provide direction for the scope and nature of the assessment. It is in this regard that the conceptual framework of systems theory and stress and adaptation (Chapter 3) is useful. Use of this framework makes it clear that the nurse must define the client's subsystems and the larger systems of which he is a part by identifying their boundaries.

A comprehensive nursing assessment requires that each of the client's subsystems and the systems of which he is a part be assessed in terms of their potential energy and the degree of boundary openness that allows them to relate to one another and to their environments. The subsystems to be assessed include the physical, emotional, intellectual, social, and spiritual aspects of the client. It is necessary to assess the number and type of stressors affecting each subsystem presently and in the past. Finally, the client's adaptations to the resultant stress must be ascertained.

Axis IV and Axis V of the third edition of the *Diagnostic and Statistical Manual of Mental Disorders* (DSM-III) address these issues. The DSM-III is the tool used by physicians to diagnose mental illness. Axes I and II of this tool provide parameters by which the individual's degree of mental health is assessed, and Axis III provides for the inclusion of physical disorders and conditions. While the American Psychiatric Association, under whose auspices this tool was developed, should be commended for its movement toward a holistic view of individuals, many psychiatric nurses have grave concern about the inclusion of assessments of psychosocial stressors and levels of adaptive functioning under the official diagnostic tool of psychiatrists. The basis of this concern is the belief that these assessments historically as well as currently fall within the province of nursing, not medical, practice.

The systems of which the client is a part that should be assessed include the client's significant others, such as family and friends, and the culture to which he belongs. In making these assessments the nurse often relies heavily on information gathered by other health care professionals, particularly the social worker. The purpose of these assessments is not only to ascertain the interrelationship of the client and other systems as they affect each other, but also to be able to develop a plan of care that is realistic in light of these resources.

The final step in the assessment phase of the nursing process is to sort and organize the data that have been collected according to themes. Themes are recurring patterns that may have different manifestations but that stem from the same source. For example, the nurse may observe that the client has an unkempt appearance, speaks deprecatingly of himself, and refuses to join in group activities that are new to him. Even though these behaviors superficially may seem to have no relationship, with a little study the nurse will learn that they all may be manifestations of a poor self-concept. The theme could then be stated as, "Presents himself as inadequate to the situation."

DIAGNOSTIC PHASE

The second phase of the nursing process is the diagnostic phase, in which the nurse formulates a nursing diagnosis. This phase of the nursing process corresponds to the formulation of a hypothesis in the problem-solving technique, is based on a synthesis of all available assessment data, and provides direction for developing a plan for nursing intervention. A nursing diagnosis differs from a medical diagnosis in that a medical diagnosis identifies the disease or illness from which the client is suffering whereas the nursing diagnosis describes the client's response (or adaptation) to an actual or potential health problem.

In recent years efforts have been made to standardize nursing diagnoses according to characteristic responses by individuals to common health problems. While standardized nursing diagnoses would undoubtedly improve communication within the nursing profession and allow for standardized plans of nursing care, many nursing leaders believe this is not a desirable or even feasible goal. Their rationale is that nursing is concerned with the uniqueness of human beings and the existence of standardized nursing diagnoses would promote standardization of nursing care, which is the antithesis of nursing itself. This argument seems to have its greatest validity in regard to psychiatric nursing, where the primary focus is on the behavior of the client, particularly as he interacts with others. Nevertheless, Table 12-1 presents a selected list of nusing diagnoses and their etiology, as approved by the Fifth National Conference on Nursing Diagnoses.

To be useful in providing direction for planning nursing care, a nursing diagnosis must be a statement that defines a theme of the client's adaptation with a potential explanation of the stressor that elicited this adaptation. A nursing diagnosis that states only the theme of adaptation is of limited use in planning care. For example, the nursing diagnosis of "anxiety" is much less useful than the nursing diagnosis of "anxiety related to role change stemming from marriage of youngest child."

The nurse frequently sees nursing diagnoses that state the theme of the client's adaptation followed by the phrase, "due to" and concluding with the postulated stressor. The use of this phrase is not recommended, particularly when psychosocial adaptations are being diagnosed. The phrase, "due to" implies a linear, cause-and-effect relationship between the stressor and the adaptation. If the client is truly viewed as a system the nurse will understand multiple stressors are affecting him at any one time and that it is impossible and inaccurate to identify a direct cause-and-effect relationship between a pattern of adaptation and a single stressor. More desirable, then, is the use of the con-

TABLE 12-1 selected nursing diagnostic categories and etiological factors*

diagnostic category	etiological factors
Anxiety	Unconscious conflict about essential values and goals of life
	Threat to self-concept
	Threat of death
	Threat to or change in health status
	Threat to or change in socioeconomic status
	Threat to or change in role functioning
	Threat to or change in environment
	Threat to or change in interaction patterns
	Situational/maturational crises
	Interpersonal transmission/contagion
	Unmet needs
Communication, impaired: verbal	Decrease in circulation to the brain
	Psychologic barriers, psychosis, lack of stimuli
	Developmental or age-related
Coping, ineffective family: compromised	Temporary preoccupation by a significant person who is trying to manage emotional conflicts and personal suffering and is unable to perceive or act effectively in regard to client's needs
	Temporary family disorganization and role changes
	Other situational or developmental crises or situations the significant person may be facing
	Client providing little support in turn for the primary person
Coping, ineffective family: disabling	Significant person with chronically unexpressed feelings of guilt, hostility, despair, etc.
	Dissonant discrepancy of coping styles being used to deal with the adaptive tasks by the significant person and client or among significant people
	Highly ambivalent family relationships
	Arbitrary handling of a family's resistance to treatment which tends to solidify defensiveness as it fails to deal adequately with underlying anxiety
Coping, ineffective individual	Situation crises
	Maturational crises

*From Kim, Mi Ja, McFarland, Gertrude K., and McLane, Audrey, M.: *Pocket guide to nursing diagnoses*, St. Louis, 1984, The C.V. Mosby Co.

TABLE 12-1   selected nursing diagnostic categories and etiological factors—cont'd

diagnostic category	etiological factors
Coping, ineffective individual—cont'd	Personal vulnerability
	Multiple life changes
	No vacations
	Inadequate relaxation
	Inadequate support systems
	Little or no exercise
	Poor nutrition
	Unmet expectations
	Work overload
	Too many deadlines
	Unrealistic perceptions
	Inadequate coping method
Family process, alteration in	Situation transition and/or crises
	Development transition and/or crises
Fear	Learned response—conditioning, modeling from or identification with others
	Separation from support system in a potentially threatening situation (hospitalization, treatments, etc.)
	Sensory impairment
	Phobic stimulus or phobia
	Environmental stimuli
Grieving, anticipatory	Perceived potential loss of significant others
	Perceived potential loss of physiopsychosocial well-being
	Perceived potential loss of personal possessions
Grieving, dysfunctional	Actual or perceived object loss (object loss is used in the broadest sense)
	Objects include people, possessions, a job status, home, ideals, parts and processes of the body, etc.
	Thwarted grieving response to a loss
	Absence of anticipatory grieving
	Lack of resolution of previous grieving response
	Loss of significant others
	Loss of physiopsychosocial well-being
	Loss of personal possessions
Health maintenance, alteration in	Lack of or significant alteration in communication skills (written, verbal, and/or gestural)
	Lack of ability to make deliberate and thoughtful judgments
	Perceptual or congitive impairment

Continued.

TABLE 12-1 selected nursing diagnostic categories and etiological factors—cont'd

diagnostic category	etiological factors
Health maintenance, alteration in—cont'd	Complete or partial lack of gross and/or fine motor skills
	Ineffective individual coping; dysfunctional grieving
	Lack of material resource
	Unachieved developmental tasks
	Ineffective family coping; disabling spiritual distress
Home maintenance management, impaired	Disease or injury of individual or family member
	Insufficient family organization or planning
	Insufficient finances
	Unfamiliarity with neighborhood resources
	Impaired cognitive or emotional functioning
	Lack of knowledge
	Lack of role modeling
	Inadequate support systems
Mobility, impaired physical	Perceptual and cognitive impairment
	Depression; severe anxiety
Parenting, alteration in: actual or potential	Lack of available role model
	Ineffective role model
	Physical and psychosocial abuse of nurturing figure
	Lack of support between or from significant other(s)
	Unmet social and emotional maturation needs of parenting figures
	Interruption in bonding process, i.e., maternal, paternal, other
	Perceived threat to own survival: physical and emotional
	Mental and/or physical illness
	Presence of stress: financial or legal problems, recent crisis, cultural move
	Lack of role identity
	Lack of appropriate response of child to relationship
Self-care deficit: feeding, bathing/hygiene, dressing/grooming, toileting	Perceptual or cognitive impairment
	Depression; severe anxiety
Self-concept, disturbance in: body image, self-esteem, role performance, personal identity	

TABLE 12-1   selected nursing diagnostic categories and etiological factors—cont'd

diagnostic category	etiological factors
Body image, disturbance in	Biophysical
	Cognitive perceptual
	Psychosocial
	Cultural or spiritual
Self-esteem, disturbance in	To be developed
Role performance, disturbance in	To be developed
Personal identity, disturbance in	To be developed
Sensory-perceptual alteration: visual, auditory, kinesthetic, gustatory, tactile, olfactory	Environmental factors
	Altered sensory reception, transmission, and/or integration
	Chemical alteration
	Psychologic stress
Social isolation	Factors contribute to the absence of satisfying personal relationships, such as:
	Delay in accomplishing developmental tasks
	Immature interests
	Alterations in mental status
	Unaccepted social behavior
	Unaccepted social values
	Altered state of wellness
	Inadequate personal resources
	Inability to engage in satisfying personal relationships
Thought processes, alteration in	Physiologic changes
	Psychologic conflicts
	Loss of memory
	Impaired judgment
	Sleep deprivation
Violence, potential for: self-directed or directed at others	Antisocial character
	Battered women
	Catatonic excitement
	Child abuse
	Manic excitement
	Organic brain syndrome
	Panic states
	Rage reactions
	Suicidal behavior
	Temporal lobe epilepsy
	Toxic reactions to medication

necting phrase "related to," which states a relationship between the two phenomena but does not rule out other factors.

Most clients have more than one nursing diagnosis. However, if the nurse identifies numerous diagnoses for the same client she should question whether she has missed a unifying theme. In other words, as the nurse gains knowledge and experience she will learn that there is usually a high degree of interrelatedness among the various nursing diagnoses and she will attempt to state them so that they are specific enough to provide direction for planning nursing care, but not so specific that the resultant plan is unnecessarily repetitious.

PLANNING PHASE

The third phase of the nursing process is developing a plan for nursing intervention. The plan for nursing intervention is derived from the nursing diagnoses and includes statements indicating the objective of the care (the nursing goal), the rationale of the objective, how the objective will be achieved (the nursing actions), and the anticipated results (the outcome criteria).

Much controversy exists about whether the objective of the care should be stated in terms of the nurse or the client. Regardless of the way in which the objective is stated the intent is the same. For example, the nursing goal "To convey a sense of worth" means the same as the client objective, "To develop a sense of worth." However, the format chosen should be used consistently.

Once stated, objectives need to be prioritized as short-term or long-term goals. Criteria for prioritization include the urgency of the situation, the amount of time required to achieve the goal, and the anticipated length of contact with the client. Unless objectives are realistically prioritized both the nurse and the client risk being continuously frustrated by failing to achieve the desired outcomes of nursing care. This is currently the case in many psychiatric hospitals that have adopted a policy of discharging clients to aftercare clinics as soon as their behavior has stabilized. As a result, the nurses in the hospital may have contact with the client for only a few weeks; there is a different nursing staff in the clinic. In these instances the hospital nursing staff is wise to limit objectives to those that can be achieved in a short period of time.

To be effective, nursing actions must be related to the goals of the care. In addition, they must be realistic in light of the resources available. Within the context of the conceptual framework of systems theory and stress and adaptation, the goals of all nursing actions are to protect the system from noxious stressors, or to increase the system's potential energy thereby enhancing its ability to adapt to the stressor, or to diminish the potency of the stressor.

Outcome criteria are statements phrased in behavioral terms that enable the nurse to assess whether the goal has been achieved. Unlike objectives, outcome criteria are always stated in terms of client behavior and are most useful when they specify the conditions under which they will occur and the time period in which they are anticipated.

The plan for nursing intervention is highly individualized for each client. However, all plans for nursing intervention should reflect the principles of psychiatric nursing as discussed in Chapter 7 of this text. See Table 12-2 for an example of a plan for nursing intervention.

IMPLEMENTATION PHASE

The fourth phase of the nursing process is the implementation of the plan of care. In implementing the plan of care, the nurse utilizes a variety of roles. These roles are discussed in detail in Chapter 2.

The following situation depicts the way a nurse carried out the plan of care shown in Table 12-2 by fulfilling a variety of roles.

TABLE 12-2   example of a plan for nursing intervention

NURSING DIAGNOSIS

Feelings of inadequacy as a male, related to developmental stressors of adolescence combined with increased familial responsibility

nursing goal	rationale	nursing action	outcome criteria
To convey a sense of worth	Adolescents' sense of worth is tenuous and fragile	Praise accomplishments, no matter how small When client verbally derogates self, disagree if appropriate without arguing	Within 1 month there will be: Increase in client's statements reflecting self-worth ("Yes, I did do that well.") Decrease in self-derogating remarks Well-groomed personal appearance, appropriately dressed

"Please take me back to the ward, Miss S., I feel sick." Tall, dark-haired 17-year-old Sam G. had walked across the dance floor and was pleading with the nurse to be allowed to leave the regular Wednesday evening dance. The dance was part of the recreational program for clients. Both Sam and the nurse knew that clients were usually encouraged to remain at the dance until it was over. She also knew that Sam had not made such a request before, and intuitively she felt that something at the dance had been upsetting to him.

Miss S. quietly made the necessary arrangements with the staff member in charge of the dance and took Sam back to the homelike unit. Then she took his pulse, temperature, and respirations to be certain that he was not physically ill. When she found that these physical signs were within the normal range, she suggested that he help her make some sandwiches. Together they went into the kitchen where they prepared a snack for the other clients who would soon be returning from the dance. Sam seemed happy to help. He and the nurse chatted and joked together. He spoke at length about his mother's illness and his family's financial problems, but he did not mention feeling ill.

After finishing the sandwiches and cleaning the kitchen, the nurse thanked Sam for his help, remarking on the speed with which he accomplished the task. They then went together into the living room and sat down on the couch. "Do you think that my face is changing?" he asked. "I just looked in the bathroom mirror, and it seems to me that my nose is getting a lot longer and uglier."

The nurse looked carefully at his face and said, "It looks just the same to me. It seems to you that your nose is getting longer?"

Soon the other clients arrived from the dance. The unit was filled with the busy noise of 25 people discussing the dance and eating the evening snack. Sam took part in all this activity but sought the nurse several times to ask questions: "Do you think you ought to call my doctor?" "Will I be able to sleep tonight?" "You think that I am going to be all right, don't you?"

Each time Sam came to ask a question, the nurse took time to listen carefully to his questions and to answer truthfully and sincerely. She did call the doctor who was on duty that evening and told him about Sam's behavior. He agreed to come to see Sam. Because the doctor was not well acquainted with him, the nurse spent several minutes telling him briefly about Sam's family problems. She pointed out that he had been anxious and tense during the evening and had seemed to cling to her and to be asking for reassurance. The doctor talked with Sam. He felt that by allowing Sam to leave the dance the nurse had been able to help him avoid an anxiety attack. The doctor told the nurse that her empathic listening and her efforts at reassuring Sam had been partially successful. The next day Sam's regular therapist was able to help him look more objectively at the problem that had been so upsetting to him. As a result of the nurse's intervention and the doctor's help Sam was able to attend the dance the following week without experiencing undue anxiety.

This example is typical of situations that nurses who work with the mentally ill frequently encounter. In her interaction with Sam the nurse used the technical nursing role by taking and evaluating his vital signs. She simultaneously engaged in the role of mother surrogate and socializing agent when she worked with Sam to prepare and serve snacks for the other clients. The therapeutic effectiveness of this activity became apparent when Sam spoke about his family's problems and then became able to communicate his concern about his physical appearance. The nurse's response to this concern reflects the role of counselor, since she listened attentively and responded in a truthful and reassuring way. The nurse displayed an understanding of the necessity for professional collaboration by calling the physician and carefully sharing with him her assessment of the client. In summary, the nurse saw this clinical situation as an opportunity to implement the plan of care through the use of a variety of nursing roles, which proved to be very helpful to the client. Without an awareness of the therapeutic potential of these activities, the nurse might have insisted that Sam remain at the dance and thereby could have contributed to the exacerbation of an acute anxiety attack.

EVALUATION OF NURSING CARE

The final phase of the nursing process is that of evaluation of nursing care. The phases of the nursing process previously cited have been described as if they were discrete entities, and the phase of evaluation is frequently seen as the last step in this process. In reality, however, all phases of the nursing process may occur simultaneously, and some form of evaluation must take place continuously. Therefore it is imperative that the nurse review the assessment of the client, the nursing diagnoses, and the plan for nursing intervention, as well as the outcome of the nursing intervention. The outcome of the nursing care should be evaluated against the outcome criteria the nurse established as she planned for the care. <u>As previously mentioned outcome criteria need to be stated in behavioral terms and as specifically as pos</u>sible.

Inherent in all aspects of evaluation is the necessity for the nurse to evaluate her own behavior and determine the degree to

TABLE 12-3   the nursing process

phase	purpose	examples of nursing action
Assessment	To collect data	Observe present behavior of the client, using all the appropriate senses
		Read client's chart and relevant texts and journals
		Interview client, his family, and other health workers
	To validate data collected from observation	Make repeated observations; discuss perceptions with others
		Read relevant texts and journals to confirm observations
	To analyze data	Sort and organize data according to themes
Diagnostic	To establish a nursing diagnosis	Synthesize all available assessment data.
		State themes of the client's adaptations and stressors
Planning	To plan for nursing intervention, using nursing diagnosis as a basis	Individualize a plan for intervention and identify the nursing goal, rationale, nursing action, and outcome criteria
		Use the principles of psychiatric nursing:
		1. The nurse views the client as a holistic being with a multiplicity of interrelated and interdependent needs.
		2. The nurse focuses on the client's strengths and assets, but does not ignore his weaknesses and liabilities
		3. The nurse accepts the client as a human being who has value and worth, exactly as he is
		4. The nurse views the client's behavior as designed to meet a need or to communicate a message
		5. The nurse has the potential for establishing a relationship with most, if not all, clients
		6. The quality of the interaction in which the nurse engages with the client is a major determinant of the degree to which the client will be able to alter his behavior in the direction of more satisfying, satisfactory interpersonal relationships
		7. The nurse views the client's behavior as the best possible adaptation he is capable of making at the time

TABLE 12-3   the nursing process—cont'd

phase	purpose	examples of nursing action
Implementation	To implement plan for nursing intervention	Function in a variety of roles while using principles of psychiatric nursing: 1. Creator of a therapeutic environment 2. Socializing agent 3. Counselor 4. Teacher 5. Mother surrogate 6. Technical role 7. Nurse therapist
Evaluation	To make planned, critical assessment of care	Review assessment data for accuracy and currency Review nursing diagnoses for accuracy and currency
	To revise or confirm plan of care	Review plan for nursing intervention Compare client's response to intervention with outcome criteria
	To make self-assessment	Evaluate own behavior Revise or confirm plan for nursing intervention based on overall evaluation

which it does or does not facilitate achievement of the goals of the plan for intervention. It should also be noted that evaluation frequently serves the purpose of identifying those aspects of care that are indeed helpful to the client and that therefore should be continued. See Table 12-3 for a summary outline of the nursing process as used in psychiatric nursing.

CONCLUDING STATEMENTS

1. The nursing process is an adaptation of the problem-solving technique and includes assessment, diagnostic, planning, implementation, and evaluation phases.
2. The assessment phase is used to collect data about the client and to organize it usefully.
3. An effective interview obtains specific information, is guided by goals, requires the use of simple, concrete and direct questions, and takes place during a specified period of time. Two major goals of an initial interview are to ascertain the client's perception of his problem and to obtain factual information about him.
4. Observation is an active, goal-directed process that utilizes all appropriate senses. The goal of observation is to deter-

mine the appropriateness and congruence of the client's appearance, behavior, and verbalizations with each other and with the situation.

5. A conceptual framework such as systems theory and stress and adaptation is necessary to provide direction for the scope and nature of the assessment. When this framework is used the client's subsystems and the systems of which he is a part are assessed for their potential energy and degree of boundary openness. In addition the stressors affecting the system and the client's adaptations are determined.

6. The final step in the assessment phase of the nursing process is to sort and organize data according to themes.

7. The second phase of the nursing process is the diagnostic phase in which the nurse formulates a nursing diagnosis. The nursing diagnosis is based on a synthesis of all the available assessment data and provides direction for developing a plan for nursing intervention. A nursing diagnosis defines a theme of the client's adaptation with a potential explanation of the stressor that elicited the adaptation.

8. The third phase of the nursing process is to develop a plan for nursing intervention. The plan indicates the objective of the care, its rationale, how it will be achieved, and the anticipated results.

9. The fourth phase of the nursing process is the implementation of the plan of care. In doing so, the nurse utilizes a variety of roles as she carries out the prescribed nursing actions.

10. The final phase of the nursing process is evaluation. This phase includes a review of the client assessment, the nursing diagnoses, the plan for nursing intervention, and the outcome of the nursing intervention in light of the outcome criteria.

SUGGESTED SOURCES OF ADDITIONAL INFORMATION

Classical

Knight, Jeane Harris: Applying nursing process in the community, Nurs. Outlook **76:**708-711, 1974.

Contemporary

Aiken, Linda, and Aiken, James L.: A systematic approach to the evaluation of interpersonal relationships, Am. J. Nurs. **73:**863-867, 1973.

Berni, R., and Fordyce, W.: Behavior modification and the nursing process, ed. 2, St. Louis, 1977, The C.V. Mosby Co.

Boettcher, Elaine, and Alderson, Sylvia: Psychotropic medications and the nursing process, J. Psychosoc. Nurs. Ment. Health Serv. **20:**12-16, Nov., 1982.

Clement, J., and Boylan, S.: Actualizing theory into practice, Perspect. Psychiatr. Care **20:**126-133, July-Sept., 1982.

Closurdo, Janette: Behavior modification and the nursing process, Perspect. Psychiatr. Care **13:**25-36, Jan.-March, 1975.

Cohen, Stephen, and Harris, Elizabeth: Programmed instruction: mental status assessment, Am. J. Nurs. **81:**1493-1518, Aug., 1981.

Dethomaso, Marita T.: "Touch power" and the screen of loneliness, Perspect. Psychiatr. Care **9:**112-118, May-June, 1971.

Gordon, Marjorie: Nursing diagnosis: process and application, New York, 1982, McGraw-Hill Book Co.

Lathrop, Vallary G.: Aggression as a response, Perspect. Psychiatr. Care **16:**203-205, Sept.-Dec., 1978.

Lipkin, Gladys B., and Cohen, Roberta G.: The uses of the interview. In Effective approaches to patients' behavior, New York, 1980, Springer Publishing Co., Inc.

Loomis, Maxine E.: Nursing management of acting-out behavior, Perspect. Psychiatr. Care **8:**168-173, July-Aug., 1970.

Lunney, Margaret: Nursing diagnosis: refining the system, Am. J. Nurs. **82:**456-459, 1982.

Mansfield, Elaine: A conceptual framework for psychiatric mental health nursing, J. Psychosoc. Nurs. Ment. Health Serv. **18:**36-41, June, 1980.

Miller, Judith F., and Hellenbrand, Diane: An eclectic approach to practice, Am. J. Nurs. **81:**1339-1343, 1981.

Moscovitz, Andrea: Orem's theory as applied to psychiatric nursing, Perspect. Psychiatr. Care **22:**36-38, Jan.-March, 1984.

Powers, Mary Ellen: Universal utility of psychoanalytic theory for nursing practice models, J. Psychosoc. Nurs. Ment. Health Serv. **18:**28-30, April, 1980.

Price, Mary R.: Nursing diagnosis: making a concept come alive, Am. J. Nurs. **80:**668-671, 1980.

Schmidt, Carolyn S: Withdrawal behavior of schizophrenics: application to Roy's model, J. Psychosoc. Nurs. Ment. Health Serv. **19:**26-33, Nov., 1981.

Schmieding, Norma Jean: Putting Orlando's theory into practice, Am. J. Nurs. **84:**758-761, 1984.

Smoyak, Shirley: Clinical practice: intuitive or based on research?, J. Psychosoc. Nurs. Ment. Health Serv. **20:**9-13, April, 1982.

Snyder, Joyce C., and Wilson, Margo F.: Elements of a psychological assessment, Am. J. Nurs. **77:**235-239, 1977.

Williams, Janet, and Wilson, Holly Skodol: A psychiatric nursing perspective on DSM III, J. Psychosoc. Nurs. Ment. Health Serv. **20:**14-20, April, 1982.

Yura, H., and Walsh, M.: Human needs 3 and the nursing process, Norwalk, Conn., 1983, Appleton-Century-Crofts.

Of particular interest

Hauser, M., and Feinberg, D.: Problem solving revisited, J. Psychiatr. Nurs., pp. 13-17, Oct., 1977.
Problem solving and creative thinking are combined in this article as a framework for addressing nursing problems in challenging situations.
Kalisch, B.: Strategies for developing nurse empathy, Nurs. Outlook **19:**714-718, 1971.
This article describes the author's experiment to develop empathy in nursing students. It is excellent for the purpose of defining the concept and discriminating between empathy and related concepts.

section IV

consumers of
psychiatric
nursing

adults with thought disturbances

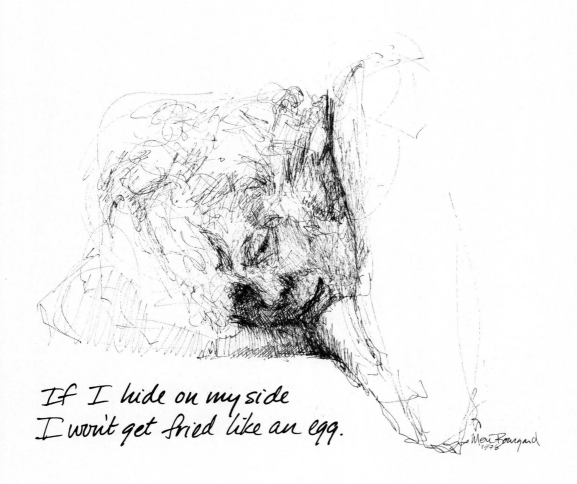

If I hide on my side
I won't get fried like an egg.

LEARNING OBJECTIVES

After studying this chapter the student will be able to:

1 Describe the symptoms exhibited by a person with the medical diagnosis of schizophrenia.

2 Discuss the dynamics of development of thought disturbances.

3 Describe behaviors the nurse is most likely to observe in adults with thought disturbances.

4 State examples of nursing diagnoses likely to be applicable to adults with thought disturbances.

5. Develop a hypothetical plan of nursing care for an adult with a thought disturbance.

The ability of an individual to deal subjectively and behaviorally with the demands of living in a highly complex society presupposes that he is able to perceive reality accurately. This is possible only if the person experiences a minimum level of anxiety and if he is able to consensually validate his perceptions with others whom he trusts. In mentally healthy people the process of consensual validation is learned early in life as a result of the development of trusting relationships with significant others. When an individual's level of anxiety is high he perceives reality in a highly personalized way that cannot be consensually validated with others. If a high anxiety level and subsequent personalized perception of reality occur often early in life they interfere with the development of basic trust. In cyclical fashion they also interfere with the accurate perception of reality even when anxiety is not heightened. Thus a pattern of reality distortion becomes established.

When an individual's distorted perceptions of reality result from and contribute to disturbed thought processes, that individual may be suffering from *schizophrenia*.

HISTORICAL PERSPECTIVE

The thought disturbance known today as schizophrenia undoubtedly has existed throughout human history. However, the deviant behavior associated with this disorder was not always viewed negatively. Some primitive societies elevated those who saw visions and heard voices to a position of prominence, believing they had supernatural powers.

The emergence of the industrial revolution and the simultaneous development of densely populated cities prevented the assimilation of persons who exhibited deviant behavior into the mainstream of society. In addition, the stressors of an increasing complex and heterogeneous society led to an increase in the incidence of deviant behavior resulting from thought disturbances.

Not until the end of the nineteenth century was formal research into the cause and nature of nervous and mental disease conducted. The pioneer of that effort was Jean Charcot (1825-1893), the great French neurologist whose clinics attracted students from every country in the world.

In 1883 Emil Kraepelin (1856-1926), a German professor of psychiatry, published the first edition of *Psychiatrie*, which in English translation changed the whole view of classifications of mental disorders in America. Kraepelin classified human behavior on the basis of symptomatology and offered a description of dementia praecox. Eugene Bleueler (1857-1939), a Swiss psychiatrist, elaborated the concept of dementia praecox and expanded it into schizophrenia in 1911. This description of schizophrenia was refined and elaborated on over the years but remained essentially the same until 1980 when the DSM-III was published. This manual attempts to describe the illness in terms more behaviorally oriented than those previously used and its multiaxial approach is designed to assess the individual holistically, not just behaviorally.

Although a necessary first step, descriptions of a disorder do not necessarily provide direction for treatment. Over the centuries many modalities have been adopted to treat persons with thought disturbances, with varying degrees of success. For example, in 1933 Dr. Manfred Sakel developed insulin shock therapy, a procedure where a series of hypoglycemic shocks are induced by injections of insulin. This treatment, as well as other somatic therapies such as hydrotherapy, have been almost completely replaced by the antipsychotic drugs and behaviorally oriented interventions, such as group therapy. These treatment modalities, while not curing thought disturbances, have proven sufficiently safe and effective in controlling their symptoms that many individuals require only limited hospitalization.

SCHIZOPHRENIC DISORDERS

Schizophrenia is classified as a *functional psychosis*. This term describes those mental illnesses in which the person's perception of reality is severely distorted because of factors other than demonstrable organic disease or intellectual deficit. Although schizophrenia is only one of several functional psychoses, it is thought to be the most serious because its onset typically occurs during late adolescence or early adulthood, earlier than the other functional psychoses. In addition, the symptoms of schizophrenia are all-pervasive, affecting all aspects of the individual's existence.

Schizophrenia appears as a distorted reaction of an individual who lacks the capacities and feelings required for effectively handling the daily challenges of reality. There is either a total lack of normal feeling tone or a distortion of the emotions. An individual with schizophrenia tends to withdraw into a world of his own subjective construction. This withdrawal is manifested behaviorally by an increasing inability to develop and maintain satisfactory interpersonal relationships. The individual frequently has great difficulty in identifying and communicating his feelings and thoughts to others, although he believes he has made many efforts to do so. Such an individual is frequently misunderstood by others, and it can be said that his communication patterns are dysfunctional.

To be diagnosed as schizophrenic, the individual must exhibit characteristic delusions, characteristic hallucinations, or other characteristic symptoms of thought impairment accompanied by blunted, flat, or inappropriate affect.

Delusions are false beliefs out of keeping with the individual's level of knowledge and his cultural group; the belief is maintained against logical argument and despite objective contradictory evidence. Delusions characteristic of schizophrenia include delusions about one's thoughts, feelings, and activities being controlled by some external force and delusions about one's thoughts being broadcast into the external world, inserted from the external world into one's mind, or removed from one's head by some external source. Religious and somatic delusions as well as delusions of grandiosity are also common.

Hallucinations are false sensory perceptions in the absence of an actual external stimulus. Although any of the five senses may be involved in a hallucinatory experience, auditory and visual hallucinations are most characteristic of schizophrenia.

Derailment (loosening of associations) is another characteristic symptom of schizophrenia and refers to a pattern of spontaneous speech in which the idea or trend of thought slips off one track onto another that is completely unrelated. As a result, the person's speech may seem unintelligible to the listener even though individual words are understood.

The term *affect* refers to the feeling tone of the individual. The schizophrenic person characteristically exhibits a blunt or flat affect, in contrast to the healthy individual whose affect conveys a feeling that is indicative of his emotional state and is congruent with the content of what he is saying. In individuals with schizophrenic disorders one observes that the feeling tone conveyed by the individual does not enhance what he is saying. It is not unusual to spend a great deal of time talking with a schizophrenic person without learning what he is feeling, despite the fact that much of the conversation was his attempt to describe his feelings. It is also not unusual for the individual to convey a feeling tone that is inappropriate to the content of what he is saying; for example he may laugh while stating how upset and sad he is because his mother just died.

Once the medical diagnosis of schizophrenia is made, the individual's behavior is further categorized into types of schizophrenia. Psychiatrists have subclassified schizophrenia into five major types, depending on the predominant patterns of behavior displayed. These subclassifications are the disorganized (hebephrenic), the catatonic, the paranoid, the undifferentiated, and the residual types. The *disorganized type* is characterized by severe personality disintegration, including hallucinations, inappropriate behavior (for example, silly laughter), and regression. *Catatonic* behavior is characterized by an acute stupor associated with a sudden loss of animation and a tendency to remain motionless in a stereotyped position; this behavior may alternate with periods of excitement and explosive overactivity. The *paranoid type* is characterized by suspiciousness and ideas of persecution or grandeur called *paranoid delusions*. The *undifferentiated type* is characterized by the prominence of psychotic symptoms that fall into more than one subtype or that do not meet the criteria for any one subtype. The *residual type* is the schizophrenic diagnosis used for individuals who no longer exhibit overtly psychotic symptoms but do exhibit inappropriate behavior characteristic of schizophrenia.

Whether it is possible to help a schizophrenic individual to reestablish himself in his family and return to his work depends on several factors:

1. The character of the prepsychotic personality. The prepsychotic personality includes the effectiveness of the individual's adaptation before becoming mentally ill, the type of interests that were maintained, and the coping mechanisms that were used.
2. The nature of the onset of the illness. Did the illness develop insidiously over a long period of time as the result of progressively more unsatisfactory methods of coping with life's problems, or was the onset rapid and precipitated by a situation external to the life of the individual?
3. The timing and nature of the treatment. Was treatment sought early in the illness, and was treatment individualized and personalized?

An individual who has adapted reasonably well to the pressures of life before becoming ill will have a better chance of recovery, at least of returning to his prepsychotic level of effectiveness, than will someone who has never adapted effectively and therefore has limited system energy. It is also obvious that someone whose illness has developed slowly and insidiously has a less optimistic future than does someone whose illness was precipitated only after experiencing great stress emanating from his environment.

Persons who receive help very soon after the development of the illness and are given individualized, skilled, and highly personalized care have a good chance of making a social recovery. This is much less true of persons who receive treatment after the illness has been fullblown for a year or more.

Authorities suggest that expectations for recovery should be in terms of social recovery and not necessarily in terms of emotional recovery. Schizophrenic individuals who have been treated may maintain a marginal adjustment, still retaining an essentially shallow affective response and shyness. They can be thought of as interpersonally fragile and may require professional help from time to time. Many schizophrenic individuals require a daily maintenance dose of one of the antipsychotic medications.

**Dynamics of
development**

If one were to ask the person with a thought disturbance what caused his illness he might respond by relating a particularly stressful event that preceded the onset of his illness by days, weeks, or months. Although not all schizophrenic persons have such events in their lives, enough experience them to make it important to distinguish between a precipitating event and causation. Although there is much ongoing debate over the cause of thought disorders, all authorities agree that the cause is likely to be a process of long standing, either physical or emotional or both. It is considered highly unlikely that a single event, either physical or emotional, no matter how catastrophic, would be sufficient to cause the drastic personality alteration seen in schizophrenia. The events reported by these persons as the possible causes of their illness are usually viewed by authorities as precipitating factors. Lay persons express this concept when they refer to the "straw that broke the camel's back." The underlying physiological and psychological structure is so fragile that the traumatic event cannot be integrated within the context of reality and the individual retreats into the illness to protect himself against total personality disintegration. It should be noted that many such individuals are unable to identify a precipitating event; instead, the onset of the syndrome is usually insidious.

Although there is no conclusive scientific proof of the cause of thought disturbances, many authorities believe that they are related to factors inherent in highly complex cultures such as that of the United States. Recent studies point to the influence of a genetic factor in schizophrenia and some authorities believe that there is likely to be a certain biochemical composition that predisposes individuals to an inadequate adaptation to stress. Credence is given to these theories by the number of schizophrenic individuals whose families report that, even as infants, these persons resisted attempts at cuddling, which set up a cyclically unsatisfying relationship between the infants and their parents. Whatever the cause it is known that most individuals who develop behavioral patterns that can be classified as schizophrenic have experienced highly unsatisfactory family relationships in their earliest formative years.

Satisfactory achievement of the first developmental task is almost always absent in the individual who develops a thought disturbance in later life. Consequently the individual develops a sense of basic mistrust rather than a sense of trust and even as a child behaves in a way that indicates his suspicion of others. This behavior in turn may elicit a conflictual response from significant others. Conflictual feedback from significant others is a potent stressor and often elicits the adaptation of massive anxiety, which in turn is a further stressor. This cyclical phenomenon characteristically results in a "not-me" self-concept whereby the individual grows up having an ill-defined sense of identity.

Although there are many theories related to the causative, or etiological, factors underlying schizophrenia, the theory that seems to have the most relevance for nursing practice is the one that postulates that faulty interpersonal relationships in the early family relationship is a major contributory factor to the ultimate development of the illness. Several theorists, the foremost of whom is Gregory Bateson, have suggested that a particular type of dysfunctional communication is present in families in which there is a schizophrenic individual. This type of communication is called the *double-bind*. A double-bind communication is one that gives two contradictory messages at the same time, thereby forcing the receiver of the messages to make a choice between at least two feelings, thoughts, or behaviors that contradict each other. An example of this type of paradoxical communication occurs when the mothering one overtly and covertly conveys to her child that to make her happy he must love her most while at the same time he must love all in the family equally. Obviously the child cannot succeed in such a situation. If such patterns of communication become the rule rather than the exception the child is likely to develop a high degree of anxiety that increasingly interferes with his ability to perceive reality accurately. It is hypothesized that the child adapts to the stress of his environment by not responding to either aspect of the message, thereby avoiding overt or covert punishment and perhaps reducing anxiety to a manageable level. Although this adaptation serves a protective function it does not enable the child to meet his needs and minimizes opportunities for the development of coping mechanisms that would be useful in other situations later in life.

It is important to understand that the initial adaptation of the child to his environment is functional in that it serves a protective purpose. Once learned however, it becomes difficult if not impossible for the growing child to alter his response in other situations in which the communication is healthy. Therefore the response that was functional in the original situation becomes dysfunctional in other situations. Furthermore the feedback given to this person is frequently negative, thereby establishing a vicious cycle that further increases the dysfunctional aspects of the communication. It is not uncommon for family members, teachers, and friends of a newly diagnosed schizophrenic person to give health personnel an account of an individual who had "always been a little different, shy, aloof," even though this may be the first time his behavior could be described as unusual enough to warrant medical attention.

The theory that faulty interpersonal relationships in early life are a major causative factor in the later development of schizophrenia has great relevance for nursing practice because it gives the nurse the opporunity to provide the client with corrective experiences in which he can unlearn the previously learned dysfunctional patterns of relating and learn healthier, functional patterns. It is often said that the most potent tool available to the nurse who works with the mentally ill is the therapeutic use of self, and it is through this use of self that the nurse provides experiences that have the potential to be corrective.

NURSING CARE OF ADULTS WITH THOUGHT DISTURBANCES
Nursing assessment

When assessing the behavior of an individual it is important for the nurse to remember that the classification of schizophrenia into five types is only of academic interest and has no practical significance from the nursing standpoint. It is valuable to recognize that the behavior of these persons is expressing a need and may fluctuate in an apparently unpredictable manner. It is necessary for the nurse to attempt to understand the needs of these persons rather than to focus on the diagnostic entities.

Behaviors the nurse might commonly observe in the person with a thought disturbance are those that relate to withdrawal (including hallucinations), feelings of suspiciousness, psychomotor retardation or overactivity, regression, social ineptitude, and unmet physical needs. Although each of these behaviors is discussed as a separate entity, it should be understood that they are all interrelated and stem from similar underlying dynamics. Therefore nursing care directed at altering one behavior will inevitably have an effect on others.

Withdrawal is characterized by retreating into a fantasy world of one's own design, termed *autism*. Autism is a form of thinking that does not take reality factors into account. The person creates a fantasy world of his own designed to fulfill needs and wishes that have not been met through the resources available in the world of reality. As such this autistic world is unique to the person and is difficult for anyone else to understand. One can understand autistic thinking to some degree by recalling the daydreaming frequently engaged in by adolescents. The process is similar in that both autistic thinking and daydreaming are designed to meet unfulfilled needs. A major difference is that the daydreamer can easily call himself back to the world of reality, whereas the individual who is engaged in autistic thinking cannot.

It is not unusual to hear someone describe withdrawn behavior with phrases such as, "I feel there is an intangible wall between us" or "I just can't seem to get through to him." A withdrawn person frequently spends most of his time by himself, seemingly ignoring persons and situations around him. He may be mute and at best speaks very little and in clipped, short phrases. Withdrawn behavior appears superficially similar to behavior resulting from depression. However, in a short time the observer will be able to distinguish between the two in that little or no feeling tone (affect) is perceived with the withdrawn person, whereas the depressed person conveys overwhelming feelings of sadness and hopelessness.

Hallucinations are common symptoms associated with withdrawn behavior. The individual experiencing hallucinations rarely offers this information spontaneously. Rather, he will be observed cocking his head to one side as if listening, staring into space as if watching something, and talking as if to someone, although no one is present.

Feelings of suspiciousness may be expressed very directly or quite indirectly. Some individuals refuse to eat because they are convinced that their food has been poisoned. This belief is an example of a delusion of persecution. Other persons may believe that those around them are talking about them and substantiate this belief by interpreting everyday events as referring to themselves (ideas of reference). More covertly some persons may show evidence of suspiciousness by such subtle clues as glancing quickly around on entering a room or, in the case of women, carrying their purse with them at all times.

Feelings of suspicousness are an adaptation to high levels of anxiety. Developing feelings of suspiciousness is an unconscious attempt to reduce anxiety to a manageable level.

Psychomotor activity refers to the level of activity of the mind and the body. It is unusual for an individual with a thought disturbance to exhibit normal psychomotor activity, that is, both mental and physical activity congruent with the requirements of the situation. Rather, the person frequently exhibits retardation or overactivity in the psychomotor realm. An extreme example of psychomotor retardation is seen in persons who are diagnosed as being in a catatonic stupor. These persons move very slowly and can take hours to walk the distance of a city block or to eat a meal. Concomitantly, they speak very slowly, which reflects an extreme slowing down of mental processes. The term *retarded* as used in this context should not be confused with the same term when it is used to refer to an intellectual deficit of a person. As previously stated, schizophrenic individuals do not suffer from intellectual impairment, although this may appear to be the case because of their temporarily diminished ability to comprehend and respond to mental stimuli. Psychomotor overactivity is manifested by loud, rapid talking (pressure of speech) and frequent rapid gross motor movements that seem aimless. Despite the quantity of activity, fine motor movements are usually impaired. This person literally finds it impossible to sit still and frequently paces, swinging his arms and talking continuously.

Regression is behavior appropriate to an age level considerably below the chronological age of the individual. Therefore regression does not refer to a specific behavior but rather to a discrepancy between the observed behavior and that expected in a healthy individual of the same age and developmental stage.

Behavior related to regression may include eating only when fed and being unable to dress oneself or carry out personal hygiene; in fact, the nurse is likely to observe disturbances in all activities of daily living.

Social ineptitude is a prominent feature of the behavior of individuals with thought disturbances. Because of the dysfunctional nature of their early childhood experiences in interpersonal relationships, these persons have not learned many of the even rudimentary social skills healthy adults take for granted. Such common occurrences as meeting people for the first time can precipitate overwhelming anxiety and may lead to highly inappropriate behavior for the situation. It is not uncommon for these persons to go to great lengths to avoid social situations and activities such as dating and team sports. Instead, they prefer to engage in solitary activities, which increases their social ineptitude and results in a cycle of withdrawal. These individuals frequently report that they have few if any friends; when they are in situations or settings where visitors or inquiries are to be expected, these two elements are in fact often lacking.

Behaviors related to unmet physical needs may or may not be related to the client's emotional problems. It cannot be overemphasized that emotional illness provides no immunity to physical illness. Therefore in the initial assessment it is imperative that the nurse determine the degree of general physical health of the client. Complaints of physical discomfort must be thoroughly investigated to determine whether they are related to physical abnormality or to the individual's emotional state.

When making the initial assessment, it is important to determine whether the person has taken any psychotropic medications and if so the kind, dosage, and frequency. The purpose of these medications is to alter emotional states biochemically, which brings about altered behavior. In addition the medications themselves may have side effects that are reflected behaviorally. It is important to differentiate between behavior induced by medications and behavior reflecting the emotional state, because the subsequent intervention differs.

Because of the nature of thought disturbances it is not uncommon to find a number of physical problems that stem from the dynamics of the emotional illness. Malnutrition is usual, either due to psychomotor retardation, suspiciousness, or generalized neglect of activities of daily living. Even though the client might not be able to tell the nurse his usual weight the nurse can observe whether or not his clothing fits properly. If an individual has been taking psychotropic medications for a period of time, especially the phenothiazines, he may be overweight, since these medications have the effect of stimulating the appetite. Obesity should not be seen as evidence of a good nutritional state; many obese people are in fact malnourished because food high in caloric value frequently has limited nutritional value.

A lack of interest in physical cleanliness and personal appearance is often one of the first changes to occur. The person with a thought disturbance may be disheveled or may be dressed bizarrely.

The individual may be confused and therefore may not spontaneously report a physical condition of long standing such as diabetes or hypothyroidism caused by a thyroidectomy, either of which may require daily supplemental medication. The nurse should be alert to indications of these and other physical conditions by observing for such evidence as scars or injection marks.

Because of psychomotor retardation or overactivity the person may have circulatory problems evidenced by peripheral edema or may be verging on a state of exhaustion.

Nursing diagnosis

As with all nursing diagnoses, the nursing diagnoses for the individual with thought disturbances are based on the themes identified during the assessment phase of the nursing process. Diagnostic categories approved by the Fifth National Conference on Nursing Diagnoses that may be specifically applicable to individuals with thought disturbances include the following:

Impaired verbal communication related to psychosis
Alteration in health maintenance related to lack of ability to make deliberate and thoughtful judgments
Alteration in health maintenance related to perceptual impairment
Impaired home maintenance management related to impaired emotional functioning
Impaired physical mobility related to perceptual impairment
Self-care deficit in feeding, bathing, hygiene, dressing, grooming, and toileting related to perceptual impairment
Disturbance in personal identity related to (to be developed)
Sensory-perceptual alteration: visual, auditory, kinesthetic, gustatory, tactile, olfactory, related to psychological stress
Social isolation related to alterations in mental status and unaccepted social behavior
Alteration in thought processes related to psychological conflicts and impaired judgment
Potential for violence directed at others related to catatonic excitement

This list of nursing diagnoses is not meant to be all inclusive or necessarily applicable to all clients with thought disturbances.

Refer to Table 12-1 in Chapter 12 for a complete list of approved nursing diagnoses.

For the nursing diagnosis to fulfill its function of providing direction for planning nursing care, the nurse may find it desirable to formulate her own diagnoses specific to the client. Examples of nursing diagnoses that stem from the assessment data just discussed could include the following:

Auditory hallucinations related to withdrawal
Delusions of persecution related to feelings of suspiciousness
Physical inactivity related to psychomotor retardation
Inability to feed self related to regression

Planning and implementing nursing care

The plan for nursing care should be derived from the nursing diagnoses and include the objectives of the care, their rationale, the nursing actions, and outcome criteria. To be effective this plan needs to be highly individualized. The suggestions that follow should be seen as general guidelines to be used if they are appropriate to the client's needs. All too often the individual is required to conform to the dictates of a set nursing care plan rather than receiving care specifically designed for him.

The objectives of all nursing care for persons with thought disturbances should relate to helping the client increase his ability to adapt to reality. If the client is allowed to continue to withdraw into his autistic world he becomes increasingly less capable of relating to others and less amenable to therapeutic interventions.

Underlying the withdrawal tendencies in persons with a thought disturbance is a consistent affective indifference or emotional impoverishment. This lack of appropriate feeling makes it difficult for the nurse to express warmth and demonstrate spontaneous interest in the client. It is helpful when the nurse understands that the individual feels lonely, isolated, and hungry for human contact but is often incapable of inviting a friendly approach from another person. Only when the plan directs the nurse to approach the individual with an accepting attitude and with friendliness can she be a source of therapeutic help.

The behavior of a person with a thought disturbance is invariably difficult to understand because it is unconsciously motivated and may have little logical relation to the immediate environmental situation. Frequently the client is out of contact with reality. This means that he is motivated by his thoughts and is not sure what is the real world and what is a result of his fantasies. Thus he may fuse or confuse his fantasy world with the world of reality. *Inappropriate* and *bizarre* may be accurate descriptive terms for much of his behavior, which is significant and meaningful only when considered from the standpoint of his emotional or instinctual needs. Although this behavior is often difficult to understand it does have real meaning for the client, and if it is closely studied the meaning often becomes obvious. One important aspect of the nursing care plan is to record what the nurse observes the client doing and saying.

Although most clients show every outward manifestation of physical maturity they are essentially struggling with many psychogenic conflicts that originated in childhood. Since their problems probably evolved at an early age from faulty emotional relationships between them and significant adults in their environment, corrective interpersonal experiences must be planned for and provided. Therefore it is highly desirable for the nurse to develop a relationship with the client in which she becomes a significant other. The nurse-client relationship is a vehicle for providing a corrective emotional experience in which the client experiences, over a period of time, the unconditional positive regard of another person who communicates in a healthy functional way.

In group settings a corrective family situation can be simulated. Often a physician assumes the role of a kindly understanding father, a nurse that of a wise, accepting mother, and other clients that of siblings. If such a simulated family experience gives the client sufficient love and acceptance over a period of time he can be helped to deal more realistically with his conflicts and can achieve some feeling of security. Calling the client Mr. Smith instead of John is a way of suggesting that he is expected to assume an adult role. Using a title that connotes respect, whatever it may be, is generally an incentive to more acceptable behavior and may convey to the client the idea that he is an important person.

The use of long and involved sentences should be avoided. Many persons with thought disturbances are easily confused and have a limited attention span. Short phrases are more effective and specific words more helpful than generalizations. For instance, *ice cream* is more meaningful than *dessert,* and *ham* is more specific than *meat.*

The nurse may be tempted to exploit the negativism displayed by some clients. She may request the client to walk backward when she assumes that he will do the exact opposite, which is the reaction actually desired. Use of negativism however in such activities as feeding the client and in giving medication may increase his confusion and encourage complete withdrawal.

Similarly making use of delusions and hallucinations to direct the client's behavior should be avoided. If, for instance, he hallucinates and believes that he hears the voice of his mother the nurse may be tempted to say that his mother just told him to eat his lunch. If the client believes himself to be John the Baptist, it might seem at first, on that delusional assumption, he can be persuaded to be more careful of his personal hygiene. The client will cease to trust the nurse when such symptoms are used to accomplish the nurse's purpose.

It is not helpful to try to explain away the individual's false ideas or argue with him about them. Such an approach will cause the individual to become increasingly hostile and suspicious. If one recognizes the significance of the delusion to the person and the fact that life is intolerable to him without this ego-saving device, the futility of trying to change the individual's ideas will become obvious. It is a wise plan to listen respectfully to the client without commenting on the content of his conversation.

If a client asks for a confirmation of his hallucinations, it is better to answer truthfully, "No, Mr. Jones, I do not see the face of Christ on the wall" or "No, Mr. Smith, your face is not that of a dog." It is wise to give honest replies that focus on reality.

Meticulous honesty and fairness on the part of the nurse are of primary importance. Should the client make a request with which it is impossible to comply, a suitable answer is, "I am sorry that I am not allowed to carry out such a procedure." Once a promise is made the nurse is obligated to carry it out. If possible all requests and questions should be answered. If no answer is possible the client should be informed that his request will be referred to an appropriate person who can give an answer or that the answer is truly not known.

When behaviors resulting from feelings of suspiciousness are prominent it is important to remember that the person is essentially shy, sensitive, and unable to relate positively to others. Because he has never learned to trust he resorts to the mental mechanisms of projection to cope with his environment and therefore places the blame for his inadequacies on people and objects about him. Hostility is frequently a dominant attitude. Insight is poor and usually the client is convinced that he is being treated illegally or without just cause. Consequently he may engage in threatening behavior, which can become dangerous to others if his anxiety becomes unmanageable.

Such a person rarely desires to enter group activity. As a defense, suspicious persons are usually aloof, sarcastic, and generally hostile toward everyone about them. This behavior is actually based on intrapersonal fear and anxiety and the nurse who truly appreciates this fact will not feel personally threatened and therefore will remain with the individual and try to allay his fear and anxiety.

Such fearful, hostile people must be approached with utmost tact and understanding. Solitary activities are more successful for them initially than are group activities.

Arguments with such individuals should be avoided since any controversy is at once integrated into the individual's delusional system. To obtain the confidence of a paranoid person requires the patient and persistent application of tact, tolerance of his hostile attitude, and a quiet consistency in establishing a relationship with him.

Because of the client's extreme sensitivity and fear of being unacceptable to others the nurse should take the initiative in stimulating his interest in social activity and recreation. It is important that the nurse know something of the client's background. With this knowledge she can initiate conversations in which he can participate. When the client develops a feeling of trust in the nurse participation in some recreational activity can then be encouraged. This may be accomplished by extending an invitation such as, "I need a partner for a game of table tennis; come and play with me." It may be best for the nurse alone to play a game with the client to help him feel secure. The nurse should provide opportunities for him to have some successful experiences. Gradually other participants can be added as he develops more confidence. These participants should be other clients and staff members who relate well with him and will promote his sense of being accepted. Staff members should be a stable group and the same individuals, including the nurse, should continue this program of socialization for several weeks or even months.

One aspect of the nurse's responsibility lies in the supervision of personal hygiene and in encouraging the client to bathe. Suspicious persons usually take at least adequate care of their own personal hygiene. However, they may make demands such as complete bathroom privacy. It is important for the nurse to help the client take responsibility for his own personal hygiene and grooming. Clients should be encouraged and helped to look as attractive as possible, since a pleasing appearance is likely to elicit the sorely needed positive reflected appraisals of others. Nurses can initiate a positive relationship by planning to help clients with all aspects of good grooming. The services of a beautician are invaluable, and it may also be of great therapeutic benefit to have female clients arrange each other's hair. Male clients should be encouraged to shave, to keep their hair well groomed, and to dress neatly.

Planning for adequate food intake for clients is a major nursing responsibility. In the case of a client who exhibits psychomotor retardation planning and cooking a meal may be temporarily beyond his ability. It is perfectly appropriate for the nurse to initiate such plans by helping him to prepare lists or by arranging to have his food preparation and intake supervised by others. In the case of an overactive patient foods that are high in caloric and protein value, that require little preparation, and that can be eaten easily are to be encouraged. Milk shakes are an example of a food that meets these criteria. The nurse's interest in the client's food intake often enhances their relationship because of the symbolic link between food and security.

Persons who retreat into a fantasy world often ignore physical illness and may offer no complaints even when the condition is a painful one. Acute mastoiditis, cystitis, lung abscess, and a broken bone in the hand or foot are examples of serious disorders that have been known to exist without complaint on the part of individuals with thought disturbances. The nurse should plan to be constantly alert to the physical condition of clients.

Standing and sitting in one position for hours may be observed frequently among persons displaying psychomotor retardation. Edema and cyanosis of the extremities are likely to develop. To avoid this the client should be encouraged to take some exercise even if it is only to walk up and down a hall.

Other physical problems may result from the chemotherapy the client may receive. It is imperative that the nurse know which medications if any, the client is taking and plan to purposefully observe for any untoward reactions.

CASE FORMULATION
a withdrawn individual

Frances B. was 19 years of age when she was admitted to the hospital. The only child of missionary parents, she was born in a mission station in Africa. Her father was a quiet-spoken man, definitely ascetic and consistent in his practice of religious teachings. The girl's mother was more practical and tolerant but was dominated by her husband. They were so busy with the work of the mission that they had little time to spend with their daughter.

During the first 5 years of her life, Frances's only playmates were native children. Toward them, she had always taken an attitude of superiority. On entering a boarding school in the United States at the age of 5, she had difficulty with her classmates. She was inclined to be too critical with them and insisted on dictating to them about personal matters. In her twelfth year she had a long siege of pneumonia, after which she lost weight and was chronically anemic and undernourished. She spent long hours in prayer and wrote endless letters to her parents, most of them consisting of long quotations from the Bible. She insisted on wearing old, worn clothing to the schoolroom and bitterly criticized classmates for not doing likewise.

Although her parents returned on furlough every 5 years, they could spend only a few days with her because they had many church meetings to attend while in the United States.

Her social behavior changed somewhat in her high school years, but she made few friends. She had a dog to which she was greatly attached, and she spent most of her free time in his company, taking long walks. She showed a preference for mathematics and biblical history.

Continued.

Frances entered the freshman year of college some 11 months before her admission to the psychiatric hospital. Although her scholastic record was good, she was known as a strange girl who avoided company, smiled a great deal to herself, and demonstrated no interest in the opposite sex. Her parents, while on furlough from Africa, visited her during the Christmas holidays, and her mother expressed fear that she was not emotionally well. She manifested little interest in their visit, in spite of the fact that she had not seen her parents for over 5 years.

During the commencement festivities she disappeared from the campus for several days; later it was learned that she had spent the time at an evangelical camp meeting. She remained on the campus during the summer months to take some advanced courses in mathematics. During this interval she roomed with two other young women in the house of one of the faculty members. The latter were in the habit of discussing their love affairs in her presence, and she suddenly manifested an unusual interest in their conversations. Among other things, she inquired about various matters of sex and how to approach members of the opposite sex. A few nights later she informed one of the girls that she saw the face of her future husband in the light fixture. She scrutinized the fixture for several hours, during which she sat in a trancelike state with a smile on her face. Early the next morning she spoke to a 13-year-old newsboy and informed him that she would marry him. When he made light of this proposal, she became upset, struck him in the face, and chased him down the street. Returning to her room, she tore out the light fixture, removed her clothing, and became unmanageable.

On being admitted to the psychiatric hospital, she refused to answer questions. She smiled to herself and identified the house physician as "Herbert." She insisted on having the window opened because "they are playing the wedding march." Her speech was incoherent; she was definitely hallucinating and stated that she was hearing voices that questioned her moral standards.

For the first few days she talked a great deal about a fantasized courtship in which she was the central character. She carried on a dialogue, at one time representing the lover, at another time the maiden. After this she entered a long period of silence, during which she was mute, resistive, and refused food. Occasionally she said, "If thy eye offend thee, cut it out." One evening she almost succeeded in enucleating her right eye with the thumb and forefinger of her right hand. She continued to talk incoherently, laughed a great deal, and made little attempt to keep her person clean.

nursing assessment

The history of Frances's life experiences gives us little information about her as a child. We do know that her father dominated both the home and the mother and placed the welfare of the mission above all else. It is quite possible that her care even as an infant was relegated to employed native women who may not have remained in the household consistently. In the development of a sense of personal security, the first 5 years of a child's life are crucial. The type of mothering person by whom the child is nurtured is of the greatest importance, especially in developing a sense of trust.

At the age of 5 years Frances B. was sent away to a boarding school. Although this was probably the best plan the parents could develop, it was apparently not helpful to the girl. Authorities believe that this period of time in a child's life is of great significance in the scheme of psychosexual development. During this period the child is beginning to identify with the parent of the same sex, has discovered that the sexual organ is a source of pleasurable sensations, and has recognized the structural difference between the sex organs of boys and girls. As has been mentioned in a previous chapter, castration fears or concern about the loss of the penis are sources of anxiety for children of this age. A boy may be concerned for fear he will be deprived of the penis as punishment, and a girl may fear that she was deprived of a penis because of some earlier punishment or accident. When a child in this age period is removed from the parents, he is apt to feel banished as a punishment for some transgression. Since sexual longings and fantasies have occupied some of the child's thoughts and since the child realizes that these are frowned on by the parents, it is natural for the child to feel that the banishment is related to "bad" thoughts.

Frances undoubtedly felt banished by being sent to boarding school. Because of her father's strict and rigid attitudes, it is quite likely that Frances was convinced that she was being punished. Even when parents are not a source of comfort and security for a child, the child mourns their loss when separated from them because they are the only significant reality known. Thus it is reasonable to believe that Frances passed through a period of loneliness and bereavement at being deprived from the only mothering person she knew.

Initially, children protest this separation by crying or by other aggressive acting-out behavior. After several days of hopelessness and withdrawal from activity, the child usually becomes detached and seems unwilling to resume a close relationship with any adult, even if the lost person returns. This detached attitude could be altered if the parent returned and remained with the child consistently. However, in

Continued.

the situation being discussed the little girl undoubtedly developed a detached attitude toward other people and attempted to isolate herself personally to avoid anxiety resulting from fear of being cast aside and abandoned a second time. Her subsequent attachment to a dog suggested that she could not trust another person with her love and therefore gave it to an animal who made no demands and gave her unconditional devotion.

After Frances had a serious illness at the age of 12, she began to spend long hours in prayer, wrote letters to her parents filled with quotes from the Bible, and wore her shoddiest clothing to school. This behavior suggests that she was seeking to gain the favor and forgiveness of her parents, who in her fantasies may have been God's representatives on earth. Undoubtedly she felt unworthy of anything better when she chose to wear old and shoddy clothing to school and again was seeking to atone for fantasized sin.

Her unusual interest in the sexual affairs of other girls of her age and the inappropriate proposal of marriage was a reactivation of the very early problem of failure to develop an integrated ego. This person developed a limited capacity to clearly evaluate the realities of the situation in which she found herself. In addition, the weak ego development made it difficult if not impossible to resolve the conflicts between the id drives (interest in sex and marriage) and demands of the superego (the incorporated standards of her parents). Likewise, she had never been able to effectively repress hostile aggressive drives and expressed these feelings freely by tearing out the light fixture.

When Frances saw the face of her future husband in the light fixture, she was exhibiting a severe mental symptom called visual hallucinations. Hallucinations are one example of the personality disintegration that takes place in individuals suffering from an active psychosis. Hallucinations, like all symptoms, meet a basic need. In this situation the face supplied an answer for her that was an outgrowth of her unconscious longing and her inability to find answers to her own sexual needs through coping adequately with the social situation.

Hallucinations are an example of being out of touch with reality. The person experiencing hallucinations is reacting to a stimulus from within the unconscious mind that is unrelated to the real situation. The behavior of such a person becomes extremely confusing when she reacts part of the time to stimuli from the real world and part of the time to stimuli from within her own unconscious mind.

nursing diagnosis

The assessment data, including present behavior, past life experiences, and an understanding of the underlying dynamics, led to the development of the following nursing diagnoses for Frances:

> Inability to develop interpersonal relationships related to fear of abandonment
>
> Violence directed toward self related to visual and auditory hallucinations
>
> Lack of attention to personal hygiene and nutrition related to feelings of worthlessness

planning and implementing nursing care for FRANCES B.

The boxed material on p. 284 is a sample nursing care plan designed for Frances. Because this client was so acutely ill on admission, all the objectives are short term.

The logical starting point in carrying out the plan was the establishment of a positive relationship with Frances. It was hoped that this relationship would lead to the development of some communication with her.

Because the nurse knew that persons with thought disturbances are highly fearful of rejection, the approach to Frances was unhurried, warm, friendly, and accepting. The nurse found it necessary to make repeated verbal overtures and to modify her own nonverbal messages to Frances before Frances was able to respond.

It was decided that the entire responsibility for the nursing care of Frances during the first weeks of her hospital experience would be assigned to a few carefully chosen nurses. This decision was made because the staff recognized that Frances needed to develop a feeling of security and to learn to trust other people. Security can be enhanced by limiting the number of individuals with whom such ill persons come in contact and by keeping their daily routines much the same for several months. In the beginning, few demands were made on Frances.

It is recognized that the attitude of the people with whom mentally ill persons come in contact during the early part of their illness has a significant effect on their recovery. Persons such as Frances require consistent acceptance, sincere interest, and constant encouragement from nurses and the other members of the professional staff.

Although communication with Frances was difficult because she used language in a highly personal way it was important for the nurse to spend time sitting with her and talking to her even though she rarely responded verbally. The nurse used simple, uncomplicated, direct statements when talking to her.

Continued.

nursing care plan for
FRANCES B.

nursing diagnosis	objective	rationale	nursing actions	outcome criteria
Inability to develop interpersonal relationships related to fear of abandonment	To assist the client to develop a sense of trust in another human being	Ability to trust is fundamental to the development of satisfactory interpersonal relationships; can be achieved only through experiencing a relationship with another human being who is accepting and meticulously consistent	Assigned nurse establishes relationship with client Approach client in a calm, friendly manner Orient client to purpose and structure of relationship Determine times and places for meeting 3 times a day for 20 minutes Convey consistent acceptance of client as an individual who has value and worth Use simple, direct statements when talking with client Sit silently with client if she is hallucinating	Within 1 month client will: Call nurse by name Show evidence of begining trust in assigned nurse by appearing for meetings on time
Violence directed toward self related to visual and auditory hallucinations	To diminish frequency of hallucinations	Hallucinations direct client to injure herself	Administer antipsychotic medication as prescribed Observe for side effects and adverse reactions to medications Reassure client about side effects Record medications given Observe for and record changes in behavior indicative of hallucinations	Within 2 weeks client will manifest behavior indicative of hallucinations only when exposed to numerous external stimuli, such as 2 persons talking to her at the same time
	To protect client from self-destructive acts	Self-destructive acts are not only physically injurious, they also contribute to client's sense of worthlessness	Restrain client as necessary Do *not* reprimand client if she attempts to injure self	Within 2 weeks client will not attempt to injure self

nursing care plan for
FRANCES B.—cont'd

nursing diagnosis	objective	rationale	nursing actions	outcome criteria
Lack of attention to personal hygiene and nutrition related to feelings of worthlessness	To assist client to assume responsibility for bathing and dressing appropriately	Personal hygiene and appropriate dress contribute to enhanced self-esteem	Establish and implement routine for bathing and dressing Bathe client as necessary Dress client as necessary Encourage client to assist with bathing and dressing	Within 2 weeks client will show interest in activities of bathing and dressing as manifested by such statements as "I'll wash my own face."
	To provide adequate nutrition	Increase resistance to physical illness Maintain physiological homeokinesis	Ascertain and serve, if possible, client's favorite foods Present food in small amounts Help client eat by providing simple directions Spoon feed if necessary Allow client to eat at her own pace Record amount eaten Encourage client to go to dining room, accompany if she indicates desire to go	Within 2 weeks client will eat 1800 calories among three well balanced meals in the dining room

These nursing interventions were related to the plan for development of a satisfactory relationship with a significant other, which would in turn decrease Frances's fears of abandonment. In addition much of her behavior was symptomatic of an individual who felt unworthy and guilty, and it was obvious that Frances's self-esteem was badly shattered. Thus the nurse's efforts were focused on trying to assist Frances to develop a more positive attitude toward herself. This was partially achieved by the attention provided for her and the sincere, interested way in which it was given. Self-esteem was also enhanced through the mechanism of assisting her to improve her grooming.

Early in Frances's hospital experience it was necessary for a

Continued.

nurse to assume a good deal of responsibility for bathing and dressing her, but in time she was encouraged to assume more and more responsibility for this activity herself. The nurses gently suggested that she would enjoy visiting the beauty parlor. At first they accompanied her on these trips and remained with her while she was there.

The dietary intake for persons who refuse food is always of great concern. Because Frances regressed when she was first admitted, the nurses tried to help her in feeding herself by making suggestions such as, "Pick up your fork" and "Put the food in your mouth." This plan was used because it was thought that she was unable to make the necessary decisions herself. However, it was eventually necessary to spoon-feed her. The nurses used an unhurried, relaxed manner and fed her from a tray in her own room.

During the spoon-feeding periods the nurses gave Frances many opportunities to take the spoon in her own hand and assume some of the responsibility for feeding herself during a part of the meal. After a few weeks she was encouraged to return to the dining room and take her meals with others.

The problem of self-destruction was especially distressing. Criticism and reprimands for this behavior were withheld because the nurses realized that it would confirm her opinion that she was indeed a bad person. The close personal attention Frances received when she was first admitted solved the problem of self-destruction during the early part of her hospitalization. However, she was helped to reestablish her own inner controls, and the nurse served as an external authority until Frances was able to accept responsibility for her own safety.

evaluation

Evaluation of the plan of nursing care and its implementation was based on outcome criteria established at the time the plan was formulated. Since the nurse knew that Frances's illness had developed slowly and insidiously, the outcome criteria she established reflected the expectation of small but significant gains. The nurse continuously reassessed the client as she provided care. As anticipated, after 2 weeks Frances was able to accept most of the responsibility for her own grooming and ate in the dining room with the other clients. In addition, days elapsed without any evidence of hallucinations and her self-destructive behavior had stopped.

After 1 month Frances showed little evidence of accepting her assigned nurse as a significant other. Although she did call the nurse by name and seemed to recognize her at most times, she rarely appeared for their meetings at the agreed-upon time. Frances's nurse was discouraged about this and arranged to have the nursing care plan reviewed at a team meeting. In view of this client's history with significant others and her progress in other areas, the team felt that the nurse's outcome criteria for this diagnosis were unrealistic in terms of time. As a result, the nurse revised this aspect of the care plan to indicate a 6-week time frame.

After 6 weeks, Frances's behavior did indicate a beginning level of trust in her assigned nurse. At that time the nurse reassessed the client's condition, developed revised nursing diagnoses, and designed a new plan of care that indicated long-term goals. She was careful to develop outcome criteria that were realistic in light of Frances's lifetime of unsatisfactory adaptation. It was anticipated that Frances could be expected to recover sufficiently to be discharged to a sheltered living situation but it was likely she would require a maintenance dose of the prescribed antipsychotic medication.

CONCLUDING STATEMENTS

1. When an individual is functioning on the basis of a grossly distorted perception of reality due to factors other than demonstrable organic disease or intellectual deficit he is said to be suffering from a functional psychosis.
2. Schizophrenia is the most serious functional psychosis.
3. To be diagnosed as schizophrenic the individual must exhibit characteristic delusions, characteristic hallucinations, or other characteristic symptoms of thought impairment accompanied by blunted, flat, or inappropriate affect. Thus schizophrenia is a thought disturbance.
4. Schizophrenia is classified into five major types, depending on the predominant behavioral patterns displayed.
5. The outlook for a person suffering from a thought disturbance depends on the effectiveness of his prepsychotic personality, the nature of the onset of the illness, and the timing and nature of the treatment he receives.
6. There is no conclusive scientific proof of the cause of schizophrenia, but the theory that seems most relevant for nursing

practice postulates that faulty interpersonal relationships in the early family relationship are a major contributory factor to the ultimate development of the illness.

7. It is believed that the development of schizophrenia is a long-standing process although the acute symptoms may appear abruptly, usually during adolescence or early adulthood.

8. Behaviors the nurse might commonly observe in the person with a thought disturbance are those that relate to withdrawal, feelings of suspiciousness, psychomotor retardation or overactivity, regression, social ineptitude, and unmet physical needs.

9. An individualized nursing care plan, based on nursing diagnoses that reflect an understanding of the assessment data, enables the nurse to select appropriate interventions that are designed to act as corrective experiences for these individuals.

SUGGESTED SOURCES OF ADDITIONAL INFORMATION

Classical

Bateson, Gregory, et al.: Toward a theory of schizophrenia. In Howells, J.G., editor: Theory and practice of family psychiatry, New York, 1971, Brunner/Mazel, Inc.

Bellak, Leopold, and Loeb, Laurence, editors: The schizophrenic syndrome, New York, 1969, Gune & Stratton, Inc.

Carl, Mary Kathryn: Establishing a relationship with a schizophrenic patient, Perspect. Psychiatr. Care **1:**20-22, March-April, 1963.

Cook, J.C.: Interpreting and decoding autistic communication, Perspect. Psychiatr. Care **9:**24-28, Jan.-Feb., 1971.

Dunham, H.W.: Sociocultural studies of schizophrenia, Arch. Gen. Psychiatry **21:**206-214, 1971.

Field, William E., and Ruelke, Wylma: Hallucinations and how to deal with them, Am. J. Nurs. **73:**638-640, 1973.

Gregory, D.: Russel and I (an experience with autism), Perspect. Psychiatr. Care **9:**29, Jan.-Feb., 1971.

Kaplan, Bert: The inner world of mental illness: a series of first person accounts of what is was like, New York, 1964, Harper & Row, Publishers.

Kline, Nathan S.: Synopsis of Eugen Bleuler's dementia praecox, New York, 1966, International Universities Press.

Lidz, Theodore, Fleck, Stephen, and Cornelison, Alice R.: Schizophrenia and the family, New York, 1967, International Universities Press.

Lipkin, Gladys B., and Cohen, Roberta G.: Effective approaches to patients' behavior, New York, 1980, Springer Publishing Co., Inc.

Peplau, Hildegard E.: Loneliness, Am. J. Nurs. **55:**1476-1481, 1955.

Robinson, Alice M.: Communicating with schizophrenic patients, Am. J. Nurs. **60:**1120-1123, 1960.

Schwartz, Charlotte Green, Schwartz, Morris S., and Stanton, Alfred H.: A study of need-fulfillment on a mental hospital ward, Psychiatry **14:**223-242, 1951.

Schwartz, Morris S., and Shockley, Emmy L.: The nurse and the mental patient, New York, 1956, John Wiley & Sons, Inc.

Schwartz, Morris S., and Will, Gwen Tudor: Low morale and mutual withdrawal on a mental hospital ward, Psychiatry **16:**337-353, 1953.

Searles, Harold: The nonhuman environment in normal development and in schizophrenia, New York, 1960, International Universities Press.

Sechehaye, Marguerite: Autobiography of a schizophrenic girl, New York, 1970, W.W. Norton & Co. Inc.

Stankiewicz, Barbara: Guides to nursing intervention in the projective patterns of suspicious patients, Perspect. Psychiatr. Care **2**(1):39-45, 1964.

Sullivan, Harry Stack: Conceptions of modern psychiatry, Washington, D.C., 1953, W.W. Norton & Co., Inc.

Contemporary

Aaronson, Lauren S.: Paranoia as a behavior of alienation, Perspect. Psychiatr. Care **15**(1):27-31, 1977.

Anders, Robert L.: When a patient becomes violent, Am. J. Nurs. **77:**1144-1148, 1977.

Anderson, Nancy P.: Suicide in schizophrenia, Perspect. Psychiatr. Care **11**(2):106-112, 1973.

Arieti, Silvano: Schizophrenia: the psychodynamic mechanisms and the psychostructural forms. In Arieti, Solvano, and Brody, Eugene B., editors: American handbook of psychiatry, ed. 2, vol. 3, New York, 1974, Basic Books, Inc., Publishers, pp. 551-587.

Arieti, Silvano: Understanding and helping the schizophrenic, New York, 1980, Basic Books, Inc., Publishers.

Bemporad, Jules R., and Pinsker, Henry: Schizophrenia: the manifest symptomatology. In Arieti, Silvano, and Brody, Eugene B., editors: American handbook of psychiatry, ed. 2, vol. 3, New York, 1974, Basic Books, Inc., Publishers, pp. 524-550.

Berckhead, Loretta: The nurse as leader: group psychotherapy with psychotic patients, J. Psychosoc. Nurs. Ment. Health Serv. **22:**24-30, June, 1984.

Berger, Milton E., editor: Beyond the double bind: communication and family systems theories, and techniques with schizophrenics, New York, 1978, Brunner/Mazel, Inc.

Cameron, Norman: Paranoid conditions and paranoia. In Arieti, Silvano, and Brody, Eugene, B., editors: American handbook of psychiatry, ed. 2, vol. 3, New York, 1974, Basic Books, Inc., Publishers, pp. 676-693.

Chamberlain, Janet: Everyman's psychosis, Perspect. Psychiatr. Care **21:**59-63, April-June, 1983.

del Campo, E.J.H., Carr, C., and Correa, E.: Rehospitalized schizophrenics, J. Psychosoc. Nurs. Ment. Health Serv. **21:**29-33, June, 1983.

Fochtman, Grace A.: Disturbances in object relations in a chronic schizophrenic patient, Perspect. Psychiatr. Care **13:**1, 13-16, Jan.-March, 1975.

Geach, Barbara, and White, James C.: Empathetic resonance: a countertransference phenomenon, Am. J. Nurs. **74:**1282-1285, 1974.

Grosicki, J., and Harmonson, M.: Nursing action guide: hallucinations, J. Psychiatr. Nurs. **7:**134, May, 1979.

Jones, Susan L.: The double-bind as a "tested" theoretical formulation—five research studies are reviewed here, Perspect. Psychiatr. Care **15**(4):162-169, 1977.

Kahn, E. Michael: Psychotherapy with chronic schizophrenics, J. Psychosoc. Nurs. Ment. Health Serv. **22:**20-25, July, 1984.

Kerr, Norine: Anxiety: theoretical considerations, Perspect. Psychiatr. Care **16**(1):36-40, Jan.-Feb., 1978.

Kerr, Norine: The destruction of "goodness" in the borderline character pathology, Perspect. Psychiatr. Care **17:**40-47, Jan.-Feb., 1979.

Koontz, Elizabeth: Schizophrenia: current diagnostic concepts and implicatons for nursing care, J. Psychosoc. Nurs. Ment. Health Serv. **20:**44-48, Sept., 1982.

Lantz, James: Adlerian community treatment with schizophrenic clients, J. Psychosoc. Nurs. Ment. Health Serv. **20:**25-30, April, 1982.

Lynch, Vincent J., and Lynch, Mary Theresa: Borderline personality, perspect. Psychiatr. Care **15**(2):72-75, 1977.

Lyon, Glee G., and Hitchins, Emily A.: Ways of intervening with the psychotic individual in the community, Am. J. Nurs. **79:**490-493, March, 1979.

McGill, C., Falloon, I., Boyd, J., and Wood-Silverio, C.: Family educational intervention in the treatment of schizophrenia, Hosp. Community Psychiatry **34:**934-938, 1983.

Maurine, Judith T.: Regressed patients in group therapy, Perspect. Psychiatr. Care **8:**131-135, May-June, 1970.

Moser, Dorothy Hale: Communicating with a schizophrenic patient, Perspect. Psychiatr. Care **8:**36-41, 45, Jan.-Feb., 1970.

Ostendorf, Mary: Dan is schizophrenic—possible causes, probable courses, Am. j. Nurs. **76:**944-947, 1976.

Pope, Harrison: Distinguishing bipolar disorder from schizophrenia in clinical practice: guidelines and case reports, Hosp. Community Psychiatry **34:**322-327, 1983.

Reid, Linda: Approahces to the aftermath of schizophrenia, Perspect. Psychiatr. Care **17**(6):257-259, Nov.-Dec., 1979.

Rosenbaum, C. Peter, and Beebe, John E., III: Psychiatric treatment: crisis, clinic, consultation, New York, 1975, McGraw-Hill Book Co., pp. 88-89.

Sarbin, Theodore R., and Mancuso, James C.: Schizophrenia, medical diagnosis or moral verdict? New York, 1980, Pergamon Press, Inc.

Schmidt, Carolyn S.: Withdrawal behavior of schizophrenics: application of Roy's model, J. Psychosoc. Nurs. Ment. Health Serv. **19:**26-33, Nov., 1981.

Schroder, Patricia J.: Nursing intervention with patients with thought disorders, Perspect. Psychiatr. Care **17:**32-39, Jan.-Feb., 1979.

Stewart, Barbara M.: Biochemical aspects of schizophrenia, Am. J. Nurs. **75:**2176-2179, 1975.

Thomas, M.: Trust in the nurse-patient relationship. In Carlson, C., editor: Behavioral concepts and nursing intervention, Philadelphia, 1970, J.B. Lippincott Co.

Tousley, Martha: The paranoid fortress of David J., J. Psychosoc. Nurs. Ment. Health Serv. **22:**8-16, Feb., 1984.

Verhulst, J., and Schneidman, B.: Schizophrenia and sexual functioning, Hosp. Community Psychiatry **32:**259-262, 1981.

White, Eleanor, and Kahn, E. Michael: Use and modifications in group psychotherapy with chronic schizophrenic outpatients, J. Psychosoc. Nurs. Ment. Health Serv. **20:**14-20, Feb., 1982.

Wilson, Janet S.: Deciphering psychotic communication, Perspect. Psychiatr. Care **17**(6):254-256, Nov.-Dec., 1979.

Of particular interest

Bateson, G., et al.: Toward a theory of schizophrenia. In Howells, J.G., editor: Theory and practice of family psychiatry, New York, 1971, Brunner/Mazel, Inc.
This classic paper presents the double-bind theory of communication patterns in families of schizophrenic clients.

Ruesch, J.: Disturbed communication, New York, 1972, W.W. Norton & Co., Inc.
Communication patterns associated with various psychiatric disorders are described and analyzed according to the author's framework of communication patterns and designing appropriate interventions.

adults
with mood
disturbances

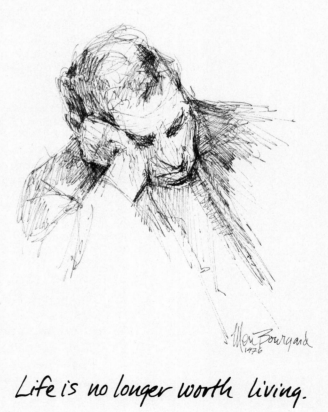

Life is no longer worth living.

LEARNING OBJECTIVES

After studying this chapter the student will be able to:

1 Differentiate between the mood states of grief and depression.

2 Discuss the dynamics of development of mood disturbances.

3 Describe behaviors the nurse is most likely to observe in an adult experiencing depression.

4 State examples of nursing diagnoses likely to be applicable to adults who are depressed.

5 Develop a hypothetical plan of nursing care for an adult who is depressed.

6 Describe those behaviors the nurse is most likely to observe in an adult who is elated and overactive.

7 State examples of nursing diagnoses likely to be applicable to adults who are elated and overactive.

8 Develop a hypothetical plan of nursing care for an adult who is elated and overactive.

All human beings are familiar with the mood states of joy and sadness. Healthy adults experience these mood states in a predictable way, usually in response to an external stimulus. Fluctuations of moods in healthy adults do not usually occur over a wide range because adults with well-integrated personalities are able to incorporate the stimulus into the total system.

However, there is great national concern about the increasing number of adults who experience disturbances in mood or wide fluctuations in mood states. Middle-aged females and the elderly of both sexes are particularly vulnerable to severe depression. The incidence of depression has been accelerating rapidly since the 1970s and shows no sign of abating. National demographic data from 1977 to 1978 indicate that over 50 of every 1000 office visits to physicians by women in the age range of 25 to 44 were for symptoms of depression.

Mood disturbances seriously interfere with the quality of life enjoyed by the affected person and his or her family. In addition, depression increases the risk of death by suicide. Nurses in all settings have a responsibility to recognize and appropriately intervene in situations where the individual is experiencing a mood disturbance.

HISTORICAL PERSPECTIVE

Mood disorders, especially depression, have been documented since ancient times. An Egyptian papyrus of 1500 BC contains a discourse on old age and says of it that "the heart grows heavy and remembers not yesterday." The Old Testament records the erratic behavior of King Saul as his moods fluctuated between elation and depression. If he were alive today this influential person would undoubtedly bear the medical diagnosis of bipolar affective disorder.

In 1896 Emil Kraepelin identified the illness known today as bipolar affective disorder and called it manic-depressive psychosis. He was among the first to recognize the cyclical nature of this disorder.

Hippocrates (460-375? BC) the greatest of the old Greek physicians, knew the symptoms of depression well and believed it resulted from a surplus of black bile, which is termed *melancholē* in the Greek language. The English word *melancholy* is derived from this Greek word.

Treatment of mood disturbances was not effective until the development of the convulsion-producing drug pentylenetetrazol (Metrazol) by Meduna followed by the introduction of electroconvulsive therapy by Cerletti and Bini in 1938. Electroconvulsive therapy was first developed as a treatment for persons with thought disorders; however, it has been found to be most effective for persons suffering from depression. Although still in use today, electroconvulsive therapy has been supplanted as a treatment for mood disorders by the psychotropic agents, specifically the antidepressant medications and lithium carbonate.

AFFECTIVE DISORDERS

Some individuals adapt to extreme feelings of anxiety, loneliness, inadequacy, and failure by overactivity, elated mood, and excessive talkativeness. The elated mood may be so pronounced and sustained that the individual expresses the belief that every good thing is possible or will soon be consumated and every wish will be fulfilled. Ideas emerge in an easy, fluid manner; thinking seems to be effortless; memory is quickened; and the individual shows a quick but superficial wit. There is an apparent sense of self-security, and fears are pushed to the background. The individual may be aggressive, cocksure in his opinions, and ready to talk with conviction on anything and everything. The ego seems to be unrestrained, and ideas pour out so rapidly and with such ease that the tongue cannot give them full expression. Hence the individual may utter only segments of ideas and may jump from one to another in a rapid barrage. He recognizes persons and objects quickly and has a tendency to argue. The person is apt to be domineering and becomes irritable, denunciatory, and hypercritical of everything that interferes with his desire for free action. He is likely to become overactive and may extend this excessive motor excitement in every direction. When limits must be set for his behavior, he sometimes becomes noisy, belligerent, and violent. His insight is always poor. This person's interest is in the outside world rather than in himself. His ideation is concerned with his environment. In fact, the individual can almost be said to be at the mercy of his environment.

Surprising as it may seem, at another time such an aggressive, overactive individual may use quite different behavior to defend against the same bad feelings. Within a few months he may be sad, may have difficulty in thinking and expressing thoughts, and may be very slow in his physical responses, or he may exhibit agitation.

Such a person may have difficulty in formulating answers, may lose his ability to concentrate, and may be unable to choose a direct line of action. The individual may be tormented by a sense of insecurity or by ideas of remorse and self-abasement or may be overcome by a sense of guilt. He may complain of a total lack of affection and of a loss of interest in the things for which he formerly had much concern. He may feel that he is lost or being punished. Such a person may have an overpowering sense of futility, a "feeling of emptiness," and a desire to retreat from everything, to seek oblivion, and to end his life. The danger of suicide is the outstanding feature of this condition, and this alone justifies the greatest caution and consideration in care and treatment.

If an individual maintains behavior marked by elation and overactivity, he is likely to carry the medical diagnosis of bipolar affective disorder, manic phase. If the behavior is predominantly characteristic of depression, the individual is said to be in the depressed phase of this illness. When the individual's behavior moves from depression to elation or from elation to depression he is said to have a mixed bipolar affective disorder.

The probability of recovery from a single episode of overactivity or depression is great. Recurrences are to be expected, although second and third attacks need not necessarily occur. An attack of overactivity in early adult life generally means more attacks later. Depressions are more likely to occur in the later years of life.

It is never safe to predict the probable duration of any given attack. There are great variations, and even the same individual may have both short and long periods of elation and depression. The average length for all untreated attacks of elation is about 6 months; for untreated depressive episodes it is generally longer. When depressive periods show a strong element of fear, anxiety, and hypochondriasis, the condition may endure for many years. Likewise, elation may become chronic, particularly in older individuals, if it is associated with organic changes in the brain such as arteriosclerosis. Current treatments, including maintenance levels of lithium carbonate as a preventive measure, have shortened the length of attacks in both elation and depression.

An outstanding feature of affective disorders is that even after repeated attacks intellectual capacities are rarely impaired. During remissions of this disorder the individual is usually able to carry on his regular occupation and live an entirely normal life.

Although a bipolar affective disorder is a common type of affective disorder, some individuals suffer from severe mood disturbances that do not meet the criteria for this diagnosis. However, the principles stated in the following discussion are applicable to all individuals with mood disturbances, regardless of their medical diagnosis.

DIFFERENTIATION BETWEEN THOUGHT DISTURBANCES AND MOOD DISTURBANCES

It is sometimes difficult for students of nursing to differentiate between the overactivity demonstrated by some individuals with thought disturbances and the overactivity that the manic individual exhibits. Both of these individuals may be physically overactive and at times both may talk excessively. The individual who exhibits catatonic behavior may fluctuate from being almost stuporous to exhibiting explosive overactivity. In such a situation the individual is probably responding to inner thoughts and feelings that are not related to reality but that are threatening, upsetting, and disturbing. This type of overactivity is especially difficult to understand because there is often disharmony between the mood and the ideas expressed. The person may smile inappropriately or laugh while speaking of the disturbing thoughts that are uppermost in his mind. He may express terrifying visual or auditory hallucinations.

In contrast, the overactivity of an individual displaying manic behavior is characterized by glib argumentative speech that may be humorous but may change quickly to sarcasm and verbal abuse. Such a person may appear to have boundless energy. He is usually irrepressible, demanding, and irritable. He frequently expresses ideas of grandeur and delusions of having great power and wealth. There is a dominant tone of euphoria even though the person may demonstrate an underlying mood of sorrow. Authorities believe that the overactivity of the manic individual is actually a defense against depression. The professional person usually finds that manic overactivity can be understood because the client maintains some contact with reality except in the most extreme examples of this illness.

Withdrawal and depression may be difficult for the beginning student of nursing to differentiate because individuals suffering from these states are usually physically inactive. However, the individual with a thought disturbance who is withdrawn demonstrates a disharmony of thought, feeling, and behavior. Although there may be a persistent mood, it has little apparent relationship to the situation in which the person finds himself or to his past experiences. In contrast, everything about the depressed individual conveys this feeling to the observer. The way the person sits, the facial expression, the voice quality, and the ideas expressed all suggest hopelessness and a sense of impending doom. Depressed individuals remain well aware of reality, and their feelings seem understandable to individuals working with them.

Some authorities believe that the attempt to differentiate these behavioral reactions is actually an artificial and unwarranted exercise. These authorities suggest that such reactions may be aspects of one broad disease entity.

DIFFERENTIA-TION BETWEEN GRIEF AND DEPRESSION

Although grief is a human condition characterized by a disturbance in mood it is a normal, common, necessary reaction to the loss of a beloved individual or object. The nurse may help the grieving person to cope with his sense of loss and guilt by encouraging him to talk about his feelings. The goal is to assist the individual to integrate this emotional reaction with similar experiences in his past and to learn from it.

Depression is a profound disturbance in mood that shares some characteristics with grief; however, it differs in many ways. Depression is not as common an expression as grief, but it occurs frequently. All nurses should be able to differentiate between the normal reaction called grieving and the pathological elaboration of grief, which is called depression. The nurse needs to recognize that normal grieving should be encouraged and that it usually terminates within a few months or a year without professional help. In contrast, depression is not self-limiting, usually does not improve without professional help, and is dangerous for the individual because of the problem of suicide.

The following listing contrasts grief and depression in terms of cause, symptoms, and outcome.

Grief (bereavement)	Depression
1. Grief is a disturbance in mood that is normal, universal, and necessary in the life experience of individuals.	1. Depression is a disturbance in mood that is a reaction to the actual, threatened, or imagined loss of a valued object, tangible or intangible. The loss, basically rooted in the individual's fantasy life, has great symbolic value. It is an overwhelming response to what the individual considers a catastrophic loss.
2. Grief is a reaction to the *real* loss of a highly valued object that may be tangible or intangible.	2. Depression is a pathological elaboration of grief. It is related to grief but is not the same.
3. Grief is a developmentally evolved adaptive process and is closely related to the ability to develop meaningful object relationships.	3. The reaction to loss in depression goes beyond grief in duration and intensity. Depression is prolonged, severe, and increasingly incapacitating in all areas of the individual's life.
4. Grief is self-limiting and gradually diminishes over a period of about a year.	4. Depression does not enter the phase of restitution within a few weeks or months and is not self-limiting. Professional help is often required.
5. Except in the early, acute stage grief is not incapacitating.	

6. The three phases of normal grieving are
  a. Shock and disbelief.
  b. Developing awareness of the pain of the loss, which eventually results in crying.
  c. Restitution, which involves the mourning experience and eventual elevation of the memory of the lost object to a degree of perfection. (This is usually completed within a year and new objects replace the lost ones.)	

DYNAMICS OF DEVELOPMENT OF MOOD DISTURBANCES

Mood deviations extreme enough to be categorized as either manic or depressive episodes have no specific causative factors that can be identified with scientific certainty. Many scientists believe that there is a hereditary factor operating because 60% to

80% of these individuals come from families in which a history of this illness exists.

Psychiatrists who accept the theoretical explanations of behavior that have been developed by the psychoanalytic school believe that extreme mood disturbances involving elation and depression are closely related to the infant's early feeding experiences. During this period the mother who provides food and attention is both an object of love and a source of frustration for the infant. Ambivalent feelings of both love and hate for the mothering person may be initiated in this early period and may be carried out throughout life. In adult life ambivalent feelings are directed toward the environment and the significant persons in the environment. Individuals who develop extreme mood disturbances such as elation and depression are thought to be reacting to the unconscious loss of a real or fantasied love object that was incorporated at an early phase of personality development. The individual first responds as if mourning for the lost love object and eventually begins to express hostility because he feels abandoned. The aggressive, overactivity of mania is thought to be a defense against the real problem of depression.

In depression the individual is thought to turn his hostility toward himself. He feels that he is at fault, that he is responsible for the loss of the love object, and that he is unworthy; thus he hates himself. He is said to be at the mercy of a punishing, sadistic superego. Such an individual has many narcissistic love needs. His adult relationships are likely to be immature and dependent. The lifelong problems with which these individuals struggle are hostility and the feelings of guilt that the hostility precipitates when their security is threatened.

NURSING CARE OF THE DEPRESSED ADULT
Nursing assessment

The individual suffering from depression expresses despair, gloom, a sense of foreboding, feelings of guilt, ideas of self-depreciation, and perhaps self-accusatory delusions. These feelings are so overwhelming that the nurse can sense them even before the person describes them. Expressions of these feelings include statements such as, "I feel worthless, rotten, no good," "Life is a struggle," or "I don't deserve to be taken care of, I'm just a burden to everyone."

The appearance of persons who are depressed is almost always unkempt and they often have not bathed recently. They lack the energy required for bathing and grooming. Furthermore, their unattractive appearance is congruent with their mood.

The reported onset of the depression is seldom associated with a specific event or loss, as is the case with persons experiencing grief. Rather, the individual will report that he has been feeling this way "for some time" and that he has lost hope of feeling better. Interestingly, some social scientists believe that the depressed person's decision to seek help has less to do with the severity or duration of his symptoms but rather reflects the fact that his social support system has been exhausted. When an individual first becomes depressed, his mood tends to elicit sympathy from friends and family. However, after many reassurances do not effect a change these people begin to back away, thereby increasing the person's sense of isolation and worthlessness. It is believed that this is the point at which the individual reaches out for help.

Regardless of the severity of the depression, the individual will almost always report changes in sleep patterns. Less severely depressed persons find they sleep for longer intervals and more frequently than usual. More severely depressed persons report they have little difficulty falling asleep but awaken in the early hours of the morning, usually between 3 and 4 AM. At that time their feelings of loneliness, overwhelming anxiety, and worthlessness are most pronounced. Time seems to move very slowly, and they believe daylight will never come. Repeated episodes of early morning wakefulness may make them fearful of going to sleep in the evening. No matter how much sleep the depressed individual has had he complains of constant fatigue. The simplest task often seems insurmountable, requiring more mental and physical energy than the person possesses.

While lay people often associate crying with depression this expression of anguish may not be present in severely depressed individuals. Sometimes these persons may sob, but tearlessly. At other times, they may not cry but their faces wear tortured expressions.

The depressed individual may exhibit psychomotor retardation where every word and action takes monumental effort. On the other hand, this individual may display agitation, often pacing the floor and wringing the hands. When agitation is present it usually indicates the presence of anxiety as well as depression.

Depressed individuals who are inactive are prone to develop physical disorders because of their inactivity. The most common of these are fecal impaction, peripheral edema, and pneumonia. Infections are frequent but the depressed person tends to ignore the symptoms of these illnesses although he almost always reports a variety of physical complaints. These complaints generally include headaches, gastrointestinal problems such as "fullness" and constipation, and chest pains. It is these complaints that prompt so many depressed individuals to visit the doctor's office.

A marked change in weight over a relatively short period of time is often associated with the client's physical complaints. Some less severely depressed persons turn to food and alcoholic beverages as a coping mechanism and thus gain large amounts of weight. Although eating and drinking may provide temporary solace, the resultant overweight becomes an additional stressor, further convincing the person of his worthlessness. Severely depressed individuals are more likely to lack appetite, as well as lacking the energy to buy and prepare food. Thus it is not unusual for them to lose a large amount of weight rapidly. They may not be aware of the amount of weight loss, but the observant nurse will make note of ill-fitting clothes.

Although not every depressed individual harbors suicidal thoughts, almost every person who attempts suicide is depressed. Consequently, the nurse should consider every depressed client as potentially suicidal unless she has reason to believe otherwise.

Some authorities believe that all individuals who contemplate suicide give clues of their intention. Common clues include a dramatic change in behavior, giving away treasured possessions, or actually talking about intentions. The common belief that a person who talks about suicide never attempts it is a fallacy. People usually talk about the thoughts that are uppermost in their minds. An individual alludes to suicide because he is thinking about it. The person who makes statements about life not being worth living, who suggests that he may not be around much longer, or who has actually injured himself should be considered at risk for suicide.

A person who is depressed is at the greatest risk for suicide after his depression has begun to lift. Many nurses who show concerned care to deeply depressed individuals relax their vigilance as the person's mood begins to lift, usually as the result of the effective use of antidepressant medications. Suicide attempts at this time are common because the individual has sufficient mental and physical energy to plan and implement a self-destructive act while still being sufficiently depressed to desire death.

Another common fallacy about suicide is that questioning the depressed individual about the presence of suicidal thoughts will give him the idea that this might be a solution to his problems. Nothing could be further from the truth. If the individual were so responsive to suggestion, it would be a relatively easy matter to suggest that life is worth living. The nurse should never hesitate to ask a depressed person if he is contemplating suicide, especially if his behavior raises that suspicion in her mind.

Nursing diagnoses

The nursing diagnostic categories and etiological factors approved by the Fifth National Conference on Nursing Diagnoses that may be applicable to individuals with mood disturbances are:

Alteration in health maintenance related to ineffective individual coping; dysfunctional grieving
Impaired home maintenance management related to impaired emotional functioning
Impaired physical mobility related to depression
Self-care deficit in feeding, bathing/hygiene, dressing/grooming, toileting related to depression
Social isolation related to unaccepted social behavior.
Potential for self-directed violence related to suicidal behavior

Based on the assessment data just described, more specific nursing diagnoses for individuals who are depressed could be formulated. Examples are:

Expressions of guilt and despair related to depression
Physical inactivity related to psychomotor retardation, or physical agitation related to psychomotor overactivity
Unkempt appearance related to lack of energy and interest in grooming
Inadequate nutrition related to refusal to eat, or inadequate nutrition related to over consumption of food and drink high in calories but low in nutritional value
Suicidal thoughts related to feelings of worthlessness and despair

Planning and implementing nursing care

The need that many inexperienced nurses feel to "cheer up" the person who is depressed is not helpful and often actually causes him to feel more guilty and unworthy than ever. When working with a depressed individual, such statements as, "Buck up," "Let's see you smile," or "There is a silver lining in every cloud" are not helpful. Gaiety and laughter have a tendency to make such a person feel more guilty and thus more morose. The nurse can be most helpful by being friendly in a kind, understanding, businesslike way. Attempts at changing his mood through logical suggestions are fruitless and should be avoided. Sometimes just sitting beside the person without trying to carry on a conversation is helpful. At others times it is effective to talk to him even though he may not answer. He will appreciate the personal interest being shown.

One of the methods by which a nurse may contribute to the care of some depressed individuals is to provide them with tasks that will help relieve feelings of guilt. Depressed individuals have been known to ask for such menial tasks as scrubbing the floor, scouring the toilets, washing dirty socks, washing windows, or scrubbing the walls. Such tasks may provide a release for the guilt of the depressed individual and a means of atonement for real or imaginary sins. Although providing such experiences is contrary to the usual recommended treatment plan, it has proved to be of great value to selected individuals. Such work assignments for depressed persons should not be carried out unless they have been approved by the treatment team.

Patience is the keynote in working with depressed individuals who are so greatly retarded in the spheres of thinking, feeling, and acting that every movement or word requires great effort and much time. The same question often needs to be asked more than once, and the nurse must wait patiently for the answer. A large part of the therapeutic value of the hospital situation lies in the fact that decisions can be made for the individual. Thus the nurse should avoid asking such questions as, "Do you want to take your bath now?" A more positive approach would be, "Your bath is ready now. I will help you with it."

Perhaps the most effective way of caring for a depressed person is to establish a simple daily schedule for him. Much encouragement and reassurance throughout each day will be required to help him follow the schedule.

These individuals often need to be supplied with extra clothing. They exercise very little and frequently become chilled without appearing to realize it. Vigilance in supplying sweaters, warm underwear, and warm stockings is important.

Encouraging depressed individuals to take pride in their personal appearance is part of their care. This is difficult because it is in opposition to their tendency toward self-depreciation. Careful supervision of personal hygiene with attention to supplying clean clothing and helping them dress neatly is important in developing pride in personal appearance. Women need to be encouraged to accept appointments at the beauty parlor, and men to go to the barbershop regularly. If a depressed individual is hospitalized because he is actively suicidal, it may be safer to ask the barber or beauty operator to come to the unit where the person is hospitalized, rather than to send him to the operator.

Many depressed individuals present a difficult feeding problem. It is helpful if the nurse can discover why food is being refused. It is not uncommon for these individuals to refuse to eat because they believe they are unworthy of receiving food. Some may say that they do not deserve food because they have not paid for it. Still others seek to destroy themselves through starvation. Many of these individuals have simply lost a desire for food, along with all the other interests they formerly had in life. Inactivity also contributes to a lack of interest in food.

Finding a way to combat the depressed individual's failure to eat depends on the reason for which the food is being refused. If failure to eat is caused by a feeling of unworthiness or the thought that the food has not been paid for, the person may be reassured by being told that the food is prepared for the group and all are expected to eat regardless of whether they pay or not. It might be helpful to provide an opportunity for such an individual to wash dishes or to do some other simple tasks to give him a feeling of "paying" for the food.

Because such individuals are susceptible to infection, it is important that their food and fluid intake be maintained. Every method of encouraging food intake should be employed. Some suggestions include providing physical exercise, serving small, attractively prepared meals, serving foods that the individual formerly enjoyed, allowing the family to bring in food, and spoon-feeding if this seems to encourage eating.

If the client is unable to sleep at night, warm tub baths, warm milk, and hypnotic drugs may be of benefit. However, treatment with antidepressant medications is usually most effective in alleviating the symptom of sleep disturbance.

An individual's need to injure or destroy himself is one of the most serious problems with which the nurse must cope. The most effective methods for dealing with this problem vary, depending on the situation and the individual. However, every nurse should be fully acquainted with some basic principles concerning care of the self-destructive individual.

Self-destructive tendencies are probably treated most effectively by developing an environment to help the individual bear the emotional pain he is suffering. Instead of removing all the potentially dangerous weapons from the environment, an attempt can be made to meet his emotional needs. This may be done by assigning a staff member, preferably a skillful psychiatric nurse, to remain constantly with the individual. The nurse helps him participate in occupational, social, and recreational activities. Subtly and appropriately, ways are identified to reassure the individual that he is a worthwhile, useful human being. The acutely depressed individual should be constantly supervised, but the focus of the supervision should be to help him deal with his feelings. The emphasis should be on supplying safe opportunities for participation in the daily routine.

Sometimes an attempt is made to ensure the client's safety by removing from his environment all the equipment with which he might injure himself. This is extremely difficult because every piece of clothing, all eating utensils, cigarettes, furniture, bathroom equipment—literally everything an individual needs in the process of daily living—could be used if the individual wished to injure or destroy himself. One client strangled herself by using a toothbrush to fashion a tourniquet from her long braided hair; another client dived headlong into the toilet and suffered a serious head wound; a third client destroyed herself by using the armholes of her knitted underwear as a noose; and a fourth client injured herself seriously by setting fire to her dress with a cigarette. If the philosophy of making the environment safe were carried to its logical conclusion, the client would be placed in an absolutely barren room with a pallet to lie on. At best this procedure of environmental control is only a preventive measure.

Depriving clients of freedom to move about may increase their self-destructive tendencies, convincing them that their worst fears are true and that they are worthless and unworthy or that they have committed an unforgivable crime and are being justly punished. An illustration of such an occurrence is an incident in which a nurse was playing cards with a young man who was actively suicidal and confined to an empty seclusion room, dressed only in trousers. As both sat cross-legged on the floor, the client over a period of hours dealt the cards a few inches to the right and the nurse unconsciously shifted her position to accommodate to the cards. This client eventually succeeded in shifting the nurse's position so that he had free access to the door through which he fled and proceeded to fling himself through a window. This incident illustrates that even with all precautions, prevention of suicide is not always possible, and its occurrence may be increased by establishing an environment that serves as a constant reminder to the client of his destructive wishes. Although there is no question that the actively suicidal client should be closely supervised, the hospital staff would be wise to emphasize the client's participation in safe activities with others rather than the environmental modifications so often unsuccessfully employed.

If individuals are able to feel that people are truly interested in them, if their needs for recognition and emotional support are being met, and if they are accompanied by workers who help them talk out their concerns, the incidence of attempts at self-destruction will be greatly lessened.

Electroconvulsive therapy

The nurse has a great responsibility in the care of the client receiving electroconvulsive therapy. This treatment is sometimes prescribed for depressed persons who have not improved after an adequate trial of antidepressant medications and whose depression manifests itself in agitated behavior. It is also used for individuals who are suicidal and for whom no other intervention has worked.

Electroconvulsive therapy is a fairly simple procedure to administer. It consists of producing a typical grand mal convulsion by applying controlled electric current. The current enters the individual's frontal lobes through electrodes placed on his temples. Breakfast is not served to the patient until after the treatment is over. Continuation of treatments depends to some extent on the individual's response to the therapy. This treatment can be successfully used for individuals who remain in the community.

When electroconvulsive therapy is to be initiated, it is the responsibility of the physician to discuss the treatment plans with the individual, to order the routine x-ray examinations and laboratory work before the treatment is begun, and to obtain the signed treatment permit. The nurse is also involved in preparing the individual for the procedure. Sometimes the person has not understood the physician's explanation when the treatment was discussed and does not understand why breakfast is withheld. The nurse may discover that he is frightened at the thought of receiving treatment. She is then confronted with the responsibility of reassuring the person and helping him to accept treatment.

Nurses should avoid using the words *electric shock* when talking about this therapy. It is much better to refer to it simply as *the treatment* when discussing it with people who are to receive it because electric shock may be frightening to a confused person and may suggest electrocution.

When reassuring the individual and encouraging him to cooperate with treatment plans, the nurse can say honestly that there will be no pain connected with the treatment and that the individual will remember nothing except the desire to sleep. It may be helpful to promise to accompany the person and to stay with him throughout the experience. If this promise is made the nurse must actually carry it out. It may also be reassuring to the individual to learn that a physician and other nurses will be with him during the actual treatment.

Sometimes the nurse is not able to reassure or convince the individual to accept the treatment. At this point the physician should be called. If the physician is unsuccessful in convincing the individual and still believes that treatment is essential, enough help should be summoned to make it possible to transport the client safely to the therapy room. After the first few electroconvulsive treatments, many individuals accept the treatment without question. However, because this treatment disturbs the memory, some individuals do not remember having had the experience and may require encouragement each time before it is given.

Before the therapy is given, the individual should be toileted. If this is not done, the person is inevitably incontinent during the treatment. Temperature, pulse, respirations, and blood pressure should be checked before the individual is allowed to go to the therapy room. If any of these findings are unusual, the physician should be notified. The treatment is usually canceled for individuals who exhibit signs of physical illness.

Because some individuals do not react to electroconvulsive therapy with a convulsion after having received sedatives, most physicians request that sedatives be withheld for 24 hours before treatment.

An airway is placed in the individual's mouth and one of the muscle-relaxing drugs is usually injected before the treatment is started. Emergency equipment is kept on hand in case the individual experiences respiratory difficulty after the treatment has been given. During and following the treatment the care of the individual is the same as that provided for any unconscious person who has just had a convulsive seizure.

After five or six treatments, patients frequently complain of confusion and loss of memory, particularly for recent events. This situation puzzles and perplexes the individual. He may fear that his memory will not return. Relatives are likely to express concern about this development unless the treatment has been carefully explained to them before it was undertaken. They should be prepared to expect such developments and to understand that the symptoms will clear up completely after the series of treatments has been concluded. They should be reassured that there will be no permanent untoward aftereffects from the treatments. Although very little is known about how electroconvulsive therapy achieves its results, it seems to break through the psychotic process and make the individual more accessible to other people. Thus after he has received a series of treatments it is frequently possible for the nurse to develop a relationship with him and to begin to help him become an active participant in group activities.

NURSING CARE OF THE ELATED, OVERACTIVE ADULT
Nursing assessment

The elated, overactive individual is easily identified even by the inexperienced nurse. This person's elation is accompanied by extreme overactivity in both the mental and physical spheres. He moves constantly and finds it almost impossible to sit or stand in one spot for more than a few seconds. His constant movement is accompanied by excessive talking. The content of his verbalizations may not be immediately understood by the listener since his thoughts occur faster than he can speak and tend to fly from

CASE FORMULATION a depressed individual

Carol B., 29 years of age, had been married 3 years and had one child 14 months of age. Family history revealed nothing significant except that her father was stolid and slow-going. He had a reputation for being a pessimist but was otherwise a stable, sober individual.

Five years before marriage Carol had had a period of nervousness and depression, which lasted about 3 months. This was precipitated by an unfortunate love affair. At that time she was attending summer school at a local university where she met a young man. He had encouraged her to believe he was greatly interested in her, but at the school outing that ended the summer session he ignored her and danced with another girl. Carol came home, said little or nothing to her parents, and the following morning was found in bed in a stupor. She had taken 12 1-grain phenobarbital tablets. She was rushed to a hospital, given emergency treatment, and then transferred to a mental health treatment center where she remained 2 weeks.

The present attack began about 6 weeks before her second suicidal attempt. Again the onset was rather abrupt. Her husband returned home from work one evening and found her sobbing. After much urging on his part, she confessed that she was crying because she was a bad mother and a poor housekeeper. The husband naturally assured her that she was quite the contrary, but this only brought more sobbing and self-depreciation. She worried excessively about a small scar on her baby's temple that was caused by chicken pox. She accused herself of "marking" the child. The family suspected that she was merely tired from her spring housecleaning and hired a helper to come in and care for the baby. Her sister-in-law was called in to act as a companion. For 3 weeks she remained at home. She complained of inability to concentrate and prayed a great deal of the time. The well-meaning sister-in-law encouraged her by suggesting that she "snap out of it," and this merely served to agitate her. She was finally taken to her parents' home in the country. On two occasions she was found walking along the country road, and when questioned as to her destination, she merely stated that she wanted to "run away from everything." Her husband came to visit her one Sunday afternoon and took her for a car ride back into the city. She requested him to stop at their home, since she wanted some extra clothes for the baby. She went to the kitchen and, before the husband could realize what she was about to do, cut both her wrists with a carving knife. She was admitted to a short-term treatment unit in a community mental health center after receiving emergency treatment for her wounds.

On the day of admission she was able to give a clear account of

Continued.

her actions but responded in a dull manner. She frequently interjected the remark that she should be dead but that she was too big a coward to take her own life. She accused herself of being a rank failure and asserted that she should never have been born. She frequently announced that there was no sense in bothering about her, since she would die the next day. She cried but did not shed many tears. She complained of a "numb" feeling in her head, of inability to sleep, and of loss of appetite. The physical examination was entirely negative.

nursing assessment

The history provides little information about the present episode of depression. However, it does provide information about the first attack, which came as a result of the failure of an interpersonal relationship of great importance to her and the loss of a beloved object—a cherished lover. At that time she attempted suicide by taking an overdose of sleeping pills.

Authorities tell us that individuals who resort to self-destruction are frequently fixated at the oral-sadistic level of psychosexual development. During the late oral period of the child's development, the loved object (the mother or the mother's breast) is unconsciously introjected.

Later in life a loved object may unconsciously represent the original object that was introjected. When an individual attempts suicide he may be seeking relief from suffering or punishment for himself, or he may be attempting to kill the introjected person.

This young woman's child was in the toilet-training period. It is at this period in the child's development that he becomes more self-assertive and begins to defy the mother. It may be that this mother viewed the change in her child from a dependent, passive organism requiring constant tender guidance to a self-assertive individual as a loss. In a sense she had lost a dependent organism and gained a demanding child. She may be overwhelmed with the new responsibilities brought about by the child's development. Thus she may blame herself for being a bad mother and a poor housekeeper and having caused a small scar on the baby's temple.

Her physical symptoms were those commonly found among depressed individuals: inability to sleep, loss of appetite, complaints of a numb feeling in the head, and crying without tears. Her emotional responses were also those frequently found among depressed individuals: inability to concentrate, self-accusatory ideas, suicidal ideas, and feelings of unworthiness. Characteristically she was able to give a clear account of all the experiences relating to her illness.

nursing diagnoses

The assessment data, including present behavior, past life experiences, and an understanding of the underlying dynamics, lead to the development of the following nursing diagnoses for Carol:

Actively suicidal related to feelings of guilt and worthlessness.
Inadequate nutrition and rest related to loss of appetite and inability to sleep.

planning and implementing nursing care for CAROL B.

The boxed material on p. 312 is an example of a plan of nursing care that could be designed for Carol B. Because she was actively suicidal individual nursing care was provided for her. Nurses or other staff members with proved ability to work successfully with depressed individuals were chosen to be with her at all times until she recovered from the acute phases of the depression. They recognized the importance of showing Carol that they cared and set about to achieve this. Their goals for her care were to protect her from her self-destructive tendencies and to encourage her to discuss her feelings about the problems that concerned her.

These staff members adopted a kind, courteous, firm, hopeful attitude toward Carol. In this way they tried to convey the impression that she was not a hopeless case as she insisted. They listened carefully to everything she said and answered her questions carefully without disputing or agreeing with her expressions of worthlessness. They accepted her silences when she did not wish to talk. They avoided using meaningless statements such as, "Cheer up," or "You know your family loves you!"

The staff members who worked closely with Carol were aware of her physical needs for food, fluid intake, and rest. They found that she ate better if served food on a tray in her room rather than going to the dining room with the other clients. If at night she wanted to sit up and talk or walk up and down the corridors the staff member who was assigned to stay with her accompanied her in these activities.

When Carol accused herself of being a rank failure, the nurse tried to help her recognize that she was improving and had demonstrated abilities and skills since coming to the treatment center. This was an attempt to improve her self-esteem.

The staff workers made decisions for Carol until she was able to make them for herself. They tried to develop a congenial pleasant living atmosphere for her. They encouraged her to become interested in some of the activities available in the occupational therapy department and accompanied her there whenever she felt well enough to go.

Continued.

nursing care plan for
CAROL B.

nursing diagnosis	objective	rationale	nursing actions	outcome criteria
Actively suicidal related to feelings of worthlessness	To protect client from self-destructive tendencies	Depressed clients who have a history of suicidal attempts are at great risk for self-destruction	Assigned nurse(s) remain with client at all times Administer prescribed antidepressant medication Observe and listen carefully for clues of suicidal intention; record same Encourage constructive activity, for example, O.T., R.T. Comment positively on accomplishments	Within 4 weeks client will: No longer express desire to kill self Acknowledge positive comments by nurse about her accomplishments, for example, by saying "thank you" Spontaneously attend O.T. and R.T. activities
	To encourage client to discuss her feelings and problems	Verbalizing feelings makes acting on them less likely Discussion of problems renders them amenable to problem solving	Reflect client's statements to encourage conversation Sit with client in silence if she does not wish to talk Convey interest in what client says Do not argue with expressions of worthlessness Avoid platitudes, such as "tomorrow will be a better day" Encourage problem solving technique	Within 2 weeks client will: Spontaneously approach nurse to express feelings Show evidence of attempting to problem solve
Inadequate nutrition and rest related to loss of appetite and inability to sleep	To increase food and fluid intake	Adequate rest and nutrition is necessary to regain physiological homeokinesis and to prevent infection	Offer small amounts of easily chewed, nutritional food at meal times Offer 6 oz. water or juice in plastic cup q2h Record amount of food and fluid taken	Within 4 weeks client will eat 3 meals a day without needing to be encouraged to do so

nursing care plan for
CAROL B.—cont'd

nursing diagnosis	objective	rationale	nursing actions	outcome criteria
	To increase periods of sleep at night	Adequate rest is essential for physiological and emotional well-being	Discourage naps during the day Remove client from environmental stimuli (for example, TV) 1 hour before bedtime Do not discuss charged issues at bedtime If client awakes at night, do not scold; be reassuring and remain with her	Within 4 weeks client will sleep from 10:00 PM to 6:00 AM without awakening

evaluation

Evaluation of the plan of nursing care and its implementation was based on outcome criteria established when the plan was formulated. Since the nurse knew that the most significant factor in alleviating the symptoms of acute depression is the prescribed antidepressant medication and that this medication requires 2 to 4 weeks to have an effect, she did not expect to see changes in Carol's behavior until then.

For several days after admission Carol remained sad and indifferent. She ate only when coaxed. She never inquired about the welfare of her child and was indifferent toward her husband during visiting hours. Although she was not particularly untidy she was rather slipshod in appearance and made no attempt to comb her hair or keep herself presentable. She took little or no interest in unit activities or in the other clients.

In the second week of Carol's hospital stay she began to show improvement. After being in the hospital for 1 month she began clamoring for discharge, insisting that she must go home to take care of her family. She was cheerful and industrious, teaching English to a small group of foreign women in occupational therapy.

Carol's nurse joined other members of the treatment team in recommending discharge to the aftercare clinic.

Continued.

one topic to another. However, with concentration the listener can usually guess the missing words and thus make sense of what the person is saying.

The appearance of the elated, overactive individual is often dramatically bizarre. Frequently he dresses in clothing that is not only inappropriate to the setting or the season, but is also very brightly colored. Females, in particular, adorn themselves with flowers in their hair, large pieces of ornate jewelry, and an abundance of sloppily applied makeup. One client appeared for admission to a Northeastern psychiatric hospital in February dressed in a long, bright yellow ball gown and a wide-brimmed straw hat. Around her shoulders she wore a foxtail stole. Her only concession to the 20° weather was a pair of checkered mittens. By the time she arrived at the hospital, this individual was almost suffering from hypothermia but had no sense of discomfort.

When the elated individual is left alone the content of his speech is likely to be jovial and humorous, often with many sexual references and puns. When his stream of talk is interrupted even by as simple and common an event as being asked a question, his good-natured banter may suddenly turn to biting sarcasm, pointed profanity, and vulgarity.

Elated individuals are very adept in discovering a physical or personality defect in the person with whom they are speaking, particularly one about which the person is sensitive. They seem to take delight in repeatedly calling attention to this defect.

As is true with many other mentally ill individuals, the elated overactive individual may be malnourished. His overactivity consumes a great deal of energy and he cannot concentrate long enough on one task to purchase, prepare, or eat food. For the same reason his hygiene needs are usually not met.

It is not unusual for the elated, overactive individual to have injuries resulting from altercations with others or from accidents. These injuries range from superficial bruises to broken ribs. However, he is unlikely to complain of discomfort. A complete physical examination must be completed as soon as possible after admission.

When asked about the nature of his problem the individual characteristically expresses little insight into the inappropriateness of his behavior or his mood. Rather, he is likely to blame a family member or friend for not understanding his circumstances. He may or may not resist treatment but when he does cooperate he goes to great lengths to make it clear that he is humoring the nurse.

Nursing diagnoses

Nursing diagnostic categories and etiological factors from the list of approved nursing diagnoses developed by the Fifth National Conference on Nursing Diagnoses that may be applicable to the individual who is elated and overactive include:

Alteration in health maintenance related to significant alteration in communication skills
Alteration in health maintenance related to complete or partial lack of fine motor skills
Social isolation related to unaccepted social behavior
Potential for violence directed at others related to manic excitement

Based on the assessment data just discussed, the following additional nursing diagnoses may be formulated as a basis for the development of a plan of nursing care:

Continuous movement and talking related to psychomotor overactivity
Inappropriate attire and inadequate hygiene related to elation
Sarcastic and profane language related to elation and overactivity
Inadequate nutrition and dehydration related to overactivity
Susceptibility to physical injuries related to hostility toward others and overactivity

Planning and implementing nursing care

Individuals suffering from elation and overactivity require skillful and tactful nursing care. Such individuals are easily irritated and angered. Whether the nurse can help elated, overactive individuals depends to a large extent on the attitude with which they are approached. The nurse's tone of voice is of primary importance. A firm, kind, low-pitched voice that carries a coaxing quality probably is most effective. The nurse who uses a loud demanding tone is quickly defeated because this approach may provoke hostile and aggressive behavior.

It is useless to attempt to hurry the elated individual because such an approach will result in anger and hostility. Thus the attitude of having all the time in the world to accomplish a procedure will be much more effective. Quiet persuasion is one of the chief aids in getting the elated individual to cooperate.

Consistent fairness and honesty in dealing with such individuals are essential if one is to maintain rapport with them over a period of time. Although they deserve and must have simple, honest explanations, long discussions and explanations should be avoided, since such activities provoke irritability.

The skillful nurse makes use of the individual's inability to maintain sustained attention by directing his thoughts away from factors in the environment that encourage his destructive tendencies, provoke his irritability, or increase his excitement.

In dealing with overactive, elated individuals the nurse must recognize that the behavior is a result of an illness and will be replaced by socially acceptable behavior when the person is well again. The inexperienced nurse may be embarrassed by the loud talking, the vulgarity and profanity, the destructive activity, and the overt sexual behavior that is apparent. However, part of the skillful care of such a person includes understanding why he needs to behave in such a way. With understanding will come acceptance of behavior.

The nurse who is accepting of the behavior of the elated individual will not scold or shame him for his unihibited actions or become angered by the pointed, biting remarks because she will understand that they are a part of his illness.

Because all elated, overactive individuals are stimulated by environmental factors one of the nurse's first responsibilities is to simplify their surroundings and insofar as possible provide a sedative environment for them. Because other people irritate the elated individual and provoke him to engage in an excessive amount of talking, it is wise to provide him with a single room. The room should be as far away from other daily activities as possible and yet easily accessible to the nurse who needs to be constantly aware of the individual and his behavior. Pictures and colorful drapes probably should be eliminated because they may be too stimulating and certainly may be destroyed in a burst of excitement. Unnecessary furniture such as a small table or a light chair may be used as a weapon if the individual becomes extremely irritated. Care must be individualized, depending on the degree of the individual's elation and the amount of his excessive energy. It is usually wise to limit the number of persons who come in contact with him. Only a few persons, chosen because of their patience and understanding approach, should be assigned to his care.

The overactive individual may react with a tremendous burst of energy for which he must find some outlet. Usually such an individual is admitted to a hospital because the outlets he has chosen for his energy have been dangerous to him or to his family. The nurse is confronted with the task of controlling or redirecting this excessive energy into more acceptable channels.

An excellent outlet for the excessive energy of individuals who are only mildly elated is writing. Most of these people are eager to write their life stories or to disclose the deficiencies of the political system to the world and thus will readily put paper and pencil to use. Many mildly elated individuals will be content to spend hours over their manuscripts.

Physical activities provided for these individuals should require large sweeping movements, since they will become annoyed and lose interest in anything requiring fine, discriminative skills. Games such as table tennis, croquet, badminton, and medicine ball are often helpful as outlets for energy, provided there is no element of competition present. In competitive games the elated patient becomes overly stimulated and excited.

It is unwise from a therapeutic point of view to threaten an excited individual or to suggest that he will be punished because of his nonconforming behavior. Such a maneuver usually results in increased hostility. If the individual is directed in an understanding and empathic way and his behavior is accepted as part of his illness it is usually possible to redirect his energy without resorting to the use of restraints. With the availability of psychotropic medications, mechanical restraint of overactive persons has been dramatically reduced.

Occasionally hospitalization is required for an individual because he is dangerous to himself or others. Intense feelings of fear, anger, hostility, or suspicion may cause individuals to strike out against other people or the environment in general. Striking out against others is dangerous. Therefore it is essential to prevent this type of behavior, if possible, and to check it if it occurs.

Usually an individual who strikes out against his environment does so because he is terrified. He may be afraid of what he believes others will do to him, or he may be undergoing terrifying hallucinatory experiences. If the latter is happening the voices may be describing what physical and mental tortures are awaiting him. It is obvious that a terrified individual can be helped only by those who are in control of their own feelings and can approach him calmly. Uncontrolled fear on the part of others is extremely upsetting to emotionally ill people.

When an individual becomes terrified, a calm, quiet staff member should assist him to a room that is away from the center of activity. The individual should remain in the quiet room until his intense feelings of fear or anger have subsided. Someone who can be helpful and can comfort the fearful individual should remain with him until he is ready to rejoin the group.

More important than managing destructive, threatening behavior is learning how it can be prevented. The first step in learning to prevent problem behavior is to discover situations that are upsetting to such individuals and to discover how to keep these from occurring. The nurse needs to learn to recognize the signs of an approaching emotional outburst and to employ measures that will help individuals to handle negative feelings without acting out against the environment. Destructive behavior on the part of terrified, angry individuals is rare where an attempt is made to recognize and meet emotional needs and where the personnel recognize the importance of developing positive interpersonal relationships with mentally ill persons.

An overactive individual often loses a great deal of weight and may become severely dehydrated. This problem is exaggerated by the fact that he frequently does not take time to eat or drink and may sleep very little. He is often oblivious to physical injury or pain. Consequently the nurse needs to be vigilantly aware of such a person's physical needs as well as his emotional ones.

Prevention of injury is one of the nurse's responsibilities. Overactive individuals may injure themselves in a burst of elation and excitement and may disregard even such a serious trauma as a broken bone.

Keeping overactive persons warmly dressed during cold weather is sometimes difficult, because clothing may be an irritating factor. Excited individuals may tear off clothing that impedes the movement of arms and legs. They often appear totally unaware of body temperature and must be safeguarded against becoming chilled.

Since constipation, fecal impaction, bladder distention, or other difficulties may be present but ignored, the nurse should observe for these conditions.

Ensuring sufficient sleep for excited individuals is another challenge. This is important because exhaustion and even death have been known to result from long-continued failure to sleep. Many of these individuals are so alert to all environmental stimuli that they sleep only 1 to 2 hours out of every 24. Some hypnotic drugs are helpful, but occasionally they may increase the individual's excitement. The problem of wakefulness usually disappears after a few days of treatment with medications.

Excited and elated individuals may not take time to sit down to eat. In such an instance it is wise to serve food that can be carried about in the hands. Sandwiches, fruit, and cupcakes are dietary items that may be "eaten on the run." Elated, overactive individuals require a high caloric intake and should have between-meal nourishment. Nurses should not disregard the need for fluids even though water fountains are usually available; the excited individual often does not take time to drink and should have water offered to him each hour.

If the individual is served food on a tray and will take time to feed himself, the equipment on the tray should be simple and unbreakable. As in every other aspect of the care of these overactive, elated persons, the nursing procedures must be individualized to meet specific needs. In some instances the elated individual may get along well in the dining room setting. However, in most instances he is so stimulated by the dining room situation that it is more helpful if he is served on a tray in his room.

Although the individual should be encouraged to carry out his own personal hygiene, he needs to be supervised closely. Some overactive, elated individuals are too ill to assume any responsibility for their physical care and may need to have much of it done by the nurse. Other less excited individuals can take a good deal of responsibility for their own cleanliness and grooming if someone skillfull directs their activities. Such individuals may become playful and mischievous in the bathroom. Because of poor judgement these individuals have been found washing their hair in the toilet bowl, throwing water about with gay abandon, or in various other ways reducing the bathroom to a shambles. It is for this reason that such individuals should not be left alone in the bathroom.

The overactive individual's mouth requires special attention, and lubrication should be applied to the lips regularly.

Since many overactive individuals require hospitalization, at least for a short time, they are available to be observed for indications of suicidal thoughts as the elation subsides.

CASE FORMULATION
an overactive individual

Maurice H., 48 years of age, was an unmarried real estate salesman who was an only child. His mother had a mental illness at 46 years of age, which was probably depression of midlife. He had been educated in private schools and earned a college degree in business administration. During his junior year in college he failed to win a scholarship and became morose, sleepless, and nervous for a period of 2 months. A few years after finishing college he entered an auto sales contest and won first prize, a trip to Hawaii. While on this trip he became overactive and insisted on eating every meal at the captain's table, where he told obscene stories and embarrassed the women passengers. He participated in frequent brawls with the stewards and complained to the purser on the slightest provocation. On disembarking he refused to return to his home city. He demanded the most pretentious accommodations at the hotel and when these were unavailable he entered into a noisy altercation with the manager that resulted in his being hospitalized because of his behavior. He remained there for 3 months and then returned to his parents' home.

The present attack began about 6 weeks before he sought help. At that time he was engaged in selling real estate in a new subdivision. He became extremely active, arose early, and approached prospective clients at bus terminals, waiting rooms, and hotel corridors. He talked in such a convincing manner that he made a good sales record in the first week. He continued to send in many deposits, bragged about his sales ability, argued noisily with his fellow salesmen, and finally was arrested because he failed to pay his fare on a city bus. He then entered a damage suit against the company for $100,000. The attorney who was approached realized the absurdities of his claims and convinced him to seek help.

Immediately after going to the mental health center he demanded to see the head physician and requested permission to use the telephone. He was fairly coherent but was circumstantial in his conversation. When asked a simple question his reply was a long, rambling, and digressive account. After being continually reminded to answer the question he did so, only to return to another long digression.

Although he believed that he was being abused he harbored no other delusional ideas and at no time was he confused or hallucinatory. His intellect was keen and his memory, particularly for trivial things, remarkable, but he had no insight into his abnormal exaltation and irritability and his judgment was poor. He made unreasonable demands of the personnel at the clinic and if refused became abusive, sarcastic, and irritable. At this time it was discovered that when a client had refused to make a down payment on a lot he had drawn the sum out of his own bank account and had forged a signature on the sales contract. This explained his amazing sales success.

He spent much of his time while in the short-term treatment unit of the mental health clinic writing letters to the mayor, various attorneys, and influential citizens. He wrote on odd pieces of paper with pencil and in a broad, sweeping hand, underlining many words and capitalizing others. Every day he met the physicians at the door of the unit and began to revile them. He particularly enjoyed arguing with the physicians, demanding evidence to prove that he was insane and consistently denying all charges of misbehavior. In a loud voice he promised to have the director of the center removed and the physicians exposed as quacks. He was suggestively lewd in his conversation with all women workers except one young woman to whom he proposed marriage.

Throughout the 4 weeks he spent in the short-term treatment unit, he was the constant focus of commotion, a chronic critic of everything and everybody about him, collecting and hoarding papers, combs, magazines, and all sorts of trash and getting into quarrels with others. Occasionally he was very agreeable and jolly, particularly if he was allowed to do all the talking. On these occasions he was fond of reciting parodies of famous poems in a quick, witty fashion. Some of these he had not quoted since his high school days.

nursing assessment　　This individual's mother suffered from a midlife depression. Too little is known about this situation to do more than suggest that the mother was unable to give her son the sense of security he required as an infant to develop into a well-adjusted adult. The mother's depression also raises the possibility of this individual having an inherited predisposition to an affective disorder.

Continued.

Maurice H. first experienced a depression at about the age of 21 when he failed to win a scholarship in college. To him this failure to achieve a prized goal represented a failure in life, and he became depressed in an unconscious effort to punish himself as his parents might have done when he failed to fulfill some expectation of theirs. For 2 months he had typical symptoms of a mild depression. He was morose, sleepless, and nervous.

A few years later Maurice won a coveted prize in an auto sales contest. This award was a trip to Hawaii that eventually resulted in Maurice's hospitalization for 3 months because of his overactivity. In this instance he probably developed anxiety over his company's high expectations. He may have reasoned that they would undoubtedly expect more and bigger sales records from him now that he had been able to achieve the award of a trip. The anxiety about being able to fulfill the future expectations of his company changed into guilt feelings that in turn caused him to feel that somehow he should be punished. To guard against the depressed feelings that arose from a sense of failure and a need to be punished, he developed overactivity and elation—the defense against depression.

Several years later he once more became involved in a competitive selling activity. His unconscious need to succeed to fulfill introjected parental expectations started the chain reaction again. Thus anxiety about succeeding caused him to be concerned about the possibility of failing, and this in turn led to the depressed feelings that accompany a loss. The loss was the anticipated failure in selling, which in his own mind had already occurred. Thus the unconscious defense against depressed feelings was again used. He became expansive, overactive, argumentative, sarcastic, irritable, made unreasonable demands, and became a constant center of commotion. In a sense, he did not give himself time to become depressed because he was too busy striking out against his environment.

Typically he was not delusional, and he did not experience hallucinations. Thus he was constantly in touch with reality. His intellect was as keen as ever, and his memory was intact.

Some inexperienced people might conclude that this man was not mentally ill. However, he was unreasonable and sometimes abusive when he did not get his own way. He also wrote letters to outside authorities because he believed he should not be undergoing treatment, and he constantly sought to expose the clinic personnel for their inefficient handling of the situation. He had no insight into his condition, and his judgment was impaired.

nursing diagnoses

The nursing diagnoses derived from the assessment data were:

Verbally hostile and physically aggressive behavior related to elation and overactivity

Inadequate food and fluid intake related to overactivity

These diagnoses were used as the basis for developing a plan of nursing care for Maurice H.

planning and implementing nursing care for MAURICE H.

The plan of nursing care developed for Maurice H. is summarized below.

The members of the staff assigned to care for Maurice were chosen carefully because his verbally hostile and physically aggressive behavior was difficult to accept. Not all staff members were able to control their feelings about his vulgar comments or to understand objectively why it was impossible for him to control his behavior. In addition, he related more positively to some individuals than to others. Finally, some staff members enjoyed working with him and others did not. All these factors were considered in the choice of individuals to work with him.

The staff decided that it would be best for him to be cared for in a unit of the treatment center where a single room was available. In such a room it was possible to eliminate all but the essential furnishings. The single room was helpful in avoiding the overstimulation that might have resulted from sleeping accommodations where he would have been involved with other clients.

nursing care plan for MAURICE H.

nursing diagnosis	objectives	rationale	nursing actions	outcome criteria
Verbally hostile and physically aggressive behaviors related to elation and overactivity	To prevent injury to client and staff To assist client to control his hostile language and physical aggressiveness	Overactivity makes client at risk to injure others or to be injured Client's language and behavior alienates him from others	Administer prescribed medication; observe carefully for signs of lithium toxicity Arrange for daily blood work and check results against norms Carefully select 3 staff to work with client per shift	Within 4 weeks client will: Be able to talk with one other person for 15 minutes without sarcasm or hostility Not attempt to hit other clients or staff unless provoked

Continued.

nursing care plan for
MAURICE H.—cont'd

nursing diagnosis	objectives	rationale	nursing actions	outcome criteria
			Reduce all environmental stimuli by: Assigning client to single room Avoiding competitive games Providing activities for him in his room Do not interrupt when client is singing or reciting Ignore client's jokes Speak in calm, direct manner using simple short sentences Do not argue	
Inadequate food and fluid intake related to overactivity	To promote adequate nutrition and hydration	Adequate nutrition and hydration necessary to regain and maintain physiological homeokinesis in light of overactivity	In addition to meals, provide high caloric nutritional snacks that can be eaten standing or walking, for example, malted milk, hamburgers Offer 6 oz. water or juice every hour Weigh weekly Observe for signs of dehydration Feed in room if client is unable to stay in dining room long enough to finish meal	Within 1 week, client will: Show signs of adequate hydration Consume sufficient calories to avoid weight loss

His recreational activities needed to be controlled because it was obvious that he became loud and disruptive when involved in competitive games. He became angry when he scored lower than other players in a game and accused them of cheating. These accusations usually brought on loud arguments and sometimes fights.

When it was necessary for the staff to intervene in such an altercation, they took advantage of his distractibility and subtly redirected his attention away from the argument to an activity that could be carried on in his room with another person, one who was able to tolerate his rapid conversation and accept his pointed criticism.

The members of the staff were careful to avoid scolding or threatening Maurice when he initiated fights with other individuals. They avoided comparing his behavior with that of other better controlled individuals or even with his own behavior on a day when he was less noisy. The staff realized that his problem behavior was part of his illness.

Maurice responded negatively to any member of the staff who attempted to speak to him somewhat sharply or who commanded him to do anything. They learned that he could not be hurried and that their approach was much more effective if they were quiet, friendly, patient, and courteous to him and used a pleasant, businesslike tone of voice. On one occasion when a staff member did order him to comply with a hospital rule, he refused and did not let the individual forget the incident.

The staff discovered that it was unwise to encourage Maurice when he was reciting or singing parodies or telling jokes. When some staff members did laugh at his jokes, he became much louder and more ribald. It was necessary for them to intervene by accompanying him to his room before he became so excited that he lost control.

In talking to this man the staff avoided getting into long, complicated discussions or giving elaborate explanations. Instead, short sentences with specific, straightforward responses to his questions seemed to satisfy him and avoid arguments.

The staff members were careful when praising him. They found that he sometimes turned the words of praise around and used them in a different context to refute a point they had been trying to make with him some time previously.

They were aware of his physical needs and realized that he frequently did not eat enough. This problem arose because his attention was distracted from the food or he left the dining room early before finishing the meal. Likewise, he sometimes had dry, cracked lips because he failed to maintain his fluid intake. Maurice was weighed every week, and when his weight had dropped below a desirable point for 2 consecutive weeks, his food was served in his room on a tray. A staff member remained with him during the meal and encouraged him to eat. Removing him from the dining room eliminated the many distracting features present in a group. At the same time he was placed on a schedule so that fluids were offered to him every hour.

Continued.

Crayons, paper, and pencils were made available to him in his room, and he was encouraged to write and sketch there in the hope that these more sedentary activities would lessen his hyperactivity. The staff members were careful to explain to him in an honest, straightforward manner why he was not encouraged to join the rest of the clients in the dining room. In like manner all other restrictions on his behavior were explained so that he could understand the reason for them and realize that he was not being rejected as a person.

evaluation

After receiving appropriate amounts of the drug lithium carbonate for 2 weeks, he gained some control of his behavior and became quieter and more amenable to suggestion. The professional staff did not believe that he was well enough to leave the hospital permanently. However, at the request of his mother he was allowed to go home at the end of 4 weeks with the understanding that he would continue taking lithium carbonate for 1 year and have the blood levels of this drug checked weekly by a physician.

Although the nurse who had primary responsibility for this client's nursing care continuously reassessed his behavior, she did not engage in a complete evaluation because Maurice was discharged after 4 weeks.

CONCLUDING STATEMENTS

1. Although grief and depression are both characterized by a disturbance in mood they differ in many ways.
2. Grief is a normal, universal, necessary and self-limiting part of life experience that is a reaction to the real loss of a highly valued object.
3. The 3 phases of normal grieving include shock and disbelief; developing awareness of the pain of the loss, which leads to crying; and restitution, which involves mourning.
4. Depression is a pathological elaboration of grief that goes beyond grief in duration and intensity and causes the individual to be increasingly incapacitated.
5. Depression is not self-limiting and often requires professional help.

6. Mood disturbances are thought to have their origins in the frustrations that occur in the late oral phase of personality development.
7. Individuals prone to the development of mood disturbances have prepsychotic personalities characterized by ambivalent, dependent, and narcissistic tendencies and have difficulty in establishing mature patterns of adult interpersonal relationships.
8. Essentially, elated, overactive individuals are venting their hostility on their environment, whereas depressed individuals have turned their hostility on themselves.
9. Depressed adults display behavior indicative of feelings of despair, gloom, a sense of foreboding, feelings of guilt, and ideas of self-depreciation. Their appearance is likely to be unkempt, they experience changes in their sleeping and eating patterns, and they report physical distress involving the gastrointestinal system.
10. The task of recognizing the potentially suicidal individual and safeguarding against the possibility of injury is one of the most important responsibilities of the nurse.
11. The elated and overactive adult displays behavior characterized by extreme overactivity in both the mental and physical spheres. His appearance is often bizarre, and the content of his speech often contains sexual references. It is not unusual for him to suffer from malnourishment and injuries.

SUGGESTED SOURCES OF ADDITIONAL INFORMATION

Classical

Beers, Clifford: A mind that found itself, New York, 1948, Doubleday & Co., Inc.

Bodie, Marilyn K.: When a patient threatens suicide, Perspect. Psychiatr. Care **6:**76-79, March-April, 1968.

Crary, William G., and Crary, Gerald C.: Depression, Am. J. Nurs. **73:**472-475, 1973.

Engel, George L.: Grief and grieving, Am. J. Nurs. **64:**93-98, Sept., 1964.

Fallon, Barbara: "And certain thoughts go through my head. . . ," Am. J. Nurs. **72:**1257-1259, 1972.

Farberow, Norman L.: Suicide prevention: a view from the bridge, Community Ment. Health J, **6:**469-474, 1968.

Jourard, Sidney M.: Suicide—an invitation to die, Am. J. Nurs. **72:**269, 273-275, 1970.

Miller, Edgar: Psychological theories of ECT: a review, Int. J. Psychiat. **5:**154-165, Feb., 1968.

McLean, Leonora J.: Action and reaction in suicidal crisis, Nurs. Forum **8**(1):29-41, 1969.

Parkes, Colin Murray: Bereavement; studies of grief in adult life, New York, 1973, International Universities Press.

Peplau, Hildegard: Themes in nursing situations, Am. J. Nurs. **53**:1221-1223, 1953.

Peplau, Hildegard: Mid-life crises, Am. J. Nurs. **75**:1761-1765, 1975.

Riley, Joan: Nursing intervention in depression, Perspect. Psychiatr. Care **5**:65-76, March-April, 1967.

Ruesch, Jurgen: Disturbed communication, New York, 1972, W.W. Norton & Co., Inc.

Rykken, Marjorie B.: The nurse's role in preventing suicide, Nurs. Outlook **6**:377-378, 1958.

Schagenhauf, G., Turpin, J., and White, R.B.: The use of lithium carbonate in the treatment of manic psychoses, Am. J. Psychiatry **123**:201-206, 1966.

Schneidman, Edwin S., Farberow, N.L., and Litman, R.L.: The psychology of suicide, Boston, 1970, Little, Brown & Co.

Ujhely, Gertrud B.: Grief and depression: implications for preventive and therapeutic nursing care, Nurs. Forum **5**:23-35, 1966.

Umscheid, Sister Theophane: With suicidal patients: caring for or caring about, Am. J. Nurs. **67**:1230-1232, 1967.

Contemporary

Akiskal, H., and Tashjian, R.: Affective disorders. II. Recent advances in laboratory and pathogenic approaches, Hosp. Community Psychiatry **34**(9):822-830, 1983.

Akiskal, H., and Webb, W.: Affective disorders. I. Recent advances in clinical conceptualization, Hosp. Community Psychiatry **34**(8):695-701, 1983.

Arieti, Silvano, and Bemporad, Jules: Severe and mild depression: the psychotherapeutic approach, New York, 1978, Basic Books, Inc., Publishers.

Bahra, Robert J.: The potential for suicide, Am. J. Nurs. **75**:1781-1788, 1975.

Bigelow, Newton: The involutional psychoses. In Arieti, Silvano, editor: American handbook of psychiatry, vol. 1, New York, 1959, Basic Books, Inc., Publishers, pp. 540-545.

Blythe, Marguerite, and Pearlmutter, Deanna: The suicide watch: a reexamination of maximum observation, Perspect. Psychiatr. Care **21**:90-93, July-Sept., 1983.

Boyajean, Anne: Fighting despair, Am. J. Nurs. **76**:77, Jan., 1978.

Busteed, Ellen and Johnstone, Charles: The development of suicide precautions for an inpatient psychiatric unit, J. Psychosoc. Nurs. Ment. Health Serv. **21**:15-19, May, 1983.

Capodanno, A., and Targum, S.: Assessment of suicide risk: some limitations in the prediction of infrequent events, J. Psychosoc. Nurs. Ment. Health Serv. **21**:11-14, May, 1983.

Diller, Julie: The psychological autopsy in equivocal deaths, Perspect. Psychiatr. Care **17**:156-161, July-Aug., 1979.

Dixon, Deborah L.: Manic depression: an overview, J. Psychosoc. Nurs. Ment. Health Serv. **19**:28-31, June, 1981.

Drake, Ronald E., and Price, Joseph L.: Depression: adaptation to disruption and loss. Perspect. Psychiatr. Care **13**:163-169, Oct.-Dec., 1975.

Harris, Elizabeth: The dexamethasone suppression test, Am. J. Nurs. **82**:784-785, 1982.

Herman, Sonya J.: Divorce: a grief process, Perspect. Psychiatr. Care **12**:108-112, July-Sept., 1974.

Hoff, LeeAnn, and Resing, Marcia: Was this suicide preventable? Am. J. Nurs. **82**:1107-1111, 1982.

Jacobson, Ann: Melancholy in the 20th century: causes and prevention, J. Psychosoc. Nurs. Ment. Health Serv. **18**:11-21, July, 1980.

Kalayam, B., and Steinhart, M.: A survey of attitudes on the use of electroconvulsive therapy, Hosp. Community Psychiatry **32**(3):185-188, 1981.

Kiev, Ari: The courage to live, New York, 1980, Lippincott & Crowell.

Laughlin, Sister Noel: Suicide: a case for investigation, J. Psychosoc. Nurs. Ment. Health Serv. **18**:8-12, Feb., 1980.

Murphy, Shirley: Learned helplessness: from concept to comprehension, Perspect. Psychiatr. Care **20**:27-32, Jan.-March, 1982.

O'Connell, Ralph: A review of the use of electroconvulsive therapy, Hosp. Community Psychiatry **33**(6):469-473, 1982.

Rosenthal, Saul H.: Involutional depression. In Arieti, Silvano, and Brody, Eugene, B., editors: American handbook of psychiatry, vol. 3, New York, 1974, Basic Books, Inc., Publishers, pp. 694-709.

Santora, D., and Starkey, P.: Research studies in American Indian suicides, J. Psychosoc. Nurs. Ment. Health Serv. **20**:25-29, Aug., 1982.

Schlesser, Michael, and Altshuler, Kenneth: The genetics of affective disorder: data, theory, and clinical application, Hosp. Community Psychiatry **34**(5):415-422, 1983.

Shmagin, Barbara G., and Pearlmutter, Deanna R.: The pursuit of unhappiness—the secondary gains of depression, Am. J. Nurs. **15**(2):63-65, 1977.

Smith, Diane M.Y.: Guided imagination as an intervention in hopelessness, J. Psychosoc. Nurs. Ment. Health Serv. **20**:29-32, June, 1982.

Stuart, Gail W.: Role strain and depression: a causal inquiry, J. Psychosoc. Nurs. Ment. Health Serv. **19**20-28, Dec., 1981.

Swanson, Ardis R.: Communicating with depressed persons, Perspect. Psychiatr. Care **13**:63-67, April-June, 1975.

van Servellen, Gwen M.: Women treating women for depression, J. Psychosoc. Nurs. Ment. Health Serv. **19**:21-24, Aug., 1981.

van Servellen, Gwen M., and Vohs Dull, Lynn: Group psychotherapy for depressed women: a model, J. Psychosoc. Nurs. Ment. Health Serv. **19:**25-31, Aug., 1981.

Vollen, Karen Helon, and Watson, Charles G.: Suicide in relation to time of day and day of week, Am. J. Nurs. **75:**263, 1975.

Weiss, James M.A.: Suicide. In Arieti, Silvano, and Brody, Eugene B., editors: American handbook of psychiatry, ed. 2, vol. 3, New York, 1974, Basic Books, Inc., Publishers, pp. 743-765.

Wright, Jesse, and Beck, Aaron: Cognitive therapy of depression: theory and practice, Hosp. Community Psychiatry **34**(12):1119-1127, 1983.

Of particular interest

Anthony, James E., and Benedek, Therese, editors: Depression and human existence, Boston, 1975, Little, Brown & Co.
This is a handy text for the student seeking to understand the origins and classifications of depressive disorders.

Kiev, A.: Somatic manifestations of depressive disorders, Princeton, N.J., 1974, Excerpta Medica Foundation.
This review of physical behaviors associated with depression is especially useful for the nurse in identifying symptoms that are related to depressive illness.

chapter fifteen

adults
with anxiety
disturbances

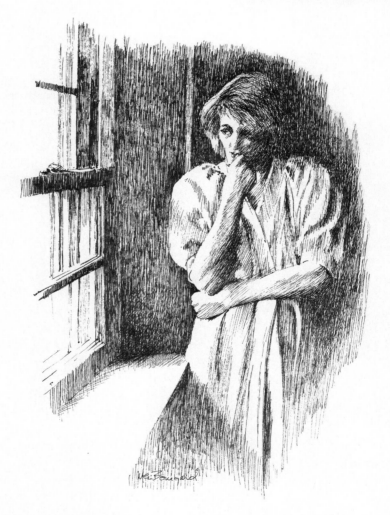

My heart is pounding so hard
and my stomach hurts so much,
I'm sure I'm going to die.

LEARNING OBJECTIVES

After studying this chapter the student will be able to:

1 Describe one example of a phobic disorder, an anxiety state, and a somatoform disorder.

2 Discuss the dynamics of development of anxiety disturbances.

3 Discuss the nursing care of adults with anxiety disturbances.

4 Discuss the types of psychotherapy and their characteristics.

5 Develop a hypothetical plan of nursing care for an adult with an anxiety disturbance.

The majority of people live relatively normal, anxiety-free lives by successfully adapting to stress and its resultant anxiety through the use of various unconscious strategies and compromises. However, there is a large group of individuals for whom these defenses are not effective. These persons must continuously focus on activities and behaviors designed to control intolerable anxiety in an unsuccessful effort to achieve a state of physical and emotional homeokinesis. In the past this group of individuals has been labeled "neurotic" by both the health care delivery system and the lay public. This term has been replaced by the more descriptive phrases of *anxiety disorders* and *somatoform disorders*.

Because individuals suffering from anxiety disturbances are in touch with reality and often recognize the inappropriateness of their behavior, many nurses have difficulty accepting them as persons in need of health care. To achieve a more understanding attitude toward these individuals, it is important to develop some knowledge about the emotional conflicts with which they struggle and the ways in which they use symptoms to cope with the anxiety that stems from these conflicts.

HISTORICAL PERSPECTIVE

Although the emotion of anxiety has been recognized since ancient Greek times the disturbances stemming directly from an inability to adapt to stress and the subsequent anxiety were not brought into focus until the early twentieth century. At that time Sigmund Freud (1856-1939) identified the role anxiety plays in the unconscious life of the individual and demonstrated how it affects his perception of reality and subsequent behavior.

During the Victorian era in which Freud practiced, many women suffered from a condition called *hysteria*. This malady manifested itself by unexplainable fatigue and weakness, "swooning," and other forms of dramatic behavior. Today these persons would be diagnosed as having an anxiety disturbance. Freud developed the technique of psychoanalysis through which he helped these patients to explore their unconscious minds for the emotional conflicts that were expressed in these symptoms. He discovered that the nature of these conflicts frequently centered on real or fantasized aggressive sexual acts. Given the culture of the day in which women were expected to assume a passive, dependent role it is understandable that they had little opportunity to resolve these conflicts and that they were expressed by symptoms indicative of passivity and dependency.

The manifestations of anxiety disturbances have changed over the years. It is a rare occurrence today to encounter an individual who exhibits the classical symptoms of hysteria, although phobic disorders are common. This change in symptomatology has led authorities to believe that the specific behaviors unconsciously chosen by the individual to express emotional conflict are determined in part by societal sanctions. For example, fainting at the sight of blood would not be culturally acceptable today, but an inordinate and irrational fear of heights evokes sympathy in this age of skyscrapers and jet travel.

The incidence of anxiety disturbances has also markedly increased over the last three decades. There is no question that this increase is related to the increased stress associated with the highly complex, postindustrial society in which we live. In fact, the last half of the twentieth century is often called "the age of anxiety."

Only persons with the severest forms of anxiety disturbances have ever been hospitalized. Therefore until recently nurses have not had much experience in providing care for individuals with less severe forms of anxiety disturbance. Since mental health care has moved into the community, however, nurses now have the opportunity and the challenge of intervening therapeutically with these individuals on an outpatient basis.

ANXIETY DISTURBANCES

Anxiety disturbances are categorized into three groups: phobic disorders, anxiety states (or anxiety neuroses), and somatoform disorders. One disturbance from each group is described below to illustrate the range of anxiety disturbances.

Agoraphobia is an example of a phobic disorder. A *phobia* is a specific pathological fear reaction out of proportion to the stimulus. The painful feeling has been automatically and unconsciously displaced from its original internal source and has become attached to a specific external object or situation. The phobia may be focused on anything that in some manner suggests death, disease, or disaster.

Agoraphobia is a fear of open spaces. The incidence of its occurrence is increasing. The individual manifests agoraphobia by expressing dread at being left alone or going out of his home. He avoids crowds and public places because he anticipates some dreadful form of collapse. Agoraphobia is particularly incapacitating because it markedly interferes with the individual's ability to live a normal life.

Obsessive-compulsive disorder is one of the anxiety states. An *obsession* is an undesirable but persistent thought or idea that is forced into conscious awareness. The thought is charged with great but unconscious emotional significance. Such a thought may include repetitive doubts, wishes, fears, impulses, admonitions, and commands.

A *compulsion* is an unwanted urge to perform an act or a ritual that is contrary to the individual's ordinary conscious wishes or standards.

It will be noted that all these intrusive ideas and compelling urges and fears appear in consciousness as thought independently self-created.

The individual who suffers from an *obsessive-compulsive disorder* is driven to think about or to do something that he recognizes as being inappropriate or foolish. There is an excessive preoccupation with a single idea or a compulsion to carry out and to repeat over and over again certain acts against his better judgment. Underlying these compulsive or obsessive states is a personality that is usually conscience-driven, sensitive, shy, meticulous, and precise about bodily functions, dress, religious duty, and daily routine.

Obsessive-compulsive disorder is a serious emotional illness because the imperative ideas so control the individual that he becomes a slave to his morbid preoccupation and can scarcely carry on his normal work and social activity. Dominating fears or phobias are the most outstanding features of this illness. The sufferer may fear dirt, bacteria, cancer, or insanity. There may be an abnormal fear of open places, narrow corridors, small rooms, running water, staircases, high places, or various animals. In fact, any object or event may serve as a phobic stimulus.

Conversion disorder is an example of a somatoform disorder. This is a purposeful although unconscious psychological mode of reaction in which the individual uses a physical symptom as a disguise in an attempt to solve some acute problem or fulfill some desire, the open or conscious gratification of which is unacceptable to the individual. Conversion represents a primitive instinctual mechanism to which a person resorts when he is incapable of adjusting through the usual methods of rational volitional activity.

The person who uses a conversion disorder unconsciously selects a set of symptoms that symbolize his problems. These symptoms are dictated by suggestion or by some previous acquaintance with persons who had the actual problem. Paralysis, blindness, and epilepsy are afflictions commonly presented by the person using conversion. The symptoms are physical, but no underlying pathophysiology can be demonstrated.

No matter what form the symptoms take, a characteristic feature of conversion is the individual's attitude of indifference toward his handicaps. There seems to be an air of contentment about the individual with conversion disorder. He seems to be more relieved than distressed, an attitude that at once suggests that he is more comfortable with the physical problem than with the mental torment.

These three examples of anxiety disturbances suggest a continuum of inability to cope with the stress of anxiety. In all instances, the original stressor is unknown to the person. However, the individual experiencing a phobic disorder is painfully aware of the anxiety it precipitates, but only when the phobic stimulus is present. In other words, the disturbance is encapsulated and the individual is able to live a relatively anxiety-free life if he can avoid the stimulus. In contrast, individuals suffering from an anxiety state such as an obsessive-compulsive disorder experience varying levels of anxiety almost continuously because the behaviors they employ as adaptations provide only temporary relief. Although this disorder is very distressing and often interferes markedly with the person's daily life, the fact that anxiety can be allowed into consciousness indicates that the system has some degree of ability to cope with the resultant stress. Finally, the individual experiencing a somatoform disorder is totally unaware of the presence of anxiety or of the fact that his physical symptoms are an adaptation to anxiety. Since there is no awareness of anxiety, it can be surmised that this individual has the least ability to cope with anxiety on a conscious level.

DYNAMICS OF DEVELOPMENT

Anxiety disturbances probably originate in the individual's early childhood experiences. Most authorities agree that the anxiety disturbance represents a conflict between two divergent drives or desires that have been repressed into the unconscious mind. It is believed that the conflict revolves around primitive impulses unacceptable to the person and his simultaneous need for acceptance by significant others.

This conflict does not necessarily cause difficulty as long as the individual has sufficient psychic energy to keep it repressed. However, when energy is diverted by the necessity to cope with other stressors the ego can no longer effect a compromise between these clashing desires and anxiety threatens to become conscious. At this point, symptoms develop as an adaptation to the emergent anxiety. This explains why symptomatology often first appears during adolescence when the individual must adapt to potent developmental stressors. In addition, the emergent, tumultuous sexuality of adolescence activates repressed unresolved sexual conflicts.

The symptoms of anxiety disturbances are designed simultaneously to alleviate the anxiety and to obscure the nature of the conflict. Thus the symptoms are socially acceptable symbols of the original conflict. For example, the compulsive handwasher is conscious of his irrational fear of germs but is totally unaware of his unconscious sexual longing for his mother. By compulsively washing his hands 10 times after toileting he experiences relief from the anxiety caused by his conflict. Unfortunately, this relief is only temporary because his action did not directly address the source of the anxiety. Thus the ritual must be repeated at frequent intervals.

It should be mentioned that an increasing amount of research indicates the probability that there is a physiological or neuro-chemical predisposition to the development of anxiety disturbances. In other words some people seem to have nervous systems that are more irritable than others, making them less able to process input to attain psychological homeokinesis. Thus a vicious cycle is established wherein the physiological manifestations of anxiety that are experienced render the individual even less able to cope with emotional conflicts. Therefore a physiological predisposition may be a necessary, although not sufficient, ingredient for the establishment of a subsequent anxiety disturbance. This theory in combination with the previously described beliefs about the dynamics of development of anxiety disturbances illustrates the inseparability of the human system and the fallacy of seeking a singular cause for this form of emotional disturbance.

NURSING CARE OF ADULTS WITH ANXIETY DISTURBANCES
Nursing assessment

Although each anxiety disturbance has its unique features it is possible to cite some commonalities about all persons suffering from anxiety disturbances. These individuals, unlike those who are psychotic, are often able to engage in the activities of daily living, hold a job, and otherwise appear fully functional. What is not known to the casual observer is that they are only able to accomplish these tasks with much difficulty. When an external stressor, particularly one that represents the loss of social prestige or love, or a threat to personal and financial security, occurs, symptoms of the anxiety disturbance are exacerbated and the individual is likely to seek help.

When seeking help the individual almost always has many physical complaints that are generally focused on the vital organs of the body. Tightness of the stomach, fast-beating heart, a feeling that the heart may suddenly stop, no appetite, loose bowels, and a heavy feeling in the abdomen are frequent complaints offered by the individual seeking assistance. Palpitation, a feeling of shortness of breath, compression sensations in the head, tight sensations in the throat, numbness in the extremities, and a constant feeling of exhaustion are other typical experiences reported by individuals suffering from anxiety disturbances. These symptoms usually frighten the person; he cannot concentrate on his work, feels depressed, and harbors fears of sudden death or insanity. Frequently many of these symptoms appear at one time and cause the individual to respond with a panic reaction or acute fear. Consequently, anxiety about the anxiety compounds the stress.

The interpersonal relationships of persons with anxiety disturbance are frequently strained. Family and friends have had much experience in attempting to reassure the client, all to no avail. Furthermore, they may have had increasing difficulty tolerating the person's idiosyncratic ways. For example, one middle-aged secretary suffering from a fear of germs was forced to share an office with several others in a typing pool. She offended her co-workers by covering her coffee mug with plastic wrap between sips to protect its contents from germs in the air. She also scrupulously cleaned her typewriter keys with a strong disinfectant every morning in case someone had touched them in her absence. When this woman's rituals became so time-consuming that she was unable to complete her assigned work, her job was threatened and she sought help from the local mental health clinic.

Nursing diagnoses

Diagnostic categories and etiological factors from the list of nursing diagnoses approved by the Fifth National Conference on Nursing Diagnoses that may be applicable to adults with anxiety disturbances include:

Anxiety related to unconscious conflict about essential values and goals of life
Anxiety related to threat to or change in socioeconomic status
Fear related to phobic stimulus or phobia

More specific diagnoses might include these:

Fear of impending physical and psychological collapse related to physiological symptoms of anxiety
Strained interpersonal relationships related to the need to adapt to the client's symptoms

Planning and implementing nursing care

Many health professionals who work skillfully and empathically with psychotic individuals find that they are not nearly so effective when giving care to those who express anxiety through physical symptoms or ritualistic behavior. A large part of the difficulty in dealing with anxious persons originates in an unconscious attitude toward persons suffering from these problems and in a failure to understand the true nature of the illness. Because such an individual is aware of his surroundings, is not carrying on a conversation with unseen people, and complains of physical symptoms that have no organic basis, some workers may feel unsympathetic toward him and may believe that he is "an attention getter" and that he could "snap out of it" if he really tried.

It is important to realize that all symptoms stemming from anxiety disturbances develop because of an overwhelming *unconscious* conflict and that the symptoms have great unconscious significance. The word unconscious has been stressed, since it is necessary to realize that the individual does not clearly understand why the symptom has developed nor what he is gaining by using the symptom repeatedly. He does realize that the symptom helps relieve unbearable anxiety and tension.

It is also important to realize that the discomfort and pain of which the individual complains is actually present even though there is no organic basis that can explain the existence of the symptoms. Experts are beginning to recognize that fear plays a significant role in causing pain. Since fear is prominent in the symptomatology of many anxiety-ridden people it is not difficult to realize that they actually feel the pain of which they complain. It is important to understand that emotionally conditioned pain is as distressing to bear as is pain that results from true physical disease.

To make an intelligent and therapeutic plan of care the health worker needs to understand the nature of the person's conflict and the meaning of his symptoms. The plan for care and treatment should be developed collaboratively by the workers who will be involved with the individual. The type of treatment required and the goals to be established should be developed in conjunction with the individual himself. Whatever the treatment goals may be, the individual requires a consistent approach from all workers with whom he will be involved.

Although many of the specific aspects of care for these individuals will need to be planned collaboratively, there are some general suggestions that apply to the nursing care of all persons suffering from anxiety disturbances.

Such individuals need a warm, friendly, empathic nurse who accepts them as people in need of help and who helps them feel that they are worthwhile human beings. Scolding or sarcastic remarks will serve only to reinforce their need to protect themselves by the use of their symptoms.

It is usually wise to listen completely and with an accepting attitude when the anxious person describes his physical symptoms. Comments should be directed toward eliciting more information about the complaints. It is important to remember that these individuals can and do become physically ill and deserve medical attention if there is any reasonable doubt about the cause of the complaint.

Some nurses ignore symptoms that stem from anxiety, and in many instances this becomes synonymous with ignoring the individual himself. Since the anxious person is using symptoms to make a bid for help or love, ignoring him increases his need to use the symptoms more frequently.

Avoid asking, "How are you today?" For anxious persons this question is often an invitation for another outpouring of physical complaints. A much more helpful way to begin a conversation might be to comment on some neutral topic that is of mutual interest.

In suggesting that an anxious person participate in some social activity, it is unwise to ask, "Would you like to go swimming with the group?" Such a question will often bring the flat answer *no* or a long recital about why the individual cannot possibly go. A more effective approach would be, "The group is going swimming. I hope that you will go with us." If the objective is to get the individual to participate in a game of table tennis, more positive results will be obtained if the tennis paddle is placed in the client's hand by the nurse, who might say, "We need one more person to play this game. Come and play." This approach is more apt to elicit participation than asking if he wishes to play.

It is helpful if the anxious individual is provided with an opportunity to succeed in the activities in which he participates. This is important because these individuals need help in building self-esteem and self-confidence. Giving deserved praise and recognition for activities performed well is one way of reassuring and encouraging them.

One of the most helpful approaches to the care of anxious clients is to assist them to develop interests outside themselves. Thus recreational and occupational therapy are significant in their treatment. Many anxiety-ridden individuals have never been able to enter into games or group activities. It is important to help them learn to play games and to participate in group activities. This provides opportunities to release tensions as well as to develop new interests. Recreational and occupational activities are usually more successful if they are focused on interests that the individual has had in the past.

The ability to encourage the anxious individual to talk about his concerns and feelings is an important aspect of his care.

The individual suffering from morbid fears and compulsions usually presents a challenging nursing problem. Some nurses who have no understanding of the forces that play a part in developing such symptoms may assume the attitude that the many maneuvers of the individual are ridiculous. Nurses have been known to force a phobic person to touch a doorknob even though it was well known that he was morbidly afraid of the dirt and germs he believed he would contact by touching the object. Other nurses have made it impossible for a client to get into the bathroom to carry out the handwashing rituals that were so important to him in releasing tensions and fears.

When phobic and compulsive individuals are not allowed to carry out the procedures they feel are necessary, they have no way of releasing tension. A high level of unreleased tension may culminate in a panic state. Nurses should make it possible for the individual to carry out the anxiety-releasing rituals he has developed. The rituals carried on by these individuals are essential for them if they are to develop a feeling of security in the situation. Because such rituals are time-consuming, time must be allowed for the individual to perform his ritualistic maneuvers.

Many health care workers, as well as the individual's relatives and friends, attempt to discuss the rituals reasonably in the hope of altering the behavior. This kind of pressure does nothing to help the individual and may actually cause him to feel more anxious and may increase his feeling of guilt.

Short-term hospitalization is usually helpful for persons who exhibit severely dysfunctional behavior because the environment is neutral, they are removed from the significant members of the family who may be the source of much emotional tension, and they are able to feel more secure where the routine is simple, makes few demands, and can be fairly accurately anticipated. Hospitalization on a medical unit may be unfortunate for some persons who have already focused most of their attention on physical symptoms that have no organic basis. Such individuals may become more tense, anxious, and fearful in a setting that emphasizes physical problems.

Some psychopharmacological agents have been helpful in reducing tension and providing the client with a degree of emotional comfort. In addition, behavior modification and desensitization are recognized as efficient and effective intervention techniques. However, the only permanent relief for persons suffering from intolerable anxiety and fear lies in discovering the basic cause of the problem and helping the individual understand the actual source of his symptoms. This is achieved through the treatment technique of psychotherapy. Psychotherapy can be conducted by any prepared mental health professional. As nurses gain additional knowledge and skill in this treatment modality they sometimes assume responsibility for its implementation.

Any procedure that promotes the development of courage, inner security, and self-confidence can be called psychotherapy. However, the traditional use of this term is limited to sustained interpersonal interactions between the psychotherapist and client where the goal is to help the client to develop behaviors that are more functional. Psychotherapy is not a fixed technique; it is more an art than a science, and its methods must be adapted and modified to fit the individual situation. In plain language, it is a form of mental exploration. It is universally acknowledged that one cannot standardize psychotherapy, that it must be individualized, and that it will vary from client to client.

Psychotherapy falls into two general types: supportive psychotherapy and "uncovering" or "insight" psychotherapy. *Supportive psychotherapy* helps the individual cope with his problems and includes such techniques as diagnosis, advice, education, guidance, counseling, assurance, and medication. *Uncovering* or *insight psychotherapy* involves exploring and bringing to consciousness the source of repressed and suppressed conflicts and experiences that operate at unconscious levels to cause anxiety. Uncovering psychotherapy gives meaning to abnormal or irrational feelings and dysfunctional behaviors.

The type of psychotherapy used is dependent on the therapist's assessment of the interrelationship of a number of variables. Chief among these variables are the extent and severity of the client's dysfunction, the client's goals, his intellectual ability, and his personal and interpersonal resources. Generally the more mentally ill the client is, the fewer resources he has, and the less intellectually capable he is, the more he will be a candidate for supportive psychotherapy. Supportive psychotherapy requires the psychotherapist to assume a direct role by offering direction and guidance. The client may not develop an understanding of the dynamics underlying his behavior, but he can learn behaviors that are more functional.

Clients who give evidence of available ego strength, a viable support system, and at least average intelligence can often benefit from uncovering or insight psychotherapy. During this type of psychotherapy, the client is encouraged to talk about his life experiences. He is encouraged to talk freely about anything that comes to his mind, as long as he relates his own ideas and concerns. This random talk allows the client to follow freely the associations that come into his mind and is accurately described as *mental ventilation*. The therapist will note that the client dismisses quickly or avoids mentioning certain occasions and events except in a superficial way. These sensitive areas are then explored more fully. The client is encouraged to talk about them more freely until they no longer cause excess emotion, a process known as *desensitization*.

The client is guided to an understanding of how his repressed feelings are related to his behavior. This is done in a simple, clear style, thereby helping the client to gain insight into the exact nature of his problem. Thus begins the process of reeducation.

It should be noted that a client who initially requires supportive psychotherapy may be able to increase his self-esteem to the point where uncovering or insight psychotherapy is indicated. A skilled psychotherapist has the ability to make this assessment and to respond accordingly.

Regardless of the type of psychotherapy employed, the client is encouraged to face his distressing problems; he is urged to think of them instead of running away from them, to become familiar with them rather than to "forget" them, and to approach their solution in a candid, open manner. He is encouraged to take an active part in his own therapy. If all goes well, he should take more and more constructive steps in the management of his own treatment. He can then answer some of his own questions and make his own decisions. The therapist measures therapeutic success by the degree to which she makes herself less and less necessary.

The most important element in any psychotherapeutic process is the relationship between the therapist and the client. The client must have confidence in the therapist and some respect for the therapist's knowledge and experience. A word of assurance alone may be the deciding factor in relieving many anxious clients of their fears. Such a relationship is dependent on a positive rapport between the therapist and the client.

A very important aspect of the therapist-client relationship is the unconscious attitude of the client toward his therapist. The therapist is cast into a variety of roles, including that of a parent. The client's attitude may be competitive or even erotic. This shifting toward the therapist of desires, feelings, and relations originally experienced by the client with his own parents, siblings, and other persons is known as *transference.* Hence every nuance of feeling, ranging from trustful dependence to open hostility, may be directed toward the therapist. When the client's attitude toward the therapist appears to be favorable, the transference is regarded as being positive. Resistant or antagonistic attitudes of the client toward the therapist imply a negative transference. The client's transference reaction to the therapist may elicit an unconscious counterresponse by the therapist. This attitude of the therapist toward the client is called *countertransference.*

The development of a transference reaction between the client and the psychotherapist is often viewed as a positive sign, for it indicates that the therapist has become significant to the client, thereby establishing the potential for the client to benefit from a corrective emotional experience. For example, if the client responds to the psychotherapist in the clinging, dependent manner that he learned in early life was necessary to maintain his mother's love, the psychotherapist can subtly but consistently encourage the client to make his own decisions while still conveying approval. Through this process the client can learn that it is possible for him to take steps toward independence without jeopardizing the highly valued relationship with the psychotherapist. The client may or may not be helped to become aware of his transference reaction and the process engaged in by the therapist to use the transference therapeutically.

A countertransference reaction is rarely, if ever, seen as hav-

**#
**

ing therapeutic potential except insofar as it provides the therapist with an understanding of the psychodynamics underlying the client's behavior. In other words, by becoming aware of her own reaction to the client, the therapist can better understand the unconscious purpose of the client's behavioral patterns. An example of a nontherapeutic countertransference is when the client behaves toward the psychotherapist as if the therapist were his parent (transference) and the psychotherapist unconsciously responds by treating the client as if he were a child for whom all decisions need to be made (countertransference). Since both transference and countertransference occur on a unconscious level, and since countertransference is not desirable, many teachers of psychotherapy require their students to undergo psychotherapy themselves as a means of discovering their own emotional vulnerabilities and increasing their own overall level of self-awareness. Whether or not a psychotherapist has undergone personal psychotherapy, supervision of psychotherapy by a skilled colleague is necessary to identify and prevent countertransference. The occurence of the transference and countertransference phenomena is a testimony to the fundamentally human nature of the psychotherapeutic process.

In summary, the success of the psychotherapeutic process depends to a large extent on the quality of the interpersonal experience between the client and the therapist. The therapy can be a success only if the therapist succeeds in motivating the client toward promoting his own well-being on his own behalf rather than to please another person. The relationship between the two must remain at a professional level and never at a social one.

**CASE FORMULATION
a ritualistic individual**

Herbert B., 47 years of age, and his wife, Jane, 46 years old, came to the community mental health center to ask for help. Mr. B. was well oriented and intelligent, had good insight, and otherwise appeared to be mentally normal. He gave the following history.

An only child, Mr. B. reported that he remembers his childhood as being uneventful. However he also stated that his mother was a meticulous housekeeper who was known in her community as a fanatic

Continued.

about maintaining correct standards of behavior and observing religious customs.

During his college days he had become emotionally upset and had worried excessively. His pastor was consulted and after several conferences he was able to resume his schoolwork and graduated at the age of 21 as an accountant. He stated that he had always been very conscientious, worried a great deal about body cleanliness, and was known for his concern about keeping his room and clothing in perfect order. He was always prompt in appearing at his office and never left his desk before 5 P.M. His fellow workers regarded him as very fussy, and his employer always remarked about the neatness of his desk and files—a comment that greatly pleased him. At home any irregularity in household routine upset him. His wife was fully aware of his rigid regard for rules and his scrupulousness. She spoke freely about the fact that their marital relations were unsatisfactory and disturbing. She had given up any hope of improving the situation by discussing it with him, because he became extremely anxious when she introduced the topic. She also stated that she was "thankful" they never had any children since she was sure that the "mess" that children normally make in the house would be intolerable for her husband.

Four months before he came to the center, Mr. B. had been assigned the responsibility of making out the income tax report for his firm, which dealt in stocks and bonds. This assignment was made on March 1 and he realized that he had but 6 weeks before the returns were to be filed. He worked under great pressure and almost every day he remained in the office until late at night. With a day to spare, he entered the final figures on a roll of paper from an adding machine. Badly in need of sleep and rest, he seized this roll, thrust it into his overcoat pocket, and dashed for the midnight bus. He intended to show the slip of paper to his wife as evidence that his job was completed. On reaching his home he could not find the roll. In a frenzy he searched his clothing and ran out on the street searching the sidewalk, but failed to find it. He was put to bed in an anxious, fearful state and remained under a physician's care for several weeks.

On returning to work he found that he had developed an overwhelming compulsion. He could no longer pass a piece of crumpled paper on the floor or sidewalk without picking it up and inspecting it. During rush hour he was greatly humiliated and embarassed by the necessity of bending over and picking up odd bits of paper. On several occasions he was knocked down by a hurrying passerby while carrying out this compulsion. A wastebasket full of discarded paper literally threw him into a panic. His only relief was obtained by waiting until after office hours when he could go over each item piece by piece. His physician recommended treatment in the community mental health center.

nursing assessment

It is significant that Herbert B.'s mother was a fastidious housekeeper and a fanatic about observing religious customs and maintaining correct standards of behavior. Undoubtedly such a mother would insist that a child achieve perfection in toilet training at a very early age. In addition, she would rear him to behave in a rigidly correct manner and would covertly encourage him to repress instinctual thoughts and desires.

A young man who at the age of 21 is known to be overly concerned about orderliness, is overly conscientious, and is worried about bodily cleanliness is already well on the road to developing compulsive symptoms to control unconscious anxiety by employing persistently repetitive acts. This behavior, like all human behavior, has purpose and meaning for the individual who employs it even though the forces producing it are unconscious. The anxiety arising from a feeling of guilt is displaced by engaging in ritualistic behavior.

In spite of Herbert's early tendencies to be upset by household irregularities he married. He and his wife managed to work out a relationship that could be tolerated. However according to his wife their sexual relationship was unsatisfactory and such an upsetting topic to her husband that she avoided discussing it. His basic problem focused, in part at least, on his unresolved conflict about his role as a marital partner. This conflict was relieved to some extent by his fastidious attitude toward his body. Such problems probably originated in the attitudes that were taught during the habit-training period.

It was not until he was 47 that Herbert's symptoms became so severe that he required treatment. This was precipitated by the loss of a scrap of paper on which was recorded a final total of a complicated accounting problem he had been assigned to complete. It is interesting that he was attempting to elicit his wife's approval for a successful task accomplished. Since he did not have her approval as a sexual partner, her approval about some other aspect of life was very necessary. The loss of the paper probably represented much more than simply the loss of a list of figures. Symbolically it must have represented the loss of love and approval. This would account for his extreme fear and anxiety. The tax report had been completed before he left the office. Thus there is little doubt that a duplicate of the

Continued.

figures could have been found. The loss must have been symbolic of the loss of something more important and irreplaceable.

In compulsive individuals the repetitive act has a symbolic significance reminiscent of a magic ritual that is designed to eradicate the possible effect of unacceptable instinctual impulses. It also represents a type of self-punishment, since compulsive acts are recognized by the individual as being unreasonable and ridiculous. In spite of the individual's partial insight, the tension and anxiety mount until the urge to repeat the act to control the tension becomes irresistible.

Like most severely anxious individuals, Mr. B. was well oriented, intelligent, and intellectually normal except for his compulsive behavior. This is an example of an individual whose personality is intact except in the one area that is involved with the compulsive behavior. However, in spite of the normal aspects of his personality, he was almost totally incapacitated by the need to examine every scrap of paper.

nursing diagnoses

The assessment data, including present behavior, past life experiences, and an understanding of the underlying dynamics, led to the development of the following nursing diagnoses for Herbert B.:

> Compulsive urge to examine scraps of paper related to anxiety stemming from unconscious conflicts
>
> Marital dysfunction related to client's inability to discuss the couple's sexual relationships

planning and implementing nursing care for HERBERT B.

The following boxed material illustrates a nursing care plan for Herbert B. After assessing his needs and formulating nursing diagnoses the nurse participated in a meeting of the mental health team that discussed Mr. B. As a result of this discussion, a collaborative decision was made not to hospitalize him. Rather, the psychiatrist prescribed diazepam and the nurse made an appointment for him to see a staff psychologist for psychotherapy three times a week. In addition, she made an appointment with him for 1 hour twice a month after one of his therapy sessions. Although the nurse's goal was not to engage in psychotherapy with this client she did have the goal of monitoring his reaction to his medication and to the family system. She was aware that as Herbert B. was able to change his behavior his relationship with his wife would also be altered.

The nurse maintained close communication with the psychologist who was engaged in psychotherapy with the client to be able to reinforce the direction he was taking and not inadvertently interfere with their relationship.

nursing care plan for
HERBERT B.

nursing diagnosis	objective	rationale	nursing actions	outcome criteria
Compulsive urge to examine scraps of paper related to anxiety stemming from unconscious conflicts	To decrease anxiety	As anxiety decreases adaptation of compulsive behavior becomes less necessary	Teach client about actions and side effects of prescribed antianxiety medication Meet twice a month with client to monitor his response to medication Keep wastebaskets out of room in which nurse and client meet Listen attentively to client's complaints	Within 1 month client will give evidence of taking medication regularly and will not experience incapacitating side effects Within 4 months client will give evidence of decreased anxiety by: Reporting a decrease in anxiety Being able to resist urge to examine scraps of paper Not developing a new compulsion
	To assist client to develop insight into underlying unconscious conflicts	Long-term relief of anxiety depends on client's becoming aware of relationship between his symptoms and underlying emotional conflict	Refer to staff psychologist for psychotherapy Meet twice a month with client's psychotherapist	Client meets regularly with psychotherapist Psychotherapist keeps nurse apprised of process of his relationship with client
Marital dysfunction related to inability to discuss the couple's sexual relationship	To increase meaningful communication between client and his wife	As couple increases meaningful communication they increase the probability of having their needs met	View family as a system Understand that as client alters his behavior system will enter disequilibrium Monitor degree of family equilibrium and report to mental health team Rehearse with client ways he might initiate conversations with his wife using techniques such as role playing	Within 4 months the client will report attempts to communicate meaningfully with his wife

Continued.

evaluation

After 4 weeks of biweekly appointments with Herbert B. the nurse was assured that he was taking his medication regularly and was not experiencing adverse reactions. Although he reported that he still felt a mild degree of anxiety almost continuously, he was able to overcome the urge to examine every scrap of paper he saw.

As Herbert B.'s behavior changed as a result of increased insight, family disequilibrium ensued. By the end of 4 months of psychotherapy Herbert B. had developed a beginning awareness of the relationship between his compulsion and his early childhood experiences, especially those with his mother. Although he still maintained his fastidious behavior he grew to understand that his fear of sexual relations with his wife was related to his unconscious association of her with his mother. He became able to consider initiating a conversation with his wife about their sexual relationship. However, the first time he introduced the subject his wife rejected his attempt by saying she did not have time to talk that evening. The nurse understood this behavior as a signal of family disequilibrium and communicated this to the mental health team. At this time the decision was made to offer this couple conjoint therapy in addition to continuing individual psychotherapy for Herbert B. It was also decided that there was no longer any reason for him to continue meeting with the nurse.

As a result of these decisions, the nurse made an appointment for Mr. and Mrs. B. with the staff social worker and made plans to discontinue her routine appointments with Mr. B. in 4 more visits. Even though she was not engaged in psychotherapy with this client, the nurse understood that their relationship was meaningful to him and must not be terminated abruptly or thoughtlessly.

CONCLUDING STATEMENTS

1. Anxiety disturbances are categorized into phobic disorders, anxiety states, and somatoform disorders.
2. A phobia is a specific pathological fear reaction out of proportion to the stimulus. Agoraphobia, a fear of open spaces, is an example of a frequently occurring phobic disorder.
3. Obsessive-compulsive disorder is one of the anxiety states. In the obsessive-compulsive disorder the preoccupation with a compelling ritual is the individual's way of defending himself against anxiety. The performance of the ritual provides a release of tension.
4. Conversion disorder is an example of a somatoform disorder. Conversion is a purposeful, unconscious reaction in which an individual uses a physical symptom as a disguise to solve some acute problem or fulfill some unacceptable desire.
5. Most authorities agree that anxiety disturbances represent a conflict between two divergent drives or desires that have been repressed. Symptoms develop when the ego can no longer effect a compromise between these conflicting desires.
6. To be helpful the nurse needs to understand that all symptoms stemming from anxiety disturbances develop because of an unconscious conflict and have great significance for the individual.
7. Individuals experiencing anxiety disturbances need a warm, friendly, empathic nurse who accepts them as worthwhile human beings who are ill and in need of help.
8. One of the most important aspects of the care of all anxious persons is to help them verbalize their concerns.
9. The ritualistic person should be allowed to carry out the anxiety-releasing maneuvers so essential to his security.
10. Psychotherapy is a sustained interpersonal interaction between the therapist and client where the goal is to help the client develop behaviors that are more functional. The two types of psychotherapy are supportive psychotherapy and uncovering or insight psychotherapy.

SUGGESTED SOURCES OF ADDITIONAL INFORMATION

Classical

Mastrovito, Rene C.: Psychogenic pain, Am. J. Nurs. **74:**514-519, 1974.
May, Rollo: The meaning of anxiety, New York, 1977, W.W. Norton & Co., Inc.

Schwartz, Morris, and Shockley, Emmy Lanning: The nurse and the mental patient, New York, 1956, John Wiley & Sons, Inc.

Sullivan, Harry Stack: Conceptions of modern psychiatry, Washington, D.C., 1953, W.W. Norton & Co., Inc.

Contemporary

Abse, D. Wilfred: Hysterical conversion and dissociative syndromes and the hysterical character. In Arieti, Silvano, editor: American handbook of psychiatry, ed. 2, vol. 3, New York, 1974, Basic Books, Inc., Publishers, pp. 155-194.

Chrzanowski, Gerard: Neurasthenia and hypochondriasis. In Arieti, Silvano, editor: American handbook of psychiatry, ed. 2, vol. 3, New York, 1974, Basic Books, Inc., Publishers, pp. 141-154.

Davis, Judith: Treatment of a medical phobia including desensitization administered by a significant other, J. Psychosoc. Nurs. Ment. Health Serv. **20:**6-8, Aug., 1982.

DiMotto, Jean W.: Relaxation, Am. J. Nurs. **84:**754-758, 1984.

Friedman, Paul, and Goldstein, Jacob: Phobic reactions. In Arieti, Silvano, editor: American handbook of psychiatry, ed. 2, vol. 3, New York, 1974, Basic Books, Inc., Publishers, pp. 110-140.

Gagan, Jeanette: Imagery: an overview with suggested application for nursing, Perspect. Psychiatr. Care **22:**20-25, Jan.-Mar., 1984.

Greenberg, William: The multiple personality, Perspect. Psychiatr. Care **20:**100-104, July-Sept., 1982.

Hagerty, Bonnie K.: Obsessive-compulsive behavior: an overview of four psychological frameworks, J. Psychosoc. Nurs. Ment. Health Serv. **19:**37-39, Jan., 1981.

Jorn, Nancy: Repression in a case of multiple personality disorder, Perspect. Psychiatr. Care **20:**105-110, July-Sept., 1982.

Karshmer, Judith F.: The application of social learning theory to aggression, Perspect. Psychiatr. Care **16:**223-237, Sept.-Dec., 1978.

Kent, Fraser: Coping with phobias, New York, 1980, Harper & Row, Publishers.

Kerr, Norine: Anxiety: theoretical considerations, Perspect. Psychiatr. Care **16:**36-40, Jan.-Feb., 1978.

Knowles, Ruth: Dealing with feelings: managing anxiety, Am. J. Nurs. **81:**110-111, 1981.

Of particular interest

Roncoli, M.: Bantering: a therapeutic strategy with obsessional patients, Perspect. Psychiatr. Care **12:**171-175, Oct.-Dec., 1974.
This article is useful in discussing an approach to one particularly challenging nursing care problem.

chapter sixteen

adults with psychophysiological disturbances

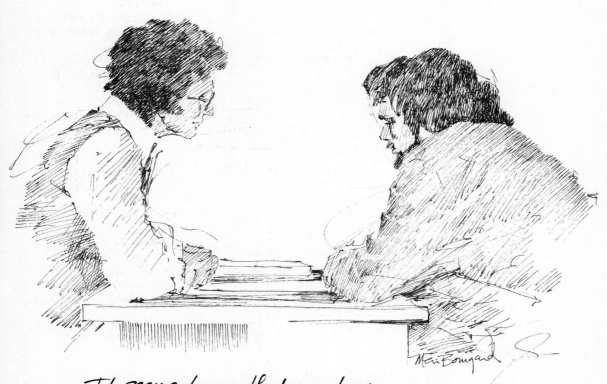

It seems to me that you have conflicting feelings about that.

LEARNING OBJECTIVES

After studying this chapter the student will be able to:

1   Describe the characteristics of psychophysiological disturbances.

2   Discuss the dynamics of development of psychophysiological disturbances.

3   Discuss the nursing care of adults with psychophysiological disturbances.

4   Develop a hypothetical plan of nursing care for an adult with a psychophysiological disturbance.

The phenomenon referred to as *somatization* is a process whereby an individual's feelings, emotional needs, or conflicts are manifested physiologically. When the need, feeling, or conflict is on a conscious level the somatization process occurs as an adaptation to the stress of the emotion. When the emotion is on an unconscious level somatization also serves the function of defending the individual against conscious awareness of the nature of the emotion. In either instance the process of somatization supports the widely accepted belief that the functions and reactions of the mind and body are inextricably related.

When the somatization process is sustained and organic changes occur, the individual is said to have a psychophysiological disturbance. Although it is important for the nurse to be aware of the emotional concomitants of all physical illnesses, it is imperative that she have some understanding of the etiological dynamics of those physical illnesses believed to be psychophysiological disturbances. Only with this understanding will the nurse be able to provide care designed to meet the individual's needs.

HISTORICAL PERSPECTIVE

Medical historians have found evidence that from the earliest times human beings have known that there is a relationship between the mind and the body. Beliefs about the nature of this relationship have changed over time however. For example some primitive people believed that deviant behavior and physical illnesses were caused by the invasion of the individual by evil spirits. This belief led to the practice of trephination, in which holes were bored into the skull of the afflicted person to facilitate departure of the evil spirit. Accompanying this surgical procedure were elaborate rituals performed by a revered member of the community known as a priest, a witch doctor, or a shaman. This procedure was sufficiently successful to justify its continued use over many centuries. Modern authorities believe that the socially sanctioned unconditional trust in the healer was the primary factor in reversing the disease process. The importance of this factor in the healing process is still seen as basic to effective intervention, whether it be physical or psychological.

Other beliefs that have supported the mind-body relationship were that deviant behavior and some forms of physical illness were caused by the individual's sinning and that a physical imbalance of body fluids or humors caused emotional problems.

Early beliefs about the mind-body relationship attempted to postulate a singular cause of either physical or behavioral malfunction. None of these early theories took a holistic view of humans as interrelated systems in which alterations in one component inevitably result in compensatory alterations throughout the entire system which, in turn, affect the entire system. Such is the case with psychophysiological disturbances.

In the past psychophysiological disturbances were referred to as psychosomatic illnesses. Unfortunately, this term has been incorrectly incorporated into the language as meaning that the physical illness is not real but rather is a product of the person's imagination designed to elicit attention and sympathy. No belief could be farther from the truth, and the health care team must never assume that persons with these disorders are not really sick or are merely looking for attention through their physical symptoms.

PSYCHOPHYSIO-LOGICAL DISTURBANCES

Psychophysiological disturbances are believed to have an emotional cause, to affect one body system, and to involve innervation of the autonomic nervous system. Affected individuals present a physical illness in which there is evidence of organic alteration. They are often acutely ill and in fact may have life-threatening exacerbations of the illness.

The individual often has little or no insight into the emotional conflicts underlying his illness and may resent any implication that such is present. Understandably he is very distressed by his physical symptoms and seeks medical treatment of them, unlike those individuals suffering from a conversion disorder. Because his symptoms interfere markedly with his ability to function and may be life-threatening he is often highly motivated to diminish or erase them. Consequently, he can be helped to identify the relationship between stressors and exacerbations of the illness even without gaining an awareness of the unconscious emotional conflict.

DYNAMICS OF DEVELOPMENT

Although there seems to be consensus among authorities regarding the major role a person's emotions play in the development of certain physical illnesses, the exact nature of that role is not yet determined. One widely accepted theory postulates that repressed conflicts are stimulated by intrapsychic or interpersonal events and lead to an overall increase in the individual's level of anxiety. An automatic physical concomitant to an increase in anxiety is innervation of the autonomic nervous system. In other words, the person who is anxious becomes physically ready to engage in flight or fight. However, since the emotional conflict that is the basis for the anxiety and the subsequent physical response is unconscious, the individual has no outlet for the physical response, as would be possible if the conflict were conscious or if the danger were external. Consequently the state of physical readiness for flight or fight does nothing to resolve the underlying emotional conflict. Should this phenomenon be sustained a cyclical pattern is established. This pattern results in physiological alterations such as a peptic ulcer, which is caused by increased gastric acid secretion and gastric hypermotility as compensatory to the initial decreased gastric acid secretion and hypomotility caused by the flight-fight reaction. As the individual perceives physical discomfort it is not unlikely that his anxiety will further increase, thereby compounding the problem. The originator of this theory is a physician named Franz Alexander, whose works on the subject remain classics in the field.

A second theory postulates that certain personality types are particularly prone to the development of certain physical illnesses. An example of this theory is the designation of a specific personality type that is considered to place the individual in a high-risk category for myocardial infarction. These persons are seen to be highly competitive and overly ambitious, and they deny any need for dependency. This personality syndrome is manifested by hard work, aggressive behavior, and a great deal of risk taking as a means of getting ahead. These persons frequently have many individuals dependent on them but no one on whom they feel they can depend.

A third theory places emphasis on the symbolism of the illness. For example a person who unconsciously feels a great deal of rage at significant others and the environment in general but for whom expression of this rage is not acceptable may develop ulcerative colitis. Since ulcerative colitis is an illness in which the person has frequent bowel movements requiring, at the very least, alterations in his and others' activities, one might say that he is symbolically defecating on those around him, a very hostile act indeed.

A fourth theory is referred to as organ weakness. This theory postulates that all humans have one body system that is relatively less healthy than are the others. If a person has underlying unconscious problems that interfere with his effective functioning but at the same time has sufficient ego strength so that a flight from reality is not necessary, this person may develop a physical illness as a means of coping with the unconscious problem. The type of physical illness developed will be determined by the body system that is most physiologically vulnerable.

Regardless of which theory or combination of theories proves to be correct they all have several concepts in common, the understanding of which will prove invaluable to the nurse in caring for persons with psychophysiological disturbances. Following are these concepts:

1. Persons who develop psychophysiological disturbances have *unconscious* emotional conflicts that increase their anxiety and interfere with their effectively meeting their needs.
2. The physical illness is a result of or an expression of this unconscious conflict and serves as a means of lowering the anxiety level.
3. The physical illness is real in that there are demonstrable organic changes that may be life threatening.

It is also generally accepted that the onset of the psychophysiological illness is associated with a real or perceived stressful life event. The physical symptoms occur as a response to this stress and mask the emotional turmoil with which the person cannot cope, thereby achieving the primary purpose of lowering anxiety. In our society, however, the individual also may experience unexpected and unintended benefits from the illness. These benefits may be such things as having one's dependency needs indirectly met, receiving attention and special consideration, or being relieved of responsibility. These benefits are *secondary gains*, which tend to unconsciously reinforce the pattern of somatization.

It is beyond the scope of this text to discuss each of the psychophysiological disturbances in depth. The student should be aware that there are many excellent references available from which much may be learned about each of these disease entities. Discussion in this chapter will be limited to the ones most commonly encountered in general nursing practice and that are illustrative of different body system involvement.

GASTRO-INTESTINAL SYSTEM

Peptic ulcer is a very common syndrome in a highly industrialized society such as the United States. The diagnosis of peptic ulcer encompasses both gastric ulcers and duodenal ulcers, although there is evidence that emotional factors play a larger role in the development of duodenal ulcers, which tend to occur more in men than in women and in younger age-groups. Duodenal ulcers stem from sustained gastric hypermotility and marked increase in gastric secretions, which eventually erodes the lining of the stomach. Clinically the individual complains of epigastric pain that occurs within 1 to 4 hours after the last meal and is relieved by eating or by taking antacids. If alterations in diet and the taking of nonprescription remedies do not help the person is likely to seek medical help, since the pain becomes severe enough that it cannot be ignored. Hospitalization may be necessary, either to establish the diagnosis through testing or for treatment. Although medical treatment is always conservative if possible, the presence of bleeding or intractable pain may indicate the need for surgical removal of the affected part of the stomach or severance of a branch of the vagus nerve. Unfortunately, when this occurs it is not uncommon for the individual to subsequently develop another even more severe form of psychophysiological disturbance.

The personality characteristics of a person who develops a peptic ulcer are those of a person who sees himself and is seen by others as strong, independent, hard-working, and unemotional. Despite their occupational successes, these persons are tormented by feelings of not having done well enough and constantly strive to achieve even higher goals. Authorities believe that underlying these behaviors are strong dependency needs in conflict with the individual's self-image that therefore cannot be directly expressed. If these needs are met, it is a result of fortuitous accident rather than goal-directed behavior.

The initial onset of the illness as well as subsequent exacerbations tend to be precipitated by stressful life events that bring the dependency-independency conflict closer to the surface of consciousness. One man experienced his first episode of duodenal ulcer attack at the time of his marriage when he left his parents' home to establish with his wife a home of their own. Despite the fact that he married an attractive, caring woman whom he loved very much, the very act of marriage abruptly changed his role from that of son to that of husband, or symbolically from child to adult. The first gastrointestinal episode was successfully treated through diet modification and medication, and the symptoms subsided. The second attack occurred after the birth of their first child, a son, 4 years later. Once again, it can be seen that the birth of a child, particularly a son with whose infantile dependency the father may have identified, put increased pressure on this man to act as a strong, responsible adult while simultaneously decreasing direct opportunities to have his dependency needs met. As in the previous attack conservative medical treatment was successful in alleviating the ulcer symptoms although they were more severe and took longer to disappear than in the initial episode. It is interesting to note that when their second child, a daughter, was born 4 years later, no exacerbation of ulcer symptoms occurred. The third and most severe episode of ulcer symptoms took place about a year after this man's father died. The father died as a result of bowel cancer, which was treated by colostomy and radiation, but which nevertheless metastasized. During the course of his illness, the father moved in with his son and daughter-in-law because of his increased need for physical care and supervision. Although the daughter-in-law provided most of the care, the son frequently willingly helped, especially with more personal tasks such as bathing. The father died in the home and during the following year the son was deeply involved in settling his father's complex estate. It was after this task was completed that he once again experienced ulcer symptoms so severe that surgical removal of two thirds of his stomach was ultimately required. It can be conjectured that the death of this man's father was unconsciously seen by him as the ultimate proof of his adulthood, which he was not able to withstand because he maintained a large reservoir of unmet dependency needs, and his father's death symbolically cut off all hope of having these needs met.

Although peptic ulcer is a common form of gastrointestinal psychophysiological disturbance other illnesses such as ulcerative colitis or chronic constipation are also seen as having a strong emotional cause.

CARDIOVASCULAR SYSTEM

A health problem of increasing incidence particularly among black Americans is that of essential hypertension. Essential hypertension is a sustained elevation of systolic and diastolic arterial blood pressure in the absence of any of the demonstrable known causes of arterial hypertension. Although persons suffering from essential hypertension may remain asymptomatic for years, if the syndrome is sustained organic alterations, particularly renal damage, may occur. Often the acceleration of the disease with resultant complications occurs in conjunction with life crises. It is believed that huge amounts of repressed rage that have no acceptable outlet are the emotional dynamics underlying the development of essential hypertension. The mental mechanism used by the individual is usually denial, since the person also has a need to conform with the expectations of others, especially authority figures, as a means of meeting his dependency needs. Feeling and expressing rage is therefore highly anxiety-producing, and the individual often has a calm, placid exterior. The frequency of occurrence of essential hypertension in the black population has led investigators to explore genetic factors simultaneously with cultural factors as major etiological predeterminants.

RESPIRATORY SYSTEM

A major psychophysiological disturbance affecting the respiratory system is bronchial asthma. Bronchial asthma is caused by bronchial obstruction that does not interfere with inspiration but causes difficulty in expiration. This results in the characteristic asthmatic wheeze that sounds so similar in all patients that it is almost diagnostic. The underlying cause of the bronchial obstruction may be an infectious process, an allergic reaction, or an idiopathic bronchospasm. When an underlying disease process such as a bacterial infection is present other symptoms such as an elevated temperature and white blood count are also present and require treatment if the asthmatic episode is to be alleviated. There are some instances, however, when there is no demonstrable physiological cause for the asthmatic episode, and it is here that emotional factors are believed to play a major etiological role in the occurrence of the illness.

The personality characteristics of the individual who suffers from asthma seem to include strong dependency needs directed toward the mother or mother figure, with simultaneous anger toward this individual, which elicits unconscious fears of abandonment. In fact, some psychoanalytically oriented authorities claim that the characteristic asthmatic wheeze is a symbolic cry for the mother. During an acute asthmatic attack the individual is a clinging, dependent person whose behavior is justified to himself and others on the basis of the life-threatening symptoms. Therefore it is not uncommon for the dependency needs of the person to be met during the acute episode, but unfortunately these temporary episodes of need fulfillment do little to alter the underlying personality dynamics, and thus future episodes are not prevented. Continued episodes of asthma result in pulmonary changes that may not be reversible and may affect the vital capacity of the person's respiratory system.

INTEGUMENTARY SYSTEM

The integumentary system serves a unique function in the ego psychology of an individual in that it is the only body system equally visible both to the person and to others. Because of this the skin represents the self to others in the environment. An awareness of this fact is reflected in such sayings as, "He's too thick- [or thin-] skinned" or "You can't tell a book by its cover."

The skin is richly endowed with sense receptors for pain, pressure, and temperature sensations. As a result, many emotional states are reflected in skin changes—the blush of embarrassment and the paling that accompany fear are examples. These common skin changes are received by others as nonverbal clues to the emotional state of the individual, frequently despite verbal reassurances to the contrary. In healthy interpersonal relationships, the skin acts as a friendly ally in communicating to others what is being felt and therefore enhances the probability of having the individual's needs met. When the skin is involved in a psychophysiological disturbance, however, it becomes a means of self-disclosure representing the individual's unconscious conflict between a repressed emotion and the simultaneous need to have this emotion known and responded to.

Numerous dermatological conditions can cause a person severe discomfort, either in the form of itching, pain, or disfigurement. Although in many instances their exact cause is unknown, an amazing number of these maladies respond well to the treatment of a dermatologist who may try a number of remedies before finding one that seems to help. Although not denying the positive benefits of the physical treatment received, many authorities believe that the major benefit is achieved from the sustained, concerned interest in the individual and his illness that is frequently shown by dermatologists and that indirectly helps to meet the person's immediate needs. Exacerbations of skin rashes and severe itching are closely related to occurrences of stressful life events to which these persons seem to respond without undue emotional upset but rather react by somatization on which they and others can focus their concern. Many psychiatrists believe that skin somatization is one of the most primitive ego defenses available and therefore are very cautious in pursuing aggressive physical and psychological treatment unless the individual is in great pain or unable to carry out activities of daily living. The rationale underlying this conservative approach is that if the person is enabled to give up this defense without a considerable increase in ego strength, he might be forced to resort to the more serious and incapacitating defense of mental illness.

MUSCULO-SKELETAL SYSTEM

The most common and severe form of psychophysiological disturbance that affects the musculoskeletal system is rheumatoid arthritis. This disease results in marked organic damage and affects not only the joints but also other tissues. Its onset may occur at any age, and it affects females more frequently than males. The personality characteristics of persons affected by this disease almost universally include masochistic, self-sacrificing behavior, which is in response to a rigid, punitive superego and a weak ego organization. Their family background frequently gives evidence of maternal deprivation, leaving them with a great many unmet dependency needs. Prior to becoming ill, these individuals indirectly express their emotional needs by being helpful and kind, willing to do almost anything for others, and thereby receiving positive feedback from their social system. Under usual circumstances therefore their dependency needs are minimally met through environmental and interpersonal support, allowing them to remain healthy until such time as this support is withdrawn. Many individuals report that an event such as the death of a spouse or the loss of a job immediately preceded the initial onset of the illness.

Treatment of these persons is exceedingly complex. Many of them reflect their emotional conflict by denying the severity of their illness and either refuse treatment or are unreliable in following the treatment regimen. Conversely, there are some who quickly become highly dependent on family, friends, and health care personnel despite the fact that their symptoms may be only mildly debilitating.

NURSING CARE OF INDIVIDUALS WITH PSYCHO-PHYSIOLOGICAL DISTURBANCES

The care of persons suffering from psychophysiological disturbances is usually directed by a physician whose emphasis is on the reduction of physical symptoms and the prevention of further organic damage. However, because of the nature of the illness, close collaboration with a psychiatrist is often necessary. Once the acute physical symptoms have abated, the psychiatrist may continue to treat the individual on an outpatient basis in an attempt to help the person deal with underlying emotional problems. The nurse is usually involved in providing care during those times when the person is hospitalized for an exacerbation of the illness or in follow-up care in the home. During her involvement, the methods the nurse uses in carrying out physical care are often pivotal factors in enhancing or impeding the overall treatment goals. The following are some suggested guidelines that should be considered in the nursing care plan for persons with psychophysiological disturbances.

The nurse must fully understand and accept the fact that these persons are physically ill and that their symptoms may reach life-threatening proportions. The nurse must not convey the attitude that she believes the individual would get better if he merely exerted more control over his emotions. During acute episodes of the illness, meeting the physical needs of the client is of primary importance, even if in so doing the nurse is supporting a dysfunctional emotional adaptation. For example, a couple whose tension-laden relationship exacerbates the wife's physical symptoms should not be encouraged to discuss their relationship during the acute episode of the wife's illness.

Most physical illnesses, regardless of cause, present a potential threat to the person's perception of himself as an independent adult. In the case of persons with psychophysiological disturbances, there often are underlying conflicts between dependency and independency needs, and the imposed dependence that results from the illness may stimulate a high degree of anxiety in the client. In such instances the nurse can be helpful if she meets the individual's needs for dependence in an indirect way while simultaneously acknowledging his status as a responsible adult. An example of such an intervention is the nurse who wisely addresses the client with a peptic ulcer as Mr. Smith instead of John. At the same time, Mr. Smith's dependency needs can be indirectly met by the nurse's administering the prescribed antacid instead of leaving it at the bedside or asking the client to ring his call light every half hour so that she can bring the medicine. By spontaneously making frequent contact with the client the nurse is indirectly saying that she is willing to take care of him without his having to assume the responsibility of asking for help. It should be noted that the administration of oral medication or food, especially milk, has great symbolic significance, since eating is the vehicle through which people have their dependency needs first met.

Many persons are not aware of the interpersonal resources available to them within their social system. Persons with psychophysiological disturbances can often benefit from help in identifying already existent interpersonal resources and in enlarging their social network, thereby increasing the possibility of having their emotional needs met by a larger variety of people.

The nurse has many opportunities to engage in conversation with the hospitalized person. She can be of emotional assistance to him if she encourages him to talk about his feelings. It must be understood, however, that many of the client's feelings are unacceptable to him and therefore acceptance of him and his feelings by the nurse is of primary importance. As in communicating with any client, the nurse is most helpful when she is accepting and nonjudgmental. Reflecting or restating what the client has said is an appropriate communication technique to employ, since a direct interpretation may be very threatening and raise the client's anxiety level and perhaps thereby increase the severity of his physical symptoms.

As is true of any client, the person suffering from a psychophysiological disturbance can be helped to feel in control of his situation by adequate explanations of what he can expect to experience during diagnostic and treatment procedures. Some clients, however , become increasingly anxious if they are given too much information and their dependency needs are best met by trusting in the judgment of their physician and nurse. Therefore the amount and nature of information offered to the client should be primarily determined by an assessment of his anxiety level. Certainly the client's questions should be answered, but the degree of elaboration should be gauged by his response to the answer rather than by the nurse's need to engage in health teaching.

The secondary gains achieved by the individual as the result of his being physically ill need to be minimized once the acute episode has passed. The nurse can be instrumental in working with him to strengthen or develop coping mechanisms that do not involve somatization.

Working with the client's family is necessary to aid them in understanding the complexity of his illness and its treatment. The effect of the family on the client and the effect the client and his illness have on the family is a process that is often explored in family therapy under the guidance of a skilled therapist.

**CASE
FORMULATION
an individual with
asthma**

Martha B. is a 25-year-old single woman who has suffered from asthma since the age of 2. Although respiratory infections have always precipitated an asthmatic attack, there have been many instances of asthmatic episodes unaccompanied by an infectious process. Martha is the only child of an attractive 45-year-old woman who has never married and who is not sure who Martha's father is. Martha and her mother live together in a well-furnished 2-bedroom apartment in a middle-class neighborhood of a large city.

Since the age of 16 Martha's mother has engaged in prostitution and became pregnant several times. For reasons that are not clear, at the time she was pregnant with Martha she decided not to have an abortion as she had done on previous occasions. After Martha was born the mother set up housekeeping in an apartment that she furnished with the child's needs in mind.

By the time Martha was 5 years old her mother had become so successful in her occupation that she no longer was a streetwalker but rather made appointments with her customers by telephone and therefore had advance notice as to when she would not be home. At those times she left Martha with her grandmother, a warm, kind woman who seemed unaware of her daughter's activities. Martha's grandmother lived alone and she was always delighted to have Martha visit. When Martha and her mother were together they seemed to enjoy each other and have a mutually satisfying relationship.

After Martha graduated from high school she took a position as a clerk in a large plastics company located in the heart of the city. She has remained with this company but has never accepted offers of promotion. Therefore her salary is essentially at the same level as it was when she was hired, because the only raises she has received were several cost-of-living increments. For this reason she feels unable to leave her mother's home and rent her own apartment.

The event preceding Martha's latest and most severe asthmatic attack was the death and burial of her grandmother. When notified of her grandmother's death, Martha responded quite stoically and, in fact, made all the funeral arrangements because her mother was out of town. On the day of the funeral Martha began to cry softly. However, by the time the family assembled at the cemetery she was severely dyspneic and had to be rushed from the gravesite to the emergency room of the local hospital. The emergency room staff were very familiar with Martha and her family situation although they did not know of her grandmother's death.

By the time Martha arrived at the emergency room she was in

acute physiological distress, gasping for air and wheezing so loudly that she could be heard throughout the waiting room. Her mother expressed genuine concern but also stated that "this couldn't have happened at a worse time since I have to leave town tonight." She begged the hospital personnel to admit Martha so she wouldn't have to worry while she was away.

nursing assessment

Martha's family situation contained all the elements sufficient for the development of idiopathic asthma. It can be conjectured that Martha's mother was in fact a very immature person lacking in self-esteem who engaged in prostitution as one means of reinforcing her feelings of worthlessness. If this were true it is likely that her decision not to terminate her pregnancy with Martha was an unconscious attempt to provide herself with a consistent person who would need and value her. Unfortunately, this rarely succeeds, since children require more attention and love than they can give during their formative developmental periods. Martha undoubtedly felt that her mother's frequent absences were a result of some failing on her part, while at the same time she experienced much anger at her mother for not providing her with the emotional support she needed. This issue could not be openly confronted since to do so would incur the risk of abandonment, thereby dooming forever the possibility of having her needs met by her mother. On the other hand the grandmother seemed able to meet some of Martha's needs, although her relationship with her own daughter was not growth-producing, as evidenced by their lack of communication.

Although she was 25 years old, it appears that Martha's developmental maturity was not congruent with her chronological maturity. Rather than struggling with age-appropriate developmental tasks, Martha's inability to establish herself in her own apartment indicates she was still struggling with dependency issues characteristic of the developmental phases of childhood. To the extent that Martha's grandmother was able to meet some of Martha's dependency needs, Martha was able to function. When the grandmother died Martha lost the only stable, consistent person in her life and was unequipped to successfully cope with this developmental stressor. Therefore her wheezing was interpreted as a desperate cry to be cared for.

nursing diagnosis

Based on the nursing assessment that included prior knowledge of the family dynamics, and an understanding of the dynamics underly-

Continued.

ing psychophysiological disturbances, the nurse formulated the following nursing diagnosis:

> Severe dyspnea related to unconscious feelings of anger at being abandoned

planning and implementing nursing care for MARTHA B.

A sample nursing care plan for Martha B. is found in the boxed material below.

The immediate objective was to restore physiological homeokinesis so Martha was given the prescribed bronchodilator by intramuscular injection. Within 10 minutes she was breathing more easily and was noticeably more comfortable. This could have been accomplished in the emergency room but in view of the family situation, the physician had decided to hospitalize her.

nursing care plan for MARTHA B.

nursing diagnosis	objective	rationale	nursing actions	outcome criteria
Severe dyspnea related to unconscious feelings of anger at being abandoned	Restore physiological homeokinesis	Although emotionally based, symptoms are life-threatening	Administer prescribed bronchodilator Observe for respiratory distress Plan physical care to conserve client's energy	Within 20 minutes of receiving medication dyspnea will decrease
	Meet client's dependency needs in a fashion appropriate to her chronological age Encourage client to express her feelings	Meeting client's dependency needs in the short term is necessary to prevent increase of physiological symptoms	Establish relationship with client by giving undivided attention Anticipate client's needs, for example, offer juice at regular intervals Listen attentively and nonjudgmentally to client's expressions of loss	Within 48 hours client will be symptom free

After her immediate physical needs were met, it was decided that Martha could benefit from constant attention from a member of the nursing staff. Therefore a student nurse who was studying the nursing care of individuals with psychophysiological disturbances was assigned to stay with Martha. While it could be argued that this intervention would result in secondary gains, it was believed appropriate during this crisis.

Under supervision of her instructor the student nurse encouraged Martha to express her feelings and was careful to respond in an empathic way even though she knew that Martha's grandmother had not intentionally abandoned her. She also attempted to meet Martha's dependency needs through such interventions as offering her liquids to drink without waiting to be asked. Although Martha was allowed out of bed, the student brought her a basin of water and a towel so she could bathe in bed if she wished.

evaluation

Martha responded so well to the interventions of medications and consistent attention that the health care team decided that she would be a good candidate for psychotherapy. This treatment option had never been offered to Martha on any previous admission, but with the loss of her grandmother it was feared that Martha would not have the resources to cope with her situation if she were not given more assistance. Martha's mother would also be invited to begin family therapy with her daughter. Although the staff were not optimistic about her agreeing to participate, they felt it was important that she be offered this help not only for Martha's well-being but for hers as well.

CONCLUDING STATEMENTS

1. The phenomenon referred to as somatization is a process whereby an individual's feelings, emotional needs, or conflicts are manifested through physical symptoms.
2. Human beings have known since the earliest times that the functions of the mind and the body are inextricably related.
3. Psychophysiological disturbances are physical illnesses believed to have an emotional cause, to affect one body system, and to involve innervation of the autonomic nervous system.
4. The person experiencing a psychophysiological disturbance may be acutely ill and have life-threatening exacerbations of the illness.
5. A number of theories attempt to explain the underlying dy-

namics of psychophysiological disturbances. All these theories have the following concepts in common:

   a. Persons who develop psychophysiological disturbances have unconscious emotional conflicts that increase their anxiety and interfere with their effectively meeting their needs.
   b. The physical illness is a result of or an expression of this unconscious conflict and serves as a means of lowering the anxiety level.
   c. The physical illness is real in that there are demonstrable organic changes that may be life threatening.
   d. The onset of the illness is associated with a real or perceived stressful life event.

6. Secondary gains are the unexpected and unintended benefits the person receives as a result of his illness that unconsciously reinforce the pattern of somatization.

7. Peptic ulcer, essential hypertension, bronchial asthma, many skin disorders, and rheumatoid arthritis are examples of common psychophysiological disturbances.

8. The nurse can be most helpful to these persons by:

   a. Skillfully meeting the person's immediate physical needs.
   b. Conveying an accepting, nonjudgmental attitude by understanding that the physical distress the individual is experiencing is not under his control.
   c. Meeting the person's dependency needs in an indirect way while simultaneously acknowledging him as a responsible adult.
   d. Helping the person to use and enlarge his interpersonal resources.
   e. Encouraging the person to talk about his feelings.
   f. Providing appropriate explanations of diagnostic and treatment procedures.
   g. Minimizing the secondary gains achieved by the individual once the acute episode of the illness has passed.
   h. Working with the person's family to aid them in understanding the complexity of his illness and its treatment.

SUGGESTED SOURCES OF ADDITIONAL INFORMATION

Classical

Alexander, Franz: Psychosomatic medicine, New York, 1954, W.W. Norton & Co., Inc.

Dunbar, Flanders: Emotions and bodily changes, New York, 1954, Columbia University Press.

Contemporary

Bahnson, Claus Bahne: Epistemological perspectives of physical disease from the psychodynamic point of view, Am. J. Public Health **64:**1034-1040, 1974.

Byrne, D.G.: Personal determinants of life event stress and myocardial infarction, Psychother. Psychosom. **40**(1-4):106-114, 1985.

Deter, H.C., and Allert, G.: Group therapy for asthma patients: a concept for the psychosomatic treatment of patients in a medical clinic, Psychother. Psychosom. **40**(1-4):95-105, 1983.

Giannini, A.J.: Psychiatric, psychogenic, and somatopsychic disorders handbook, New Hyde Park, N.Y., 1978, Medical Examination Publishing Co., Inc.

Haggarty, J.: The psychosomatic family: an overview, Psychosomatics **24:**615-623, July, 1983.

Haggarty, J., and Drossman, D.: Use of psychotropic drugs in patients with peptic ulcer, Psychosomatics **26:**277-284, Feb., 1985.

Jackson, Bettie: Ulcerative colitis from an etiological perspective, Am. J. Nurs. **73:**258-261, 1973.

Krcek-Frank, Roseanne: Psychosomatic problems in the People's Republic of China, J. Psychosoc. Nurs. Ment. Health Serv. **18:**15-18, Dec., 1980.

Krishnan, K., France, R., and Houpt, J.: Chronic low back pain and depression, Psychosomatics **26:**299-302, Feb., 1985.

Matussek, P., Agerer, D., and Seibt, G.: Aggression in depressives and psoriatics, Psychother. Psychosom. **43:**120-125, March, 1985.

Minuchin, Salvador: Families and family therapy, Massachusetts, 1974, Harvard University Press, pp. 240-254.

Reckless, J., and Fauntleroy, A.: Groups, spouses, and hospitalization as a trial of treatment in psychosomatic illness, Psychosomatics **13:**353-357, June, 1972.

Rimon, R., and Laakso, R.L.: Life stress and rheumatoid arthritis, Psychother. Psychosom. **43:**38-43, Jan., 1985.

Santonastaso, P., Canton, G., Giovanni, B.A., and Zamboni, S.: Hypertension and neuroticism, Psychother. Psychosom. **41:**7-11, Jan., 1984.

Sarason, I., Sarason, B., Potter, E., and Antoni, M.: Life events, social support, and illness, Psychosom. Med. **47:**156-163, March/April, 1985.

Starkman, M., and Appelblatt, N.: Functional upper airway obstruction: a possible somatization disorder, Psychosomatics **25:**327-333, April, 1984.

Weiner, H.: What the future holds for psychosomatic medicine, Psychother. Psychosom. **42**(1-4):15-24, 1984.

Karasu, Toksoz: Psychotherapy with physically ill patients. In Karasu, Toksoz, and Bellak, Leopold, editors: Specialized techniques in individual psychotherapy, New York, 1980, Brunner/Mazel, Inc.

Wittkower, Eric D., and Warnes, Hector: Psychosomatic medicine: its clinical applications, New York, 1977, Harper & Row, Publishers, Inc.

Wolf, S.: Peptic ulcer, Psychosomatics **23:**1101-1105, Nov., 1982.

Of particular interest

Wittkower, Eric D., and Warnes, Hector: Psychosomatic medicine: its clinical applications, New York, 1977, Harper & Row, Publishers, Inc. *This useful text contains an exceptionally good series of articles on the major physiological manifestations of psychological dysfunction.*

chapter seventeen

adults with
substance
dependence

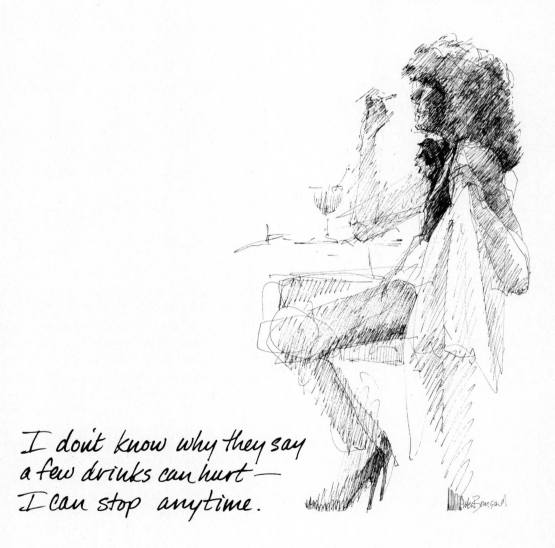

*I don't know why they say
a few drinks can hurt—
I can stop anytime.*

LEARNING OBJECTIVES

After studying this chapter the student will be able to:

1 Differentiate between substance abuse and substance dependence.

2 Define physical and psychological dependence.

3 Describe the characteristics of alcohol dependence. ✓

4 Describe the short-term treatment of the alcohol-dependent individual.

5 Describe the way in which Alcoholics Anonymous helps alcohol-dependent individuals maintain a life free of alcohol use.

6 Describe the characteristics of heroin dependence. ✓

7 Discuss the use of methadone as a treatment of heroin-dependent individuals.

8 Describe the effects of barbiturate dependence. ✓

9 Discuss the effects of amphetamine dependence. ✓

10 Describe the effects of use of cocaine, hallucinogens, and marijuana.

11 Discuss the treatment of drug-dependent individuals.

Very few human behaviors have consequences as far reaching as do those of the substance-dependent individual. In addition to affecting his own physical, emotional, and social well-being, the behavior of the substance-dependent individual affects the well-being of his family and that of the society at large. For example, industry has documented that alcoholism is one the primary reasons for the loss of time and productivity both on the assembly line and in the executive suite. Therefore alcohol dependence has become a significant factor in the economic health of the nation.

Criminal activity is an integral aspect of drug dependence. Hard drugs must be procured from an illegal source, thereby contributing to the maintenance of organized crime. In addition, the price they command often causes the individual to resort to criminal activity to obtain sufficient funds to maintain his dependence. Even when the drug-dependent individual does not have to engage in criminal activity to support his dependence, he most certainly must spend money better used for other purposes. As a result, it is not unusual for his family to have inadequate food, clothing, and shelter. As the substance dependence increases, the source of legally gained income inevitably is cut off, usually because of the individual's inability to maintain his job.

Another complexity surrounding substance dependence is the inevitable involvement of the individual with both the legal and health care systems. This overlap in social systems is not unique to these disorders but the nature of the overlap is problematic since the goals of the legal and health care systems are diametrically opposed. The goal of the legal system is to punish the offender, while the health care system views the individual as a person in need of help. This conflicting view of the same behavior developed, in part, because of lack of definitive information about the nature of substance dependence. Until research documents these behaviors as an illness or society is willing to legalize dependence, the substance-dependent individual will remain caught between the divergent purposes of these two systems.

HISTORICAL PERSPECTIVE

The nontherapeutic use of mind-altering substances is as old as the history of humanity. The Old Testament gives an account of Noah who became drunk on wine and apparently collapsed. The New Testament abounds with cautions against intemperance in many activities, including the drinking of alcoholic beverages. Thus it must be concluded that alcohol abuse was common in those days.

Historical reference to substance abuse is not limited to alcohol. American Indians used hallucinogenic substances as an integral aspect of religious rituals. In the 19th century cocaine was widely used throughout the civilized world, as was opium.

It was not until the twentieth century however that the incidence of substance dependence became great enough to cause national concern. The Harrison Act of 1914 regulated drug traffic for the first time and provided for the licensing of certain groups such as physicians who could legally dispense these drugs for medicinal purposes. In the early 1920s the Volstead Act was passed, which made the sale of alcoholic beverages illegal. This law was ultimately repealed because it did little to curb the consumption of alcoholic beverages but it did contribute to the development of crime syndicates that trafficked in the illegal manufacture and sale of liquor. The effect of the Harrison Act was similar to that of the Volstead Act, namely, addicts were forced to turn to illegal sources to obtain drugs. Governmental response has not been the same, however. Rather than legalizing mind-altering drugs as had been done with alcohol, stricter laws aimed at both the user and the supplier continue to be passed.

The number of alcohol-dependent persons in this country has always been great. Alcoholism has existed in most ethnic groups at all socioeconomic levels. In contrast, prior to World War II heroin addiction was most prevalent among Caucasians in the southern United States. Since the war the highest incidence of this type of drug dependence is found in northern urban areas among the Black and Hispanic cultures. In fact, almost 50% of the heroin addicts today are in New York City.

The use of mind-altering drugs reached epidemic proportions in the 1960s and 1970s among lower- and middle-class adolescents and young adults in urban and suburban areas throughout the entire country. It appears that the level of drug usage among this group reached its peak in the 1970s. However, there has been a concomitant rise in alcohol usage among adolescents and young adults. In fact, alcohol abuse or dependence is the most frequent psychiatric disorder reported for males from 18 to 65 years of age in three Eastern cities for the period of 1980 to 1982.

Of most recent concern is the increased use of cocaine. Prior to the 1980s cocaine was used primarily by those in the entertainment industry and young, upwardly mobile, middle-class, highly educated white males. Because of a glut of cocaine smuggled into the United States, its price has dropped markedly, now making it within the economic reach of even lower income wage earners. Its availability, relatively low cost, and association with celebrities combine to make cocaine a fashionable drug.

Although many persons are highly critical of governmental policies concerning alcohol and other drugs, the ineffectiveness of the government in controlling the availability of these substances does not explain their appeal to such a large segment of the society. As is true of many other forms of mental illness, it is believed that the stress of twentieth century life is a prime factor in creating the conditions requisite to the flourishing of alcohol and drug dependence.

SUBSTANCE ABUSE AND DEPENDENCE

The third edition of the Diagnostic and Statistical Manual of Mental Disorders (DSM-III) differentiates between abuse of alcohol and drugs and dependence on these substances. Substance abuse is difficult to determine because whether it exists or not is often a subjective opinion that depends on the situation. In general, the term refers to the use of any substance for other than therapeutic purposes. However, the individual who, for example, habitually uses over-the-counter sleeping aids because of insomnia certainly is using this medication for therapeutic purposes but also could be considered to be abusing it.

In contrast, substance dependence is more easily determined. There are two types of dependence, physical and psychological. Physical dependence is reflected by a physiological adaptation to the substance so that the body must have it to function asymptomatically. Furthermore, tolerance to the substance increases with physical dependence, requiring the individual to increase the dosage to achieve the same effect. Physical dependence, however, is not conclusive until symptoms of withdrawal can be demonstrated. When an individual becomes physically dependent on a substance the focus of his concern quickly shifts from using it as an adaptation to an emotional problem to needing it to prevent the emergence of physiological symptoms of withdrawal. Thus physical dependence ensures self-perpetuation.

Psychological dependence is believed to be learned behavior in which the individual genuinely believes he cannot function without the substance. The thought of its potential unavailability causes high anxiety and unremitting efforts to obtain it. Psychological dependence on a substance is one of the reasons why so many physically dependent individuals continue to crave the substance even after they have been physiologically withdrawn from it.

Most substances are likely to produce physical dependence if taken consistently over even a short period of time. However, all substances can create psychological dependence in susceptible individuals. Either type of dependence is deleterious to the physical, emotional, and social functioning of the individual and, as previously stated, often brings the person to the attention of the health care and legal systems.

ALCOHOL
DEPENDENCE

Alcohol is a central nervous system depressant. The amount required to produce a demonstrable effect varies according to the interrelationship of such variables as the percentage of alcohol in the beverage, the tolerance the individual has developed to the substance, his physical and emotional state of health, and the nature of the environment in which he is drinking. In addition, the amount and type of food in the stomach constitute a major factor that affects the rate of absorption. Hard liquor drunk by a person unaccustomed to alcohol who is emotionally upset, has not eaten all day, and is in the company of persons who are accepting of intoxication is certain to produce a very rapid effect.

Once alcohol is absorbed into the bloodstream it affects all body tissues but its immediate effects are caused by its action on the brain. At a level of 0.05 percent of alcohol in the blood, inhibitions are diminished and the individual is likely to say and do things that would be unacceptable to him if he were sober. Interestingly, there is a societal norm that, to a point, excuses the behavior of an individual who has been drinking on the grounds that he has been drinking. This cyclical thinking is based on the belief that the behavior of a person when drunk is not a reflection of him but rather a manifestation of the alcohol. The reality is that the impulses acted on emanate from the person and the alcohol merely removes the barriers to their implementation.

At a level of 0.10 percent of alcohol in the blood, motor and speech activity is impaired. It is for this reason that there has been a recent national campaign against driving a motor vehicle when drinking.

Alcohol dependence may take many forms and has many causes. One individual may be a *chronic alcoholic,* which means that he drinks excessively and is incapacitated most of the time. Another person may be referred to as a *periodic* or *cyclic alcoholic,* which means that he drinks excessively during certain periods of his life but during other periods may not drink at all. A third type of alcoholism is exhibited by an individual who drinks large quantities of alcohol daily over a period of years. At first he may not seem to be seriously affected by this overindulgence. Slowly and insidiously, physical, mental, and emotional deterioration occurs. Eventually this person may be described as suffering from alcoholic deterioration. No matter what type of alcoholism is being considered, the problem is thought to have as one of its bases some emotional conflict, frustration, or feeling of inadequacy. In addition to emotional factors, much current research is being conducted to determine if there is, in fact, a physiological component that differentiates the alcoholic from others who are able to drink alcohol without deleterious effects or a subsequent craving to do so. One theory states there is a physiological inability to absorb and/or eliminate the substance. Another theory has postulated an allergic type of reaction among some people. If it can be demonstrated that the development of alcohol dependency requires the existance of certain physiological factors it would clearly place the responsibility for treatment of these individuals within the domain of the heath care system.

Each alcohol-dependent person is a unique individual with problems that are characteristically his own. Many alcohol-dependent individuals use alcohol in somewhat the same way that psychotic individuals use psychotic symptoms. That is, they escape from reality through alcohol, whereas some psychotic individuals escape from reality through the use of their symptoms. When some alcoholics are deprived of alcohol, they may substitute psychotic symptoms such as withdrawal from reality, depression, or a paranoid reaction.

Sometimes alcohol is used to cover symptoms of mental illness. Thus some people who are labeled as alcoholics are actually suffering from a depression or anxiety state. Such persons are clearly in need of the care and treatment usually provided in a mental health treatment center.

Many alcoholics are described as having oral personalities. This suggests that they are fixated at an early stage of emotional development. This early stage of emotional development is called the oral-dependent period and is characterized by infantile emotional reactions. Such individuals receive many of their emotional satisfactions from the intake of food and fluids by mouth. They find it difficult to function as independent adults and unconsciously want to be dependent on a strong person, much as they once were on a mother figure. In general, the alcohol-dependent individual is an unhappy, distraught person unable to cope with the stresses of daily living. Whether these factors are causes or effects of his alcoholism is not clear.

Short-term, immediate treatment of the alcohol-dependent individual is focused on withdrawing him from this substance and assisting him to attain or regain physical health. This is accomplished by symptomatic treatment of the anxiety, tremors, nausea, and diaphoresis that accompany withdrawal. Seizures and delirium tremens are serious, life-threatening conditions that may occur during detoxification.

Delirium tremens is an acute reaction to the withdrawal from a heavy and consistent intake of alcohol for a period of several weeks without an adequate intake of food. In an individual who has been a chronic alcoholic for several years, delirium tremens may be precipitated by a head injury or a surgical procedure without the individual's having taken alcohol at the time of its appearance. Delirium tremens consists of confusion, excitement, and delirium. It is usually of relatively short duration and does not cause a profound and permanent change in the personality.

The delirium is preceded by loss of appetite, restlessness, and insomnia. Slight noises cause the patient to jerk with fear, and moving objects lead to great excitement and agitation. Gradually, consciousness becomes clouded, friends are no longer recognized, and shadows on the wall appear as insects or crawling animals. The person becomes terrified, picks imaginary threads off the bedclothing, feels and sees nonexistent insects on his skin. There is a ceaseless fumbling and picking movement of his fingers and hands. The person's face has an anxious or terrified expression, and his eyes are bloodshot. His skin is moist with perspiration; his tongue and lips are tremorous. His pulse is rapid and weak, and there is always some elevation of temperature.

Anticonvulsant and sedative medications, along with high potency vitamins and copious amounts of clear liquids, are employed during this phase of treatment, to both prevent and treat seizures and delirium tremens. Because of the serious physiological disequilibrium the person experiences as he goes through withdrawal from alcohol, this procedure is best carried out in a hospital by staff who are knowledgeable about the varied problems involved.

Despite the magnitude of the problem of alcohol dependency in the United States, few specific long-term measures of helping these individuals refrain from drinking have been developed. One method that has been used with mixed results is called the *aversion treatment*. This treatment consists of allowing the individual to drink a good deal of his favorite alcoholic beverage, after which an emetic drug is administered. In a few minutes the person becomes acutely nauseated and spends approximately an hour vomiting and retching. The treatment is administered two or three times a week until he develops such an aversion to alcohol that he begins to gag at the sight of the alcoholic beverage toward which the aversion has been developed. This treatment does not help the individual solve any of his basic emotional problems, although some therapists have combined the treatment with psychotherapy. The aversion treatment does keep some individuals away from alcohol for several months, and some are able to give it up permanently. Many individuals substitute some other form of emotional support for alcohol and may begin the use of drugs, particularly the barbiturates, after giving up the use of alcohol.

The drug disulfiram (Antabuse) has been used successfully to treat some alcohol-dependent individuals. It functions something like the aversion treatment in that the individual who takes a specific amount of disulfiram daily will become nauseated when he takes even a small amount of alcohol. This drug is helpful as long as the individual is under close supervision and takes the drug regularly. Away from supervision some individuals stop taking the drug. The drug is considered to be dangerous in some instances, and a few individuals have suffered adverse reactions from it.

The only potentially effective long-term treatment of the alcohol-dependent individual requires that he accept the fact he is an alcoholic. This step is often the most difficult to achieve since the defense mechanism of denial is universally employed by the alcohol-dependent person. If he is able to acknowledge to himself and others that he cannot cope with his life without the help alcohol provides and that he needs assistance he may be able to be helped by psychotherapy.

Mental health professionals have had less success in treating the alcohol-dependent individual than has the lay organization known as Alcoholics Anonymous. Alcoholics Anonymous was founded in 1935 by two alcoholics and usually admits to membership only individuals who are themselves alcoholics. It has had a dramatic development and today numbers more than 160,000 members throughout the world. Alcoholics Anonymous offers the alcoholic answers to his emotional needs because it uses psychological principles that have been recognized as being effective in helping troubled people. Alcoholics Anonymous also has two affiliated groups. One is for their spouses and the other for their teenaged children.

Because membership is limited to individuals who themselves have been unable to control the problem of alcohol, members have a good deal of sympathy, patience, and understanding for each other. They work in teams of two or three and call on known alcoholics who are in need of help. Through the program of the organization they are able to meet the alcoholic's dependency needs by seeking him out, encouraging him, helping him find a job, accompanying him to meetings of the organization, and helping him develop a sense of personal value and worth. Membership requires that each individual admit that he is powerless over alcohol and is in need of help from a power greater than himself. He searches out his own past errors and, having admitted them to another human being, undertakes to make amends for them. He strives to follow a simple code of living that eventually becomes a philosophy of life. The organizational meetings include tesimonials by the members concerning their struggles with alcohol and their eventual triumph.

Alcoholics Anonymous offers an experience in group participation and the use of group support. This organization is able to assist its members to develop a new emotional orientation toward life and to begin to meet the problems of life without the aid of alcohol. Many physicians refer alcoholic patients to this organization for help. Most social agencies work closely with Alcoholics Anonymous, and it is generally accepted as the most helpful approach to the problem of alcoholism available at this time. The following life story of one member will serve to point up the effectiveness of the work of this group.

Mr. White, a successful 34-year-old shoe salesman, was the father of 4 children ranging in age from 2 to 10 years when his wife was killed in an automobile accident. When this tragedy struck the White family they were living in a modest home they had started to purchase. Mrs. White's parents lived in the same neighborhood and were able to help Mr. White with the care of the children. However, he was responsible for their total care after he came home from work each evening and all day on Saturday and Sunday. In addition, he found that he had to plan meals, direct the housekeeper who came in for a few hours each day, and make many decisions that were entirely new to him about the care of the home and the children. Mr. White missed the golf games he had formerly enjoyed on Sunday afternoons. In many ways he felt overwhelmed by the responsibility of being both mother and father to 4 children. He felt lost without the advice and counsel he had grown to seek and expect from his wife.

In spite of his apprehension, he planned ways to make it possible for him to carry this added responsibility. At first, neighbors and fellow workers were concerned and asked often about how things were going. Occasionally someone invited the family out for a meal so that once in a while he was relieved of having to prepare the evening meal. However, in a few months people began to take his tragic plight for granted and no longer seemed concerned about him or his family.

It was about 6 months after the death of Mrs. White that he began stopping at a bar for a drink after work. Soon he found that the companionship in the bar was so pleasant that he lingered longer than he should and drank more than he had intended. Frequently the children were crying when he arrived home because they were hungry and there was no one at home to prepare the evening meal. The 10-year-old daughter did all she could and eventually began assuming the responsibility for cooking supper. This made it possible for Mr. White to spend many more evenings away from home and frequently to return inebriated. Soon his paycheck began to dwindle. He no longer worked efficiently, and his commissions decreased. Eventually he was fired from his job. Things grew progressively worse for the White family. After Mr. White lost his job, the unpaid grocery bills began to accumulate. The housekeeper stopped coming. Mr. White drank more and more to ease his anxiety, loneliness, and feelings of guilt.

Two members of Alcoholics Anonymous knocked on the front door one evening when Mr. White was lying on the couch sleeping off the latest bottle of whiskey and the children were finishing a meager supper of cereal and milk. When the knock came the 10-year-old daughter opened the door somewhat fearfully. She answered the questions about the grocery bills and her father's job. The visitors explained that they planned to find a home for the children until Mr. White was well enough to care for them. They told her that they were planning to place her father in a hospital for a few days until he felt like working. These plans were carried out. The children were placed in a foster home, and Mr. White was admitted to a general hospital in which Alcoholics Anonymous maintained a unit for the use of their members who were in need of physical care. He remained in the hospital for 2 weeks. During this time he received vitamin therapy and a normal diet. Members of Alcoholics Anonymous visited him regularly and discussed his problems. They talked about the ways in which the organization could help him. When he was ready to leave the hospital, friends from Alcoholics Anonymous helped him find a job, and for a few days they accompanied him to and from work. They also began taking him to the organizational meetings where he became interested in other men who needed help with problems much like his own. As time went on Mr. White was able to reestablish his home and to resume the care of his children. Eventually he remarried and was able to establish a home from which he received the emotional satisfactions that he needed. Thus he was helped to give up alcohol permanently.

DRUG DEPENDENCE

Although alcohol is technically a drug, the term *drug dependence* refers only to those chemicals taken in forms other than drinking. Some drugs are injected directly into the bloodstream, others are ingested in the form of pills, while still others are absorbed through the mucous membranes of the nose or mouth. Marijuana is smoked.

Opiate dependence

Opiates are central nervous system depressants. Morphine, heroin, and codeine are derivatives of opium; demerol and methadone are synthetic substitutes. Although some opiate-dependent persons use morphine or demerol most do not have access to these drugs and use heroin, which is readily available on the streets of large cities.

These drugs are parenterally administered and produce a temporary state of well-being; troubles appear to be trifling and remote and there is a comfortable sense of complete relaxation. The individual feels "normal," which means he feels as if his basic needs have been met. He feels sexually satisfied, full of food, free from anxiety and pain, and is not concerned with aggressive feelings. Ever-increasing amounts are necessary to produce this exhilaration, so that the heroin user may require as much as 15 to 20 grains daily. Unfortunately, when the effects wear off and sufficient amounts are not immediately available, certain *withdrawal symptoms* promptly appear. Tears, sneezing, coryza, yawning, great irritability, and restlessness become quickly evident. Within 24 hours this is followed by abdominal cramps, vomiting, and diarrhea. To these distressing symptoms are added headache, sweating, and pains in the muscles and joints of the lower extremities. Finally, on the third day of abstinence the nervous irritability is so pronounced that the individual becomes hysterical, noisy, and threatening; he frequently throws and destroys objects within his reach. Within a week, however, all these painful withdrawal reactions disappear.

Most heroin-dependent individuals are undernourished, either because they have anorexia or because they cannot afford to purchase enough food. Heroin dependence does not cause mental deterioration but the treatment that addicts receive from society causes them to deteriorate socially. Contrary to general opinion, the addict is not a fiend or a criminal. He is in fact an inadequate, immature individual who shrinks from authority and commits crimes to obtain money to buy the drug. Whenever a heroin-dependent individual obtains an adequate dose he may expose his addiction with an abnormal euphoria and contentment or even a sleepy languor. The pupils may show a telltale "pinpoint" constriction, and in most instances the arms and thighs are scarred or pigmented by the hypodermic needle.

The heroin-dependent individual is generally emotionally immature and unstable and has developed few effective methods of coping with stress other than reliance on the drug. It is important to understand that the reality with which these individuals must cope contains few elements conducive to positive mental health. They are often members of a cultural minority and live in ghetto-type surroundings with little realistic hope of changing their circumstances. They become easy prey to drug pushers as early adolescents or sooner. Once "hooked" they must continue to live close to the source of drug supply, which means that the heroin-dependent individual is compelled to associate with the people who smuggle the drug into the country and the pushers who sell it. It should be noted that few, if any, smugglers or pushers are themselves dependent on heroin but actively support its use by others.

In addition to the heroin users found in the slums of big cities a growing number of physicians and nurses are dependent on morphine and demerol, which they illegally obtain from hospitals or fraudently written prescriptions. State licensing authorities and professional organizations are actively involved in not only punishing these persons but also in facilitating their treatment.

Until recently it was thought to be absolutely necessary to treat the opiate-dependent person in a closed institution to prevent the concealed continuance of the habit. Currently dozens of treatment centers treat drug-dependent individuals, especially heroin addicts, on an outpatient basis. These centers usually provide the drug methadone as a replacement for heroin.

Withdrawal of opium derivatives has been made more humane through the use of methoadone, which is a substitute for the opiate on which the individual is dependent. The use of methadone has been a somewhat controversial method of treating drug addiction. This is partly because methadone has been declared to be a narcotic by the Federal Bureau of Narcotics. However, some authorities believe that the use of methadone in treating former heroin addicts holds the best hope for halting their criminal activities and for making them self-supporting citizens. It has been used more or less successfully with large groups of heroin addicts in several large cities.

In the use of methadone the individual loses his heroin dependency by becoming addicted to the "substitute," methadone. The user then requires regular doses of methadone daily.

This treatment has at least two advantages: (1) it is relatively inexpensive—an individual can be maintained on methadone for a few cents a day and (2) an individual who is on methadone does not lose his ability to function normally—he can usually hold a job and function as a responsible citizen. Today most large cities have methadone clinics where several hundred individuals go to receive the daily dose of methadone. Most clinics require proof that the individual is not continuing to use heroin by requiring him to produce a urine specimen free of the drug. Methadone as a treatment for heroin addiction continues to be controversial but because of its advantages it is used widely.

Unless the individual who is dependent on an opiate or one of its derivatives is highly motivated to give up the habit, he is likely to return to it after treatment. Sooner or later most of these individuals gravitate into the habit of seeking their former associations, visiting old haunts, and finding life more tolerable when they resume use of the drug and regain the artificial sense of security it affords.

Barbiturate dependence

Barbiturates are central nervous system depressants and include phenobarbital, pentobarbital (Nembutal), secobarbital (Seconal), and methaqualone (Quaalude). They are legally prescribed treatments for insomnia and epilepsy. Their effect is similar to that achieved by drinking alcohol. In some respects barbiturate dependence is more dangerous than dependence on alcohol because large numbers of pills can be and are taken at the same time by suicidal people although it is unlikely that a sufficient amount of alcohol could be consumed at one time to result in death. In addition, the mental confusion caused by both alcohol and barbiturates often leads to these substances being used together, resulting in accidental death.

Early stages of intoxication are manifested by muscular incoordination with ataxia, dizziness, nystagmus, slurred speech, and sluggish mentality. The person acquires many bruises by falling or stumbling against walls and furniture. In more profound barbiturate intoxication, there are varying degrees of stupor, speech is incoherent, memory is defective, and hallucinations may appear. When aroused, the person is usually very irritable and resistive. He presents the symptoms of a person suffering from delirium. Recovery may be slow and may leave in its wake a mild degree of permanent brain damage.

Treatment of persons dependent on barbiturates must begin with *gradual* withdrawal of the drug. Sudden, complete withdrawal is often fatal. Individuals who present themselves voluntarily for detoxification are also treated with a high-calorie, high-vitamin diet. Persons who are in a coma caused by barbiturate overdose must be treated aggressively with dialysis to lower the level of barbiturates in the blood.

Amphetamine dependence

Amphetamines are central nervous system stimulants. Numerous chemical compounds fall in this category, the most common of which are racemic amphetamine sulfate (Benzedrine) and methamphetamine (Desoxyn). In the past these drugs have been legitimately used in small doses under medical supervision to treat depression and curb appetite. Individuals who take these drugs solely to become "high" take from 6 to 200 times the daily dose usually prescribed by a physician. Intravenous amphetamines are called "speed" in street language.

The physiological effect of these drugs is to raise the blood pressure, sometimes to dangerous levels. Large doses have been known to cause immediate death, accounting for the saying among drug users that "speed kills."

Individuals who use amphetamines think these drugs increase their physical energy, sharpen their physical and sexual reactions, and increase their confidence. Thus a period of frantic activity results from the ingestion of large amounts of amphetamines. This is followed by a great letdown in which the fatigue and depression are so tremendous that the addict is apt to seek release by taking the drug again. Chronic use of amphetamines can lead to a schizophrenic-like psychosis with paranoid features. This reaction is a result of the drug and is not related to the premorbid personality. In addition, prolonged use at high dosages can lead to massive, irreversible brain damage that may result in death. The use of amphetamines today is not as great as it was in the 1970s, probably because of the drug's deserved reputation as highly dangerous.

Cocaine usage

Cocaine, a central nervous system stimulant, is commonly believed not to cause physical dependence. However, in 1983 the National Institute on Drug Abuse declared cocaine to be a "powerfully addictive" substance linked to cardiac arrests, seizures, and respiratory ailments. This agency has received reports of cocaine-related illnesses that have doubled in number since 1980. Cocaine-related deaths have tripled since that time.

Whether or not cocaine causes physical dependence it almost always causes psychological dependence. It acts in much the same way as do amphetamines but has a shorter duration of action. It is taken by "snorting" or intravenous injection and produces an unusually potent euphoria that serves as a major reinforcement of its use.

Because the public generally believes cocaine to be a safe drug and its price is relatively reasonable, it is being used by an increasing number of people.

Hallucinogen usage

Lysergic acid diethylamide (LSD or acid) and polychloridated biphenyl (PCP or angel dust) are powerful hallucinogens. LSD was first used in research studies in an attempt to discover the cause of schizophrenia. PCP is legally used as an animal anesthetic. Ingestion of reasonably small doses of either substance produces temporary hallucinations and other schizophrenic-like symptoms. The user experiences waves of color, and vibrations seem to pass through the head. Individuals believe that they have had an almost mystical experience in which the nature of emotional conflicts becomes clear.

Although there is little evidence that the use of these drugs causes physical dependence, they are dangerous for several reasons. First, these substances cause some individuals to believe they have supernatural powers, and more than one person has been killed in an attempt to fly. Second, for reasons that are not clear a "bad trip" sometimes occurs. This adverse reaction is manifested by very frightening perceptions instead of the desired peaceful experience. The bad trip that occurs from the use of PCP sometimes brings to the surface long-repressed mental conflicts and psychotic reactions. "Flashbacks" in which the user experiences hallucinations days or weeks after using a hallucinogen can occur with either LSD or PCP.

Marijuana usage

Until recently marijuana was an easily obtained and relatively inexpensive drug. It is a crude preparation from the whole *Cannabis sativa* plant, which grows wild in Mexico and is easily cultivated in the United States. It is usually absorbed into the body through the smoking of cigarettes called *reefers*. Hashish is prepared by scraping resin from the tops of the hemp plant. The active ingredient in both marijuana and hashish is tetrahydrocannabinol, with hashish being much more potent.

Inhalation of marijuana causes a state of exhilaration or euphoria. Under its influence the user feels light in body, as if he were floating through space, and his general behavior is not unlike a mild mania. Marijuana is not an aphrodisiac but it can lower inhibitions and intensify sexual pleasure. It seems to make many users temporarily passive, in contrast to alcohol, which frequently releases aggression. Marijuana affects the individual's sense of time but not his motor and perceptual skills. Users become psychologically dependent on it but may not become physically addicted as with morphine.

Currently a great deal of attention is being given to marijuana by the government because its use has risen dramatically. Official arguments have been carried on in the press concerning the relative dangers of marijuana and the appropriate penalties that should be or should not be levied against people who use it. Unfortunately, there is a limited amount of research on which to base a scientific, unbiased judgment concerning the immediate dangers of smoking marijuana or the eventual outcome of long-term use of this drug. Many of the research findings have been contradictory. Certainly the present laws controlling its use are inequitable, as well as widely unenforceable.

TREATMENT OF DRUG DEPENDENT INDIVIDUALS

In the past the United States government maintained one treatment center for drug-dependent individuals at Lexington, Kentucky. It was called the National Institute of Mental Health Clinical Research Center. In such a specialized hospital everything possible was done to help drug-dependent individuals break their habit and become useful, productive citizens. Many individuals were treated at Lexington several times. Unfortunately, the personality of some drug addicts is so faulty that many were not able to function without the emotional support the drug provides. When the programs at this facility proved ineffective the hospital was closed.

Many communities have organized facilities for treating individuals who suffer from drug dependence. As in all situations that involve the emotions, it is necessary to discover why this kind of unusual emotional support is needed and then attempt to supply the support in more positive ways while at the same time helping the individual to give up the drug.

Some authorities believe that a more realistic approach to the problem of drug dependence would be to supply each drug-dependent individual with a minimum weekly supply of the drug on which he is dependent. This practice, it is argued, would make the illegal traffic in drugs unprofitable. It is thought that this practice of supplying a small amount of the drug to the addict each week would aid in cutting down the crimes that addicts now commit to obtain drugs. It would make it possible for the addict to purchase adequate food and maintain his physical health at an optimum level instead of denying himself food to purchase the drug, as he frequently has done in the past.

As is true with the treatment of alcohol-dependent persons, the most effective long-term treatment for drug-dependent individuals is conducted by a self-help group called Synanon. This organization sponsors residential centers in many large cities. These centers are usually under the direction of a trained professional worker, who may have one to two other professionally trained people to assist him. Most of the therapy as well as the work required to maintain the center is done by the drug-dependent individuals who are there to be helped or by those who have been helped and who stay on to make a contribution to the work.

In these situations, drug-dependent individuals who sincerely want to stop the drug habit live with other people struggling with similar problems. The house is usually organized along the lines of communal living, with each person accepting a share of the work necessary to keep the house liveable and to prepare the meals. Several group sessions are carried on each week, during which members of the group are supportive to each other but are very straightforward in demanding that the group members face their rationalizations, evasions, personal problems, and social deceptions. If a member returns to drugs, he is expected to leave the group. This realistic but supportive approach has apparently helped many drug-dependent individuals to give up drugs and return to school or to a job.

CASE FORMULATION: a heroin-dependent individual

David S. is a 24-year-old, single man who was admitted to a long-term residential drug rehabilitation program, following a 2-week inpatient stay on a detoxification unit for withdrawal from heroin. David began using marijuana and then heroin when he was a junior in high school because his 14-year-old girlfriend refused to date him any longer. About the same time, David was sent by his mother, who lived in New York City, to attend high school in a distant southern city because his parents were getting a divorce.

According to David, marijuana made him feel excited, stimulated, and happy. Everything seemed more pleasant, and he enjoyed his daydreams. He was also sexually stimulated by the drug. About the same time, he tried taking barbiturates, which made him sleepy. Because he did not enjoy their effect, he did not continue them. He got drunk a few times, but alcohol failed to produce the calmness and contentment he was seeking. Since marijuana did not completely satisfy him either, he was convinced that his willpower would be great enough to allow him to stop using this drug when he wanted to be free of it.

David first took heroin in the vein. He described feeling a "flash," which was accompanied by a flush of blood from the abdomen to the head and a feeling of happiness. Although the "flash" passed away, a constant feeling of euphoria remained. For the first time in his life he experienced a feeling of deep contentment. He said, "It didn't

Continued.

affect my intellect, only my emotions. I was happy and content." From that time on he took heroin to assist him in facing any situation that caused him to be tense or anxious. Heroin helped him feel independent of his mother and reduced his nervousness when he was out with a girl. Although heroin gave him a feeling of contentment, it lessened his sexual desire and made it impossible for him to reach a sexual climax.

After David discovered the contentment heroin could achieve for him, he became involved in crimes to support his drug habit. As his need for larger and larger quantities of heroin grew, making his habit more costly, his crimes became more frequent and more serious. His mother repeatedly intervened to keep him out of jail by paying his fines. He entered several colleges but because of his drug habit was never able to stay in any of them for more than a semester.

Finally David tried to withdraw himself from heroin. He thought he could achieve this by himself, since he had been withdrawn twice before in treatment centers. He was not able to accomplish his goal and finally at 24 years of age signed himself into a detoxification unit in the hope of stopping the drug so that he could return to college. He had set for himself the goal of becoming an engineer.

Following the 2-week detoxification program, staff members recommended to David that he admit himself to a long-term residential treatment setting, due to the chronic nature of his difficulties and his past inability to remain abstinent when confronted by stressful life events.

The residential drug rehabilitation program was staffed by a variety of professional and nonprofessional staff, including recovered drug addicts. The staff worked with David to develop a plan of care designed to meet his individual needs and enhance his strengths. On admission to the center, David was drug free. He appeared undernourished, but was in no acute physical distress. He initially gave evidence of being highly motivated and tested in the superior range on a standardized intelligence test.

During the admission interview, David recounted the following information about his early childhood. He stated that his parents were married when his mother was 16 years old. David was their first child, and he recalled his mother often reminding him that his birth had been traumatic for her. During his formative years his father suffered from tuberculosis and spent many months in a sanitarium. David remembered that when he was 3 and 4 years old his mother fondled his genitals when she bathed him. As he grew older, she allowed him to observe her dressing and bathing but scolded him if he evidenced interest in her body.

nursing assessment

David's history reveals a number of factors that potentially contributed to his addictive behaviors and his reliance on heroin for a sense of well-being. He described the feelings of happiness, contentment, relief of anxiety, and independence that he experienced when using heroin.

David's relationship with his mother was a highly ambivalent and conflicted one. From the time he was a child he had been given the message that he was unwanted and unloved. Owing to her own difficulties in adjustment, David's mother was unable to provide him with a healthy environment in which to develop and grow. Her sexually provocative behaviors contributed to David's poor psychosexual adjustment and his anxieties in relation to intimacy with women. David's attempts to separate from his mother were unsuccessful. Her continual interventions on his behalf with the police enabled him to continue his addictive behaviors while maintaining his unhealthy and dependent relationship with her. The absence of a healthy male role model further hindered David's ability to develop effective adaptations to stress. He seemed to rely solely on drugs for a sense of well-being and autonomy and used drugs to deal with all anxiety-provoking situations.

David failed to develop a healthy sense of self as an autonomous male individual. His dependence on drugs may have been a substitute for the dependence he experienced in relation to his rejecting and controlling mother. The adaptation was dysfunctional in that his use of drugs further impeded his ability to negotiate the adolescent tasks of separation and identity development.

David appeared undernourished, probably due to his use of funds to purchase heroin rather than food. His work history was poor, as was his school performance, and he had begun to rely on stealing to purchase heroin. David's strengths included his superior intelligence, as well as his apparent motivation to remain free of drugs and to pursue a career. His willingness to commit himself to a long-term rehabilitation center indicated his emerging recognition of the severity of his drug dependence and his desire for change.

Continued.

nursing diagnosis

The nursing diagnoses derived from the assessment data were as follows:

> Malnourishment related to inadequate food and fluid intake
>
> Ineffective coping methods related to long-term reliance on drugs to cope with stressful life events
>
> Inability to develop and maintain healthy relationships with the opposite sex, related to fear of rejection and psychosexual conflicts

planning and implementing care for DAVID S.

The plan of nursing care for David S. is summarized in the box on p. 395. The team working with David consisted of a variety of professional and nonprofessional members and included a primary nurse, the team psychiatrist, a psychiatric social worker, and an occupational therapist. In addition, David attended Synanon meetings daily. These meetings were held each evening at the center and were attended by several recovered drug addicts, one of whom served as David's sponsor.

The staff members assigned to David were mature individuals experienced in the treatment of clients with substance dependence. They approached David in a hopeful, caring, and supportive fashion, while clearly maintaining boundaries of separateness and setting firm limits. The initial task of treatment was to assist David to recognize and accept his heroin addiction as a problem, thereby breaking through the massive defense of denial common to drug-dependent individuals. Despite David's high motivation to be drug free, the treatment team expected that David eventually would express ambivalence in relation to treatment, and they would need to help him remain abstinent at that time. Finally, treatment would focus on assisting David to develop alternative coping methods to handle stressful life events and uncomfortable feelings to prevent a return to reliance on drugs as a coping style.

The treatment approach consisted of a variety of modalities, including group therapy; peer groups; milieu therapy; peer pressure; recreational and expressive-creative therapies; and assistance with developing social and vocational skills. A contract developed by David and the team outlined mutual expectations for treatment participation. In addition, David was expected to do his share of housekeeping and meal preparation as outlined by the community in weekly meetings. David agreed to the plan as written and was given his final copy of the contract. He agreed to remain in the program for 1 year, to remain drug free as evidenced by daily urine screens, and to follow the contract as written. David was assigned a primary nurse whose plan was to establish a supportive but firm relationship, to develop a climate of acceptance that allowed for the expression of feelings, and to facilitate David's full participation in the program as outlined. Violation of the treatment plan would constitute grounds for immediate review and potential discharge.

nursing care plan for
DAVID S.

nursing diagnosis	objective	rationale	nursing actions	outcome criteria
Malnourishment related to inadequate food and fluid intake	To increase client's nutritional status	Malnourishment predisposes client to physical illness	Monitor client's intake, encouraging three well-balanced meals each day Supplement daily meals with high-calorie nutritional snacks between meals	Within 1 week client will gain 5 pounds Within 1 month client will show evidence of adequate nutrition in hair, skin, eyes, and mucous membranes
Ineffective coping methods related to long-term reliance on drugs to cope with stressful life events	To assist client to abstain from drug use	The use of drugs is indicative of wavering motivation and represents regression to past dysfunctional coping styles	Convey a caring but firm attitude Conduct daily urine screens for drugs Encourage daily participation in Synanon groups Encourage frequent meetings with sponsor Offer positive appraisals for abstinence	Within 2 weeks client will: Obtain urine for drug screens without reminder, and remain drug free Attend Synanon meetings daily without reminder
	To assist client to recognize and accept his drug addiction as a problem	The defense mechanism of denial will strongly impede an addicted individual's ability to develop new behaviors and coping styles	Convey hope and support while confronting emerging evidence of the use of denial Encourage participation in Synanon, peer groups, and community discussions	Within 2 weeks the client will: Willingly attend Synanon, peer group, and meet with sponsor daily without reminder Initiate discussions of behaviors related to addiction and the negative impact of these behaviors on life goals

Continued.

nursing care plan for
DAVID S.—cont'd

nursing diagnosis	objective	rationale	nursing actions	outcome criteria
	To assist the client to develop alternative coping methods to deal with stressful life events and uncomfortable feelings	Long-term therapeutic success of a drug-dependent individual is highly dependent on the development of new coping styles to replace drug use	Accept expressions of fear related to loss of heroin as a coping method Assist with the exploration of new coping styles Encourage and monitor attendence of biweekly group therapy Encourage participation in expressive activities (that is, art, music, poetry)	Within 1 month the client will: Begin to discuss ways to deal with uncomfortable feelings Plan and begin a creative project Attend group therapy without reminder
	To assist client to develop and follow through with career and educational plans	Successful performance in educational endeavours will afford a sense of independence and mastery, and enhance self-esteem and ability to cope	Discuss educational and career interests, conveying hope and support Offer positive appraisals for success Refer to vocational counselor	Within 1 month the client will Initiate discussion related to career plan Meet with vocational counselor
Inability to develop and maintain healthy relationships with the opposite sex, related to fear of rejection and psychosexual conflicts	To assist client to develop a sense of trust in close relationships as well as the belief that identity can be simultaneously maintained	Ability to trust is vital to the development of an intimate relationship, as is the conviction that one will survive as a separate and autonomous individual	Establish trusting relationship, conveying support and acceptance of client as an individual with value, in daily meetings Encourage autonomous and healthy behaviors and independent decision making	Within 2 weeks the client will initiate conversation in meetings with primary nurse
	To assist client to explore and discuss anxieties related to intimate relationships with women	Verbal exploration of psychosexual conflicts will diminish anxiety and enhance the probability of their resolution	Encourage discussion by use of reflective listening, conveying acceptance and support	Within 2 weeks the client will identify feelings and fears related to intimacy

evaluation

David's participation and progress were reviewed by all staff members with David present on a biweekly basis. While he made steady progress, his course of treatment was not without difficulty. After 2 months at the center, it was felt that David was ready to handle an all-day pass to visit with his mother. David had verbalized the hope that he could use some of his new knowledge and behaviors, and that the meeting would go well. On David's return, his urine drug screen revealed that he had used marijuana while on pass, despite his earlier denial of any drug use. He began to challenge staff when confronted and vehemently denied that the action had any meaning, stating, "It doesn't mean anything . . . it wasn't heroin, just pot. What's the big deal?" David was confronted by his peers in group therapy the following day and became withdrawn, sullen, and nonverbal for several weeks. He then began to discuss his fears related to a "life without drugs" with his primary nurse, who encouraged him to discuss and explore these issues in the various groups he attended. David accused the nurse of being rejecting, just like his mother, by her suggesting that he take his problems elsewhere. The nurse remained accepting of these feelings and encouraged David to discuss them. Gradually he began to use groups and peers for increased support and became particularly close to a group of men close to his age. They relied on one another for support and encouragement.

Each new anxiety-producing circumstance David confronted led to a desire to return to drug use. As he began to explore career avenues, his anxiety again increased, as did the desire to rely on drugs. David feared each new step toward an independent and drug-free existence. He often expressed the feeling that others were "forcing" him to quit drugs and was frequently reminded by peers that he had voluntarily chosen to make a commitment to treatment.

David slowly continued to progress toward recovery. He gradually developed an interest in pottery and became quite skilled. He began to expand his support network and develop new relationships. He became particularly helpful with individuals new to the program. In addition, he began to discuss and explore his angry but dependent feelings toward his mother. He began to attend a local university part-time to pursue his interest in engineering and was permitted increased time away from the center in an effort to encourage independent living and to confront stress while support was available.

As the time of David's discharge drew near, many separation issues arose. David's fears about living independently emerged in full force. He angrily stated that he felt as if he was being "thrown out."

Continued.

He expressed the wish to remain longer. David was assisted in coping with these feelings by peers and staff. He was encouraged to continue his involvement with support groups in the community, and contracted to volunteer at the center once a week. At the time of discharge, staff members were hopeful that David had made much progress and would continue to make gains with available supports, meetings with his sponsor, and weekly visits to his therapist. He had not made much progress in the area of heterosexual relationships and continued to be quite anxious and fearful when he contemplated dating and intimacy. It was hoped that David would begin to explore this issue in the future with his therapist.

CONCLUDING STATEMENTS

1. As is true of many other forms of mental illness, it is believed that the stress of twentieth century life is a prime factor in creating the conditions requisite to the flourishing of alcohol and drug dependence.
2. *Substance abuse* refers to the use of any chemical substance for other than therapeutic purposes. *Substance dependence* refers to physical or psychological reliance on a substance.
3. *Physical dependence* is reflected by a physiological adaptation to the substance, indicated by a tolerance to the substance and symptoms of withdrawal when the substance is not taken. *Psychological dependence* exists when the person believes he cannot function without the substance. Either type of dependence is deleterious to the physical, emotional, and social functioning of the individual.
4. An alcohol-dependent individual may drink excessively all the time, or he may drink to excess only periodically, or he may drink large quantities of alcohol daily over a period of years.
5. No matter what type of alcoholism is being considered, the problem is thought to have as one of its bases some emotional conflict, frustration, or feeling of inadequacy. In addition a growing amount of research is focused on identifying physiological factors that differentiate the alcoholic from others who are able to drink alcohol without deleterious effects or a subsequent craving to do so.

6. Short-term treatment of the alcohol-dependent individual is focused on withdrawing him from the substance and assisting him to attain or regain physical health. This is achieved by symptomatic treatment and prevention of seizures and delirium tremens.

7. The only potentially effective long-term treatment of the alcohol-dependent individual requires that he accept the fact he is an alcoholic. This is difficult to achieve since these individuals characteristically use the defense mechanism of denial.

8. Alcoholics Anonymous is a lay organization that has had much success in helping alcoholics maintain a life free of alcohol use. They assist persons in developing a sense of personal value and worth through individual and group support.

9. Heroin is an opiate derivative readily available on the streets of large cities. It is a central nervous system depressant that creates a sense of total well-being in the user.

10. The heroin-dependent individual is generally emotionally immature and unstable and has developed few effective methods of coping with stress other than reliance on drugs.

11. Once heroin dependency has been established the individual must continue to live close to the source of drug supply, compelling him to associate with the people who illegally smuggle the drug into the country and sell it.

12. Methadone is a synthetic opiate substitute widely used as a treatment for heroin dependence. Although it has had some success as a treatment, its use is controversial since the individual becomes dependent on it and must have daily doses.

13. Barbiturates are central nervous system depressants and have an effect very similar to that of alcohol. Barbiturate dependence can be very dangerous because of the possibility of lethal overdose.

14. Amphetamines are central nervous system stimulants that affect the user by increasing his physical energy, sharpening his physical and sexual reactions, and increasing his confidence. This "high" is followed by tremendous fatigue and depression.

15. Cocaine is a central nervous system stimulant with effects similar to those produced by amphetamines. It is widely believed that this drug does not cause dependence but in 1983

the National Institute on Drug Abuse declared it "powerfully addictive." The incidence of its use is on the rise.

16. Hallucinogens produce temporary hallucinations and an almost mystical experience. They can be dangerous because people under their influence may believe they have supernatural powers and can injure or kill themselves by attempting such feats as flying.

17. Inhalation of marijuana causes a state of exhilaration or euphoria. Many research findings about this drug are contradictory.

18. No effective means of long-term treatment of drug-dependent individuals has been developed, although Synanon, an organization similar to Alcoholics Anonymous, is having the most success.

SUGGESTED SOURCES OF ADDITIONAL INFORMATION

Classical

Barbee, Evelyn L.: Marijuana a social problem, Perspect. Psychiatr. Care **9:**195-199, Sept.-Oct., 1971.

Caskey, Kathryn K., Blaylock, Enid V., and Wauson, Beryl M.: The school nurse and drug abusers, Nurs. Outlook **18:**27-30, Dec., 1970.

Condon, Alice, and Roland, Arelene: Drug abuse jargon, Am. J. Nurs. **71:**1738-1739, 1971.

Fort, Joel: Comparison chart of major substances used for mind alteration, Am. J. Nurs. **71:**1740-1741, 1971.

Kimmel, Mary E.: Antabuse in a clinic program, Am. J. Nurs. **71:**1173-1175, 1971.

Kromberg, Carol J., and Proctor, Judith Betz: Evaluation of a day program, Am. J. Nurs. **70:**2575-2577, 1970.

Morgan, Arthur James, and Moreno, Judith Wilson: Attitudes toward addiction, Am. J. Nurs. **73:**497-501, 1973.

Pearson, Barbara A.: Methadone maintenance in heroin addiction, Am. J. Nurs. **70:**2571-2574, 1970.

Contemporary

Berger, Fred: Alcoholism rehabilitation: a supportive approach, Hosp. Community Psychiatry **34**(11):1040-1043, 1983.

Betemps, Elizabeth: Management of the withdrawal syndrome of barbiturates and other central nervous system depressants, J. Psychosoc. Nurs. Ment. Health Serv. **19:**31-34, Sept., 1981.

Bissell, L., and Jones, R.: The alcoholic nurse, Nurs. Outlook **29:**96-104, Feb., 1981.

Boyd, Carol, and Mast, Deborah: Addicted women and their relationships with men, J. Psychosoc. Nurs. Ment. Health Serv. **21:**10-13, Feb., 1983.

Brodsley, Laurel: Avoiding a crisis: the assessment, Am. J. Nurs. **82:**1865-1873, 1982.

Burkhalter, Pamela K.: Nursing care of the alcoholic and drug abuser, New York, 1975, McGraw-Hill Book Co.

Butz, R.H.: Intoxication and withdrawal. In Estes, Nada J., and Heinemann M. Edith, editors: Alcoholism: development, consequences, and interventions, ed. 2, St. Louis, 1982, The C.V. Mosby Co.

Carruth, Beatrice F.: Modifying behavior through social learning, Am. J. Nurs. **76:**1804-1806, Nov., 1976.

Carruth, Georgia R., and Pugh, June B.: Grieving the loss of alcohol: a crisis in recovery, J. Psychosoc. Nurs. Ment. Health Serv. **20:**18-21, March, 1982.

Chafetz, Morris E., Hertzman, Marc, and Berenson, David: Alcoholism: a positive view. In Arieti, Silvano, and Brody, Eugene B., editors: American handbook of psychiatry, ed. 2, vol. 3, New York, 1974, Basic Books, Inc., Publishers, pp. 367-392.

Chavigny, Katherine: Self-esteem for the alcoholic: an epidemiologic approach, Nurs. Outlook **24:**636-639, 1976.

Cohn, Lucille: The hidden diagnosis, Am. J. Nurs. **82:**1862-1864, 1982.

Detzer, Eric, Carlin, Albert S., and Muller, Bart: Detoxifying barbiturate addicts: hints for psychiatric staff, Am. J. Nurs. **76:**1306-1307, 1976.

Dickinson, Sister Corita: The alcoholic an unperson? Nurs. Forum **14:**194-203, 1975.

Ditzler, Joyce: Rehabilitation for alcoholics, Am. J. Nurs. **76:**1172-1175, 1976.

Elliott, Barbara, and Williams, Etna: An employee assistance program, Am. J. Nurs. **82:**586-587, 1982.

Estes, Nada J.: Counseling the wife of an alcoholic spouse, Am. J. Nurs. **74:**1251-1255, 1974.

Foreman, Nancy Jo, and Zerwekh, Joyce V.: Drug crisis intervention, Am. J. Nurs. **71:**1736-1739, 1974.

Fortin, Mary L.: A community nursing experience in alcoholism, Am. J. Nurs. **80:**113-114, Jan., 1980.

Fortin, Mary: Detoxification, then what? A community nursing course in alcoholism, Am. J. Nurs. **80:**113-114, 1980.

Fultz, John M., et al.: When a narcotic addict is hospitalized, Am. J. Nurs. **80:**478-482, March, 1980.

Gibson, Deborah E.: Reminiscence, self-esteem and self-other satisfaction in adult male alcoholics, J. Psychosoc. Nurs. Ment. Health Serv. **18:**7-11, March, 1980.

Haglund, R.M.J., and Schuckit, M.A.: The epidemiology of alcoholism. In Estes, Nada J., and Heinemann, M. Edith, editors: Alcoholism: development, consequences, and interventions, ed. 2, St. Louis, 1982, The C.V. Mosby Co.

Jefferson, Linda, and Ensor, Barbara: Help for the helper: confronting a chemically impaired colleague, Am. J. Nurs. **82:**574-577, 1982.

Johnson, Vernon E.: I'll quit tomorrow, San Francisco, 1980, Harper & Row, Publishers.

Kurose, K., Anderson, T., Bull, W., Gibson, H., Grubb, P., Krefetz, N., Naqvi, A., and Smith, M.: A standard care plan for alcoholism, Am. J. Nurs. **81:**1001-1006, 1981.

Loweree, F., Freng, S., and Baines, B.: Admitting an intoxicated patient, Am. J. Nurs. **84:**616-618, 1984.

McCoy, S., Rice, M., and McFadden, K.: PCP Intoxication: psychiatric issues of nursing care, J. Psychosoc. Nurs. Ment. Health Serv. **19:**17-23, July, 1981.

McDermott, Sister Raphael: Maintaining the methadone patient, Nurs. Outlook **18:**22-26, Dec., 1970.

Mann, George: Recovery of reality: overcoming chemical dependency, San Francisco, 1980, Harper & Row, Publishers.

Marks, Vida L.: Health teaching for recovering alcoholic patients, Am. J. Nurs. **80:**2058-2061, 1980.

Mitchell, Carol Edgerton: Assessment of alcohol abuse, Nurs. Outlook **24:**511-515, 1976.

Mittleman, Hollace, Mittleman, Roger, and Elser, Bernard: Cocaine, Am. J. Nurs. **84:**1092-1095, 1984.

Mueller, John F.: Treatment for the alcoholic: cursing or nursing? Am. J. Nurs. **74:**245-247, 1974.

Naigle, Madeline: The nurse and the alcoholic: redefining an historically ambivalent relationship, J. Psychosoc. Nurs. Ment. Health Serv. **21:**17-25, June, 1983.

Nyswander, Marie: Drug addiction. In Arieti, Silvano, and Brody, Eugene B., editors: American handbook of psychiatry, ed. 2, vol. 3, New York, 1974, Basic Books, Inc., Publishers, pp. 393-403.

Pilette, Wilfred: Caffeine: psychiatric grounds for concern, J. Psychosoc. Nurs. Ment. Health Serv. **21:**19-24, Aug., 1983.

Pugh, June B.: My love: the story of an addiction, J. Psychosoc. Nurs. Ment. Health Serv. **20:**22-24, March, 1982.

Scherwertz, Priscilla: An alcohol treatment team, Am. J. Nurs. **82:**1878-1879, 1982.

Schickit, Marc: Alcoholism and other psychiatric disorders, Hosp. Community Psychiatry **34:**1022-1027, 1983.

Schloemer, Nancy, and Skidmore, Jacquelyn: Opiate withdrawal with clonidine, J. Psychosoc. Nurs. Ment. Health Serv. **21:**8-14, Oct., 1983.

Seixas, F.A.: The course of alcoholism. In Estes, Nada J., and Heinemann, M. Edith, editors: Alcoholism: development, consequences, and interventions, ed.2, St. Louis, 1982, The C.V. Mosby Co.

Smith, James: Diagnosing alcoholism, Hosp. Community Psychiatry **34**(11):1017-1021, 1983.

Smith, Thomas M.: The dynamics in time-limited therapy with methadone-maintained patients, New York City V.A., Perspect. Psychiatr. Care **16:**28-33, Jan.-Feb., 1978.

Spring, Gottfried, and Rothgery, Jean: The link between alcoholism and affective disorders, Hosp. Community Psychiatry **35**(8):820-823, 1984.

Twerski, A.: Early intervention in alcoholism: confrontational techniques, Hosp. Community Psychiatry **34**(11):1027-1039, 1983.

Weist, J.K., Lindeman, M., and Newton, M.: Hospital dialogues, Am. J. Nurs. **82:**1874-1877, 1982.

Yearwood, Alma C., and Hess, Susanne K.: How can an alcoholic change in 28 days? Am. J. Nurs. **79:**1436-1438, 1979.

Of particular interest

Estes, Nada J., and Heinemann, M. Edith, editors: Alcoholism: development, consequences, and interventions, ed. 2, St. Louis, 1982, The C.V. Mosby Co.

The authors provide a comprehensive literature review on the problem of alcoholism. It is an excellent resource regarding various aspects of the problem.

Mann, George: Recovery of reality: overcoming chemical dependency, San Francisco, 1980, Harper & Row, Publishers.

This is a complete report on the nature, effects, treatment, and prevention of chemical dependency. It includes personal histories and the latest information on diagnostic and treatment methods for alcoholism and other dependencies.

Symposium on alcohol and drug abuse, Nurs. Clin. North Am., Sept., 1976.

Chemical dependency is the focus of several articles in this collection. It is useful in providing the reader with several relevant perspectives on the problem.

chapter eighteen

adults
whose behavior
is antisocial

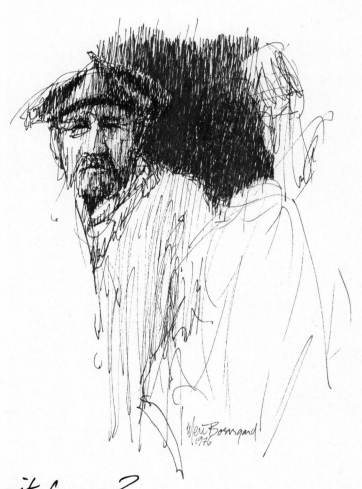

What's in it for me?

LEARNING OBJECTIVES
After studying this chapter the student will be able to:

1 Define antisocial behavior.

2 Discuss the changing view of homosexuality as a sexual preference.

3 Discuss the prevention and treatment of sexual deviance.

4 Describe the characteristics of the adult who engages in antisocial acts.

5 Discuss the dynamics of development of antisocial behavior.

6 State examples of nursing diagnoses likely to be applicable to adults who engage in antisocial acts.

7 Develop a hypothetical plan of nursing care for an adult who engages in antisocial acts.

Certain individuals engage in behaviors that are in opposition to the values and principles on which their society is built. Such behaviors are often termed antisocial. The causes of antisocial behaviors are even less clearly understood than are the causes of behaviors associated with disturbances in thought or mood. Antisocial behaviors are somewhat unique in that their very existence is considered an assault on the fundamental values of society. This does not mean that the individual, his family, and his immediate associates do not suffer as a result of his behavior; rather, the nature of the individual's behavior is such that it threatens the community at large by opposing the social order, even though few people may be directly involved. Examples of such behavior are antisocial acts and sexual deviations.

HISTORICAL PERSPECTIVE

Certain individuals engage in a number of antisocial acts, such as persistent lying, "conning" others, recklessness, and a general failure to accept the social norms of lawful behavior. Such individuals were labeled "sociopaths" or "psychopaths" in the past. Although this terminology is no longer used, the characteristics and numbers of these persons remain the same as they have throughout history. It is unfortunate that no enlightened understanding or effective treatment has been developed to assist these individuals to achieve a more satisfactory adaptation.

Historically, some nations have viewed sexual deviations entirely as a moral and legal problem rather than as a health problem. Now there is reason to believe that an understanding of the psychological causes of sexually deviant behavior is beginning to develop. Some positive changes in attitude can be observed in the treatment of these individuals by the courts, professional people, and law enforcement officers. Today there seems to be a beginning recognition of the fact that individuals who display sexually deviant behavior may suffer from a personality defect caused by factors beyond their control.

The third edition of the *Diagnostic and Statistical Manual of Mental Disorders*, published in 1980 by the American Psychiatric Association, describes a number of sexual deviations under the general category of Psychosexual Disorders. Included in this general category are voyeurism, pedophilia, fetishism, transvestism, and exhibitionism, which are discussed later in this chapter. *Homosexuality,* which involves the sexual attachment and love for an individual of the same sex, was once classified as a psychosexual disorder. However, homosexuality was eliminated from the DSM III as a diagnostic category. Instead the diagnostic category of Ego-dystonic Homosexuality was included. This psychosexual disorder is characterized by a pattern of homosexual arousal that the individual describes as subjectively distressful and unwanted. Thus treatment is not indicated for those homosexual individuals who recognize and accept their sexual choice.

The marked change in the thinking of most mental health professionals in regard to homosexuality may be attributed to a number of factors, and reflects changing attitudes in contemporary society. For example, the last decade has seen rapid development in the study of and research in human sexuality, the results of which have begun to alter traditional concepts of sexuality in general. In addition, the concern for human rights that has emerged in the past few decades has paved the way for many minority groups to demand equality, including the homosexual community.

Currently, homosexual or "gay" individuals are encouraging the attitude of recognizing and publicly admitting that their choice for a sexual relationship is someone of the same sex. Another significant aspect of the "gay rights" movement is its struggle to improve the legal status of homosexuals. They are slowly achieving equal rights in the areas of housing and jobs. Many individuals with a homosexual orientation carry on well-adjusted and productive lives. They bitterly resent traditional theories, which hold that homosexuality develops out of negative early childhood experiences. Recent studies of a large group of homosexuals have shown that many are capable of effective functioning in the business and professional world. Earlier studies focused attention on poorly adjusted homosexual individuals who had sought psychiatric help. Psychiatry has come to recognize that the process of labeling a homosexual individual as abnormal and deviant can have a profoundly negative impact on the individual's life and life choices. Today's clinical research reflects more acceptance of homosexuality as a lifestyle, and addresses more contemporary issues, such as therapy for the homosexual couple.

ADULTS WHO ENGAGE IN SEXUAL DEVIATIONS

The sexually deviant individual is one who gets sexual satisfaction by immature methods throughout adult life. Normal sexual development in the human being is a slow and complex psychobiological process. As Freud has postulated, the sexual instinct passes through several stages of growth, and an arrest or fixation at immature levels may cause serious distortions of the total personality. The various sexual deviations are, therefore, malconditionings or incomplete expressions of the psychological accompaniments of sexual activity. Apart from the explanations offered by psychoanalysts, little is known about the cause of most deviations in sexual behavior. In general, society looks with antipathy and disfavor on individuals who practice sexual deviations, and in some instances expresses violent resentment. However, sexually deviant individuals tend to repeat their particular deviation even after experiencing cruel, inhuman punishment and suffering.

As more psychological understanding of the personalities of individuals who have failed to achieve a mature psychosexual development is achieved, there is a growing belief on the part of specialists that the psychopathology underlying their problems is basically related to otherwise uncontrollable anxiety. Usually sexual deviation is only one manifestation of a deep-seated emotional dysfunction of long duration. All individuals who use a deviant outlet to achieve sexual satisfaction exhibit a pattern of behavior that is repeated compulsively without reason or logic. It is not a substitute for normal sexual relations but is carried on to meet a specific unconscious need, which the individual himself does not understand.

The following is an example of such behavior. A respected middle-aged married citizen of a small midwestern town was arrested for *voyeurism* (for being a Peeping Tom). He admitted that for most of his life he had been peeping at night into the bedroom windows of his neighbors. Unfortunately he was not apprehended for many years, and when he was finally caught, the anger of the townspeople was so great that he and his family were forced to leave the community.

Examples of sexual deviations

In addition to voyeurism, some of the other sexual deviations, or psychosexual disorders, categorized in the third edition of the *Diagnostic and Statistical Manual,* include pedophilia, fetishism, tranvestism, and exhibitionism.

Pedophilia is the technical term used to describe a pathological sexual interest in children. It is a sexual deviation of adults, characterized by both acts and fantasies of engaging in sexual activity with children as a preferred or exclusive way of achieving sexual excitement. It is a subject that has received, both directly and indirectly, increased attention in the media. Regardless of whether the incidence of pedophilia has actually risen in recent years or simply has received more public attention, it is clear that the sexual exploitation of children is currently perceived as a major social and moral problem.

Many individuals believe that practices such as child pornography potentially reflect and contribute to the sexual exploitation of children, who are a vulnerable population in a rapidly changing world. In addition, it is feared that the large number of missing and kidnapped children reported in recent years may be victims of sexual exploitation and then perhaps murder.

The adult who engages in pedophilia usually feels inadequate sexually. There is an immature or improperly fixated sexual preference, which may be due to basic defects in psychosexual development or to underlying psychopathology such as depression. Often the individual is afraid to approach an adult, for fear of being rejected or of being sexually inadequate. Thus the individual approaches a child sexually in the unconscious hope that he will be accepted by a less discriminating person. His behavior is apt to frighten the child, who usually cries out for help. The cry frightens the offender, who may flee. Unfortunately, some offenders have in fact injured or killed the child to keep from being apprehended.

Fetishism occurs in men who may unconsciously fear genital heterosexual contact due to castration fears that developed early in life. For these men sexual feeling is attached to some inanimate object that may have belonged to a woman for whom the individual once developed admiration, or the object may simply have a female association. The fetish may be a glove, a shoe, a brassiere, or some other very personal feminine object. Since contact with the object usually leads to orgasm, the use of the fetish is a substitute for genital heterosexuality.

Transvestism occurs when an individual has a deep-seated urge to dress in the clothing of the opposite sex. In some persons this urge may be one of several manifestations of a profound personality disturbance involving homosexuality with a paranoid ideation.

Exhibitionism occurs when the individual has an uncontrollable urge to exhibit the genitalia to others, usually members of the opposite sex. This symptom is thought to occur in persons who are defending themselves against guilt and fear of punishment arising out of unconscious incestuous wishes. For example, the male exhibits the penis to reassure himself that it is still intact and that he has not been punished for his incestuous desires. Exhibition of the genitals may also serve to demonstrate sexually aggressive feelings.

Prevention and treatment of sexual deviance

Sexually deviant behavior, like all human problems with a psychological origin, should be prevented so that treatment becomes unnecessary. An important step in prevention is effective sexual education for all children. Currently, much discussion is being carried on thoughout the United States concerning sex education. The arguments focus on who should provide it and where it should be given. Some lay people are attacking the efforts that have been made in some schools to provide adequate sex education. The schools introduced this instruction because there was evidence that sex education was not being adequately provided elsewhere. Certainly children require accurate and complete sexual information if they are to develop wholesome, mature attitudes. Most authorities agree that such information can be taught most effectively in schools by individuals who are educationally prepared to provide such information. Most people also agree that this teaching should be reinforced and elaborated by the parents in the home.

Not only is adequate sex education essential, it is also necessary to provide positive parent-child relationships and a healthy family environment in the early formative years for children to achieve mature psychosexual development. Because children identify sexual roles at an early age, they need the influence of adults of both sexes to establish an identification with an adult of the same sex. Thus the family pattern established in homes is crucial to the healthy emotional development of children. During their formative years they need guidance from mature adults in redirecting aggressive impulses into constructive and socially acceptable channels.

It would be helpful if early corrective experiences could be provided for children who seem to be developing social reactions that vary greatly from those expected from others of their peer group.

Established sexually deviant behavior is difficult to treat successfully because the problem arises out of the individual's personality structure. By the time an individual comes to the attention of professional workers who can provide treatment, the personality structure has developed. The individual seeks sexual satisfaction in a deviant way because his psychosexual development has been arrested or has regressed to an immature and less threatening level. Thus sexually deviant behavior is a deeply ingrained part of the individual's personality. In addition, he has little understanding of it, and since it temporarily satisfies his sexual needs, he is loath or unable to substitute more mature behavior.

One available treatment method that may be able to assist the individual to make a profound alteration in his personality adaptation is psychoanalysis. This treatment is expensive, involves a great deal of time and personal commitment on the part of both the individual and the analyst, and consequently is available only to a limited number of people. Success is entirely dependent on the sincere interest of the individual in changing his sexual orientation. Although individuals who practice sexually deviant behavior are interested in avoiding involvement with the legal authorities, they are not always interested in profoundly altering their sexual orientation.

If competent psychiatric treatment is available, if the individual is highly motivated to change his lifelong pattern of adaptation, and if he is prepared to continue therapy for a prolonged period of time, some positive changes in sexual orientation may be achieved.

Some individuals who practice sexually deviant behavior are sentenced to prison terms because some aspect of their behavior is considered damaging to the morals of others. Prison environments have a negative influence on these individuals. In spite of this, it is sometimes necessary to confine some of them in corrective institutions if they have committed serious social offenses.

When an individual who exhibits sexually deviant behavior requests psychiatric help and willingly accepts treatment, some authorities believe that it is therapeutically valuable to hospitalize him. In this way the individual's therapist can supervise his environment. Another advantage of hospitalization is that it removes the individual from the environment in which sexually deviant behavior was his code of expression. In time, with competent psychiatric help, the individual may be able to redirect his sexual and aggressive drives so that his personal and social functioning may be improved.

Nurses and other staff sometimes behave as if the individual who has a history of sexual deviation is a social outcast. When they habor such feelings, they inevitably treat the person in a cold, unfriendly manner. Such feelings on the part of a member of the professional treatment team tend to destroy much of the therapeutic effect the group is attempting to achieve. Such attitudes suggest that the individual holding them fails to realize that the sexually deviant person is not entirely responsible for his problem.

Sexually deviant individuals deserve a friendly, accepting climate in which they are treated with respect and consideration. In addition, they require the establishment of firm limits that are fairly and consistently enforced. Since the nurse has a good deal of responsibility for developing the climate in the treatment situation, her understanding of the client's problem and her attitude toward him are of major importance. He needs to have a well-planned schedule of daily activities available so that he can avoid lethargy and boredom. He needs help in becoming an active participant in some aspects of the planned schedule of activities.

ADULTS WHO ENGAGE IN ANTISOCIAL ACTS

Individuals who engage in antisocial acts are persons who have a long history of dysfunctional behavior in the areas of interpersonal relationships and occupational endeavors. In addition, they often have a criminal record, may be dependent upon alcohol or drugs, and frequently engage in sexually deviant behavior. What is so outstanding about these persons, however, is not their history or even their behavior, but rather the initial impression they make. Even when his past is known, such an individual easily impresses a stranger with his articulate expression, his ability to rationalize or justify his behavior, his fantasized exploits, and his general appearance. The casual acquaintance quickly succumbs to this charisma and becomes his staunch supporter.

Behind this effective facade of charm is a personality that is incapable of valuing other people. Rather, this person views others as objects to be manipulated to achieve his purposes. These individuals are characterized by a total lack of responsibility and an inability to conform to even the minimal moral and legal standards of society if these conflict with the fulfillment of their desires. They possess poor judgment and insight, do not profit by experience or punishment, and are notoriously unreliable. They consciously fabricate stories to impress the listener and have an uncanny ability to rationalize contradictions in their stories. In addition, they seem incapable of experiencing guilt or remorse for their behavior, although they will express these feelings if they believe it will be to their advantage to do so.

For reasons that are unknown this personality disturbance occurs almost exclusively in men. In addition, these persons are always of at least average intelligence, with many having superior intellectual abilities. Because of their criminal behavior many of these persons are found in the jails and prisons of the country. It is unlikely, however, that the professional criminal suffers from an antisocial personality. A successful life of crime requires long-range, careful planning. This is impossible for an individual with an antisocial personality because his behavior is characterized by impulsiveness and a low tolerance for frustration.

Dynamics of development

The reason that individuals who engage in antisocial acts are unable to develop satisfactory social relationships is unknown. The defect seems to lie in the emotional and volitional aspects of the personality rather than in the intellectual areas.

Studies of the histories of these individuals reveal that they were emotionally impulsive and maladjusted children. In fact, adjustment difficulties before age 15 is one criterion of this diagnosis. Some authorities believe that careful history taking would indicate antisocial behavior before age 12 in most, if not all, individuals who engage in antisocial acts as adults. These adjustment difficulties include poor school performance related to frequent truancy, petty crimes including thefts and arson, and a uniform lack of satisfactory relationships with family, peers, and authority figures.

These individuals have apparently failed to develop a socialized superego. The personality appears to be dominated by the primitive demands of the id. The ego has failed to establish a mature identity or to evolve socially useful adaptations and controls. In some way these individuals have failed to make a positive identification with parents or parental substitutes who could have provided the love, security, recognition, and respect that a child requires if he is to develop into an emotionally healthy adult. Failure to make a positive identification and to develop socially acceptable controls on his own behavior may have been the result of faulty parent-child relationships.

Social scientists who have conducted longitudinal studies of these individuals report that they frequently come from home environments in which there is only one parent, who is likely to be alcohol or drug dependent or who has an antisocial personality, or both. As a result, the child has little or no supervision and the rules of conduct that are established are enforced inconsistently. The child is, in essence, left to fend for himself, often on the streets of the slums of large cities.

Although these familial factors are present often enough to be noteworthy, it is important to understand that not every child who is a product of such a background develops an antisocial personality. Furthermore, some adults who engage in antisocial acts do not have this family background. Therefore it must be concluded that there are other, as yet unknown, factors that are necessary for the development of an antisocial personality.

NURSING CARE OF ADULTS WHO ENGAGE IN ANTISOCIAL ACTS
Nursing assessment

Whatever its cause, it is generally accepted that this disturbance has its origin in early childhood and that the adult manifestations are merely more serious continuations of a life-long pattern of antisocial behavior.

Individuals who engage in antisocial acts are rarely admitted to hospitals for the primary purpose of treating their personality defect. Rather, they are more commonly found on the streets of the slum sections of large cities, in jails and prisons, or in private psychiatric hospitals where their families have placed them because of their embarrassing behavior. In other words, the nurse is likely to come in contact with these persons only secondarily to the personality disturbance. Therefore identifying such a person becomes a particular challenge. He may be a patient in a general hospital because of a physical illness, or he may present himself to private or public relief agencies.

The nurse should always suspect this personality disturbance when an individual has a life-long history of dysfunction, in the absence of a psychosis. This is particularly true when he is able to convincingly explain his history on the basis of deficiencies in others or unfortunate circumstances. She should also be alert to the possibility of the existence of this phenomenon when the individual exhibits little motivation to change or alter those behaviors that are severely dysfunctional, but rather focuses his concern on relatively unimportant minutiae.

Of almost diagnostic significance is the nurse's reaction to the person. Despite all she may know about him, this individual is able to "con" the inexperienced nurse into defending and supporting his antisocial actions and believing that she alone can help him. These feelings are termed a *rescue fantasy* and nurses, who are inclined to be nuturing, are particularly vulnerable to the development of this phenomenon.

Nursing diagnoses

Nursing diagnoses approved by the Fifth National Conference on Nursing Diagnoses that may be applicable to adults who engage in socially offensive behavior are:

Social isolation related to unaccepted social behavior
Social isolation related to unaccepted social values
Social isolation related to inability to engage in satisfying personal relationships
Potential for violence directed at others related to antisocial character

In addition to these approved diagnoses, the following may also be applicable:

Inadequate impulse control related to inadequate or inappropriate ego development

Inability to profit from experience related to the lack of a socialized superego

Low tolerance for frustration related to inadequate coping mechanisms

Disregard for authority related to the lack of a socialized superego

Planning and implementing nursing care

Some nurses feel that an individual who behaves in an antisocial way is a criminal and therefore should not be treated within the health care system. Other nurses believe that little, if anything, is wrong with these persons and therefore they do not require treatment. Both these extreme attitudes can prove detrimental to the individual who engages in antisocial acts.

Although the current trend is to keep as many individuals as possible out of institutions, many authorities still believe that persons who engage in antisocial acts require hospitalization if they are to be treated with any hope of success. The institution should provide a friendly, accepting, humane environment, where firm, reasonable, consistent limits and controls are placed on behavior. A permissive atmosphere is usually not helpful for these individuals. They need to be helped to develop a socialized superego, and such growth may be fostered by an organized, structured, controlled environment.

The treatment goals should include helping them to accept and use more socially approved attitudes and standards in their relationships with other people. To achieve this they must be helped to trust other people. It is hoped that this can be achieved through the development of a therapeutic relationship with one of the members of the professional treatment team. Since the psychiatrist is usually the ultimate authority in the treatment team, it would probably be helpful if the therapeutic relationship could be developed with a psychiatrist who could provide the necessary discipline.

The treatment goals can be promoted through a system of rewards and prohibitions, with socially acceptable behavior being rewarded with privileges and less acceptable behavior being responded to by the withholding of privileges.

If the antisocial behavior has developed out of negative social and cultural influences, the individual should be helped to seek a more acceptable social situation. Certainly he should be encouraged not to return to the same environment.

Because the individual who engages in socially offensive behavior is often attractive, intelligent, and an interesting conversationalist, he easily gains control of the situation by manipulating others. It is helpful to remember that although these individuals are usually clever in manipulating others, they frequently use extremely poor judgment. They are likely to be troublemakers among other clients and have been known to organize psychotic individuals for the purpose of accomplishing their antisocial plans.

Although the nurse can be most effective if she uses a helpful, friendly approach when dealing with the individual who exhibits antisocial behaviors, she also needs to be constantly alert to the possibility of his attempting to gain control of the situation. The clinical team should identify approaches they believe will be most effective in dealing with this individual and should list the responsibilities that he will be expected to fulfill. When these decisions have been made, it is of primary importance for all hospital personnel to be consistent in carrying them out and in holding the individual to fulfilling his obligations.

These individuals do not profit by being scolded or lectured. Such an approach is never helpful and will serve only to arouse angry feelings. Since it is thought that these individuals learn little from experience, punishing them accomplishes nothing. Limits must be set on their behavior, since they frequently indulge in temper tantrums or destructive activities to achieve their objectives.

When the individual is demonstrating antisocial behavior, it is important to treat him in such a manner that he will know that the staff want to help him even though he cannot be allowed to continue the behavior he is exhibiting.

Individuals with antisocial attitudes need a variety of challenging activities throughout the day. They are likely to plead for special privileges, but the nurse should be cautious about granting such requests. Like all other individuals they should be rewarded for acceptable behavior. If possible, these individuals should be placed in situations in which they can obtain socially acceptable satisfactions. Thus success in some type of industrial therapy is ideal. It is essential to insist these individuals fulfill the responsibilities expected of them, since they are likely to co-operate only at their own convenience.

Because many of these individuals lack a well-developed social conscience, they usually function poorly in group activities. However, insofar as possible, it is suggested that they be helped to accept a role in some of the available group functions.

Individuals with antisocial attitudes vary greatly in emotional needs and personality limitations. Their care in the treatment center should be designed to help them with their individual problems and to make it possible for them to cultivate a more socially acceptable approach to living.

Due to the personality characteristics of the antisocial individual that result in behavior that is superficially pleasing, staff misjudge this group of persons more often than any other with whom they come in contact. Inexperienced staff are likely to feel that a perfectly normal person is being detained for treatment without justification; in this case it is important that a more experienced health professional be consulted for clarification.

CASE FORMULATION
an individual with antisocial behavior

James B. is a 30-year-old, unmarried man who was admitted to the state psychiatric hospital after being arrested for vagrancy and following children as they walked to school in the morning. He is the oldest child of a woman who divorced his father after many episodes of abuse to both her and the child. Shortly after leaving her husband, James' mother took him and his two younger siblings to live in a rooming house, the only accommodations she could afford. Within a week she was befriended by another tenant, an unemployed, alcohol dependent man 20 years her senior. This man moved in with the Bs, ostensibly to save money, and within a month convinced Mrs. B. to move with him to the rural area in which he had been reared. Even though they had no financial resources they were successful in renting a rundown shack on several acres of land. This property was owned by an absentee landlord. It was in this environment that James remained until he was 15 years old.

Continued.

Upon moving to the rural community, the family was befriended by well-meaning members of the local church. However, James was unable to curb his antisocial behavior, which included truancy, dismembering a dead cat, setting small fires in the bedrooms of the home, and stealing money from Sunday School offerings. Amazingly, he was never held back in school even though he was functionally illiterate. In fact, his teachers routinely appeared at the home on Christmas Eve with many gifts for all the children. When his mother asked to have him repeat a grade, the school authorities stated their belief that such an action would hinder the progress the teachers felt he was making.

James became involved with the law for the first time at age 12 when he volunteered to solicit money for a church benevolence. He was successful in collecting 70 dollars, which he spent on candy, cigarettes, and arcade games. The minister of the church brought legal charges against James, who was placed on 1 year's probation in the custody of his mother, although Mrs. B. was incapable of controlling him.

When James was 15 years old the landlord evicted the family from their home because they had not paid rent for the past 3 years. The landlord indicated he would have been willing to wait for the rent if they had maintained the house and land. However, since the house was in a state of extreme disrepair and the acreage was strewn with garbage and machine parts, he felt he had no choice but to evict them. The Social Service Agency to whom the family was well known found them an apartment in a community 20 miles away. On the trip to this apartment the family stopped in a public rest area. James ran out of the back door of the rest room and hitchhiked 400 miles to a large metropolitan area. His mother never notified the police that he was missing and they have not seen each other since.

Upon arriving in the city, James quickly became prey to a "pimp" who fed, housed, and clothed him in return for his services as a prostitute for businessmen whose sexual preference was young boys. He was so endearing that several businessmen gave him money and personal gifts, in addition to the fee they paid for his services. When his "pimp" discovered this extra source of income, he was so enraged that he almost beat James to death.

James fled this situation and since then has been drifting in the "skid row" section of another large city. He has a lengthy criminal record for petty crimes and has been committed to a psychiatric hospital four times.

Upon admission, he appeared malnourished but was in no acute physical distress. The mental status exam indicated no psychosis or organic disturbance. He stated he was following the children to protect them from predators.

nursing assessment

This case history demonstrates rather clearly many of the characteristics of an individual who is said to possess antisocial behaviors. As a young child James was severely abused by his father and probably a witness to this man's abuse of his mother. It is not unreasonable to assume that he adapted to his fear through repression. James' mother seemed incapable of providing the support or structure necessary for a child to develop in a mentally healthy way. The fact that she became involved with an older, unemployed, alcohol-dependent man indicates her poor judgment.

James' childhood behavior indicates a wide range of antisocial behaviors. Of significance is the fact that despite these behaviors and his lack of academic achievement, there is evidence James was well liked by his teachers. It is also significant that his first known act of stealing occurred in defiance of the church that had befriended him and his family.

Certainly this man failed to develop a socialized superego. Thus his behavior was dominated by instinctual demands, he failed to develop a constructive identity, and he had not incorporated socially useful controls. Like other individuals who are said to possess antisocial behaviors, he seemed incapable of conforming to social or legal standards. Even though he was previously treated at several psychiatric hospitals he did not profit by this experience or by his encounters with the law.

Despite his dirty clothing and malnourished physique, the nurse found him quite charming and convincing in his explanations of his behavior.

nursing diagnoses

The nursing diagnoses derived from the assessment data were:

Malnourishment related to inadequate food and fluid intake
Antisocial behaviors related to lack of inpulse control
Lack of guilt or anxiety related to unsocialized superego

These diagnoses were used as the basis for developing a plan for nursing care for James B.

planning and implementing nursing care for JAMES B.

The plan of nursing care developed for James B. is summarized in the box beginning on p. 420. It should be noted that no psychotropic medications were prescribed.

The team psychiatrist assumed primary responsibility for James'

Continued.

treatment in the belief that this client would respond best to the member of the team who has the most authority.

The nursing staff who gave care to James B. were mature, experienced individuals. They strove to develop a friendly, accepting, humane environment while at the same time established firm, consistent, reasonable controls. Because they had previous experience working with clients who engaged in antisocial behaviors, they were alert to James' manipulative behavior and were not fooled by his charm.

James was assigned a single room to prevent his influencing other clients in private. A schedule of activities, which included O.T. and R.T., and reading classes, was developed. A plan of specified rewards and withholding of privileges was designed to accompany each activity, and was implemented depending upon James' participation. A copy of this schedule and reward structure in the form of a contract was given to James. He and the psychiatrist both signed it. This contract specified that no excuses would be accepted as reasons for James' lack of attendance at the scheduled activities.

evaluation

The contract specifying James' behavior was reviewed by all staff and rigidly adhered to. He showed little difficulty in fulfilling the terms of the contract and therefore received a number of awards. For example, he was allowed to stay in the day room and watch the television until midnight for each activity he attended and participated in

nursing care plan for
JAMES B.

nursing diagnosis	objectives	rationale	nursing actions	outcome criteria
Malnourishment related to inadequate food and fluid intake	To increase client's nutritional status	Malnourishment predisposes client to physical illness	Make sure client eats 3 well balanced meals each day as served in cafeteria Supplement meals with high calorie, nutritionally sound snacks (for example, malted milk) 3 times/day until 20 pounds have been gained	Within 1 week client will gain 5 pounds Within 1 month client's hair, skin, eyes, and mucous membranes will show evidence of adequate nutrition

nursing diagnosis	objectives	rationale	nursing actions	outcome criteria
Antisocial behaviors related to lack of impulse control	Teach impulse control through behavior modification techniques	Structured, consistently enforced schedule reinforced by rewards can enable client to control behaviors	Assign to a single room Plan schedule of activities designed to increase number of skills Enforce client's participation in scheduled activities by rewards and withholding privileges as specified in contract	Within 2 weeks client will attend and participate in three of the four scheduled daily activities spontaneously and without complaint
			Do not allow staff to be drawn into client's manipulation (for example, all requests for privileges must be made directly to Dr. F; all decisions about nursing care to be made by Ms. R.)	Within 1 month client will give evidence of attempting to gain rewards by altering behavior
Lack of guilt or anxiety related to unsocialized superego	To increase sense of responsibility for accountability for own actions	Assumption of responsibility and accountability for own behavior is necessary for development of a socialized superego	As situation arises teach client socially acceptable behaviors and consequences to himself and others of ignoring these. For example, stealing other client's property hurts both persons	Within 1 month client is able to repeat consequences to himself and others of his behavior
			Enforce rewards and withholding privileges as outlined in contract with meticulous consistency	Within 1 month client gives evidence of attempting to gain rewards by altering behavior

for a week. This resulted in his staying up late for 4 nights a week.

An unanticipated negative outcome of James' treatment was the fact he bragged to other clients about how special he was as evidenced by his private room and television privileges. Three weeks

Continued.

after admission he found his room ransacked and his few personal belongings gone or destroyed. Another client quickly admitted he had done this to "teach him a lesson." James was very distraught and apparently fearful about this event and a number of nursing staff freely sympathized with him.

At this point, a team conference was called to evaluate James' progress and current status. The absolute necessity of pointing out the part James played in this incident was stressed. His apparent distress and fear were viewed as ungenuine and as an attempt at manipulation. In addition, the contract was revised to make it more stringent. It was the team's consensus that the only real progress James had made in 3 weeks was a return to a sound nutritional status.

James remained in the hospital for another 3 weeks before he was discharged to a transitional living situation. Although his presence on the unit created identifiable tension some staff were sad to see him leave. His behavior on the unit had become more acceptable, but the staff had little hope he would be able to maintain this level of functioning in the community.

CONCLUDING STATEMENTS

1. Antisocial behaviors are somewhat unique in that their very existence is viewed as an assault on the fundamental values of society. Antisocial behaviors include sexual deviations and antisocial acts.
2. The sexually deviant individual is one who gets sexual satisfaction by immature methods throughout adult life.
3. Little is known about the cause of most deviations in sexual behavior.
4. Homosexuality was once categorized as a psychiatric disorder, but is no longer classified as such. Treatment is indicated only for Ego-dystonic Homosexuality, in which the individual describes homosexual arousal as distressful and unwanted and seeks assistance.
5. Homosexuality occurs frequently and many individuals with

a homosexual orientation carry on well-adjusted, productive lives.

6. Sexually deviant behavior may be prevented by effective sexual education of children and by the provision of positive parent-child relationships and a healthy family environment in the early formative years.

7. Established sexually deviant behavior is difficult to treat successfully. However, if competent psychiatric treatment is available, if the individual is highly motivated to change his lifelong pattern of adaptation, and if he is prepared to continue therapy for a prolonged period of time, some changes in sexual orientation may be achieved.

8. Individuals who engage in antisocial acts have a history of dysfunctional behavior in the areas of interpersonal relationships and occupational endeavors, often have a criminal record, may be dependent upon alcohol or drugs, frequently engage in sexually deviant behavior, and charm strangers with their articulateness.

9. Although the dynamics of development of antisocial behavior are unknown, it is generally accepted that this disturbance has its origin in early childhood and that the adult manifestations are merely more serious continuations of a life-long pattern of antisocial behavior.

10. Individuals with antisocial behaviors are treated most successfully in a situation that provides an organized, structured, controlled environment.

11. Treatment goals for individuals who engage in antisocial behaviors include helping them to accept more socially approved attitudes and standards in their relationships with other people.

12. Individuals who engage in antisocial acts need to be rewarded for acceptable behavior.

SUGGESTED SOURCES OF ADDITIONAL INFORMATION

Classical

Dannels, Joann C.: Homosexual panic, Perspect. Psychiatr. Care **10:**106-111, July-Sept., 1972.

Lion, John R., editor: Personality disorder: diagnosis and management, Baltimore, 1974, The Williams & Wilkins Co.

Shaw, C.R.: The Jack-Roller: a delinquent boy's own story, Chicago, 1930, University of Chicago Press.

Contemporary

Barile, Linda: A model for teaching management of disturbed behavior, J. Psychosoc. Nurs. Ment. Health Serv. **20**:9-11, Nov., 1982.

Cohn, Lucille: They all felt wounded, J. Psychosoc. Nurs. Ment. Health Serv. **19**:24-36, July, 1981.

Gross, Mary Jane: Changing attitudes toward homosexuality, Perspect. Psychiatr. Care **16**:70-75, March-April, 1978.

Horowitz, June A.: Sexual difficulties as indicators of broader interpersonal problems (as reflected in psychotherapy groups), Perspect. Psychiatr. Care **16**:66-69, March-April, 1978.

Lawrence, John C.: Homosexuals, hospitalization, and the nurse, Nurs. Forum **14**:305-317, 1975.

Levine, Martin P., editor: The sociology of male homosexuality, New York, 1980, Harper & Row, Publishers.

Marmor, Judd, editor: Homosexual behavior: a modern reappraisal, New York, 1980, Basic Books, Inc., Publishers.

McNiff, Martha A.: Nursing in a psychiatric prison service, Am. J. Nurs. **73**:1586-1587, 1973.

Morrison, Elizabeth: Lesbians in therapy, J. Psychosoc. Nurs. Ment. Health Serv. **22**:18-22, Aug., 1984.

Raymond, Janice G.: The transsexual empire, Boston, 1980, Beacon Press.

Roache, Margaret Olson: Humanistic learning, Am. J. Nurs. **74**;1453-1456, 1974.

Rouslin, Sheila: A psychoanalytic view of homosexuality: an interview with Joseph Geller, M.D., Perspect. Psychiatr. Care **16**:76-80, March-April, 1978.

Shindul, Judith, and Snyder, Marie: The legal side: legal restraints on restraints, Am. J. Nurs. **81**:393-394, 1981.

Silverberg, Robert: Being gay: helping clients cope, J. Psychosoc. Nurs. Ment. Health Serv. **22**:18-25, Feb., 1984.

Socarides, Charles W.: Homosexuality. In Arieti, Silvano, and Brody, Eugene B., editors: American handbook of psychiatry, ed. 2, vol. 3, New York, 1974, Basic Books, Inc., Publishers, pp. 291-315.

Thomas, Sandra P.: Bisexuality: a sexual orientation of great diversity, J. Psychosoc. Nurs. Ment. Health Serv. **18**:19-27, April, 1980.

Tripp, C.A.: The homosexual matrix, New York, 1976, W.W. Norton & Co., Inc.

Of particular interest

Frosch, James P.: The treatment of antisocial and borderline personality disorders, Hosp. Community Psychiatry **34**(3):243-248, 1983.
This article provides the reader with a summary of trends in the literature addressing approaches to the borderline and antisocial personality disor-

ders. The author also addresses the difficulties that clinicians encounter when diagnosing the various personality disorders.

Reid, William H.: The antisocial personality: a review, Hosp. Community Psychiatry **36**(8):831-837, 1985.
The author provides an excellent discussion of the antisocial individual, including accurate diagnosis, psychodynamic theories, and treatment.

populations
at risk

adolescents

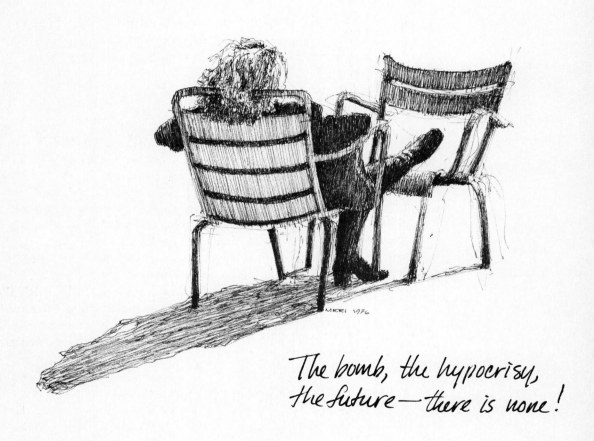

The bomb, the hypocrisy,
the future — there is none!

LEARNING OBJECTIVES

After studying this chapter the student will be able to:

1 Discuss three major developmental tasks of adolescence.

2 Discuss the sociocultural factors that impede mentally healthy resolution of the developmental tasks of adolescence.

3 Describe common behavior disturbances of adolescence.

4 Discuss the dynamics of development of behavior disturbances of adolescence.

5 Describe the characteristics of an adolescent suffering from the eating disorders of anorexia nervosa and bulimia.

6 Discuss the dynamics of development of eating disorders in adolescence.

7 Describe the characteristics of a potentially suicidal adolescent.

8 Develop a hypothetical plan of nursing care for adolescents who exhibit behavior disturbances, suicidal behavior, or eating disorders.

Adolescence is the term used to describe the period of life that falls between the ages of 12 and 18. This period spans the developmental phase between childhood and adulthood that is marked by intense biological, cognitive, intrapsychic, and interpersonal changes. One of the major tasks of adolescence is separation from the family as a means of establishing an independent identity and assuming an adult role in society. This struggle for independence is often awkward and at times, stormy as the individual experiences confusion and fear regarding his ability to master the tasks of this stage. The adolescent wrestles with the desire to stay close to protective parental figures and the simultaneous desire for freedom and autonomy. This ambivalence is often manifested by continual conflicts between the adolescent and his parents.

The adolescent is engaged in an intrapsychic struggle in an attempt to establish a new psychological equilibrium. In addition, the individual is exerting much effort to control new desires and impulses that come about as a result of biological maturation. The outcome of these struggles is largely dependent on the success with which earlier developmental tasks have been achieved.

Today's adolescent confronts this critical developmental period during a time of great stress generated by the highly complex postindustrial society in which he lives. The stresses of contemporary Western culture may contribute to the distress, alienation, loneliness, and despair that at times characterize the adolescent experience. The number and severity of emotional problems of adolescents continue to increase. Adolescent suicide has been described as an epidemic in the United States; the rate has tripled in the last 20 years. Self-destructive behaviors such as drug abuse, alcoholism, eating disorders, and sexual promiscuity are also on the rise.

The study of adolescence as a distinct developmental period is a relatively new specialty in the fields of psychiatry and nursing. There is much disagreement among authorities regarding the cause, prevention, and treatment of emotional disorders in adolescence. This specialty requires more attention than can be provided within the scope of this text. However, the topic deserves attention because nurses in numerous settings continue to confront the challenges of and opportunities for involvement in the prevention and treatment of emotional problems of adolescence.

HISTORICAL PERSPECTIVE

The study of adolescence as a distinct developmental stage did not come about until after World War I, and more notably in the post–World War II years. The concept of adolescence has been termed a product of the twentieth century. Adolescence is not a distinct biological fact; rather, it is a culturally determined phenomenon.

A number of factors led to interest in adolescence as a distinct stage. In preindustrial societies the progression from childhood to adulthood was a smooth one with limited choices. Children gradually took over the tasks and chores required to meet the basic needs of the family. With the advent of the industrial society, numerous social changes postponed the age at which the passage into adulthood occurred. A decrease in infant mortality and the lengthening of the average lifespan led to an extension of the period of childhood. Industrialization and expanding technology required increased education and training, and a separation of the child from the adult began to occur as youth entered educational institutions. The placement of adolescents into educational settings delayed their entry into the workplace, where it was feared they would compete with the growing population of adults for a limited number of jobs. Thus the prolongation of adolescence served an economic function as well.

The student role set adolescents apart as a distinct and separate population. In addition, the post–World War II baby boom created a very large subgroup of adolescents in the 1960s and 1970s. A distinct adolescent culture emerged, and an interest in their unique development as well as their distinct problems led to a more careful examination of this specific age group. Although a number of Freud's papers commented on adolescence, his major contributions were specific to childhood development. In contrast, Anna Freud further broadened the understanding of this population in her papers on adolescence and ego defense mechanisms. Erikson built on Freud's theory by defining the adolescent developmental task of identity vs. role diffusion.

Early theorists described adolescence as extremely turbulent, chaotic, and unstable by nature. More recent studies indicate that normal passage through adolescence may be much less turbulent than was originally thought. Fluctuations in mood are common, but feelings such as depression and anxiety are thought to be transient and related to external stressors. There is much controversy about which behaviors constitute normal adolescent growth and development. Unfortunately, much understanding of this population has been derived from studying those who were disturbed. More research with varied groups of adolescents is needed if the prevention and treatment of adolescent disorders are to be effective.

BEHAVIOR DISTURBANCES OF ADOLESCENTS

Adolescence is the period of transition from childhood to adulthood, marked by multiple changes and numerous developmental tasks. Biologically, there is an acceleration of growth and the emergence of secondary sexual characteristics. The adolescent experiences an awakening of powerful sexual urges that he must learn to control. At the same time he is faced with the task of separating from his family and establishing an independent identity. There is much ambivalence, as the adolescent is torn between the wish to retain the love and protection of his parents and his desire to become independent and self-directed. Socially, adolescence is a time of preparation for the adult role, and relationships developed during childhood must be renegotiated.

Adolescence is a time when individuals normally experience fluctuations in behavior, changes in mood, and a certain amount of emotional disequilibrium because many disruptions occur and early attachments must be relinquished. Studies reveal that many lesser disturbances of adolescence may correct themselves in time. Depression, anxiety, and anger are commonly experienced and are often related to external situational factors. However, some behavior disturbances may be predictive of continued difficulties in adult emotional adjustment, occupational success, and intimate relationships. They may, in fact, be precursors to major mental illness. Recent investigations show that, because of this uncertainty, it is wise to take adolescent disturbances seriously.

A small number of adolescents may develop serious emotional disturbances. Some may develop the characteristic symptoms of schizophrenia, including withdrawal, bizarre ideation, hallucinations, ideas of reference, and feelings of unreality as described in Chapter 13.

Some research indicates that depression and bipolar disorders may be more common in adolescence than previously thought. Recognition and treatment of these disturbances have been described in Chapter 14. Treatment skills similar to those used with adults are used for adolescents with these illnesses. Of particular concern in recent years is the rise in the adolescent suicide rate, which is discussed later in this chapter.

Disturbed adolescents often manifest problems in behaviors that reflect and symbolize difficulties with the specific developmental tasks of this stage. As the adolescent struggles with issues of separation and emancipation from parents and the establishment of a personal identity, difficulties may be manifested by dysfunctional behaviors. Extreme forms of rebelliousness, such as juvenile delinquency, truancy, running away, and substance abuse often represent the fear, ambivalence, and confusion that such adolescents feel about assuming the adult role. Dysfunctional behaviors may occur as the result of the adolescent's effort to establish a separate identity. Substance use and abuse may reflect an attempt to rebel against the adult world; it may also represent the adolescent's attempt to self-medicate deep emotional conflicts and anxieties. Overly passive, compliant, and conforming behaviors may be indicative of a high degree of anxiety related to independent behavior or an overreliance on the approval of others to define a sense of self.

Sexual promiscuity and unwed teenage pregnancy are topics of much concern in recent years. Adolescence is a time of rapid physical maturation, and the individual experiences intense sexual urges. The eventual tasks of this stage include the mastering of sexual impulses and separation from parents. Problems with these tasks are often evident in difficulties with intimacy and sexuality. Sexual promiscuity may be viewed as the manifestation of difficulties in mastering sexual urges, as well as a means for the adolescent to act out depressed, anxious, and angry feelings. The adolescent of today receives confusing and contradictory messages about sexual behavior. Although the postwar years brought the sexual revolution with its increased openness and sexual permissiveness, there are simultaneous and conflicting messages that condemn and forbid such behavior. Needless to say, such confusion sets the stage for difficulties with the tasks of this stage.

Statistically, the out-of-wedlock birthrate has increased dramatically in the last quarter century. Although there are many individual differences among unwed, pregnant teenagers, it has been suggested that this phenomenon may represent an attempt to establish independence from parents by replacing that relationship with another parent-child relationship.

Eating disorders are another group of behavioral disturbances that typically arise in adolescence. They are discussed in more depth later in this chapter.

DYNAMICS OF DEVELOPMENT

The behavior disturbances of adolescence appear to be related to multiple factors. These causes are as diverse and numerous as are the behaviors manifested by disturbed adolescents.

Clearly, the successful completion of earlier developmental tasks will influence the adolescent's ability to progress successfully through this stage. If the individual is not adequately equipped to confront the demands of adolescence, difficulties may be manifested by numerous dysfunctional behaviors. Factors that facilitate healthy development of the adolescent include a warm and supportive family environment where efforts toward autonomy are encouraged, close peer group affiliation with other healthy adolescents, and a community concern for the adolescent population. Relationships with supportive school teachers can offer the adolescent healthy adult role models outside of the home as he attempts to break the dependence on that environment. The absence of a safe and secure environment in which new behaviors can be tested can make healthy resolution of this developmental phase difficult.

As stated previously, many social factors are seen to influence the development of the adolescent in today's world. Some may contribute to the behavioral disturbances seen in this group. Much has been written about the sense of alienation and the increased stress faced by adolescents in contemporary culture. The rules are no longer clear. The fragmentation of familial and social institutions leads to confusion about values and identity. Where the progression from childhood to adulthood was once relatively smooth with limited options, today the choices abound. Where roles were once dictated, today's adolescent must determine who he is and how he will fit into the society. Factors such as these may contribute to the steady rise of disturbances in the adolescent population.

External stressors or traumatic events may further threaten or delay healthy adolescent development. The loss of a parent through death or divorce might occur at a time when the adolescent is struggling with ambivalent feelings toward loved ones, and such an event might lead to strong feelings of guilt, depression, or anger. In today's mobile society where relocating is common an adolescent may be faced with the difficult task of developing strong group ties in an unfamiliar town or city. Any such event may add to the existing stressors the adolescent normally experiences, and may potentially contribute to the conflicts that manifest themselves in disturbed behavior.

NURSING CARE OF THE ADOLESCENT WITH BEHAVIOR DISTURBANCES
Nursing assessment

The adolescent with behavior disturbances can usually be recognized by extremes in behavior. Because normal adolescents appear to experience transient periods of depression, anxiety, and general fluctuations in mood and behavior, identification of disturbed behavior is often difficult. It is important to look for the prolonged, persistent, and crippling effects that accompany the behavior of the disturbed adolescent.

Adolescents who are severely mentally disturbed exhibit the same symptoms as do adults with the same disturbances. The depressed adolescent, then, appears unkempt and lethargic and describes feelings of guilt and low self-esteem. There may be clues of suicidal ideas as well as multiple physical complaints. The adolescent who develops symptoms of schizophrenia develops the behaviors that characterize that disorder, such as withdrawal, bizarre ideation, ideas of reference, and hallucinations. The anxious adolescent is inordinately preoccupied with physical complaints and sensations, experiences disturbed interpersonal relationships and is plagued by unrealistic fears.

Behavior disturbances specific to adolescence often take the form of *acting-out behaviors*, a term used to describe the displacement of desires and emotions onto a particular situation in the form of a behavior. Disturbed adolescents often have a difficult time verbalizing emotions such as anxiety, fear, and depression. Thus they may act out these feelings in dysfunctional behaviors such as aggression, juvenile delinquency, sexual promiscuity, drug and alcohol abuse, and truancy. Recent findings indicate that a persistent pattern of such behaviors should alert the professional to the likelihood of serious difficulties in adjustment. As stated previously, it is better to be overly cautious with adolescents than to ignore behavior that often signals serious disturbances. One adolescent girl was suspended from school for acts of open verbal rebellion, truancy, and drug use. When the social supports available to her were withdrawn because of her suspension, she overdosed on a bottle of pills in an attempt to commit suicide. When treated at the local mental health clinic, she was found to be seriously depressed, and her rebellious acts were determined to be an effort to fend off her painful emotions.

As more is learned about the normative behaviors for adolescent development, assessment skills will continue to improve.

Nursing diagnoses

The nursing diagnoses for adolescents with behavioral disturbances are based on the data gathered during the assessment phase. In some cases the diagnostic categories and etiological factors include those previously discussed in the chapters on the major psychiatric disorders, such as schizophrenia, depression, and bipolar disorders.

Diagnostic categories approved by the Fifth National Conference on Nursing Diagnoses that may be specifically applicable to this population include:

Social isolation related to inabiity to engage in personal relationships

Potential for self-directed violence related to suicidal behavior

Anxiety related to situational or maturational crises

Ineffective family coping, disabling, related to highly ambivalent family relationships

The nurse may formulate more specific diagnoses based on the assessment of the individual client. Examples of nursing diagnoses more specific to the previously discussed assessment data could include:

Sexual promiscuity related to feelings of low self-esteem and worthlessness

Social withdrawal related to fears of rejection

Truancy related to fears of failure

Planning and implementing nursing care

The nursing care plan for the adolescent with behavior disturbances is derived from the nursing diagnoses. Adolescents, like other consumers of psychiatric nursing care, are individuals with unique needs, problems, and strengths. The nurse should be cautious about labeling adolescents as all alike and should appreciate the negative consequences of such a practice.

Treatment of the adolescent requires collaboration among the therapist, the child care workers, the school, the nurse, the family, and the social worker in identifying the individual's problem and helping him to cope with it.

To facilitate and provide corrective experiences, the nurse who works with the behaviorally disturbed adolescent must be aware of the developmental tasks of this period. Group activities and cohesiveness should be encouraged, as they serve to facilitate independence from parental figures, development of social skills, and efforts to establish identity. Peer group pressure can be an effective means to facilitate behavioral change.

At the same time the nurse must be aware of the necessity of providing safety and security for the adolescent group. This can be achieved, in part, through the use and enforcement of group norms and rules that prohibit aggression, substance abuse, and other acting-out behaviors. Consistency is imperative with this group, as is clear limit setting. The goal is to provide safety in a firm but caring manner. The environment must be safe and secure if the adolescent is to test out new, more functional behaviors.

The adolescent is experiencing rapid physiological growth, which has numerous physical and psychological implications. Adolescents require adequate space for the discharge of excess energy, and efforts should be made to provide that space within the limitations of the setting. In addition, nutritional needs are great.

The adolescent with symptoms of substance abuse often needs specific, structured treatment, which is frequently delivered in settings designed for this purpose. If the individual has become drug or alcohol dependent, a detoxification and abstinence period must be undertaken before rehabilitation can occur. The adolescent must then develop alternative, more functional ways of coping with stress. The involvement of the family is necessary to repair the disruptions that the behavior often creates and to examine the stressors in the home environment and familial relationships.

Disturbed adolescents often have particular difficulty with the tasks of mastering sexual impulses and establishing healthy heterosexual relationships. Nurses must be aware of their own sexuality and be able to provide role modeling and guidance in this area. The nurse may assess and discuss the sexual activities of adolescent clients to determine the nature and meaning of this behavior, as well as to determine whether or not precautions are being taken to prevent unwanted pregnancy. Unwed pregnancy is often a very traumatic experience for the teenage girl because social supports are often withdrawn and she often must leave school. In such cases the nurse must collaborate with school officials to facilitate continued growth and development opportunities for the pregnant teenager. Counseling of the pregnant teenager should be designed to address the needs and concerns specific to this situation. It is suggested that the pregnant teenager be provided a peer group of girls of similar age, with role models for nurturance and childrearing if the infant is to be kept, with educational and career facilities, with physical care, and with opportunities for recognition of and involvement with the father when possible.

Recently abortion has become a controversial topic. Pro-life advocates and proponents of abortion are polarized and antagonistic. The implications of this controversy are many for unwed, pregnant teenage girls. Those who opt for abortion may be consumed with guilt and remorse after the pregnancy has been terminated and may face constant reminders of the implications of their decision. If teenagers experiencing unwanted pregnancies are to be assisted, they must be provided with viable options that allow for their continued development. Issues such as continued education must be addressed. The responsibilities and involvement of the fathers must be taken into consideration and emphasized in both prevention and intervention plans.

There continues to be much controversy among authorities over the appropriate treatment setting for adolescents. It is suggested by many that the inpatient treatment setting should be utilized only for the more seriously disturbed adolescent. Because knowledge of how to treat behaviorally disturbed adolescents is evolving rapidly it is likely that the literature will soon delineate more conclusively appropriate settings for various conditions.

The nurse who works with the adolescent is faced with the exciting challenges of this rapid time of growth, as well as with the frustrations that go along with intervening with this population. Staff members can expect to be viewed, at times, as parental authority figures and thus become the target of much ambivalence, hostility, and anger. If the nurse remains objective but accepting, and firm but caring, the adolescent may eventually learn that anger and ambivalence do not destroy a relationship and that people with different beliefs and frames of reference can genuinely care for each other. Under the best circumstances, the adolescent may be able to use newly acquired skills to achieve a healthy separation from his parents and to develop an independent adult identity.

EATING DISORDERS: ANOREXIA NERVOSA AND BULIMIA

The incidence and awareness of the eating disorders known as anorexia nervosa and bulimia have risen dramatically in recent years. Both disorders most commonly begin in adolescence and young adulthood and primarily affect females. Although much has been written on eating disorders in recent years in both professional and popular literature, there is disagreement among authorities about the cause and treatment of these disorders.

Anorexia nervosa is the term used to describe a disorder characterized by extreme weight loss, behavior designed to effect weight loss, an intense fear of fat, a distorted body image, and peculiar patterns of eating and handling food. The term *anorexia* is a misnomer in that it means loss of appetite. However, the anorectic rarely experiences loss of appetite until late in the illness.

Bulimia is the term used in the *Diagnostic and Statistical Manual of Mental Disorders* (DSM-III) to describe a disorder marked by episodic, uncontrolled, and rapid consumption of food over a short period of time (binge eating), inconspicuous eating during a binge, and termination of the binge by abdominal pain, sleep, social interruption, or self-induced vomiting. The bulimic individual makes repeated attempts to lose weight by severe dieting, fasting, laxative abuse, or self-induced vomiting. She is aware of the fact that her eating behaviors are abnormal and is plagued by self-deprecating thoughts and depressed moods.

Dynamics of development

Anorexia nervosa was first described in the literature by Richard Morton in 1689, who termed it *nervous atrophy.* In 1874, 200 years later, William Gull defined anorexia nervosa as a distinct psychological disturbance and gave it its name. It has only been in recent years, however, that interest in this disorder has intensified.

Bulimia has only recently been recognized as a distinct and specific disorder. Binge eating was first described by Stunkard in 1959, who reported case descriptions of this behavior. In very recent years bulimia has reached epidemic proportions, particularly among the young female college population. The DSM-III defines bulimia as a distinct disorder with specific clinical features.

Early psychodynamic theorists suggested anorexia nervosa symbolized a wish to be pregnant and fantasies of oral impregnation, which the individual rejects by starvation. Today a number of theories exist that propose other possible causes of this disorder. It seems that an understanding of bulimia and anorexia nervosa demands an openness to numerous views because the study of these disorders is relatively new and the causative factors are likely to be many.

Some theorists propose a behavioral perspective and suggest that these behaviors are learned patterns. Others utilize a psychodynamic framework and suggest that these behaviors reflect a developmental arrest in the very early years of childhood around issues of trust, autonomy, and separation-individuation. Family theorists propose that the behaviors take place within the context of disturbed family relationships, faulty communication, and lack of boundaries between family members.

Social theorists point to the dramatic rise in the incidence of these disturbances in recent years. Some relate this rise to societal pressures to be thin, to the changing role of women and the conflicting messages given to females, and to the absence of a clear set of values and norms that guided the behavior of adolescents of previous generations. Still others believe that these disorders are biological in origin, or that a biological predisposition exists.

There is general consensus among experts that an appropriate model for the treatment of these disorders must integrate biological, psychological, and social perspectives. These disorders manifest themselves in disturbances in all subsystems. The symptoms are physiologic, psychologic, and social. Appropriate interventions clearly must address the whole person, and a plan of nursing care must be individualized to meet the needs of the client.

NURSING CARE OF CLIENTS WITH ANOREXIA AND BULIMIA
Nursing assessment

The individual with anorexia usually comes to the attention of the health care system after a drastic reduction in weight. Therefore she has an emaciated appearance. She has drastically reduced her total food intake, most specifically those foods containing carbohydrates. There are ritualistic and bizarre eating habits, such as hiding and hoarding foods, collecting recipes, dawdling and methodically rearranging food on the plate, and refusing to eat with family or in public. These individuals have an intense fear of getting fat, despite their often emaciated appearance. Symptoms of depression are often evident, such as sleep disturbances, crying spells, and suicidal ideation. They usually have amenorrhea and a lack of interest in sexual activity. The individual often engages in excessive exercising and is preoccupied with food and weight loss. Physical signs include hypothermia, bradycardia, dependent edema, dehydration, hypotension, and lanuga, a fine downy hair covering the body. Laboratory tests reveal electrolyte imbalances, including hypokalemic alkalosis secondary to self-induced vomiting and laxative abuse. These individuals are often withdrawn and socially isolated. They are described by family members as having been perfect children with above-average scholastic achievement and fear of failure.

The individual with bulimia often appears healthier than the client with anorexia because the behavior is generally less incapacitating. This person is usually of normal body weight or slightly overweight and reports frequent fluctuations in weight. The individual with anorexia is often shy and withdrawn but the client with bulimia is frequently an extrovert. The individual will often report low self-esteem and self-loathing, symptoms of depression, and a fear of losing control. She is able to describe the binge episodes and will report frequent attempts to lose weight through fasting or severely restricted diets, laxative abuse, or self-induced vomiting. There is usually an excessive fear of fat and a preoccupation with weight and weight loss. At times, other self-destructive behaviors such as suicide attempts, kleptomania, and sexual promiscuity are present. Individuals with bulimic behaviors are often described as perfectionists, high achievers scholastically and professionally, and highly dependent on the approval of others to maintain self-esteem. They fear rejection and loss of control. Physical signs usually relate to the behaviors of self-induced vomiting and laxative abuse and include electrolyte imbalances, cardiac irregularities, edema, dehydration, swollen salivary glands, broken blood vessels in the eyes, tooth decay from erosion of the enamel, broken nails and scars on the knuckles from self-induced vomiting, and general gastrointestinal distress. The individual with bulimic behaviors often describes a loss of control. If the binge-purge behaviors are excessive, the victim becomes socially isolated and dominated by these behaviors. Family relationships are often strained and disturbed, and the family feels helpless, angry, and rejected.

Nursing diagnoses

Diagnostic categories and etiological factors from the list of nursing diagnoses approved by the Fifth National Conference on Nursing Diagnoses that may be applicable to individuals with eating disorders include:

Alteration in health maintenance related to ineffective individual coping
Anxiety related to situational and maturational crises
Ineffective family coping related to situational or developmental crises
Impaired verbal communication related to psychological barriers

More specific diagnoses might include the following:

Extreme weight loss related to fear of fat and distorted body image

Sense of powerlessness related to difficulties with autonomy

Social isolation related to dysfunctional coping behaviors

Altered nutritional status related to starvation and purging behaviors

Planning and implementing nursing care

Individuals with eating disorders pose specific challenges to professionals, who often feel frustrated and helpless in their efforts to nurture those who reject their attempts. Food and eating are quite symbolic in this culture, often representing love and nurturance. Individuals with eating disorders have conflicts that specifically focus on these symbols, and their behaviors may be viewed by some as rejecting and hostile. In caring for clients with such disorders, one must keep in mind the powerful sense of ineffectiveness that seems to grip them, and work toward building a relationship of collaboration and trust.

Numerous treatment modalities have evolved to treat clients with anorectic and bulimic behaviors. The nursing care plan should be developed in collaboration with the client in an effort to capitalize on strengths as well as to intervene in dysfunctional behaviors. The meanings of the behaviors must be understood if a therapeutic plan is to be developed. Although diverse opinion exists as to the most appropriate method of treatment, there is general consensus that consistency and agreement among the health care workers must exist for treatment to be effective. Thus collaboration and communication within the team is imperative for the effective care of these clients.

Immediate interventions and short-term goals generally focus on a restoration of normal nutritional status because complications of malnourishment may be serious and eventually lead to death. The various inpatient treatment programs are derived from a number of models, including those based on behavioral interventions where positive reinforcements are used to reward weight gain and/or stabilization, and an appropriate intake of a balanced daily diet. During this phase of treatment it is imperative that staff offer support as well as consistency. An attitude of firm caring has been found helpful. In addition, treatment must address such potentially dangerous behaviors as suicidal ideation and other acting-out behaviors that sometimes exist.

Long-term goals and interventions are aimed at the underlying issues as previously discussed, as well as at the establishment of more functional coping mechanisms and healthy relationships. In an attempt to help the individual develop a sense of autonomy the nurse might help the client plan and test new independent behaviors. The client with an eating disorder often possesses a sense of ineffectiveness. The nurse might assist the individual to identify and express these feelings and then facilitate situations in which the client might achieve a sense of mastery and success. One treatment unit offers art and poetry therapy, which gives the client the chance to express feelings while simultaneously experiencing a sense of achievement when projects are completed.

Group therapies and support groups are often utilized to assist individuals to improve social skills and reduce the social isolation they experience. These groups also encourage autonomous and independent behavior in a population that is struggling to separate from family and achieve identity. Group cohesiveness and activities often faciliate this process.

Family therapy is often employed with clients and their families to try to alleviate family stress and achieve effective communication and healthy relationships. The nurse might individually encourage the client, as well, to identify family stressors and recognize the dysfunctional behaviors previously used to cope with stress.

Educational groups are utilized in the treatment of these individuals. Information is provided about healthy nutrition, the physical consequences of anorectic and bulimic behaviors, and the social pressures exerted on women of today to remain unhealthily thin. In addition to providing information, it is likely that such groups facilitate sharing and help these individuals to recognize that they are not alone in their struggles.

Psychotherapy with a qualified individual is aimed at helping the individual to discover the underlying causes of her problems and the source of the anorectic and bulimic symptoms. In addition, some psychopharmacological agents have been shown to be helpful in the treatment of these disorders.

Nurses who work with individuals who have anorexia nervosa or bulimia can tell many stories about the challenges and frustrations they confront. Many of the issues that arise are similar to those already discussed in treating the adolescent population. The individual is ambivalent, confused, and in conflict about the task of separation and often manifests his conflict in anger directed at the nurse. In addition, the individual often rejects the nurse's efforts to nurture. Nursing is a predominantly female profession, faced with the same issues that all women in our society are confronting. Thus there may be a tendency for the nurse to identify with the female who is experiencing an eating disorder. This is especially true of young nurses who have only recently made the passage into adulthood. On the other hand, the very nature of the profession puts the nurse in an ideal position to develop new insights about the feminine nature of eating disturbances. Therefore nursing is in the position to make many contributions to the understanding of these individuals.

ADOLESCENT SUICIDE

Suicide is one of the major causes of death for persons between the ages of 10 and 24. The adolescent suicide rate has increased rapidly in the last two decades. It is frightening to realize that authorities believe that the real incidence of adolescent suicide is even greater than the statistics indicate.

Authorities on adolescent development are defining this problem as catastrophic and epidemic. Understanding of and knowledge about adolescent suicide remains limited, and experts are struggling to define methods of prevention and intervention. Much of what was said in Chapter 14 about the individual contemplating suicide applies to the suicidal adolescent as well. However certain factors are unique to the adolescent population.

Dynamics of development

Although the shocking rise in the incidence of adolescent suicide is recognized, the causes of such behavior are not clearly understood. Studies of adolescent suicide behavior indicate individual, familial, and sociocultural issues as factors influencing this behavior.

Some studies indicate a familial tendency toward suicidal behavior, which possibly is learned. Major psychiatric disturbances such as depression and schizophrenia seem to be linked to suicidal attempts in some adolescents. An impulsive personality trait has also been identified in some adolescents who have attempted or committed suicide. It has also been suggested that adolescents do not have a clear and realistic sense of death or of the finality of the act of suicide. Therefore suicidal behavior may be an effort to express anger or hostility toward loved ones or to make others feel sorry for real or imagined offenses.

Confusion over emerging sexual impulses and gender identity is common during adolescence, and suicide may represent an effort to resolve such conflicts. Substance abuse has also been linked to teenage suicide.

In terms of family dynamics a number of factors seem to relate to suicidal behaviors. Such factors include broken homes, family disorganization, overly strict parental discipline, lack of communication, and suicidal behavior in family members.

Much attention has been focused recently on the sociocultural factors that contribute to suicidal behavior in adolescence. The dramatic rise in incidence points to the influence of social change. A number of researchers cite the fact that violence has become acceptable in our society, and that the adolescent has become numb to violence. In addition, authorities point to increased family mobility and rootlessness that lead to a sense of alienation and loneliness at a time when group affiliation is vital. Social isolation often precedes a suicidal act.

A number of authorities discuss the prevailing stress found in our Western culture as a factor contributing to the incidence of adolescent suicide. In addition, adolescents in our society do not really have a place—they are neither child nor adult. They are often segregated into educational institutions where strong relationships with adults are lacking at a time when guidance and support are required.

It is also believed that the media have, at times, sensationalized or romanticized the act of suicide. Such idealization of the act may contribute toward suicide among those already contemplating the act. For example, epidemics of suicide have been reported in certain schools, reflecting the communicable nature of the behavior. If suicide is glorified or seen as a plausible method of coping with the life crises of adolescence, the number of suicides is likely to increase.

Although studies of suicidal behavior in adolescents indicate that it is determined by numerous and diverse individual, familial, and social factors, one factor is almost always present. This central issue is a sense of invisibility—a feeling that one is not recognized or appreciated, and a belief that one has very little impact on the world around him.

NURSING CARE OF THE SUICIDAL ADOLESCENT
Nursing assessment

It is believed that many adolescents contemplating suicide give clues of their plans and intentions. Some of these clues and behaviors have been identified in Chapter 14. The nurse must be sensitive to such clues, which include preoccupation with themes of death, the expression of suicidal ideas, and the giving away of valued possessions. For example, one adolescent boy worked part-time for years to buy a sports car. The day before he attempted suicide he offered the car to his older brother.

Changes in sleeping patterns are often noted. The suicidal adolescent sleeps either too much or too little. Changes in eating patterns and resultant weight gain or loss may occur. A withdrawal from family and friends is common. The individual often has changes in school performance including lowered grades and truancy. Extreme fluctuations in mood, such as outburts of anger alternating with crying spells, often occur. Finally, drug or alcohol abuse is often found in suicidal adolescents.

A previous suicidal attempt increases the likelihood of a later attempt. In addition, the recent suicide of a friend or family member increases the probability that the adolescent will act on his suicidal impulses.

Although clues to suicide are often given by the potentially suicidal adolescent, the nurse must be cautioned that the absence of clues does not eliminate the possibility of suicidal behavior. If any suspicion of suicidal ideas is present it is far better to risk confronting these than to ignore this potential problem.

Nursing diagnoses

The nursing diagnostic and etiological factors approved by the Fifth National Conference on Nursing Diagnoses that may be applicable to the suicidal adolescent include:

Potential for self-directed violence related to suicidal behavior
Social isolation related to inability to engage in satisfying interpersonal relationships
Ineffective individual coping related to maturational crises

More specific nursing diagnoses based on the assessment data given may be formulated as follows:

Suicidal thoughts related to a sense of ineffectiveness and worthlessness
Social isolation related to fear of rejection and despair

Additional diagnoses may be formulated to address the more specific problems of the suicidal adolescent. If the individual is manifesting symptoms characteristic of the major psychiatric illnesses, such as depression or schizophrenia, the nursing diagnoses discussed in previous chapters are appropriate.

Planning and implementing nursing care

The nurse caring for the suicidal adolescent should be familiar with the principles outlined in Chapter 14 on the care of the suicidal adult. An environment that facilitates a sense of worthiness and conveys a caring attitude is vital. There should be opportunities for the suicidal adolescent to participate safely in activities that enhance a sense of mastery and self-esteem. The individual must be safe and secure while able to engage in adolescent group activities. The therapeutic relationship offers the opportunity for the suicidal adolescent to express and explore feelings in a climate of empathy and concern.

The plan of care for the suicidal adolescent must be derived from the nursing diagnoses. Each suicidal adolescent will have unique problems and strengths, and the plan of care must reflect these differences.

In the event of a successful adolescent suicide the nurse must deal with the anguish of many affected individuals. At times the nurse may be able to offer assistance to family members, school counselors, and others involved. It has been said that the true victims of suicide are the survivors. Surviving family members experience intense remorse and feelings of guilt. In addition, such a crisis will magnify any existing problems in marital and family relationships. The principles of crisis intervention, as outlined in Chapter 22, are useful in such situations. Siblings must be observed carefully because suicide in one family member may precipitate such behavior in others.

The nurse may also be consulted by school officials concerned about the potential epidemic nature of the problem. Education that focuses on the realistic aspects of death and the impact of the behavior on loved ones is often enormously beneficial. Peers must be helped through the grieving process and the stages of shock and denial, developing awareness, and eventual acceptance.

It is imperative that the nurse be concerned with the prevention of adolescent suicidal behavior. As nurses assume roles in varied settings many opportunities for involvement in this aspect of care present themselves. Research indicates that early recognition of the warning signs is vital. Once again, education seems to be a valuable tool. The nurse may be asked to collaborate with school officials and other professionals in providing education about suicide, as well as assistance for adolescents in coping with stress and depression.

Experiences that offer the adolescent opportunities to develop a sense of belonging and mastery might be the best way to prevent suicidal behavior. Recreational activities and centers, clubs, and church groups may help prevent the desperate sense of loneliness and alienation that contributes to all of the disturbances of adolescents. Ongoing adult involvement in the lives of adolescents enhances the probability of successful resolution of this developmental phase, and nurses have a responsibility to provide some of this involvement.

CASE FORMULATION
a behaviorally disturbed adolescent

Jennie B., a 15-year-old girl, was referred to the community mental health center by the school counselor with the approval of her mother. She came to the center willingly and described herself as unhappy, upset, and without friends. The school counselor was concerned about Jennie, who had entered the school as a new student only a few months earlier. Her concern focused on the following problems: Jennie had made no friends, was receiving failing grades, was absent from school almost half the time, and was involved in almost no school clubs or extracurricular activities.

Jennie talked freely to the nurse at the mental health center and stated she could not study because she did not sleep well at night. She described nightmares that frightened her and kept her awake, the content of which featured an older man who molested her sexually.

In discussing her family she spoke of the frequent fights between herself and her mother over her mother's drinking and her mother's boyfriend. About a year ago Jennie's mother and father had separated, and they were in the process of getting a divorce when she came to the clinic. After her parents separated, Jennie's father moved to another city and rarely found time to come back and visit with his three children, of whom Jennie was the oldest. She blamed her mother for the separation and the move from their old neighborhood and the school she had attended all her life.

Jennie's two brothers had become her responsibility since her mother's interest in her boyfriend had increased. Thus she was expected to supervise her younger brothers, get their meals, and do the laundry. With this amount of work expected of her, Jennie stated she was too tired to attend school more than half the time. Jennie's brothers did not follow her directions and resented her attempts to supervise them. Thus there was conflict among the children in this family and no adult to act as a buffer in such conflicts. Jennie felt unloved and unwanted.

Her mother's boyfriend was a large, middle-aged taxi driver who teased Jennie a good deal. She told the nurse that she disliked him intensely and stated that she was afraid of him. In addition, she did not want anyone taking her father's place in the home because she loved her father very much.

Jennie was somewhat smaller in stature than most girls of her age. Her breasts had not yet begun to develop, and she was extremely sensitive about this fact. She viewed her flat-chested appearance as a serious defect that made her different from other girls. Also, she had not yet begun to menstruate, which increased her belief that she was different and lacking in feminine appeal. Unfortunately, Jennie was not physically attractive because her hair was dull and unkempt and her complexion sallow.

Jennie's mother was invited to come to the clinic to discuss the treatment plans for her daughter. She found it difficult to arrange a convenient time, because she held a part-time job. However, she finally kept the appointment and gave much of the same information about the family situation as did Jennie. However, Jennie's mother stated that the conflict among the children was caused by Jennie's attempt to boss her brothers. She felt that Jennie's resentment of her boyfriend was the cause of many of their disagreements and declared that her dates were none of her daughter's business. According to her mother, Jennie was her father's favorite child, but he did not deserve her devotion.

Jennie's developmental history, as related by her mother, was uneventful except that she had been enuretic until the age of 9. This problem reappeared after the separation of the parents and was present even now. Her mother also reported that Jennie had responded to discipline by having temper tantrums. These began when she was being toilet trained and continued until she was 9. Although

Continued.

she no longer had what could be described as temper tantrums, she did fly into rages. These rages seemed to be related to the mother's boyfriend and the approaching divorce. The mother stated that because of her job and home responsibilities she had not been able to work with the school counselor.

nursing assessment

Jennie appeared to be experiencing difficulties in resolving the tasks of normal adolescent development, as a number of factors impinged on her life. Such factors included the loss of a close relationship with her father, a recent move, increased responsibilities at home, family conflicts, a perceived lack of attention and love, and the recent presence of her mother's boyfriend whom Jennie feared and resented. All of these factors might have contributed to the difficulties in adjustment that Jennie was experiencing. Adolescence is a time when the individual experiences ambivalent feelings toward the parents, which include a desire for love and affection along with a seemingly conflicting desire for autonomy and emancipation from the parents. The loss of her father at such a time might have made Jennie feel abandoned and guilty. In addition, her mother did not appear able to provide the love and support required during this period. Jennie might be blaming her mother for the loss of her father.

Jennie moved at a time when peer relationships and group involvement are important, and she found it necessary to enter a strange school and develop new relationships—something she had always found difficult. Her responsibilities at home might have prevented her from performing well at school, establishing successful relationships with peers, and engaging in extracurricular activities, which are all potential sources of self-esteem for adolescents. Jennie had not developed the physical characteristics of a woman and felt different and unloved.

Jennie's mother might have been ill-equipped to offer Jennie the love and support she needed for the successful resolution of earlier developmental tasks. The presence of enuresis and temper tantrums in childhood might have indicated the anger and frustration that Jennie felt toward her mother in early years and an effort to gain control and autonomy. The reappearance of enuresis when Jennie's father left home might represent the revival of these old childhood feelings toward her mother because Jennie now blamed her for the loss of her father.

Jennie's behavior disturbances reflected the difficulties she was experiencing with the tasks of adolescent development. Her rages might have reflected feelings of rejection and were directed toward her mother for saddling Jennie with home responsibilities, withholding love, and introducing an unwanted man into the home. The increase in Jennie's nightmares might relate to the introduction into the family of her mother's new boyfriend. Her social isolation might indicate feelings of low self-esteem and a fear of competition and failure. These feelings of inadequacy seem to have been reinforced by Jennie's slow sexual development.

nursing diagnoses

The assessment data lead to the following nursing diagnoses:

> Anger and verbal hostility related to feelings of rejection
> Social isolation related to low self-esteem and fear of competition and failure
> Poor school performance related to disturbed family relationships
> Poor hygiene related to poor body image and feelings of worthlessness

planning and implementing nursing care for JENNIE B.

The plan for nursing care for Jennie is summarized in the box on p. 450.

Jennie was admitted to a residential treatment setting for adolescents with behavior disturbances where many opportunities for corrective experiences were available. After assessing her needs and formulating the nursing diagnoses, a plan of care was developed. An appointment was made for a physical examination to determine any specific cause of her slow sexual development. The examination revealed no significant findings.

A trusting therapeutic relationship was established with Jennie's primary nurse, who treated Jennie with respect and dignity and listened carefully to whatever she said. Her opinions were accepted, and the nurse avoided judging and moralizing.

The nurse attempted to convey a firm and caring attitude. She encouraged Jennie to function independently by establishing fair and reasonable limits while also praising autonomous behaviors, encouraging participation in extracurricular activities, and including Jennie in decisions regarding her care and treatment.

It was felt that Jennie's problems at school were a partial reflection of her problems at home. Continued efforts were made to involve Jennie's mother in treatment, although her resistance indicated that Jennie might have to learn to accept her mother's limitations and develop independent coping skills to deal with family stress.

Finally Jennie was encouraged to participate in age-appropriate activities, in an effort to assist her to develop healthy peer relationships and a sense of belonging.

Continued.

nursing care plan for
JENNIE B.

nursing diagnosis	objective	rationale	nursing actions	outcome criteria
Anger and verbal hostility related to feelings of rejection	To assist client to direct anger and hostility into socially acceptable activities	Verbal hostility leads to further conflicts and increases the client's sense of unworthiness and feelings of rejection	Encourage participation in age-appropriate expressive and physical activities, for example, sports, art, music, and physical exercise Comment positively on successful participation	Within 1 month client will: report talking to mother for 15 minutes without verbally hostile behaviors spontaneously and independently participate in alternative activities
	To encourage client to explore feelings	Discussion of problems often renders them amenable to problem solving	Utilize reflection to encourage expression of feelings Convey acceptance of angry feelings Convey interest Encourage problem solving	Within 1 month client will: spontaneously express feelings of anger show evidence of problem-solving behaviors
Social isolation related to low self-esteem and fear of competition and failure	To encourage the client's involvement in age-appropriate occupational and recreational activities	Social success with peers will enhance self-esteem and facilitate successful mastery of developmental tasks	Encourage participation in activities, for example, clubs, church groups, recreational and occupational therapies Accept feelings of frustration Comment positively on successful participation	Within 2 weeks client will: spontaneously involve self in one group activity weekly report success in one activity
	To encourage the client's involvement in adolescent group therapy	Discussion of concerns with other adolescents facing similar difficulties will enhance sense of belonging The expression of feelings may render them more amenable to problem solving	Refer to group therapy Encourage biweekly attendance Comment positively on attendance and involvement Accept expressions of frustration and fear	Within 2 weeks client will: attend group therapy biweekly spontaneously express her feelings

nursing care plan for
JENNIE B.—cont'd.

nursing diagnosis	objective	rationale	nursing actions	outcome criteria
Poor school performance related to disturbed family relationships and low self-esteem	To facilitate interest in school subjects and assignments To encourage independent functioning To encourage the identification of family stressors and encourage problem-solving techniques	Successful performance in school helps to enhance self-esteem and sense of mastery Separation from family is a developmental task of adolescence; successful resolution will enhance worthiness Identification of stressors will facilitate problem solving techniques and increase the likelihood of functional resolutions	Discuss school topics with client and encourage and reinforce interests; offer positive appraisals for success Suggest and encourage involvement in extracurricular activities View the family as a system Recognize that as client's behavior alters the system will enter disequilibrium Assist with identification of stressors in family	Within 1 month client will: report interest in school topic earn improved school grades identify family stressors and demonstrate efforts to problem solve
Poor hygiene related to poor body image and sense of unworthiness	To encourage improved hygiene	Good hygiene and dress may enhance self-esteem	Encourage client to engage in daily routines of hygiene and grooming Offer compliments for improved appearance	Within 2 weeks client will show interest in grooming, for example, combing hair, age-appropriate dress

---

evaluation

Evaluation of the plan of nursing care and its implementation was based on the outcome criteria developed in the planning phase.

Jennie made steady progress in the residential treatment setting, where ample opportunities were provided for healthy relationships and corrective experiences with both adults and peers. Her rages disappeared, and verbal hostility diminished. A tutor assisted Jennie to focus on school work, and improvement was noted. It seemed that her external controls improved, and her self-esteem was enhanced.

Discharge to outpatient services was recommended, where Jennie would continue in psychotherapy with a clinical nurse specialist.

CONCLUDING STATEMENTS

1. The treatment of emotional disorders in adolescents is recognized as an area of specialization in both psychiatry and nursing.
2. There is even less agreement among authorities concerning the cause, prevention, and treatment of emotional problems of adolescents than there is concerning similar problems among adults.
3. Understanding normal personality growth and development is essential before disturbances of adolescence can be understood.
4. The major developmental tasks of the adolescent include separating from parents, understanding and controlling emerging sexual impulses, and achieving an identity.
5. Causes of the increase in the number of adolescents with behavior disturbances are many and varied, but appear to relate to some of the basic problems in our culture.
6. Many of the disturbed behaviors of adolescents represent attempts to defend against anxiety.
7. Treatment of the adolescent with behavior disturbances requires an individualized care plan developed to express the unique needs, problems, and strengths of the person.
8. The therapeutic treatment setting for the adolescent must provide for safety and security, while allowing adequate space for the discharge of excess energy as well as opportunities for autonomous behaviors and healthy peer group activity.
9. Nurses working with the behaviorally disturbed adolescent need to examine their feelings, attitudes, and behavior to design and implement therapeutically effective treatment.
10. The nurse needs much self-understanding to deal therapeutically with hostile and provocative behavior.
11. Behavior disturbances in adolescence can be transient in nature and related to external factors. However, recent literature indicates that a pattern of persistent disturbed behavior often indicates more serious disturbances.
12. Anorexia nervosa is a disorder occurring most commonly in adolescents and is characterized by extreme weight loss, behavior directed toward weight loss, an intense fear of fat, distorted body image, and peculiar ways of handling food.
13. Bulimia is a disorder commonly occurring in late adoles-

cence and young adulthood, marked by episodic, uncontrollable, and rapid consumption of food over short periods of time (binge eating), and termination of the binge by abdominal pain, sleep, social interruption, or self-induced vomiting.

14. Suicides among adolescents in this country have rapidly increased in the last two decades; it is felt that the rising incidence may reflect sociocultural factors and stressors.

SUGGESTED SOURCES OF ADDITIONAL INFORMATION

Classical

Bowlby, John: Separation anxiety: a critical review of the literature, J. Child. Psychol. Psychiatry **1**:251-269, 1961.

Contemporary

Beard, Margaret: Interpersonal trust, life events and coping in an ethnic adolescent population, J. Psychosoc. Nurs. Ment. Health Serv. **18**:12-20, Nov., 1980.

Bloom, Michael: Adolescent-parental separation, New York, 1980, Gardner Press, Inc.

Buchanan, Diane, and Rogers, Ann: A comprehensive treatment program: an inpatient, interdisciplinary approach, J. Psychosoc. Nurs. Ment. Health Serv. **18**:42-45, July, 1980.

Calderone, Mary: On the possible prevention of sexual problems in adolescence, Hosp. Community Psychiatry **34**(6):528-530, 1983.

Caplan, Gerald: Child and adolescent psychiatry. In Arieti, Silvano, editor: American Handbook of psychiatry, ed. 2, vol. 2, New York, 1974, Basic Books, Inc., Publishers, pp. 3-397.

Ciseaux, Ann: Anorexia nervosa: a view from the mirror, Am. J. Nurs. **80**:1468-1470, 1980.

Dambacher, Betty, and Hellwig, Karen: Nursing strategies for young drug users, Perspect. Psychiatr. Care **9**:201-205, Sept.-Oct., 1971.

Danziger, Sharon: Major treatment issues and techniques in family therapy with the borderline adolescent, J. Psychosoc. Nurs. Ment. Health Serv. **20**:27-34, Jan., 1982.

Doyen, Lisa: Primary anorexia nervosa: a review and critique of selected papers, J. Psychosoc. Nurs. Ment. Health Serv. **20**:12-18, June, 1982.

Evans, David: Explaining suicide among the young: an analytic review of the literature, J. Psychosoc. Nurs. Ment. Health Serv. **20**:9-16, Aug., 1982.

Fox, Kathleen: Adolescent ambivalence: a therapeutic issue, J. Psychosoc. Nurs. Ment. Health Serv. **18**:29-33, Sept., 1980.

Freeberg, Sandy: Anger in adolescence, J. Psychosoc. Nurs. Ment. Health Serv. **20**:29-31, March, 1982.

Gilead, Maggie, and Mulaik, Jane: Adolescent suicide: a response to a developmental crisis, Perspect. Psychiatr. Care **22**:94-101, July-Sept., 1983.

Gispert, Maria, Brenich, Paul, Wheeler, Kirk, and Krieger, Laurie: Predictors of repeat pregnancies among low income adolescents, Hosp. Community Psychiatry **35**(7):719-723, 1984.

Hart, Nancy A., and Keidel, Gladys C.: The suicidal adolescent, Am. J. Nurs. **79**:80-84, 1979.

Hodgman, Christopher: Current issues in adolescent psychiatry, Hosp. Community Psychiatry **34**(6):514-521, 1983.

Huberty, David J., and Malmquist, Jeffrey D.: Adolescent chemical dependency, Perspect. Psychiatr. Care **16**:21-27, Jan.-Feb., 1978.

King, Dorothy A.: Anorexic behavior: a nursing problem, J. Psychiatr. Nurs. **71**:11-17, May-June, 1971.

Mellencamp, Astred: Adolescent depression: a review of the literature, with implications for nursing care, J. Psychosoc. Nurs. Ment. Health Serv. **19**:15-20, Sept., 1981.

Moore, Judith, and Coulman, Mary: Anorexia nervosa: the patient, her family and key family therapy interventions, J. Psychosoc. Nurs. Ment. Health Serv. **19**:9-14, May, 1981.

Puskar, Kathy: Structure for the hospitalized adolescent, J. Psychosoc. Nurs. Ment. Health Serv. **19**:13-16, July, 1981.

Richardson, Thomas: Anorexia nervosa: an overview, Am. J. Nurs. **80**:1470-1471, 1980.

Schmidt, Ann Marie: Adolescent female rape victims: special considerations, J. Psychosoc. Nurs. Ment. Health Serv. **19**:17-19, Aug., 1981.

Schmidt, Mary P.H., and Duncan, Beverly A.B.: Modifying eating behavior in anorexia nervosa, Am. J. Nurs. **74**:1646-1648, 1974.

Tiedt, Eileen: The adolescent in the hospital: an identity-resolution approach, Nurs. Forum **11**(2):120-140, 1972.

Wilbur, Cornelia, and Aug, Robert: Sex education, Am. J. Nurs. **73**:88-91, 1973.

Of particular interest

Fagin, Claire M., editor: Readings in child and adolescent psychiatric nursing, St. Louis, 1974, The C.V. Mosby Co.
This excellent book outlines the role of the nurse in relating therapeutically with adolescent clients and makes use of clinical examples to assist the reader in application.

Wilkinson, Teresa: Childhood and adolescent psychiatric nursing, Oxford, England, 1983, Blackwell Scientific Publications, Ltd.
This comprehensive text is a valuable resource for the nurse working with adolescent clients. The author examines developmental needs and issues common to this population and utilizes the nursing process to offer relevant suggestions for intervention.

chapter twenty

populations
at risk

the elderly

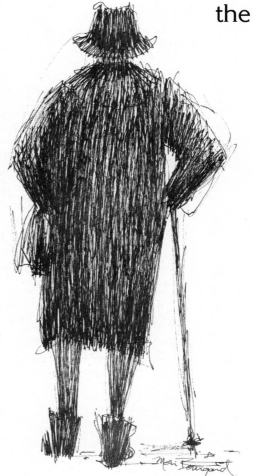

*I have no regrets about the past,
but it's lonely without him.*

LEARNING OBJECTIVES

After studying this chapter the student will be able to:

1   Describe some social forces that affect the mental health of the elderly in present society.

2   Discuss some common experiences and behaviors of elderly persons encountered by the nurse in any setting.

3   Describe some of the behavior disturbances associated with aging.

4   Discuss the dynamics of development of suspiciousness, depression, and confusion in elderly persons.

5   State examples of nursing diagnoses likely to be applicable to elderly persons with behavior disturbances.

6   Discuss nursing interventions appropriate for elderly persons with behavior disturbances.

7   Describe the symptoms exhibited by a person with the medical diagnosis of Alzheimer's disease.

8   Discuss the dynamics of development of Alzheimer's disease.

9   State examples of nursing diagnoses likely to be applicable to clients with Alzheimer's disease.

10 Develop a hypothetical plan of nursing care for an elderly person with Alzheimer's disease.

Old age is an integral part of the life cycle, not one stage separated from the rest of life. Unfortunately, the United States is a youth oriented society and the elderly are viewed as a homogeneous group to which predominantly negative characteristics are ascribed. For example, a common but erroneous belief is that once a person has reached the arbitrarily established age of retirement he becomes at best, useless, or at worst, a burden to his family and to society. It is also believed that individuals over 65 or 70 years of age inevitably become forgetful and confused. While the elderly share much in common with each other, as do persons in any other developmental stage, the reality is they are also individuals who continue to adapt in the ways they have learned in earlier years. Elderly individuals still have the potential to learn and grow. Survival with esteem—not mere physical survival—is the goal of the aged person.

When any age group is viewed separately from the society in which it lives an incomplete and inaccurate assessment is obtained. Because of this society's negative attitudes toward aging, it is impossible to understand the aging process without also understanding the impact of society on the elderly.

The aged are beset by the same social problems as the young, but their options for dealing with such problems are more limited. One example is economic inflation during which the value of savings and pensions is eroded and there are very few opportunities for employment even if an older person were physically able to hold a job. In our society the elderly as a group are poor. In certain groups—American Indian and blacks—over 75% of the elderly live below the poverty level. Poverty not only deprives persons of the means to fulfill their basic needs adequately, it also deprives them of a powerful social tool. It takes money to look one's best and to attend many social functions.

Another example of a social phenomenon that affects the elderly is the change from small stable communities to large mobile urban centers. This change affects people of all ages and often results in a feeling of powerlessness. Older persons in particular are left without family to help cope with the bureaucracies necessary to survival in a complex society. The result often is a sense of alienation and worthlessness.

The accelerating rate of social change, as well as technological change, has subjected human beings to an unprecedented need to adapt. The ability of the elderly to make effective adaptations is dramatically impeded by a society that puts no value on age. Simple cultures value older persons because it is this group that passes on the legends of the culture. In contrast in an industrialized society mythology that remains important is written down, printed, and sold. Therefore in an industrialized society characterized by the nuclear family and printed and electronic communication media, there is no role for the elderly. In a society such as this it is obvious that the achievement of Erikson's psychosocial task of aging—the achievement of ego integrity versus despair—might be difficult to achieve, especially since the negative attitudes of society toward aging have often been internalized by the elderly themselves.

It is important for all concerned citizens to confront and challenge events in the culture that support devaluation of the aged.

If health care personnel, particularly nurses, are to promote the mental health of the elderly, it becomes imperative for them to understand the interaction between the inevitable characteristics of the aging process and the characteristics of the culture. This interaction may very well result in the symptomatology associated with the organic mental disorder of senile dementia, to be described later in this chapter.

HISTORICAL PERSPECTIVE

Throughout history there has always been an occasional individual who has lived to reach the age of 80, 90, or even 100. However, never before has the life expectancy of the average individual been as long as it currently is. For example, white males born in 1900 had a life expectancy of 48 years; white females born in the same year had a life expectancy of 51 years. In contrast, white males born in 1978 had a life expectancy of 70 years and white females had a life expectancy of 78 years. Therefore, until the twentieth century it was the unusual individual who lived beyond 50 years of age. Many women died in childbirth; the general population was vulnerable to epidemics of respiratory infections and other communicable diseases; and there were few effective treatments for such life-threatening illnesses as cancer and cardiovascular disease. In addition occupational hazards took their toll and the death rate from accidents was high. These factors combined with few preventive measures resulted in what is now seen as a short life expectancy. Therefore illnesses associated with old age were rarely experienced and poorly understood.

Because of the increased life expectancy and effective treatment of illness and injuries, the number of persons 65 years of age or older is larger than ever before. It is projected that more than 13% of the total population will be over age 65 by the year 2005, representing a 60% increase in this age group from 1980. As the number of people who live longer increases there is a concomitant increase in the health care needs of this population, including mental health needs. Until recently it was assumed that a person who lived long enough would eventually become "senile" and that the symptoms of confusion and regression associated with this diagnosis were inevitable outcomes of the aging process. As the total number of persons in this age group increases this assumption can no longer be made without being validated by research. Not surprisingly, recent research is demonstrating that only 1% of all mental problems of the elderly result from functional mental illnesses. The remaining 99% of the behavior problems are associated with physical disorders such as small strokes, hypothyroidism, and brain tumors. Over 50% results from Alzheimer's disease, a dementia that frequently occurs in the later years of life.

Dementia is a term used to describe organic mental disorders characterized by deterioration of intellectual abilities, with impairment in memory, abstract thinking, cognition, judgment, and impulse control. Personality and behavioral changes result from this disease process and an organic factor is assumed to be its underlying cause. Dementia may be reversible or progressive in nature, depending on the specific cause. *Senile dementia* is the term used to describe a progressive degenerative, irreversible dementia with onset after age 65. Authorities report that the diagnosis of senile dementia is often misapplied to those suffering from functional psychiatric disorders such as depression and from dysfunctional behaviors resulting from the normal process of aging interacting with the inordinate stressors experienced by the elderly. Thus it is essential that the assessment of elderly individuals manifesting these symptoms be multidimensional and include psychosocial and environmental factors as well as biophysiological aspects.

Alzheimer's disease, which is discussed in depth later in this chapter, is a degenerative, progressive, irreversible syndrome first discovered in 1906 by a German neurologist, Alois Alzheimer. Dr. Alzheimer treated a 51-year-old woman who exhibited all the symptoms associated with senility of the elderly. He became curious about her symptoms in light of her young age. After her death he examined her brain and discovered that parts of it contained clumps of twisted nerve-cell fibers that he called "neurofibrillary tangles." Although he did not understand what caused these abnormal nerve-cell configurations, he felt certain their existence created the patient's behavior. Alzheimer's disease was assumed to be rare and to affect only the relatively young, leading to it being called a "presenile dementia."

With the advent of the electron microscope in the 1960s, scientists discovered the same neurofibrillary tangles in elderly persons diagnosed as having senile dementia. Thus it is now concluded that Alzheimer's disease is not rare and confined to the relatively young, but rather accounts for over 50% of the cases of dementia in the aged.

THE AGING PROCESS

The elderly population is a diverse group. Elderly persons have as many individual differences as do those in earlier developmental stages. The negative stereotyping that has been applied to elderly individuals has recently been described as "ageism," a term representing the discriminatory practices against the elderly in our culture. The stereotype that describes all elderly persons as irritable, forgetful, rigid, regressed, and confused is a distorted and limited view. Most elderly individuals can be healthy and productive, and continue to learn and grow when they are allowed to do so.

There is no exact definition of old age. It is a developmental stage defined by complex physiological, psychological, and sociological factors. It has been defined by some gerontologists as the period marked by the relinquishing of midlife roles (career, parenting), combined with the view of oneself as being elderly.

Although elderly persons are individuals with diverse needs and strengths, they share some commonalities as do persons in other developmental stages. Physiological changes often occur as a result of normal aging, but the rate of change varies with each individual and with each organ system. These changes include increasing perceptual difficulties, diminished psychomotor abilities, and memory deficits that are reflected by difficulty in recall. However, these physiological changes appear to create little difficulty in the achievement of life goals for most elderly persons.

In contrast, sociological and psychological changes profoundly affect the aged person and often include such factors as retirement and loss of adequate income, family reorganization, and the discriminatory practices that devalue the elderly in our culture. As a result of normal aging the characteristic personality of the individual often becomes more prominent. Thus the suspicious individual may become even more so in old age. Habitual ways of behaving continue, as do social skills, verbal skills, judgment, and comprehension.

The major developmental task of this stage as previously discussed in Chapter 4 is described by Erikson as ego integrity vs. despair. The mentally healthy elderly individual accepts the inevitability of death, and feels satisfied with the uniqueness and achievements of his life.

The elderly exhibit a number of characteristic behaviors while confronting the tasks of aging. The nurse caring for the elderly in any setting can offer assistance and enhance this process by recognizing the normal tasks and facilitating their resolution. The following are experiences and behaviors of the elderly frequently encountered by the nurse, with suggestions for possible interventions.

Life review

Life review is the process of thinking about the meaning of one's life. Most authorities believe that life review is a nearly universal occurrence as older persons face the prospect of impending death. On the one hand, life review facilitates achieving closure to one's life. On the other hand, it leads to personal growth by bringing unresolved crises to consciousness, allowing them to be talked about at length in such a way as to facilitate their resolution.

The life review process involves almost obsessive reminiscence—remembering the significant events, people, and places in the past that helped to shape and provide meaning to the individual's life. When an individual is engaged in life review, he finds this to be an all-engrossing task. Small wonder that he has little interest in the events of the present, while the events of the past are recalled and recounted in minute detail.

Because it is likely that all elderly people reminisce whether alone or with another person, it is vital that the nurse facilitate this process as a means of providing interpersonal feedback. Furthermore, planning for nursing intervention will become more individualized to the needs of the client if the life review process is used both as an aspect of assessment and as a means for intervention. At the very least, the nurse giving care to an elderly person must allow time to actively listen to his reminiscences and provide appropriate feedback.

Loneliness

More than any other group, aged persons often experience loneliness. Moustakos observes:

Elderly citizens in our society are particularly affected by the social and cultural changes and by the separation, urbanization, alienation, and automation in modern living. There is no longer a place for old age, no feeling of organic belonging, no reverence or respect or regard for the wisdom and talent of the ancient. Our elderly citizens so often have feelings of uselessness, so often experience life as utterly futile. Old age is fertile soil for loneliness and the fear of a lonely old age far outweighs the fear of death in the thinking of many people. Loss of friends and death of contemporaries are realities. The mourning and deep sense of loss are inevitable, but the resounding and lasting depression which results and the emptiness and hopelessness are all a measure of the basic loneliness and anxiety of our time.*

To combat the loneliness of the elderly, nurses need to reach out consistently to the older person. Five minutes daily for 5 days is a louder message of concern and caring than is 20 to 30 minutes once in a while. Attempts to involve the older person in a relationship must be persistent. Nurses need to be aware of their own feelings of loneliness that may be triggered by the loneliness they sense in the older person. Younger nurses in late adolescence often experience profound loneliness as they seek their own identity and thus often want to move away from others who are experiencing loneliness. Therefore the withdrawal of the older person may evoke a mutual feeling of withdrawal in the nurse. The nurse must be conscious of her own feelings and aware of her needs when she is tempted to withdraw from the older person.

Loss and grief

When a major interpersonal loss occurs, physical changes that the individual had not been previously aware of are often brought to awareness and perceived as losses. This phenomenon, in turn, intensifies the significance of the interpersonal loss. For example, it is not unusual to hear an elderly women remark, "If my husband had died 10 years ago, I could have managed this house by myself, but now I'm not physically able to keep the place up."

The need to grieve for losses may not be seen as necessary by the older person, and grieving may be avoided because of the pain associated with this process. Many aged persons develop physical problems rather than grieving thereby directing their attention and the attention of others away from the loss and its attendant emotions to the somatic concerns. Consequently, the crisis of the loss is not resolved.

The older person's limited energy level and reluctance to ex-

*Moustakos, Clark: Loneliness, Englewood Cliffs, N.J., 1961, Prentice-Hall, Inc., p. 26.

perience pain and resentment allow him to deal with these feelings only in small, manageable doses. The nurse must observe for signs that the older person has had enough for now. The willingness to return again and again to the painful area both by the nurse and by the older person provides for the resolution of the crisis. One 89-year-old man who had experienced a major illness was talking about the loss of his mother when he was 7 years old. He paused and said, "There are losses that everyone expects as they go through life and those you get through. However, there are losses that you feel that, in some way, you caused or that it was your fault, and those are much harder to bear. And the worst losses are those that refresh old wounds—they bring the pain of other losses to the surface. These are very hard losses to bear."

The nurse can be most effective in helping the elderly person resolve his grief about a major interpersonal loss by:

1. Assisting the person to accept the pain of the loss by validating that it is appropriate to feel pain over losses.
2. Encouraging the expression of sorrow and sense of loss by commenting on nonverbal communication, such as a shaky voice or teary eyes.
3. Facilitating the expression of hostility by viewing it as a sign of the older person's feeling of vulnerability.
4. Facilitating the expression of guilt. When the person says, "If only I had done . . . ." it is helpful if the nurse restates this comment by saying, "I sense you blame yourself for . . . ." Only if the person is able to acknowledge that he feels guilty can the reality of the situation be explored.
5. Assisting the older person to talk about the person who has died. Asking questions about how they met and the experiences they shared is most facilitative of helping the bereaved person to relive meaningful experiences.

The process of grieving over a major interpersonal loss may take as long as 2 years in the elderly. Signs that the individual is beginning to resolve his grief in a healthy way include indications that he is beginning to see himself as separate from the deceased person. The most common indicator of this differentiation is a movement away from talking about "we" to referring to "I." In addition, the healthy resolution of grief is indicated by behaviors indicating adaptations to an environment that acknowledges the absence of the deceased person. For example, the widow who disposes of her husband's clothing to use his closet for storing her sewing materials has made a constructive environmental adaptation that acknowledges the death of her husband. Finally, the person who is successfully resolving his grief over a major loss is able to form new relationships that are mutually satisfying and rewarding.

BEHAVIOR DISTURBANCES OF THE ELDERLY

Like younger individuals, elderly persons have widely varying needs and strengths. Most elderly persons are able to lead active and productive lives, and continue to grow and learn during this developmental period. A person who has successfully completed earlier developmental tasks has a higher possibility of successfully completing the task of aging, and a helpful and supportive environment certainly contributes to its successful resolution. Nevertheless, difficulties sometimes arise. Many of the cognitive and behavioral impairments associated with the aging process actually result from a combination of physiological, social, psychological, and environmental stressors encountered by the individual within the context of a culture that does not value the elderly. Therefore it is imperative that a holistic perspective be employed when assessing the elderly person.

A small number of elderly individuals develop emotional disturbances. Some may manifest the characteristic symptoms of depression, which often go unrecognized in the elderly person. The physiological symptoms of depression—constipation, slow movements, insomnia—are expected signs of age so they tend to be ignored. Apathy and lack of interest in the environment are characteristics of depression in the aged but are stereotypically viewed by most persons as characteristic of the aging process itself.

The frequency of depression in the elderly appears to be significantly greater than in other age groups. There is a decided increase in the severity and the number of depressions in the aged and a close relationships between physical illness and depression. The aged seem better able to tolerate the loss of a loved one or of their prestige than the loss of their physical health. The nurse who helps older persons maintain and sustain an interest in controlling those factors that keep them healthy, such as diet, helps to prevent depression.

Suicide prevention is an important aspect of nursing care when working with the depressed elderly (see Chapter 14).

Nurses must be aware that some elderly, physically ill persons are unwilling to see any alternative except death. The fear of the process of dying, experiencing unremitting pain, being alone, and not being in control of their lives are frequently cited factors in the choice of suicide as means of coping. Several life-threatening methods used by older people are refusal of medication, failure to follow prescribed medical regimes, and refusal to eat or drink.

Extreme suspiciousness or outright paranoia is frequently encountered in older person, particularly in those individuals who were not trusting in their earlier years. When this personality structure is compounded by the hearing and sight losses that accompany aging, the person is likely to misinterpret others and the environment and conclude that the world and the people in it are hostile. To be sure, all persons experience instances in which they are the object of hostility or discrimination, but the suspicious elderly person overgeneralizes these isolated events so that his view of the environment becomes consistent with his preconceived ideas of persecution. The necessity for change that accompanies relocation sets a fertile stage for the onset of a paranoid reaction in the elderly. The following case illustrates such a situation.

Mrs. Daniels is a 75-year-old widow who had lived by herself in the inner city apartment she shared with her husband until his death 5 years ago. Mrs. Daniels's daughters who live in the suburbs became increasingly concerned about their mother's safety in the inner city. They prevailed on her to move and finally, after 6 months, were able to convince her that she would be better off living in a newly constructed apartment complex for senior citizens in a better section of the city. Shortly after she moved Mrs. Daniels began to suspect that people were stealing her belongings. She also began hearing voices that told her they were going to "get her" in retaliation for the way she had behaved when she was a child. Mrs. Daniels told her daughters about these experiences. The community mental health nurse was called in to assess the situation.

At times the elderly person exhibits the symptom of *confusion*, which may be related to a variety of etiological factors. Dealing creatively with aged persons who are confused is a challenge for nurses. When confusion is sudden and acute the assessment process includes determining its cause. However, confused persons are in obvious need, and often the nurse must take action before a thorough assessment can be made.

Dynamics of development

The behavior disturbances of the elderly appear to be related to a wide variety of factors. The social stressors and economic pressures encountered by those entering old age are believed to play a major role in late life disturbances.

The successful completion of earlier developmental tasks will enhance the older person's ability to progress successfully through this life stage. Factors that appear to contribute to a healthy existence for the elderly include a helpful and supportive environment, a sense of belonging, a sense of autonomy and control over one's life, the ability to communicate one's thoughts to others, a feeling that one is respected, and a sense that one is loved.

Many social factors appear to contribute to the behavior disturbances manifested by elderly individuals, some of which have been previously discussed in this chapter. The devaluation of the elderly in this culture clearly has an impact on the older person's sense of self-worth. The sense of alienation that accompanies the loss of the extended family in modern technological society leads to increased stress. A change in economic and social status often accompanies retirement, contributing further to a sense of alienation, powerlessness, and worthlessness.

The elderly person is faced with multiple losses that appear to contribute to difficulties in adjustment. There is frequently a loss of loved ones, of valued roles, and of physical health that appear to contribute to the symptoms of depression, confusion, and suspiciousness. The acceleration of loss, personal change, and social change can create an inordinate amount of stress in the elderly person.

Finally, many elderly persons manifesting behavior disturbances are suffering from physical disorders, such as brain tumors, hypothyroidism, small strokes, vitamin deficiencies, chronic alcoholism, and Alzheimer's disease.

NURSING CARE OF THE ELDERLY PERSON WITH BEHAVIOR DISTURBANCES
Nursing assessment

The nursing assessment of the elderly individual must be comprehensive and thorough, and include physiological, neurological, cognitive, behavioral, psychosocial, and environmental aspects. It is imperative that the nursing assessment be multidimensional. Nursing interventions are derived from the nursing assessment and resultant nursing diagnoses and vary widely depending on the identified cause of the disturbance.

A comprehensive physical examination includes medical, drug, and nutritional history. Pulmonary and cardiovascular functioning should be assessed. Extensive laboratory tests, such as urinalysis, complete blood count, and blood serum tests for electrolyte disturbances, are essential. A neurological assessment is done as well. Mental status is assessed in the areas of orientation, memory, abstract thinking, judgment, language and perception, and concentration. When confusion exists it is helpful to note when the individual appears most confused. For example, some persons become more confused when left alone for long periods of time or with oncoming darkness.

It is also helpful to observe the elderly person's behavior. Behaviors indicative of memory loss or forgetfulness, poor social judgment and performance abilities, changes in personality such as withdrawal or hallucinations, and lack of orientation to time, place, and person should be taken seriously. Sleeplessness, restlessness, or agitation may be noted and may be indicative of both depression and organic disease.

Finally, it is imperative that psychosocial and environmental factors be assessed. Recent loss or life change frequently precipitate behavioral disturbances. Relocation can potentially contribute to confusion or suspiciousness. An assessment of these factors includes an exploration of family and social relationships in order to determine available support systems or potential stressors.

Nursing diagnoses

The nursing diagnoses for the elderly with behavior disturbances are based on the data gathered during the assessment phase of the nursing process. Diagnostic categories approved by the Fifth National Conference on Nursing Diagnoses that may be applicable to this population include:

Social isolation related to inadequate personal resources
Potential for self-directed violence related to suicidal behavior
Fear related to sensory impairment
Disturbances in self-concept related to psychosocial factors

The nurse may formulate more specific diagnoses based on the assessment of the particular client. Examples of nursing diagnoses more specific to the previously discussed assessment data could include the following:

Confusion related to loss of spouse and living alone
Disturbances in self-concept related to loss of job

Depression related to multiple personal losses
Suspiciousness related to recent relocation and deficits in sight
  and hearing

Planning and implementing nursing care

The nursing care plan for the older person with behavior disturbances is derived from the formulated nursing diagnoses. The nurse should remember that older persons, like those in younger developmental stages, are individuals with varying strengths and needs. The care plan should reflect this recognition.

Treatment of the elderly person can be a challenge to the nurse and pose an opportunity for creativity. The nurse engaged in the care of the elderly client should be aware of the developmental tasks of this period to enhance the client's ability to successfully complete this stage. A variety of interventions can be utilized to address the needs of the older person manifesting behavior disturbances.

The nurse caring for the depressed or suicidal elderly person should be familiar with the principles outlined in Chapter 14. The therapeutic relationship will offer opportunities for the elderly person to begin to express and explore feelings, and reestablish a sense of self-worth. The individual must feel safe and secure and the environment should convey empathy and concern. In addition to intervening therapeutically on an individual basis with the elderly depressed person, group activities are often very useful in helping to alleviate depression. Although traditional group psychotherapy is rarely appropriate, remotivation groups and other quasi-social, task-oriented groups have been successfully used by nursing personnel in helping the depressed older person.

Confused persons are in obvious need of intervention. The nurse might attempt to orient the confused person by introducing herself and proceeding in the least threatening manner to elicit only the information needed to help with the immediate problem. For instance, the nurse might say, "My name is Miss Jones. You seem afraid of something on the wall, Mrs. Smith. Would you tell me what is frightening you?" Hospitalization for any reason is also a time of high risk for confusion and therefore an appropriate time for the nurse to begin preventive intervention. While all persons need to know what is going to happen to them when they are hospitalized, when aged persons are hospitalized, knowledge and support are critical to the prevention of confusion and to keeping the elderly person accessible to intervention when confusion does occur. Demands placed on elderly persons who are hospitalized should be kept to a minimum. Young technicians need to learn that x-ray films, blood tests, and other tests cannot be hurried because this creates a situation where the older client feels highly anxious, incompetent, and out of control.

As the older person loses the ability to hear all tones accurately and communication becomes a problem, there is a greater risk of his not perceiving the reality of a given situation. Neurological status should be thoroughly assessed in acute confusion and periodically assessed in chronic confusional states. Of course vital signs, electrolyte balance, and blood urea nitrogen level are baseline assessments for any person who has a sudden onset of confusion. Prevention of confusion and early intervention with individuals who are confused are cardinal principles to follow with elderly persons. Remembering that the elderly person has adaptive responses to shut others out, one should make persistent efforts to maintain contact. If possible, a calm, consistent persistence over a period of time is the best therapy, although this is not always possible. All staff members should be aware of basic strategies of care. For example, the elderly individual should be approached slowly to avoid startling him. He should be called by name at all times, and the nurse should use her name often. Elderly persons who close their eyes often are not asleep. The nurse needs to get as near as possible to keep eye contact at the person's level. Touch contact should be initiated carefully and gently, perhaps by taking the individual's hand at first. If he pulls away, attempts to establish touch contact should be made later.

Lighting should be strong without glare and natural light is preferable to artificial light. Elderly persons should have eyeglasses, hearing aids, and any other needed support appliances readily available. All unnecessary stimuli should be closed out when the nurse is trying to engage the confused elderly person in conversation. If the person is frightened, someone should stay with him. This is where a member of the family could be very helpful if this person understands what is expected and receives some positive reinforcement.

Basic reality orientation is very helpful and should be part of the therapeutic relationship from the beginning. For instance, the nurse might say, "You are in the hospital for your broken hip, and in a few minutes we're going to help you sit in a chair where you can watch the Today Show." It is important to keep the routine in the hospital as near to the home lifestyle as possible. The more the lifestyle is changed, the greater the risk of confusion. Medications, especially those for control and sedation, should be used with caution, and systematic monitoring for response to treatment should be frequent.

Whatever the elderly person is able to do alone should be encouraged and help given only to ensure success with the task. Food should be placed so that the older person can see it and smell it. The confused elderly person often needs to be told what the food is. If he is not eating well high caloric drinks offered frequently help to maintain nutrition. The nurse should encourage the family to help with nutritional problems because they may know and be able to supply some favorite foods.

Family members may be very helpful if they are taught how to deal with the individual who is confused. The family should be made aware that it is not helpful to withhold information from the aged, confused person. Sometimes family members and staff members think they are sparing the older person's feelings. In reality, the person almost always knows that something is amiss but does not know how to deal with mixed communication and thus becomes more confused, often acting bewildered. During acute confusional states individuals need to know what day it is, where and when the meals are served, where the bathroom is, and what time of day it is—morning, afternoon, or evening.

It is truly a fine thing to see a nurse model creative care of a confused elderly person. Often she must use her whole being to explore the meaning of the behavior of a confused individual and to respond in a way that is helpful and dignified to him. Modeling excellence in terms of caring for aged, confused persons is the best way to teach staff and families.

Appropriate intervention goals when working with older persons who are exhibiting unwarranted suspiciousness include reducing the individual's anxiety level by establishing a relationship with him, helping him to restructure his environment to maximize his sense of control, and minimizing his sight and hearing deficit by the use of prosthetic devices or by adapting the environment to better accommodate the sensory loss. Throughout all these interventions the consistent presence and availability of the nurse is of inestimable value in helping the aged person give up his feelings of suspiciousness.

Nursing care of the elderly manifesting disturbances in behavior can be an exciting and challenging opportunity for the nurse. It is a relatively new field, and much new and relevant research is being generated in this specialty area. Numerous opportunities are available for the nurse who chooses to care for the elderly, including the chance to relate to those individuals who have contributed much to our society and continue to have much to share.

ALZHEIMER'S DISEASE

Alzheimer's disease is a progressive and irreversible disorder affecting up to three million Americans. It is estimated that 7% of those over 65 years of age in the United States are severely disturbed by this disease. It is the fourth leading cause of death among our elderly. Although the literature on this disease has been relatively sparse, it has recently attracted increased attention and research efforts.

Alzheimer's disease is a degenerative brain disease that is devastating for victim and family alike. Its onset is insidious, and there follows a uniformly progressive deterioration. Early signs include loss of memory, difficulty with language, poor attention span, and personality changes. Later, poor judgment, confusion, agitation, incontinence, and severe personality changes are evident. Finally, the individual is no longer able to walk or to control elemental functions, and gradually sinks into coma and death.

Alzheimer's disease most commonly occurs after age 65 but may occur as early as age 40. It is a form of *dementia*, which is the term used to describe organic mental disorders marked by a deterioration of intellectual abilities, impaired memory, abstract thinking, cognition, judgment, and impulse control. When dementia occurs after age 65 and is irreversible in nature it is termed *senile dementia*. Senile dementia is said to result in a gradual and orderly development of the following symptoms:

1. Loss of memory for recent events. The happenings of today are hazy, whereas minute details of events of early life are readily recalled.
2. Increased difficulty in comprehension. Important events

are no longer significant if they do not directly affect the life of the individual.

3. Tendency to reminisce. Dwelling on the life and achievements of early years occurs, with a desire to recount them frequently.

4. Intolerance of change. An alteration in routine is likely to precipitate tension and irritability.

5. Disorientation. The year is frequently forgotten and then the day of the month, but the day of the week, which more directly dictates the routine of the individual's life, is generally retained.

6. Restlessness. There is a desire to be up and about, to travel from relative to relative, sometimes resulting in the individual's getting lost.

7. Insomnia. There is a tendency to get up in the late hours of the night or early morning and to wander aimlessly about the house.

8. Failure of judgment. An aversion to taking on new responsibilities and a tendency to withdraw into apathy and indifference occur.

Alzheimer's disease accounts for over half the cases of dementia in the elderly. The remainder of the cases appear to be related to cerebrovascular disease, thyroid disease, vitamin deficiencies, drug reactions, chronic alcoholism, and brain tumors. Thus some of the dementias manifested by elderly individuals are related to reversible causes and can be treated. It must be remembered, as well, that many of the above symptoms occur as a result of emotional and social stressors, and are not indicative of dementia, a disease process that must be etiologically related to a specific organic factor. To view these symptoms in isolation from the cultural context in which they occur is to artificially separate emotional problems from the stressors that are likely to cause their development. To separate emotional problems from social problems is a mistake with any age group, but to do so with the aged is to completely misunderstand the process of aging in our society.

Dynamics of development

Senile dementia was once blamed on impaired blood circulation to the brain, and was felt to be an inevitable consequence of aging. Today it is known that Alzheimer's disease accounts for over half the reported cases. The causes of Alzheimer's disease are unknown. However increased research is beginning to provide some important clues. Biopsy of the brain tissue reveals neurofibrillary tangles and neuritic plaques. In addition, recent research reveals that victims of Alzheimer's have reduced levels of acetylcholine, possibly related to a loss of neurons in the basal ganglia.

It is felt that genetics may play a role in Alzheimer's disease. Children of victims have a 50% risk of developing the disorder. Although the causes of Alzheimer's disease remain unclear, it appears that there may be several related causes. There is a current commitment to research efforts in this area in both the public and private sectors.

NURSING CARE OF THE INDIVIDUAL WITH ALZHEIMER'S DISEASE
Nursing assessment

The nursing assessment of the individual with Alzheimer's disease incorporates many of the principles outlined in the previous section on behavior disturbances of the elderly. Assessment would include biological, psychological, social and environmental factors. Other disorders must be ruled out, including depression and other functional psychiatric disorders, vitamin and mineral deficiencies, electrolyte disturbances, drug intoxication, chronic alcoholism, organ-specific causes, infections, brain tumors, and reactions to stress from life events. Many of these disturbances are reversible with appropriate interventions.

The onset of Alzheimer's disease is gradual and insidious. Signs of deterioration frequently go unnoticed for some time, and are first detected by those closest to the individual. Early signs include diminished energy and withdrawal, memory impairment, language difficulties, and poor attention span. Gradually the individual may become confused and manifest poor judgment. There may be severe personality changes and the eventual appearance of disorientation, restlessness, agitation, combativeness, and paranoid ideas. Finally, there are gait disturbances, incontinence, abnormal reflexes, and seizures; the individual ultimately becomes helpless and bedridden.

The course of Alzheimer's disease from onset to death ranges from 2 to 20 years, with the usual course being 5 years. In the early stage of the illness the individual is aware of his deterioration and is likely to experience a severe depression. Both the individual and family are devastated. Families of the victims must witness the deterioration of their loved one, who gradually does

Nursing diagnosis

not recognize them and who eventually behaves like a total stranger.

The nursing diagnoses for individuals with Alzheimer's disease are based on the data collected in the assessment phase, and reflect the stage of progression of the disorder. Diagnostic categories applicable to this population that have been approved by the Fifth National Conference on Nursing Diagnoses include the following:

Alteration in thought processes related to physiological changes
Alteration in health maintenance related to cognitive impairment
Self-care deficit related to cognitive impairment
Potential for violence directed toward others related to organic brain syndrome

More specific diagnoses may be formulated by the nurse based on the assessment of the individual client with Alzheimer's disease:

Inability to perform activities of daily living related to cognitive deterioration
Impaired physical mobility related to cognitive impairment
Potential to harm self and others related to alteration in thought processes
Impaired verbal communication related to organic brain syndrome

Planning and implementing nursing care

The nursing care plan for the client with Alzheimer's disease is derived from the nursing diagnoses and the interventions address the specific needs identified. Many nursing interventions applicable to the elderly with behavior disturbances are also appropriate here. However, intervention approaches must reflect the stage of disease progression. The client who enters a long-term health care facility has usually progressed to a later stage of the disease, and cognitive impairments are likely to be severe.

The nurse attempts to improve the cognitive functioning of the individual through communication techniques and sensory stimulation. The therapeutic relationship can provide a forum for the discussion of feelings, opinions, and the facilitation of daily life decisions. In the early stages of the disease both individual and group techniques can be utilized. Group discussions can focus on stimulating topics and encourage active participation. The creative therapies are useful, including art, creative writing, and poetry. Later in the disease process more individual approaches are indicated.

Memory impairment can be impeded through the use of environmental aids and clues. One family utilized signs to remind their relative of routine tasks and safety factors. Simple lists may be of assistance, as well, in the early phase. Precautions can be taken to ensure environmental safety, such as installing gates, rearranging furniture, and removing dangerous objects.

Encouraging life review is a frequently utilized therapeutic tool. By assisting the individual to reminisce, long-term memory is stimulated and the opportunity to resolve earlier life crises is made available. The client with symptoms of the later stages of the disease is assisted by many of the interventions discussed in relation to the confused elderly person. Clear and consistent communication is utilized. The individual is approached calmly, and always addressed by name. Basic reality orientation is helpful. Interventions for sleeplessness include warm baths, soft music, warm milk, light exercise, and a small amount of wine. When the individual is agitated it is important to be aware of safety factors. At times small doses of antipsychotic agents are utilized for acute disturbed states and extreme restlessness. In such cases low doses of Navane and Haldol are recommended. Care must be taken in the administration of these medications because of the prolongation of drug elimination in the elderly.

The nurse caring for the client with Alzheimer's disease must be aware that the disease is progressive and irreversible. The individual will eventually become bedridden and helpless, and it will be necessary to meet his most basic needs. In the course of the disease process the client may become quite agitated and combative. The nurse must be prepared to intervene, and to accept these behaviors in a nonjudgmental fashion. The nurse must continue to afford the individual the respect and dignity that she would show to any client.

The families of the victims of Alzheimer's disease are in desperate need of assistance and support. Efforts should be made to maximize their strengths, allow for the expression of feelings, provide education, and mobilize social supports. The nurse can help the family to prepare for the time when the institutionalization of their loved one may be necessary. The Alzheimer's Disease and Related Disorders Association (ADRDA) is an organization with 120 chapters in the United States that has much to offer the victims of Alzheimer's disease and their families. These services include hot lines, self-help groups, and respite care programs. The nurse can educate the family about this organization and other local services.

CASE FORMULATION: a victim of Alzheimer's disease

Mr. Chall is a prominent 65-year-old attorney who was admitted to a local inpatient mental health facility for a diagnostic work-up. He had recently been experiencing memory loss that had seriously affected his professional performance, until he had felt forced to take a leave of absence. He admitted that he had been attempting to disguise these difficulties for some time, but lately had been finding these attempts more and more difficult. He described finding himself standing in the middle of a room at home having no idea why he was there or how he got there.

In addition, Mr. Chall was finding it more and more difficult to conduct conversations and found himself practicing and rehearsing. He described having to think carefully about every word he said. He reported feeling depressed and wishing to withdraw from social interactions.

Although Mr. Chall was known for his pleasant personality his wife reported recent disturbing changes. He had begun losing his temper at his wife and daughters at the slightest provocation. The family felt that they had to "walk on eggs" when he was nearby.

Mr. Chall had always been most meticulous about his personal hygiene and grooming. Recently, however, he had begun to find routine tasks more difficult. His wife noted that his grooming was often poor. At times he dressed in the same suit for a number of days in a row and his shirts and ties were spotted with food stains. Such behavior was highly unusual for such a meticulous man.

Both Mrs. Chall and his family were extremely concerned. After a thorough assessment and diagnostic work-up, he and his family were informed that he had the medical diagnosis of Alzheimer's disease. Upon learning of the diagnosis Mr. Chall became deeply disturbed and manifested further evidence of withdrawal behaviors. The family was devastated, and turned to the staff for support and assistance.

nursing assessment

Mr. Chall appeared to be experiencing many of the behaviors manifested by individuals in the early stages of Alzheimer's disease. Fading memory was evident as were attempts to mask this symptom. Mr. Chall was experiencing difficulties with language, and some trouble with the performance of the routine tasks of daily living. These symptoms were impairing his work and social life.

Personality changes were among Mr. Chall's predominant symptoms. Abrupt temper tantrums were noted by the family members, despite a previously pleasant personality. Feelings of depression and a desire to withdraw from social interactions were reported by Mr. Chall.

As a result of Mr. Chall's behaviors, the family was experiencing a very difficult time. Both Mr. Chall and his family were further devastated when the diagnosis of Alzhemier's disease was learned.

nursing diagnoses

The assessment data lead to the following nursing diagnosis:

Alteration in thought processes related to memory impairment and cognitive deterioration

Difficulties in verbal communication related to organic brain disease

Lack of attention to personal hygiene related to cognitive deterioration

Withdrawal and anger related to cognitive disease process and diminished sense of self-worth

Alteration in family process related to impairment of family member

planning and implementing nursing care for MR. CHALL

The plan of nursing care for Mr. Chall is summarized on p. 478. Interventions were based on the present behaviors. However, the progressive nature of this disorder must be kept in mind and appropriate revisions made as changes in Mr. Chall's status occur. It was decided that Mr. Chall would return home in 2 weeks, allowing time for the family to prepare to offer the needed support and assistance. Long-term plans were postponed for the present time, although the potential inevitability of placement in a long-term care facility was recognized.

A therapeutic relationship was established with Mr. Chall's primary nurse, who treated him with respect and dignity and approached him in a clear, consistent fashion on a regular basis. Mr. Chall was en-

Continued.

nursing care plan for
MR. CHALL

nursing diagnosis	objective	rationale	nursing action	outcome criteria
Alteration in thought processes related to memory impairment and cognitive deterioration	To assist the client to maintain environmental contact and interaction	Environmental contact and cognitive stimulation can slow the process of deterioration and enhance dignity and self-worth	Establish therapeutic relationship with client Interact with client in a clear, consistent manner Assist with the development of memory aides (signs, lists) Provide reality orientation and sensory stimulation Ensure client safety	Within 2 weeks the client will: List routine daily tasks Develop appropriate memory aids
Difficulties in verbal communication related to organic brain disease	To facilitate and enhance the client's ability to maintain communication with others	Verbal communication can stimulate cognitive functioning and contribute to a sense of belonging and esteem	Accept and respect client's attempts to communicate Encourage discussion of life review and present day events Encourage participation in group discussion Facilitate family discussions and interactions	Within 2 weeks the client will: Spontaneously discuss daily events with the nurse Actively participate in group discussions
Lack of attention to personal hygiene and grooming related to cognitive deterioration	To assist the client to perform tasks of bathing and dressing	Adequate hygiene and appropriate dressing will help to sustain dignity and self-worth	Establish and implement bathing and dressing routine Encourage client to perform own hygiene as able Assist with dressing as necessary	Within 2 weeks the client will: Follow the established bathing and dressing routine Accept assistance as needed
Withdrawal and anger related to cognitive disease process and diminished sense of self-worth	To encourage the client to discuss his feelings and problems	Ventilating feelings in a supportive context will assist the client to work through feelings of grief and loss	Meet regularly to allow client opportunity for ventilation Convey empathy and support Utilize reflective listening techniques to facilitate conversation Sit in silence and offer acceptance if the client does not wish to talk	Within 2 weeks the client will spontaneously discuss feelings and recent losses with the nurse

nursing care plan for
MR. CHALL—cont'd.

nursing diagnosis	objective	rationale	nursing action	outcome criteria
Alteration in family process related to the impairment of family member	To assist the family to cope with the present crisis and to prepare for and accept prognosis	Resolution of present crisis will render family more able to offer their loved one the necessary support and prevent further disequilibrium in family system	Meet with family members weekly Offer education and refer to local support services Offer support and encourage the expression of feelings Facilitate problem solving	Within 2 weeks family will be able to discuss present and future plans for the care of Mr. Chall

couraged to communicate his feelings and his interests to the nurse, who listened in a caring, supportive, and interested manner. Mr. Chall was encouraged to review his life's achievements and memories, as well as to discuss his present-day concerns and ideas. Participation in a discussion group was encouraged, where stimulating topics were explored. In addition, Mr. Chall was encouraged to participate in creative therapies, such as art and creative writing.

The nurse assisted Mr. Chall to develop memory aids, to help him to recall daily tasks and routines. He developed lists and reminders to help him structure his daily activities. It has been found that such aids are very successful in improving self-care and autonomy.

A daily routine was planned to assist Mr. Chall with bathing and hygiene. Clothes were laid out the night before, with the assistance of the nurse when necessary.

Finally, the nurse directed some of her energy toward the needs of the family who felt devastated as a result of Mr. Chall's deterioration and poor prognosis. Education was provided, as was support and assistance with crisis resolution. The family was referred to the local chapter of the Alzheimer's Disease and Related Disorders Association, an organization that could provide much support and assistance in planning for the future.

evaluation

Evaluation of the plan of nursing care and its implementation was based on the outcome criteria developed.

Mr. Chall showed some improvement while in the inpatient setting. He reported that he felt less depressed, although he continued to feel embarassed and fearful of social interactions. However, he was able to discuss the feelings related to the loss of his health, and continued his efforts to communicate with others. Mr. Chall found the memory

Continued.

aids extremely helpful as reminders for the tasks of the day, and felt more control over his actions as a result. He continued to experience changes in mood, including mild temper tantrums.

The family became involved in the local chapter of ADRDA and reported that they were receiving much assistance from this organization. Although unable to make long-term plans, they received many helpful suggestions about how to best provide for Mr. Chall's needs once he returned home. It was felt by the nursing staff that the family continued to experience denial related to Mr. Chall's prognosis, but that with the support of the services they had engaged they would eventually come to terms with the inevitability of Mr. Chall's deterioration and death. At the time of Mr. Chall's discharge, the family appeared able to receive him warmly into the home for the present. They were advised to utilize the recommended support services as they took on the physical and emotional task of caring for their loved one.

CONCLUDING STATEMENTS

1. Elderly persons have as many individual differences as do those in younger stages. In addition, there are commonalities of experience for elderly individuals in our society.
2. Social forces in our culture affect the mental health of the elderly, including the negative attitudes held toward aging.
3. Life review is a nearly universal occurrence in older persons as they face the prospect of impending death. Nurses need to facilitate this process as a means of providing interpersonal feedback.
4. More than any other group, aged persons often experience loneliness. Nurses need to be aware of their own feelings of loneliness that may be triggered by the loneliness they sense in the older person.
5. The elderly are subject to an inordinate number of losses to which they adapt in varied ways.
6. The need to grieve for losses may not be seen as necessary by the older person and may be avoided because of the pain associated with this process.

7. The nurse can be most effective in helping the elderly person resolve his grief about a major interpersonal loss by:
   a. Assisting the person to accept the pain of the loss by validating that it is appropriate to feel pain from losses.
   b. Encouraging the expression of sorrow and sense of loss by commenting on nonverbal communication, such as a shaky voice or teary eyes.
   c. Facilitating the expression of hostility by viewing it as a sign of the older person's feeling of vulnerability.
   d. Facilitating the expression of guilt.
   e. Assisting the older person to talk about the person who has died.
8. Suspiciousness or outright paranoia is frequently encountered in older persons, particularly in those who were not trusting in their earlier years.
9. Appropriate intervention goals when working with older persons who are exhibiting unwarranted suspiciousness include reducing the individual's level of anxiety, helping him to restructure his environment to maximize his sense of control, and using appropriate measures to minimize his sight and hearing deficits.
10. In addition to the nurse's intervening therapeutically on an individual basis with the elderly depressed person, group activities are also very useful in helping to alleviate depression.
11. An index of risk for precipitating confusion in elderly persons is the amount and rate of change they have experienced.
12. When aged persons are hospitalized, knowledge and support are critical to the prevention of confusion and to keeping the elderly person accessible to intervention when confusion does occur.
13. *Senile dementia* is a term used to describe the progressive, degenerative organic mental disorders of old age marked by deterioration of intellectual abilities with impairment in memory, abstract thinking, cognition, judgment, and impulse control.
14. Alzheimer's disease is an irreversible progressive and degenerative dementia that accounts for over 50% of the dementias of old age.
15. Appropriate nursing interventions for victims of Alzheimer's

disease address the cognitive deterioration, and include communication techniques and sensory and environmental intervention. In addition, the family is included in the nursing plan of care. They are offered the support and education needed to care for their loved one, to develop future plans, and to work through the grieving process.

SUGGESTED SOURCES OF ADDITIONAL INFORMATION

Classical

Bancroft, Anne Vandermay: Now she's a disposition problem, Perspect. Psychiatr. Care **9:**96-102, May-June, 1971.

Browne, Louise J.: Reality therapy for the geriatric psychiatric patient, Perspect. Psychiatr. Care **10:**135-139, July-Sept., 1972.

Burnside, Irene Mortenson: Grief work in the aged patient, Nurs. Forum **8:**416-427, 1969.

Burnside, Irene Mortenson: Group work among the aged, Nurs. Outlook **17:**68-71, June, 1969.

Burnside, Irene Mortenson: Gerontion: a case study, Perspect. Psychiatr. Care **9:**103-109, May-June, 1971.

Burnside, Irene Mortenson: Loneliness in old age, Ment. Hyg. **55:**391-397, 1971.

Burnside, Irene Mortenson: Touching is talking, Am. J. Nurs. **73:**2060-2063, 1973.

Burnside, Irene Mortenson: Listen to the aged, Am. J. Nurs. **75:**1801-1803, 1975.

Levine, Rhoda L.: Disengagement in the elderly—its causes and effects, Nurs. Outlook **17:**28-30, Oct., 1969.

Mead, Margaret: The right to die, Nurs. Outlook **16:**20-31, Oct., 1968.

Stone, Virginia: Give the older person time, Am. J. Nurs. **69:**2124-2127, 1969.

Yalom, Irvin D., and Terrazas, Florence: Group therapy for psychotic elderly patients, Am. J. Nurs. **68:**1690-1694, 1968.

Contemporary

Alfano, Genrose J.: There are no routine patients, Am. J. Nurs. **75:**1804-1807, 1975.

Botwinick, Jack: Aging and behavior: a comprehensive integration of research findings, New York, 1978, Springer Publishing Co., Inc.

Bowe, Frank: Rehabilitating America, New York, 1980, Harper & Row, Publishers.

Bozian, Marguerite W., and Clark, Helen M.: Counteracting sensory change in the elderly, Am. J. Nurs. **80:**473-478, March, 1980.

Brink, T.L.: Is TLC contraindicated for geriatric patients? Perspect. Psychiatr. Care **15:**129-131, 1977.

Britnell, J., and Mitchell, K.: Inpatient group psychotherapy for the elderly, J. Psychosoc. Nurs. Ment. Health Serv. **19:**19-24, May, 1981.

Buchanan, Dale: Psychodrama: a humanistic approach to psychiatric treatment for the elderly, Hosp. Community Psychiatry **33**(3):220-223, 1982.

Bumagin, Victoria E., and Hirn, Kathryn F.: Aging is a family affair, New York, 1980, Lippincott and Crowell.

Burnside, Irene Mortenson: Psychosocial nursing care of the aged, ed. 2, New York, 1980, McGraw-Hill Book Co.

Busse, Ewald W., and Pfeiffer, Eris, editors: Mental illness in later life, Washington, D.C., 1973, American Psychiatric Association.

Carty, Rita: Patients who cannot hear, Nurs. Forum **11**(3):290-299, 1972.

Chaisson, M., Beutler, L., Yost, E., and Allendar, J.: Treating the depressed elderly, J. Psychosoc. Nurs. Ment. Health Serv. **22**:25-30, May, 1984.

Chamberlin, Adaline B.: Providing motivation, Am. J. Nurs. **78**:80, Jan., 1978.

Cohen, Stephen, and Bunke, Sister Erica: Programmed instruction: sensory changes in the elderly, Am. J. Nurs. **81**:1851-1880, 1981.

Cumming, Elaine, and Henry, W.E.: Growing old: the process of disengagement, New York, 1979, Basic Books, Inc., Publishers.

Dresen, Sheila E.: Staying well while growing old: autonomy; a continuing developmental task, V, Am. J. Nurs. **78**:1344-1346, Aug., 1978.

Dupuis, Pamela H.: Old is beautiful, Nurs. Outlook **18**:25-27, Aug., 1970.

Ettlinger, R., Binkowski, N., and Zaiser, A.: A senior citizens' center and a geriatric transitional house at a state psychiatric hospital, Hosp. Community Psychiatry **35**:1029-1033, Oct., 1984.

Frenay, Sister Agnes Clare, and Pierce, Gloria L.: The climate of care for a geriatric patient, Am. J. Nurs. **71**:1747-1750, 1971.

Gage, Frances Boland: Suicide in the aged, Am. J. Nurs. **71**:2153-2155, 1971.

Galton, Laurence: The truth about senility—and how to avoid it, New York, 1980, Lippincott & Crowell.

Gioiella, Evelyn: Give the older person space, Am. J. Nurs. **80**:898-899, May, 1980.

Gresham, Mary L.: The infantilization of the elderly: a developing concept, Nurs. Forum **15**:195-210, 1976.

Hayter, Jean: Patients who have Alzheimer's disease, Am. J. Nurs. **74**:1460-1463, 1974.

Held, Martin, Ransohoff, Paul, and Goehner, Patricia: A comprehensive treatment program for severely impaired geriatric patients, Hosp. Community Psychiatry **35**:156-163, Feb., 1984.

Hirschfeld, Miriam J.: The cognitively impaired older adult, Am. J. Nurs. **76**:1981-1984, 1976.

Hirschfeld, Miriam: Care of the aging holocaust survivor, Am. J. Nurs. **77**:1187-1189, July, 1977.

Kalish, R.A.: Late adulthood: perspectives on human development, Monterey, Calif., 1975, Brooks-Cole Publishing Co.

King, Kathleen S.: Reminiscing psychotherapy with aging people, J. Psychosoc. Nurs. Ment. Health Serv. **20**:21-25, Feb., 1982.

Limandri, Barbara J., and Boyle, Diana W.: Instilling hope, Am. J. Nurs. **78**:78-79, Jan., 1978.

McMordie, William R., and Blom, Sharon: Life review therapy: psychotherapy for the elderly, Perspect. Psychiatr. Care **17**:162-166, July-Aug., 1979.

Moritz, Derry A.: Understanding anger, Am. J. Nurs. **78**:81-83, Jan., 1978.

Niland, Maureen: Understanding the elderly, Nurs. Forum **9**:273-289, 1972.

Putnam, P.A.: Orienting the young to the old, Nurs. Outlook **22**:519-521, 1974.

Schwab, Sister Marilyn: Caring for the aged, Am. J. Nurs. **73**:2049-2053, 1973.

Simpson, S., and Wilson, L.: Meeting the mental health needs of the aged: the role of psychiatric emergency services, Hosp. Community Psychiatry **33**:833-836, Oct., 1982.

Teusink, J. Paul, and Mahler, Susan: Helping families cope with Alzheimer's disease, Hosp. Community Psychiatry **35**:152-156, Feb., 1984.

Vander Zyle, Sharon: Psychotherapy with the elderly, J. Psychosoc. Nurs. Ment. Health Serv. **21**:25-29, Oct., 1983.

Vladeck, Bruce C.: Unloving care, New York, 1980, Basic Books, Inc., Publishers.

Whitehead, J.A.: Psychiatric disorders in old age: a handbook for the clinical team, New York, 1974, Springer Publishing Co., Inc.

Wilkiemeyer, Diana S.: Affection: key to the care for the elderly, Am. J. Nurs. **72**:2166-2168, 1972.

Of particular interest

Busse, E.W., and Pfeiffer, E.: Behavior and adaptation in late life, ed. 2, Boston, 1977, Little, Brown & Co.
Assessing mental functioning of the elderly individual is an important facet of this collection of articles on gerontology.

Butler, Robert N., and Lewis, Myrna I.: Aging and mental health: positive psychosocial approaches, ed. 2, St. Louis, 1977, The C.V. Mosby Co.
This text is an excellent resource for evaluating the biopsychosocial functioning of the elderly individual. It is especially valuable for initial assessment of the individual and for community- and institutionally-based treatment.

Hospital and Community Psychiatry: Special issue on mental health and aging, **33**:entire issue, Feb., 1982.
This entire issue addresses topics relevant to mental health and aging.

chapter twenty-one

populations
at risk

the physically ill

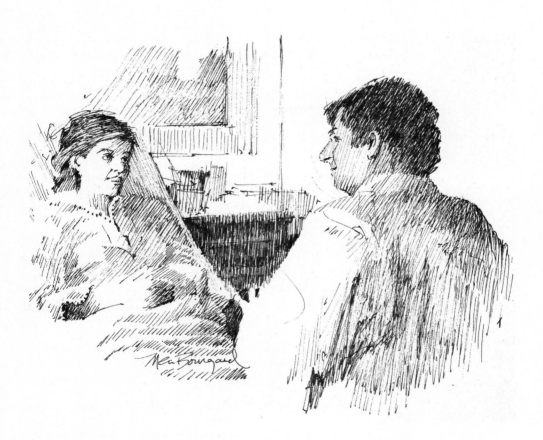

I didn't think anyone in this busy place had time to just sit and talk!

1 State some general guidelines for meeting the emotional needs of physically ill persons.

2 Describe common emotional reactions precipitated by the use of mechanical devices in the treatment of the physically ill.

3 Describe common emotional reactions precipitated by organ transplants.

4 Describe common emotional reactions precipitated by the loss of a body part.

5 Describe common emotional reactions precipitated by cardiac surgery.

6 Describe common emotional reactions precipitated by an untoward obstetrical experience.

7 Describe common emotional reactions precipitated by an abortion.

8 Discuss the emotional aspects of death and dying as described by Kübler-Ross.

It was stated earlier that sound interpersonal skills are foundational to all nursing practice. This belief implies that knowledges and skills regarding interpersonal relationships should be an integral part of the nurse's entire educational program. Nevertheless, it is apparent that all too often the emotional needs of the physically ill are given little attention and that student nurses frequently look to their psychiatric nursing experience to provide them with direction in giving more comprehensive care to the physically ill. Therefore this chapter is devoted to helping the nurse develop an understanding of some common emotional needs of the physically ill individual, although no situation in this chapter can be discussed in depth.

HISTORICAL PERSPECTIVE

Before the current advances in the medical and nursing sciences nurses could do little to assist physically ill individuals other than helping them meet their most basic physical needs. The time-honored nursing actions of bathing and feeding patients certainly must have met many of their emotional needs as well.

As medical science developed physicians delegated to nurses

procedures that they no longer had time to perform. An example of such a procedure is the assessment of vital signs. Some nurse authors believe that as an occupation nursing eagerly embraced these delegated technical procedures in an attempt to gain higher status by mimicking physicians. Whether this interpretation is true or not it is a fact that current nursing care of physically ill persons is characterized by the execution of an increasing number of highly technical procedures, often to the neglect of attempts to meet the person's emotional needs. In fact, it is not unusual for a patient to report that the most understanding person he encountered while in the hospital was an aide or cleaning lady.

Growing dissatisfaction with nursing care provided in general hospitals has been the subject of numerous studies. These studies indicate that only a few complaints are related to physical care. The large majority of dissatisfactions have to do with the failure of professional nurses to establish satisfying interpersonal relationships with individuals receiving their services. The nurse is frequently said to lack warmth, to fail to give individuals a feeling of being important human beings, to fail to listen empathically to the concerns of individuals being cared for, or to fail to ask enough questions to gather the necessary data to make wise decisions about individual needs.

Many physically ill individuals are in a state of crisis precipitated by the nature of their illness or its treatment, or both. Consequently nursing has a tremendous opportunity to promote the mental health of a large number of persons if it will reclaim its heritage of meeting the emotional needs of the physically ill.

GUIDELINES FOR MEETING THE EMOTIONAL NEEDS OF THE PHYSICALLY ILL

Physically ill individuals display a variety of feelings, which may include intense anxiety, hostility, depression, elation, fear, anger, and sorrow. These are the same feelings that may be expressed by the mentally ill. Perhaps one of the few differentiations that can be made between the reactions of these two groups is the presumed ability of the physically ill to maintain conscious control of behavior and to use better judgment than do individuals who are mentally ill. However, even these expected differences are not always observed.

It is often difficult and more challenging to recognize and cope with the emotional needs of the physically ill than it is to work effectively with the emotional needs of the mentally ill. Because part of a mentally ill individual's problem is his lack of emotional control, he sometimes expresses needs openly and directly. The emotionally ill individual's needs may be difficult to understand, but their existence is obvious. Because he is said to be mentally ill, the nurse realizes that part of the task is to help him cope with his emotional problems. In contrast, the physically ill individual usually tries to control his feelings and to solve his own problems. Nurses frequently expect this individual to cope with his own emotional problems. They sometimes fail to recognize that in addition to his need for physical care the physically ill person needs the same acceptance, understanding, and concern as does the mentally ill person.

Good physical care is always the starting place in meeting the emotional needs of physically ill persons. The nurse can demonstrate a caring attitude about the individual by an unhurried approach, attentive, perceptive listening, and anticipation of physical needs. It is also important that the nurse not respond to the client's anger with an angry response. The nurse will not be tempted to respond in an angry manner if she understands the frustration and fear that are the basis for the client's outburst. Likewise, she will not attempt to minimize the client's concerns by using hollow phrases such as, "Tomorrow will be a better day."

The very occurrence of a physical illness serious enough to warrant hospitalization interrupts the normal life-style of the individual and his family. As a result some degree of stress is produced to which the individual and his family may or may not be able to adapt successfully. In addition any physical illness for which hospitalization is necessary forces the individual to assume a dependent role that may be disturbing to him. Although society's view of masculinity and femininity is becoming less stereotyped, a dependent role is still seen as particularly problematic for men, who are often expected to portray an image of strength and independence and who may see physical illness as an expression of weakness. Inability to accept the forced dependency required in many hospitals is one reason for the uncooperative behavior of some individuals.

The modern hospital is a highly organized creation of a mechanized world. Regardless of the nature of the illness that brings the individual to the hospital, he is expected to submit to a variety of procedures without always understanding what they are or why they are being done. He often believes they are being performed without his consent or without his having been given any explanation about them. Many procedures that seem commonplace to health professionals, such as enemas, catheterizations, and intravenous injections, may be viewed by others as intrusions into their bodies. Not only may the individual have no understanding of the reasons for the procedure, he may also feel that he has lost control over his body. At the same time, he frequently is covertly given the messge by personnel that he should be thankful to them for performing these procedures. This conflict may result in an increase in his anxiety level, which, paradoxically, decreases the effectiveness of the procedure itself. Therefore it is imperative for the individual's physical and emotional well-being that the nurse provide him with an opportunity to explore his feelings about the procedure as well as giving him an appropriate explanation of its nature.

Although the individual may have signed an operative permit, he is not likely to realize that this may cover a variety of tests and procedures before the actual operation is undertaken. The physician may have explained the preoperative tests, but the anxiety level of many individuals is so high that they are unable to comprehend what the physician is saying. Even when individuals are able to concentrate on the physician's words, they do not always understand the full meaning of them, and the preoperative procedures may still come as a shocking surprise. It is not difficult to understand that a newly admitted surgical patient may be frightened and feel that he has lost his identity. Such a situation could be eased if nurses understood the importance of giving reassurance, if they could identify the basis for the anxiety, and if they were skillful in giving emotional support. Sometimes reassurance requires only a few minutes of time spent listening, answering questions, and recognizing that the individual is a unique human being reaching out for understanding and help.

Sometimes the results of hospital procedures, especially surgical procedures, precipitate an emotional crisis. Such a crisis is overwhelming for a person who has already developed the feeling that he is lost, forgotten, and reduced to a childlike state of dependence in the hospital. These feelings may actually impede his recovery and may cause him to view his hospitalization as an extremely traumatizing experience.

EMOTIONAL REACTIONS PRECIPITATED BY THE USE OF MECHANICAL DEVICES

Currently developments in biomedical science have provided several life-sustaining devices that make it possible to prolong the lives of many individuals who would be doomed to death otherwise. Among these devices are hemodialysis machines and cardiac pacemakers.

The hemodialysis machine is likely to produce a more profound emotional response from the individual than the pacemaker. The individual who must rely on such a machine recognizes how dependent he is on the device for life itself. He also becomes aware of the fact that his activities are circumscribed by his need to be attached to the machine for 8 to 10 hours, two or three times each week. This schedule interferes with his work, his ability to make a living, his social life, and his family life.

Dependency on a mechanical device to sustain life in the case of both the pacemaker and the hemodialysis machine creates anxiety in almost all individuals who are so involved. It causes many individuals to feel dehumanized and to be concerned about the maintenance of their personal autonomy. In addition the individual may be resentful and angry, or he may be depressed and respond by being tearful, disinterested in his surroundings, and uncommunicative. On the other hand, the individual may express his anger and frustration at the situation by speaking sharply to the nurses or to his family. He may express fear by demanding constant attention and that the nurse remain with him at all times. He may express his disturbed emotional feelings by being critical of the hospital or clinic where he must go for the dialysis. He may fear that the device will fail to function properly and thus end his life abruptly.

Pacemakers do not interfere with the individual's activities as much as do hemodialysis machines, but they sometimes cause great anxiety and fear because it is possible for them to stop working properly without giving adequate warning. Individuals who must rely on either of these devices realize they will never be completely well again and must look forward to a long-term reliance on mechanical assistance.

Because the hemodialysis machine must be attached to the

individual so often, a permanent arteriovenous shunt is frequently implanted in an arm or leg to provide access to an artery or vein whenever necessary. Individuals with these shunts have been known to tear them out, losing a great deal of blood. This action is usually considered a suicidal gesture: the rate of suicide among individuals who resent their dependence on hemodialysis machines is high.

Family members have been taught to operate portable dialysis machines and thus free the individual from constantly returning to a hospital or clinic to have his blood cleansed. However, this practice makes it necessary to teach a family member to operate the machine and to require that the family member be available when the treatments are scheduled. This amount of dependence on another person is also cause for hostility and resentment among some individuals and has not provided the solution to the time-consuming dialysis procedure that it was originally intended to do.

Individuals who must rely on mechanical devices often feel that they have lost control of their bodies and of their destinies. This may lead to a loss of confidence and self-esteem. Such a loss of confidence results in behavior that requires emotional support and understanding.

In summary, the currently available life-saving biomedical devices are capable of improving the physical health of the individual but do not always improve emotional health. Specifically, those individuals who must rely on hemodialysis machines are chronic worriers. They worry about all the daily problems of living that confront everyone. They require nurses who are skilled in understanding that their behavior is sometimes an expression of anger, fear, and depression brought on by their resentment of being dependent for life on a mechanical device and being unable to control the situation. They require a great deal of reassurance and emotional support.

EMOTIONAL REACTIONS PRECIPITATED BY ORGAN TRANSPLANTS

Organ transplants are viewed by medical scientists as providing a viable alternative for individuals with seriously damaged organs, especially hearts and kidneys. As increasingly effective drugs are developed to combat the problem of tissue rejection, the number of organ transplants is likely to increase.

Almost from the initiation of organ transplant surgery, it was recognized that providing an organ for an individual from the body of another could be an emotionally disturbing experience both for the person donating the organ and the recipient. Thus psychiatric evaluation of the donor as well as the recipient was begun soon after some of the earliest kidney transplants were performed. Since there were more individuals awaiting transplant surgery than there were appropriate organs available it was possible to choose the organ recipients carefully. Thus those who were thought to be able to accept an organ from another individual without being emotionally disturbed were chosen. Likewise donors should be stable individuals before agreeing to supply an organ for another. One mother who donated a kidney to a son was heard to shout at him, "What do you expect from me? Wasn't it enough that I gave you life? Do you also demand a part of my body?"

Organ transplant procedures are long and involved surgical techniques. Individuals who are the focus of such procedures are aware of their physical condition and that they are seriously ill. They realize that without a transplant their lives would end within a short time and that the only hope for the future lies in the replacement of the damaged organ. Thus they are willing to undergo the procedure even though they recognize the seriousness of the situation and the possibility that the organ may be rejected. These individuals are understandably fearful of what the future will bring. Although many of the recipients of such surgery have been able to cope successfully with their anxieties and fears a few have responded with full-blown psychiatric reactions. There are few situations in which an individual is placed under so much tension as when he undergoes an organ transplant. Nurses working with these individuals need to be sensitive to their emotional difficulties, to be realistically reassuring, and to provide as much emotional support as the individuals require. The individual should be encouraged to discuss his concerns and fears about death, dependency on others, and loss of self-esteem.

The fact that an individual who was close to death would grieve over the loss of a useless body part comes as a surprise to many nurses. Nevertheless, such is often the case and if she is to be helpful the nurse must help the individual go through the grieving process. In general, the nurse needs to express concern for the individual and interest in his future welfare.

EMOTIONAL REACTIONS PRECIPITATED BY THE LOSS OF A BODY PART

Every person has a mental image of his own body that is called the *body image*. This body image may be realistic or it may be part of the individual's wish-fulfilling fantasy about himself. To a large extent, an individual functions within the boundaries of this unconscious image. A young man once said in a hopeless voice, "I can never marry. What woman would want a man with one short leg?" This man's body image was so misshapen and ugly that he could not accept it. Because he could not accept his own body he was convinced that no one else could. He was especially convinced that no woman could want him as a marriage partner. Although he was reasonably attractive, his reaction to all aspects of life was in keeping with this attitude of being worthless and of having an unacceptable body.

Some people maintain an unrealistic image of themselves that was realistic at an earlier period in their lives. For example, it is not uncommon to hear a large, matronly woman ask a saleswoman for a size 12 dress. Without making a comment the understanding clerk brings out the required large size and helps the customer try on the garment.

Surgical removal of a breast or the uterus are among the most emotionally disturbing surgical procedures that women must face. It is unfortunate that many nurses have not been helped to understand the meaning these experiences have for some women and have not been assisted in helping with the feelings precipitated by such surgical procedures.

Although people respond in highly individual and unique ways to the same surgical procedures, almost all women unconsciously feel that they have been mutilated by a breast amputation or the removal of the uterus. If given an opportunity after such a surgical procedure, many women will express feelings about not being a whole woman or about being of less value to the world than they were before the operation. They may express fears about losing the acceptance of their marital partners.

Many women pass through a period of mourning for the lost part of the body. Nurses need to understand the realistic reasons that underlie the frequent tears shed by women hospitalized in a gynecological unit of the hospital and should accept this as an expression of a normal emotional response about an extremely upsetting experience. Crying is probably one of the most helpful ways of expressing grief. Unfortunately, some women cannot cry about this kind of problem. Instead, they sometimes repress their feelings of despair and sadness and respond in other ways that may be more difficult for the nurse to understand and cope with. After breast surgery one woman turned her face to the wall, refused to see any visitors, and requested that even her husband be excluded from the room.

Sadness and mourning may be expressed in a reaction that appears to an observer as an outburst of anger. The individual may respond as does a child when something of value is taken away. This response may be an expression of underlying depression, but the external reaction is one of anger at having lost something that was highly valued. Another frequent response to such a surgical loss is an unconscious feeling on the part of the woman that she is being punished for some real or fantasized transgression that may have occurred years before. This feeling may lead the woman to respond as if she were unworthy of attention from friends or relatives.

The possible reasons for the many emotional reactions to breast amputation and hysterectomy are as varied as the women who require these procedures. The important thing for the nurse to remember is that these experiences are difficult for women to accept, that individuals respond to them in highly individual ways, depending on their life situation and personality, and that the nurse needs to demonstrate an understanding and caring attitude about the woman and her feelings.

Women are not the only people who are unable to accept an altered body image. All individuals who submit to disfiguring surgery of any type have a variety of fears that focus on their concern about being acceptable to other people, especially to their sexual partners. Operations involving amputation of a leg of disfiguring facial surgery are especially difficult for individuals to accept. However, it has been noted that people are able to accept body mutilation more readily when the location is such that it is evident to everyone. This phenomenon may result from the fact that something that is obvious must be recognized and talked about. Some individuals refrain from mentioning a problem that is hidden under clothing. They are therefore burdened with a tremendous amount of unresolved sensitivity for years. Perhaps the much joked about American habit of discussing one's operation and exhibiting the surgical scar at social gatherings has some psychologically healing attributes. It is therapeutic to help individuals discuss the way they feel about the surgical procedure they have experienced.

Nurses should avoid censuring individuals who blame the surgeon for their disfigured bodies. It is a natural human response to relieve anxiety by blaming someone else for an unhappy situation that the individual cannot control with his usual defenses.

One example of this kind of reaction was a man who was hospitalized for plastic reconstruction of a thumb that was lost in an accident involving high-voltage electricity. After several skin grafts and months of hospitalization, the man was disturbed when he saw the reconstructed thumb. It was many times larger than a normal thumb and was covered with short hair because the skin graft had been taken from the patient's thigh. He had expected a normal-looking thumb and had looked forward to having a functioning hand as a reward for the long period of boring hospitalization. He was bitterly disappointed and disgusted at the appearance of the thumb. He remarked to the nurse, "Look at that! It's obscene. I am going to sign myself out of this hospital and have my own doctor cut this thing off." The nurse reported this reaction to the head nurse who said, "He should be ashamed of himself for criticizing his doctor, who is the best plastic surgeon in this part of the country. The doctor has worked terribly hard on that thumb."

The individual did leave the hospital against medical advice. He was angry and disappointed. If someone had explained that the surgeon planned to shape the thumb to normal proportions after the body had established effective circulation to the new tissues, he might have been helped to wait for a few more weeks for the surgeon to complete the delicate and tedious work. Unfortunately, the nurse with whom the client had developed a positive relationship did not know enough about plastic surgery to use the opportunity to be helpful at the time when he needed reassurance. This incident highlights the importance of the nurse's possessing and using scientifically correct knowledge concerning the nature of the illness and treatment.

A colostomy is another emotionally disturbing experience for individuals. In our culture the emphasis placed on cleanliness and fastidiousness in personal hygiene creates a serious conflict for those who find it medically necessary to resort to a colostomy.

Cultural attitudes toward toileting, which are taught early in a child's life, sometimes cause the adult to rebel at the thought of caring for a colostomy. Probably no surgical procedure has the potential for presenting individuals with more emotional and social problems than does a colostomy. Although hundreds of individuals have been able to adjust successfully to colostomies, the nurse should not forget that the person who is just beginning to cope with the problems presented by the loss of normal bowel function has many hurdles ahead of him. Individuals who have undergone a colostomy worry about their acceptability to their friends and their sexual partners. Persons who have received support in working through their feelings about their colostomies report that they have been able to maintain satisfying sexual relations. Unfortunately, others find that it becomes emotionally impossible for them to do so.

It is helpful if individuals with colostomies are encouraged to express their feelings, attitudes, and questions about their condition. Individuals are not helped by nurses who insist on the light, gay approach and refuse to involve themselves in serious conversation about these problems. The person with a colostomy deserves a nurse who will give his situation thoughtful, empathic, realistic consideration.

Such procedures as colostomy operations are performed only when they are necessary to save the individual's life. The nurse cannot alter the problems that such an operation presents, but she can help the individual to talk about the problem, to accept the reality of this situation, and to learn all he can about his condition so that he can handle it as effectively as possible. The following clinical report illustrates the effect that a colostomy can have on some fastidious people.

A fastidious man who understood English poorly entered the hospital with a diagnosis of far-advanced carcinoma of the rectum. He had suffered a great deal before coming to the hospital and was grateful when surgery relieved the pain. A colostomy opening was established. His physical recovery was rapid. When he was discharged, he left many gifts for the hospital staff. In every way he appeared to be happy and grateful. The surgeon had attempted to explain the seriousness of the problem to the patient before surgery. The hospital staff believed that the man understood the nature of his operation and the need for a permanent colostomy. One week after discharge he returned to the surgical clinic and requested admission to the hospital to have the colostomy opening closed. Again the surgeon explained the nature of the operation and the permanent character of the surgery. The individual left the clinic without appearing to be upset. The next day the newspapers carried a notice of his suicide.

The problems experienced by this individual undoubtedly grew out of his language handicap and his attitude toward the importance of physical cleaniness. Although his response to the colostomy was unusual, many individuals will admit that in the beginning of their experience with a colostomy, they occasionally wondered if life was worthwhile under such circumstances. Of particular significance in this situation was the individual's lack of expression of any negative feelings. If the health care personnel truly understood and appreciated the huge emotional significance of a colostomy, they would have viewed this man's behavior as an untoward response and could have intervened in a way that might have prevented the suicide.

Surgical operations on the male genitourinary tract sometimes cause severe emotional conflicts. Occasionally such an operation precipitates a psychotic reaction. The following clinical report presents an example of such a situation.

A middle-aged gentleman who was a devoted church member was admitted to a surgical unit because of symptoms of prostatic hypertrophy. A successful operation was performed to relieve the distressing symptoms. Within 1 or 2 days he was complaining of suggestive pictures on the walls of his room, which he said the hospital authorities had placed there for the purpose of tormenting him. The nurses were confused by these complaints because no pictures were hanging in his room. A psychiatrist was called to talk with the individual who told the psychiatrist that the annoying pictures were of young nude women. The gentleman stated that a man of his principles should not be surrounded by such lewd art.

The psychiatrist concluded that the individual was not able to accept the fact that a man of his social standing would indulge in such an active fantasy life dealing with sexual material. To relieve his own anxiety about his unconscious sexual longings, which were dramatically brought to light by his complaint about the nude pictures, he unconsciously used the mechanism of projection. It was much more acceptable to him and safer from the standpoint of self-esteem to blame the hospital for hanging pictures of nude women around the room than to accept the explanation that the pictures represented his own fantasies.

This unusual reaction was undoubtedly precipitated by the surgical procedure, but it would not be accurate to say that the procedure caused the response. During most of this individual's life he probably had exerted a great deal of emotional energy to repress unacceptable sexual thoughts. The emotional crisis presented by the surgical experience was apparently enough to make it impossible for him to continue to repress his unacceptable thoughts.

EMOTIONAL REACTIONS PRECIPITATED BY CARDIAC SURGERY

Individuals respond to life-threatening situations uniquely, depending on the coping mechanisms they have developed and the attitude of personal security they maintain. In view of this, it is difficult, if not impossible to predict how a specific individual will respond to any surgical procedure, especially one that is potentially as dangerous as cardiac surgery.

No matter how well the individual appears to be anticipating the procedure, the nurse must realize that cardiac surgery is a major crisis and that the person is struggling to control feelings of anxiety and fear. He cannot avoid being concerned about the possibility of death and the separation from family and friends.

Individuals who have accepted the fact that they must undergo cardiac surgery have come to this decision after months or years of cardiac symptomatology. They may have been semi-invalids because of these symptoms, or the surgery may have been planned in the hope of preventing future invalidism. Thus the individual's fear of the outcome of the procedure is coupled with his anticipation of great improvement in his health in the immediate future.

The nurse assigned to the individual before cardiac surgery should be prepared to anticipate any number of reactions, depending on the individual's personality. He may deny the seriousness of the situation and avoid discussing it. This attitude probably suggests that he finds it difficult to bear the burden and thus copes by avoiding the topic. A different person may discuss his fears, may become tearful, and, by identifying many personal needs, may insist that the nurse stay with him. A third individual may appear to be angry and sarcastic and may be critical of the way the nurse performs the necessary nursing procedures. Each of these individuals deserves a calm, empathic nurse who is a good listener and who understands that the emotional response the individual is exhibiting is his way of coping with a situation that presents him with a personal crisis. The nurse should encourage him to express his feelings and concerns and should respond to his questions in an honest, straightforward manner without alarming him. The individual deserves to be assured that he will be cared for by a team of physicians and nurses who are knowledgeable, skillful, and deeply interested in his welfare and comfort.

After the surgical procedure the individual will be helpless and dependent for a short time. As he becomes aware of his dependence on others and on mechanical devices, he may respond in a variety of ways. He may be depressed and hopeless or angry and sarcastic. The postsurgical response is dependent to a large extent on the coping mechanisms the individual has used in the past.

Just as in the presurgery period, these patients require a quiet, calm, reassuring nurse who listens carefully to their comments and encourages them to express their anxieties and concerns. Reassurance is essential for these individuals, as is focusing on the reality of the improvement they are making.

Recent experimentation in replacing the heart with a mechanical pump has been the subject of much publicity. The emotional reactions of the recipients and their families have been scrutinized as closely as have their physical responses. To date there is little reason to believe that these persons react differently than do any others with major cardiac surgery. However, it will be important to observe how these individuals and their families cope with the stressors of their condition while living in the community.

EMOTIONAL REACTIONS PRECIPITATED BY AN UNTOWARD OBSTETRICAL EXPERIENCE

Many nurses choose to work in obstetrics because the obstetrical unit is said to be a happy place. In talking about their work, obstetrical nurses frequently emphasize the great happiness of mothers and fathers when a new baby is born. It is true that there is much happiness among new parents, but nurses should not overlook the fact a few new mothers are emotionally distressed and in great need of understanding and reassurance because they have delivered imperfect babies or their babies have failed to survive. Young mothers who deliver imperfect babies may be as troubled as mothers whose babies are stillborn.

Production of perfect babies has traditionally been thought to be one of the most important tasks performed by women. When a woman fails in this effort, she sometimes wonders about her effectiveness and her intrinsic value. Therefore mothers of imperfectly formed babies or premature infants are frequently distressed by doubts concerning their own adequacy as women and by guilt about their responsibility for the existence of the problem. It may surprise some nurses to learn that almost all mothers whose babies are born prematurely or congenitally imperfect respond with questions that reflect concern about themselves. They ask questions such as, "What did I do to cause this?" or "Why has this happened to me?" Since the cause of prematurity and many congenital imperfections is not fully understood, scientific explanations of these events often cannot be given. Even when scientific explanations are available, they do little to remove the personal sense of failure these mothers often feel.

Guilt causes people to feel uncomfortable. When a mother feels guilty about her baby's imperfections, she may reject it outright or may spend the rest of her life punishing herself for failing to give her child a perfect body. This punishment might take the form of slavishly serving the child in an attempt to make up in every possible way for the child's poor start in life. This reaction is one of the disguised forms that rejection may take.

As in many other situations, the nurse cannot alter the reality of the difficult situation but can encourage the mother to talk about her feelings. If the mother can be helped to discuss some of these feelings, she may come to feel less guilty and may be able to clear away some of the emotion about the problem so that constructive steps can be taken and solutions can be planned.

Some women who have set high achievement goals for themselves find it particularly difficult to accept an imperfect baby. The following clinical report demonstrates this point.

An English professor from a large midwestern university found that she was pregnant for the first time at the age of 40. She and her husband were moderately happy about this new development in their lives. However, they were sorry to have to give up their plans for a sabbatical leave and a trip abroad. When the baby boy was born, he had a bilateral harelip and a cleft palate. When the nurse brought the baby to the mother, she looked at him and said, "That can't possibly be my child," The nurse assured the mother that it was her little boy. She said to the nurse, "Don't bring that baby in here again. I won't have a baby that looks like that!" In 5 days the mother left the hospital without asking to see her baby again. The father arranged for a nurse to help him take his son to a distant city where he had an appointment with a famous surgeon who specialized in repairing harelips. Within a few weeks the mother began to experience overwhelming feelings of anxiety and guilt for which she saw no cause. These feelings became so intense that she sought professional help. Through psychotherapy this mother eventually was able to understand the highly personalized meaning that the birth of her imperfect baby had for her.

EMOTIONAL REACTIONS PRECIPITATED BY AN ABORTION

Few situations in a woman's life have such a potential for producing a variety of emotional responses as does abortion. The response on the part of the woman involved is a highly individual one dependent on many factors. Some of these factors include her religious beliefs and cultural background. Some religious groups are explicit in their teaching against abortion, whereas others are more inclined to leave such a decision to the woman and her physician. Some cultures emphasize the relationship between a woman's intrinsic value to society and her ability to produce children; others place more importance on the quality of life that can be provided for the mother and child. Another factor is the woman's relationship with the father. If the relationship is a stable one and the man agrees that abortion is a wise decision, the reaction of the woman may be less emotionally distressing than if he wishes her to maintain the pregnancy. If the pregnancy is unwanted because of the circumstances surrounding conception (such as rape) or if by genetic counseling techniques the fetus has been identified as being seriously defective, the opportunity for abortion may be greeted with relief.

Some individuals may be convinced that they have discarded the early religious instructions that they received and the attitudes taught within the family about such controversial questions as abortion. However, these attitudes are difficult to discard and may greatly influence the woman's emotional response even though they are not recognized consciously.

Many women are able to accept an abortion without experiencing any untoward emotional reaction. However, it is not uncommon for certain individuals to express feelings of serious personal loss, deep regret, shame, guilt, a loss of self-esteem, and sadness. Such individuals may have difficulty in sleeping, experience a loss of appetite, exhibit a lack of interest in their home and work, express resentment toward the man involved, and cry frequently.

Unless the nurse visits in the home or works with women in a clinic situation there is little opportunity to be helpful to these individuals since abortion is usually a procedure that is completed within an 8- or 10-hour period and usually does not require overnight hospitalization.

If opportunities are available, it is helpful to encourage the woman to discuss her feelings and how she perceives the situation. In certain individuals an abortion may precipitate a crisis. In this case the person should be treated as any other individual who is overwhelmed by a problem of daily living.

Women anticipating an abortion should have an opportunity to think the situation through with the help of a nurse therapist. Because abortion is irreversible, alternatives should be thoroughly explored before a choice is made.

EMOTIONAL ASPECTS OF DEATH AND DYING

No discussion of the emotional needs of the physically ill would be complete without addressing the needs of the individual who is dying. With the development of complex medical technology the ability to prolong life has increased. This ability has raised questions about the quality of life and in the opinion of some has contributed to the unconsciously held belief that death occurs only as a result of the failure of the individual or the health care team to "try hard enough."

It is important for all health care personnel to understand that death is an inevitability and that dying persons have a right to be treated humanely. The specter of a dying person surrounded by machines and technicians so that the family cannot even reach him is frightening. The opposite often occurs as well, namely, that the terminally ill person is figuratively abandoned. Individuals in this situation are often relegated to rooms farthest away from the nurse's station, receive only cursory attention from medical and nursing staff, and may have few visitors.

The nurse must be concerned about remedying both of these extreme situations. Nursing, more than any other health care profession, has the opportunity and the obligation to assist the dying person and his family to achieve a satisfactory resolution of this last phase of life. To fulfill this responsibility the nurse needs to develop an understanding of the emotional needs of the terminally ill person.

Dr. Elisabeth Kübler-Ross, a pioneer in thanatology, has studied the responses of hundreds of terminally ill persons. Her subjects included persons of all ages, socioeconomic levels, and cultural backgrounds. These persons also represented a wide variety of illnesses and injuries, both acute and chronic. Regardless of their differences, Dr. Kübler-Ross found that all dying persons progress through a similar process of emotional response. Her formulation, which is probably familiar to most nurses, delineates five stages of dying.

Denial is the initial response caused by the person not being able to deal emotionally with the reality of his impending death. To deal with the intense anxiety that this news engenders, the person uses the ego defense of denial. As a result, persons in this stage often express the belief that a mistake has been made in laboratory reports or that the physician is incompetent. As with any person who is using the defense of denial, the nurse will be most helpful if she understands that this defense is operative because the individual has sustained a massive emotional assault that he cannot handle directly without endangering the integrity of his personality. Consequently, the wise nurse intervenes in a manner that allows the individual to maintain this defense while simultaneously not avoiding the reality of the situation. For example, the nurse would not encourage a person who is in this stage of the dying process to make plans for his funeral but she would encourage him to take his medications as they were prescribed. Because the reality of the situation is such that the individual soon becomes sicker, the length of this stage is relatively short in individuals who are mentally healthy. It should be noted that illnesses that initially do not have symptoms that cause incapacitation, such as chronic lymphocytic leukemia, may enable even mentally healthy persons to cling to the denial of the fact that they are dying.

Anger characterizes the second stage of the dying process. During this stage individuals often feel as if they are victims of fate, circumstances, medical incompetence, or a vengeful God. Their thoughts and verbalizations center around the question of, "Why me?" They fear the dependency their illness creates and often resent their family and the health care workers who try to be of help. Since feeling and expressing anger are not acceptable to many people, some dying persons may express their anger in covert, rather than overt ways. Most nurses recognize the anger and underlying anxiety in terminally ill individuals who complain about everything and everyone. Only the sensitive, insightful nurse recognizes the same dynamics in the individual who expresses his anger in passive ways, such as "forgetting" to take his medication and then asking the nurse what he should do.

Bargaining is the third stage of the dying process characterized by the individual attempting to gain more time by trading off "good" behavior. Most commonly, the dying individual bargains with supernatural powers—God, fate, or whatever higher Being he believes can effect a change in his condition. Bargaining takes the form of, "If you (let me live until Christmas) then I (will bequeath half of my money to the church)." The behavior that the person "trades off" is highly individualized and is probably related to earlier unresolved conflicts. The bargaining stage is helpful to the dying person in that it temporarily eases his anxiety and enables him to deal with the pain and dependence that may accompany his illness.

The *depression* stage follows bargaining. Depression begins when the reality of the situation can no longer be ignored and the uselessness of denial, anger, and bargaining is apparent. The depression that the individual feels is a response to an overwhelming sense of anticipated loss—the loss of his entire world. At this stage the dying person looks and acts depressed and often has no need to talk with others about how he feels. He must use his energy to confront the fact that what is done is done, and what is undone will remain so. Because he is depressed, the person in this stage of dying makes few demands. Consequently his behavior is often misinterpreted as "cooperative."

Acceptance is the final stage of the dying process when the individual has come to peace with himself about the fact that his death is imminent. Acceptance is characterized by an affective void; the person is not happy, nor is he depressed. His interests, even in his own care, narrow. During this time only those persons who are most significant to him are able to elicit a positive response. The presence of others is merely tolerated. This does not mean, however, that the dying person cannot receive comfort from the nursing interventions of a warm, caring nurse. It does mean that the most effective interventions are likely to be nonverbal in the form of physical comfort measures delivered in a competent, compassionate way.

Understanding the emotional needs of the dying person is of value to the nurse only if she is able to combine this knowledge with self-awareness. Since death and dying are not viewed by our culture as natural phenomena, nurses, like most people, have been taught since early childhood to avoid the subject. This cultural attitude may be compounded by the nurse's own developmental stage. The developmental stages of adulthood and middle age are the stages most nurses are in and may prove to be particularly problematic in regard to the issues of death and dying. The stage of adulthood, especially early adulthood, is a time when people view all things as being possible. As a result, the nurse in this stage may be prone to view the terminally ill person as representative of the failure of the health care team. The nurse who is dealing with the developmental tasks of middle age may be actively dealing with the awareness of her own mortality reinforced by the declining health of her parents. The terminally ill person may represent the nurse's vulnerability to the prospect of her own death.

In either instance, the nurse may feel anxious and guilt ridden and avoid dealing with her feelings by avoiding the patient. During those times when the nurse cannot avoid the person, she avoids the reality of the situation by assuming a false air of cheerfulness, by changing the subject when the person or his family start to talk about death, or by not answering the client's questions. Other nurses may respond angrily to the dying person, as if his dying were his fault. This counterproductive response seems especially justifiable to the nurse when the dying person's poor health habits, such as smoking, have obviously contributed to his terminal illness. Only if the nurse can be helped to explore and confront her own feelings about the dying process will she be able to give the skilled, compassionate care the dying person deserves.

SELF-HELP GROUPS

The nurse should make an effort to become aware of the increasing number of community-based organizations designed to provide information and support to individuals and their families who have experienced certain medical or surgical procedures or the death of a family member. For example, there are Ostomy Clubs throughout the country whose members are people who have had ileostomies or colostomies and who meet regularly to discuss with each other the ways in which they have solved the problems they encounter. In some parts of the country similar groups are available for persons who have undergone mastectomies, laryngectomies, abortions, or myocardial infarcts. By being aware of the availability of these organizations in the community the nurse will be able to inform others of them. Although these clubs are not designed to substitute for medical supervision, the value of the support and understanding that can be gained from persons who have had similar experiences is inestimable in helping individuals and families to regain or attain a state of positive mental health.

CONCLUDING STATEMENTS

1. The large majority of complaints made by individuals concerning their hospital care have to do with the failure of professional nurses to establish satisfying interpersonal relationships with them.
2. Good physical care is always the place to start in meeting the emotional needs of physically ill persons.
3. Any physical illness that requires hospitalization forces the individual to assume a dependent role that may be disturbing and may cause him to react with what is sometimes called uncooperative behavior.
4. People who are newly admitted to general hospitals may feel frightened and may develop a sense of having lost their identity.
5. Individuals who must rely on mechanical devices, such as hemodialysis machines and pacemakers, often feel that they have lost control of their bodies and of their destinies.
6. Providing an organ for an individual from the body of another can be an emotionally disturbing experience, both for the person donating the organ and for the recipient. There are few situations in which an individual is placed under so much tension as when he undergoes an organ transplant.

7. Every individual has a mental picture of his body, which is called the body image and which may be realistic or part of the individual's wish-fulfilling fantasy about himself.

8. Surgical removal of a breast or the uterus are among the most emotionally disturbing surgical procedures a woman may be called on to accept.

9. Although people respond in highly individual and unique ways to the same surgical procedures, almost all women unconsciously feel they have been mutilated by amputation of a breast or the removal of the uterus.

10. All individuals who submit to disfiguring surgery of any type have a variety of fears that focus on their concern about being acceptable to other people, especially their sexual partners.

11. In this culture the emphasis placed on cleanliness and fastidiousness in personal hygiene creates a serious emotional conflict for individuals who find it medically necessary to resort to a colostomy.

12. The nurse is being therapeutic when she helps individuals to talk about the way they feel regarding the surgical procedure that they have experienced.

13. Mothers of imperfectly formed or premature babies may be distressed by doubts concerning their own adequacy as women or by guilt concerning their own responsibility for the existence of the problem.

14. As in many other situations, the nurse cannot alter the reality of the difficult situation for the new mother with an imperfect baby but can encourage her to talk about her feelings and help to lessen her guilt. This may make it possible for the new mother to view the problem realistically and to plan solutions.

15. It is important for all health care personnel to understand that death is an inevitability and that dying persons have a right to be treated in a humane manner.

16. Dr. Elisabeth Kübler-Ross has delineated five stages in the dying process: denial, anger, bargaining, depression, and acceptance.

17. Understanding the emotional needs of the dying person is of value to the nurse only if she is able to combine this knowledge with self-awareness.

18. The value of the support and understanding that can be gained from participation in self-help groups is inestimable in helping individuals and families regain or attain a state of positive mental health.

SUGGESTED SOURCES OF ADDITIONAL INFORMATION

Classical

Francis, Gloria M.: Cancer: the emotional component, Am. J. Nurs. **69:**1677-1681, 1969.

Kübler-Ross, Elisabeth: On death and dying, New York, 1969, Macmillan Publishing Co., Inc.

Larsen, Virginia A.: What hospitalization means to patients, Am. J. Nurs. **61:**44-47, May, 1961.

Martin, Harry W., and Prange, Arthur J.: The stages of illness—psychosocial approach, Nurs. Outlook **4:**168-171, March 1962.

Mead, Margaret: Understanding cultural patterns, Nurs. Outlook **4:**260-262, May, 1956.

Quint, Jeanne C.: The impact of mastectomy, Am. J. Nurs. **63:**89-92, Nov., 1963.

Van Bree, Nancee S.: Sexuality, nursing practice, and the person with cardiac disease, Nurs. Forum **14:**397-411, 1975.

Velazquez, Janet M.: Alienation, Am. J. Nurs. **69:**301-304, 1969.

Contemporary

Aadalen, Sharon Price, and Stroebel-Kahn, Florence: Coping with quadriplegia, Am. J. Nurs. **81:**1471-1478, 1981.

Billings, Carolyn: Emotional first aid, Am. J. Nurs. **80:**2006-2009, 1980.

Blackwell, B., Galbraith, J., and Dahl, David: Chronic pain management, Hosp. Community Psychiatry **35**(10):999-1008, 1984.

Brigman, C., Dickey, C., and Zegeer, L.: The agitated aggressive patient, Am. J. Nurs. **83:**1408-1412, 1983.

Brolin, Rose Homan, and Auld, Margaret E.: Hodgkin's disease, Am. J. Nurs. **74:**1982-1986, 1974.

Bowlby, John: Loss, New York, 1980, Basic Books, Inc., Publishers.

Boyle, Mary A., and Cinca, Rudy L.: Amyotrophic lateral sclerosis, Am. J. Nurs. **76:**66-68, 1976.

Bragg, T.L.: Psychological response to myocardial infarction, Nurs. Forum **14:**383-395, 1975.

Breu, Christine, and Dracup, Kathleen: Helping the spouses of critically ill patients, Am. J. Nurs. **78:**50-53, Jan., 1978.

Burgess, Helen A., et al.: When a patient on lithium is pregnant, Am. J. Nurs. **79:**1989-1990, Nov., 1979.

Cantor, Robert C.: And a time to live, New York, 1980, Harper & Row, Publishers.

Copp, Laurel Archer: The spectrum of suffering, Am. J. Nurs. **74:**491-495, 1974.

Covelli, Pat: Borrowing time, Philadelphia, 1980, J.P. Lippincott Co.

Cressy, Mary K.: Psychiatric nursing intervention with a colostomy patient, Perspect. Psychiatr. Care **10:**69-71, April-June, 1972.

Dafflitti, Judith Gregorie, and Swanson, Donna: Group sessions for the wives of home-hemodialysis patients, Am. J. Nurs. **75:**633-635, 1975.

Davidson, Shirlee and Noyes, Russell: Psychiatric nursing consultation on a burn unit, Am. J. Nurs. **73:**1715-1718, 1973.

Davis, Marcella Z.: Socioemotional component of coronary care, Am. J. Nurs. **72:**705-709, 1972.

Ellis, Rosemary: Unusual sensory and thought disturbances after cardiac surgery, Am. J. Nurs. **72:**2021-2025, 1972.

Featherstone, Helen: A difference in the family, New York, 1980, Basic Books, Inc., Publishers.

Finesilver, Cynthia: Reducing stress in patients having cardiac catheterization, Am. J. Nurs. **80:**1805-1807, 1980.

Foster, Sue, and Andreoli, Kathleen: Behavior following acute myocardial infarction, Am. J. Nurs. **70:**2344-2348, 1970.

Francone, Carol A.: My battle against Wilson's disease, Am. J. Nurs. **76:**247-249, 1976.

Garfield, Charles A.: Stress and survival: the emotional realities of life-threatening illness, St. Louis, 1979, The C.V. Mosby Co.

Gluck, Miriam Mandsager: Group therapy in a pain management program, J. Psychosoc. Nurs. Ment. Health Serv. **18:**21-25, Nov., 1980.

Grace, Mary Jo: The psychiatric nurse specialist and medical surgical patients, Am. J. Nurs. **74:**481-483, 1974.

Hagin, Joan M.: Infant death: nursing interaction and intervention with grieving families, Nurs. Forum **13:**371-385, 1974.

Heusinkveld, Karen Billars: Cues to communication with the terminal cancer patient, Nurs. Forum **11:**103-113, 1972.

Howard, Marianne, and Corbo-Pelaia, Sally: Psychological after-effects of halo traction, Am. J. Nurs. **82:**1838-1843, 1982.

Jansson, Diane P.: Student consultation: a liaison psychiatric experience for nursing students, Perspect. Psychiatr. Care **17:**77-82, March-April, 1979.

Lambert, Vickie A., and Lambert, Clinton E.: The impact of physical illness and related mental health concepts, Englewood Cliffs, N.J., 1979, Prentice-Hall, Inc.

Lerner, Gerda: A death of one's own, New York, 1980, Harper & Row, Publishers.

Levinger, Gloria: Working through recovery after mastectomy, Am. J. Nurs. **80:**1118-1120, 1980.

Lindenmuth, J., Breu, C., and Maloaley, J.: Sensory overload, Am. J. Nurs. **80:**1456-1458, 1980.

Lopez, Kay, and Seastrunk, Jay: Temporal lobe epilepsy: a new entity in psychiatry, J. Psychosoc. Nurs. Ment. Health Serv. **18:**10-15, 1980.

Loxley, Alice Keating: The emotional toll of crippling deformity, Am. J. Nurs. **75:**1839-1840, 1972.

Lucas, Mary Jane, and Folstein, Marshal: Nursing assessment of mental disorders on a general medical unit, J. Psychosoc. Nurs. Ment. Health Serv. **18:**31-33, May, 1980.

McLachlan, Eileen: Recognizing pain, Am. J. Nurs. **74:**496-497, 1974.

Marszalek, Ellen Jean, and Solomen, Janet S.: A breast counseling service, Am. J. Nurs. **81:**1658-1659, 1981.

Neu, Carlos: Coping with newly diagnosed blindness, Am. J. Nurs. **75:**2161-2163, 1975.

Nobel, Mary Ann: Communication in the ICU: therapeutic or disturbing, Nurs. Outlook **27:**195-198, March, 1979.

Norman, S. and Brown, T.: Seizure disorders, Am. J. Nurs. **81:**984-994, 1981.

Perron, Denise M.: Deprived of sound, Am. J. Nurs. **74:**1057-1059, 1974.

Pisarcik, Gail, et al.: Psychiatric nurses in the emergency room, Am. J. Nurs. **79:**1264-1266, July, 1979.

Reix, Laura: Managing a life with chronic disease, Am. J. Nurs. **73:**261-264, 1973.

Richardson, Karolee: Right brain-left brain: the nurse consultant and behavior change following stroke, J. Psychosoc. Nurs. Ment. Health Serv. **20:**37-39, May, 1982.

Rowan, A. James: Diagnosis and treatment of epilepsy, Hosp. Community Psychiatry **34:**540-547, 1983.

Schneider, Judith Simpson: Hopelessness and helplessness, J. Psychosoc. Nurs. Ment. Health Serv. **18:**12-21, March, 1980.

Santopietro, Mary-Charles S.: Meeting the emotional needs of hemodialysis patients and their spouses, Am. J. Nurs. **75:**629-632, 1975.

Schneidman, Edwin: Voices of death, New York, 1980, Harper & Row, Publishers.

Severin, Nelda K., and Becker, Robert E.: Nurses as psychiatric consultants in a general hospital and emergency room, Community Ment. Health J. **10:**261-267, Fall, 1974.

Smith, Dorothy: Survival of illness: implications for nursing, New York, 1981, Springer Publishing Co., Inc.

Stewart, Rege S.: Psychiatric issues in renal dialysis and transplantation, Hosp. Community Psychiatry **34**(7):623-628, 1983.

Streltzer, Jon: Psychiatric aspects of oncology: a review of recent research, Hosp. Community Psychiatry **34**(8):716-724, 1983.

Tatelbaum, Judy: The courage to grieve, New York, 1980, Lippincott & Crowell.

Trusley, Martha: The use of family therapy in terminal illness and death, J. Psychosoc. Nurs. Ment. Health Serv. **20:**17-22, Jan., 1982.

Tucker, Catherine: Complex partial seizures, Am. J. Nurs. **81;**997-1000, 1981.

Weinstein, Leslie J., Chapman, Mary M., and Stallings, Mary A.: Organizing approaches to psychiatric nursing consultation, Perspect. Psychiatr. Care **17:**66-71, March-April, 1979.

Whitman, Helen M., and Lukes, Shelby J.: Behavior modification for terminally ill patients, Am. J. Nurs. **75:**98-101, 1975.

Williams, Margaret A.: Cultural patterning of the feminine role—a factor in the response to hysterectomy, Nurs. Forum **12:**379-387, 1973.

Zahourek, Rothyln, and Jensen, Joseph S.: Grieving and loss of the newborn, Am. J. Nurs. **73:**838-839, 1973.

Zahourek, Rothlyn: Hypnosis in nursing practice—emphasis on the "problem patient" who has pain—part 1, J. Psychosoc. Nurs. Ment. Health Serv. **20:**13-17, March, 1982.

Zahourek, Rothlyn: Hypnosis in nursing practice—emphasis on the "problem patient" who has pain—part 2, J. Psychosoc. Nurs. Ment. Health Serv. **20:**21-24, April, 1982.

Of particular interest

Kübler-Ross, Elisabeth: Questions and answers on death and dying, New York, 1974, Macmillan Publishing Co., Inc.
This is a classic book about the process of death and dying. It contains the author's formulation of the stages of the dying process. It is essential reading for all students of nursing.

Simenon, Georges: The bells of bicetre, New York, 1965, The New American Library Inc.
This book is recommended for every student and every member of the therapeutic team. It is concerned with the experiences and reactions of a patient hospitalized after a cerebrovascular accident.

section V

interventions in psychiatric nursing

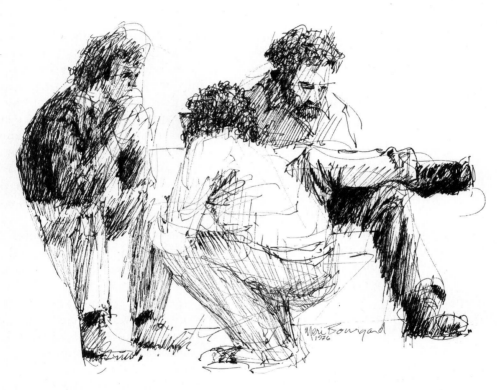

What is it about getting on a bus
that frightens you?

1 Define the term crisis.

2 Differentiate between developmental and situational crises.

3 Discuss the characteristics of a crisis state.

4 Discuss the sequential phases of a crisis state.

5 State the goal of crisis intervention.

6 Discuss in sequence the steps of crisis intervention.

Crisis intervention is a subject of interest to all health professionals. It is a technique that is used successfully by persons with a variety of backgrounds to aid individuals and families in understanding and effectively coping with the intense emotions that characterize a crisis. Once the client is able to deal with his emotions, he often is able to make appropriate decisions regarding behavior that may be required for resolution of the problems that surround the crisis. Although the responsibility for crisis intervention does not fall into the province of any one health care discipline, a discussion of it is included in this text because nurses are often in the position to engage in this technique or to counsel other health care workers in its use. Furthermore, nurses who work with the mentally ill are expected to have particular expertise in the understanding and management of emotional problems and are often looked to by their colleagues as consultants in crisis states.

HISTORICAL PERSPECTIVE

As is true of many other contemporary innovations in American psychiatry, crisis theory and intervention had their foundation in the experiences of the military during World War II. During that war there were more psychiatric casualties than physical, even after an attempt had been made to screen out those persons with a history of mental illness. Many of the seeming casualties, however, were precipitated by the soldier's experiences in combat. Some of these soldiers were treated close to the front, primarily because of a shortage of personnel and the inaccessibility of other treatment settings. Much to the surprise of all, those who received immediate, reality oriented, supportive intervention and were returned to combat as soon as possible fared better emotionally than did their counterparts who were evacuated to treatment centers and treated with psychoanalytically oriented interventions.

After the war the techniques used so successfully were applied with equal success to civilians who were victims of diasters. Perhaps the most famous of these was the fire in 1942 at the Cocoanut Grove, a nightclub in Boston. The emotional reactions of the survivors of this diaster were studied in depth over a period of years by Eric Lindemann. His findings about the symptoms and management of acute grief remain the classical work in the field.

Despite its use earlier, crisis intervention did not become a recognized treatment modality until the 1960s. During that time Gerald Caplan made numerous contributions to the literature on the subject and was instrumental in developing a theory to explain the manifestations of a crisis in essentially healthy people as well as postulating intervention techniques. Since that time numerous others from all health care disciplines have contributed to the growing body of knowledge about the subject.

DEFINITION OF CRISIS

The term *crisis* is often used by lay persons to describe a situation or a feeling state. It is not unusual to hear an individual say about an event, "It was a crisis." If in fact the event referred to was a turning point in a situation, the use of the term is correct according to the dictionary definition of the word. When referring to a feeling state, persons often report that they are in a crisis when they are very upset. Almost always this is an incorrect use of the word according to its technical definition.

Mental health authorities define a crisis as *a state of disequilibrium resulting from the interaction of an event with the individual's or family's coping mechanisms, which are inadequate to meet the demands of the situation, combined with the individual's or family's perception of the meaning of the event.* Therefore a crisis refers to an interactional process among these three variables that is reflected in the feeling state of the individual or family. Although anxiety usually underlies the feeling state, the individual may feel depression, anger, fear, or any other of a wide range of emotions. However, it is not the emotion that is unique to a crisis, nor is it the event. Rather, it is the meaning of the event to the individual or family and their inability to cope with it that produces the crisis. Therefore not every person who is anxious, depressed, angry, or fearful is in a crisis, nor does a traumatic event necessarily produce a crisis in those whom it affects.

Health professionals are greatly interested in crisis intervention for a number of reasons. First, more people are voluntarily seeking mental health care for problems that are not necessarily indicative of long-standing dysfunction. In the past, because of the social stigma associated with mental illness, mental health counsel was sought only if the person was severely disturbed and exhibiting bizarre symptoms such as hallucinations or delusions. Although there is still more stigma associated with mental illness than with physical illness, society is gradually becoming more accepting of the value of mental health treatment so a larger number of people voluntarily seek help for less severe problems. These problems are often individual or familial crises.

Second, as professionals have gained more experience in dealing with persons in a crisis, they have realized that former unresolved crises often emerge to consciousness in conjunction with the present crisis. Therefore intervention can be directed toward both the present and past situations, providing a unique opportunity to help the client resolve long-standing problems in a relatively short period of time.

Finally, crisis intervention is of great interest to mental health professionals because it provides a specific opportunity to prevent mental illness and to promote mental health. Prevention of mental illness is achieved by helping the client to use already established coping mechanisms that he has successfully used in the past or by assisting him in developing new, healthy defenses. If this can be achieved the necessity for the client to resort to pathological defense mechanisms, even mental illness, can be avoided.

Promotion of mental health through crisis intervention has been documented by researchers who have engaged in follow-up studies of individuals and families who have experienced crises. It has been demonstrated that there are three possible outcomes of a crisis state: (1) the client may reintegrate at a lower or less healthy level of functioning than the one prior to the crisis, (2) the client may reintegrate at the same level of functioning as previously, probably as a result of completely repressing the crisis situation and its attendant emotions, or (3) the client may reintegrate at a higher, healthier level of functioning than the level prior to the crisis experience. This last possible outcome was a startling realization at the time it was first described because the goal had always been prevention of mental illness. The idea that people could actually grow and benefit from an emotionally traumatic experience opened vast potential for increasing the level of mental health in a large population. In fact some authorities see a crisis as a catalyst that disturbs old habits, evokes new responses, and becomes a major factor in charting new developments. Therefore the challenge that a crisis provokes may bring forth new coping mechanisms that serve to strengthen the individual's adaptive capacity and thereby, in general, to raise his level of mental health.*

Research studies have further documented that, although any one of the three outcomes can occur with or without skilled intervention, resolution of the crisis resulting in a lower level of functioning or the same level of functioning is more likely to occur without intervention, and resolution of the crisis resulting in a higher level of functioning is more likely to occur with intervention. Consequently, to promote mental health as well as to prevent mental illness, an increasing number of communities have established crisis intervention centers. These centers may take the form of mental health emergency rooms, suicide prevention clinics, family guidance clinics, or telephone crisis services. Whatever the name, these centers are always staffed by personnel skilled in crisis intervention.

TYPES OF CRISES

Two types of events may precipitate a crisis state: developmental and situational events. It should be understood, however, that very few events inevitably produce a crisis state in all persons. If the reader reviews the definition of crisis, it will be clear that the nature of the event is only one factor in the production of a crisis. In addition to the event, the other two necessary factors are the personalized meaning of the event to the individual and family, and the nature and extent of their coping mechanisms. These must interact in such a way as to produce a state of

*Rapaport, Lydia: The state of crisis: some theoretical considerations. In Pared, Howard J., editor: Crisis intervention: selected readings, New York; 1965, Family Service Association of America.

disequilibrium. For example, a hysterectomy may be well received by a 50-year-old unmarried career woman who sublimates her maternal needs through the children of friends and relatives and whose emotional energy is directed toward her profession. Another 50-year-old woman experiencing the same surgical procedure may be plunged into a state of crisis because her identity unconsciously has been formed around her role as mother and homemaker, and the hysterectomy marks the end of her childbearing years, thus threatening her sense of self. To take this example one step further, the same career woman may enter a state of disequilibrium or crisis if she loses her job or retires, whereas the homemaker might respond to a loss of her outside job with an inner sense of relief.

Nevertheless, two types of events have been described that are likely to precipitate a crisis state in many individuals and families. The first event is the *transition period between developmental phases.*

Developmental crises are well documented. The reader will remember that each stage of development has its own developmental task, the achievement of which requires the individual to emphasize certain behaviors and to minimize others. Consequently, the family as a unit is called on to adjust and adapt to the changes experienced by each of its members. Although these changes in individuals are most pronounced during infancy and early childhood, they occur throughout the entire life cycle. Therefore any family unit is likely to have members who represent at least two different developmental stages. Many families have members who may be experiencing one of five or six different developmental stages, each stage having its own needs and manifestations. When this is the case, it is common to find family disequilibrium occurring because behaviors that meet the needs of one or more of its members may be in direct opposition to the needs of other members. An increasingly common example of such a situation is the phenomenon of adult children who return to the home of their parents to live after having been away for a few years. This phenomenon is occurring more often today, related in part to problems in the society at large. A scarcity of jobs and economic inflation make it difficult if not impossible for some young adults to become economically independent. Nevertheless the young adult is developmentally ready to work on establishing his independence but is in a position of dependence on his parents. On the other hand, his parents are developmentally ready to address their generativity needs by engaging in civic-type activities, not by nurturing a family. It does not take much imagination to appreciate the nature and extent of the family disequilibrium that may result from this situation.

Developmental crises are characterized by their predictability. For example, behavioral scientists know that a young married couple will have new demands placed on them when their first child is born. No matter how eagerly they may anticipate this event, many young parents react with depression and frustration when the dependency needs of the infant cause them to alter their previous spontaneous life-style. During midlife this couple may go through an anxiety-laden period when they question the value of the direction they have taken in their marriage, family, and work. Finally, the same couple might become depressed and frustrated once again when they find that their long-anticipated freedom from responsibility for childrearing is limited by the financial and physical limitations of old age. Although the transition from one developmental phase to another is always fraught with a certain degree of increased individual and familial tension, these transitional periods can be prevented from becoming crises through the use of anticipatory guidance.

Anticipatory guidance is primarily an educative process that helps prepare the individual and family for behavioral changes likely to occur in the near future. This process has been greatly aided by the proliferation of information about behavior during each developmental phase now available in newspapers, magazines, and paperback books. Therefore many families successfully engage in their own anticipatory guidance without requiring the assistance of health care professionals.

Public health nurses are in a unique position to provide anticipatory guidance. As they visit families in their homes, they have the opportunity to assess the entire family situation, even though they might be present to give care to only one member. For example, the nurse might counsel the mother of a 2-year-old in regard to the meaning of his negativistic behavior while visiting the home to administer a parenteral diuretic to the grandmother. The opportunities for anticipatory guidance by nurses are not limited to home visits. The nurse is in a position to assess the family dynamics when a member is hospitalized for a physical illness and visitors seek out the nurse to covertly ask advice about their problems rather than those of the patient. The astute nurse will recognize these clues and respond in a helpful way.

The second type of event that may combine with other factors to produce a state of crisis is called *situational*. By definition most situational crises cannot be as accurately predicted as can developmental crises. Situational events that can precipitate a state of crisis include such major catastrophes as the unexpected death of a family member due to accident, the loss of a home through fire or flood, and sudden widespread economic depression as occurred in the 1930s. The event does not have to be as catastrophic as these to precipitate a state of crisis. Any event, no matter how minor or even how desirable it may superficially appear, may combine with the individual's or family's perception of it to produce a situation that is felt to be *hazardous* to the equilibrium of the system. If the event is perceived as hazardous, and the individual or family does not have adequate coping mechanisms available to ward off such a threat, a state of crisis will ensue. Although most people would understand why a family might enter into a state of crisis after their home was burned in a fire that killed their infant daughter, few lay people would understand why a family might enter a state of crisis after the father receives a major promotion to the position for which he has been striving for many years. In this example, the promotion might represent a threat to a satisfying life-style, a change in social class and social group, and increased responsibility for all family members. Therefore although the family would undoubtedly gain many things they desire and have worked for, to do so they must give up the familiarity of the life they have known, and they may not have immediately available the coping mechanisms necessary to make a smooth adjustment.

Whether the type of event that precipitated the crisis is developmental or situational the characteristics of the crisis state remain essentially the same.

CHARACTERISTICS OF A CRISIS STATE

A crisis state is not seen as an illness but rather as an upset in the steady state of the system. The behaviors engaged in by those experiencing the crisis sequentially express feelings of being overwhelmed and an inability to cope, followed by attempts to cope, that may or may not be successful. Massive amounts of *free-floating anxiety* underlie these behaviors. The anxiety may be perceived as such, or it may take the form of depression or anger at various points in the crisis state. Since great amounts of anxiety cannot be sustained by the human being without serious damage to the personality organization the individual consciously and unconsciously actively seeks to reorganize his personality in such a way that he rids himself of this unbearable emotion. Therefore *a state of crisis is self-limiting*, usually from 4 to 6 weeks in length. It is almost always resolved in this time frame, although not always in the healthiest way. If new more adequate coping mechanisms are not developed within this time period, the individual is likely to repress the events and emotions surrounding the crisis to avoid further personality disorganization, which would result from prolonged maintenance of a high level of anxiety. Thus a pseudoresolution to the state of crisis is achieved.

As previously discussed, a crisis state seems to be a response to an event, whether developmental or situational, that is perceived as hazardous. Consequently, a crisis state is highly individualized, and an event that may precipitate a crisis in one individual or family may not necessarily have the same effect on another individual or family. Hazardous events are further categorized into three groups: (1) those that represent a *threat* to fundamental instinctual needs or to the person's sense of integrity, (2) those that represent a real or perceived *loss*, and (3) those that represent a *challenge*.

Another characteristic of the crisis state is that *it rarely affects an individual without also affecting those significant others who comprise the individual's social support system*. In most instances, this system is the family group. Therefore it is usually inappropriate to view an individual as being in a state of crisis without also taking into consideration the fact that it is highly likely that the family is also in a state of crisis. This point has numerous implications for intervention. Obviously any resolution to the crisis achieved by an individual in isolation from his previously established social system may be short-lived if it is not workable within the system as a whole.

Because of the mobility of the population in this country and the subsequent demise of the large, extended family, many persons have developed support systems that are not limited to and in fact may not include, family members. Therefore it is important to recognize that friends and neighbors may serve as significant others to an individual even though these persons may not be relatives in the traditional sense. This social pattern is increasingly seen in older persons whose spouses have died and whose married children live at a great distance. In all instances, the individual being counseled should be the one who defines his significant social system, not the mental health worker who may be misled into making assumptions based on traditional societal patterns.

PHASES OF A CRISIS STATE

Whether it be an individual or a family that is in a state of crisis, the crisis seems to run through a series of definable, although overlapping, phases.

The initial phase is that of *denial*, which usually lasts for a period of hours. Denial is a defense mechanism that the mind unconsciously employs to protect itself from the sudden assault of intense anxiety. Denial is evident in the situation where a 55-year-old executive calmly returns to his usual business activities after being informed by the corporate president that he has been fired. In most mentally healthy persons, the reality of the situation quickly becomes apparent and leads into the next phase of crisis, which is characterized by increased tension.

During the phase of *increased tension*, the persons involved make valiant efforts to continue their activities of daily living but do so while attempting to cope with ever-increasing amounts of anxiety. During this phase, therefore, the individual or family remains functional although those who know them can easily see indications of increased tension in the form of hyperactivity or psychomotor retardation. A common example of this phase is seen in persons who are successfully making funeral arrangements for a loved one who has just died unexpectedly. The phase of increased tension is followed by disorganization.

During the phase of *disorganization*, those in a crisis seem to "fall apart." They can no longer continue with activities of daily living, become obsessively preoccupied with the event, and may remember earlier events they thought they had forgotten and that, unbeknownst to them, have a symbolic link to the current situation. It is during this phase that the person in a state of crisis is consciously flooded by a great deal of anxiety and fears that he may be "losing his mind." The fact that he is in a state of crisis may or may not be apparent to him. If it is not, as is often the case, it is usual for the person to become highly anxious about his anxiety, thereby compounding the problem. Therefore it is during this phase that most persons seek professional help, if this has not been done previously.

The next phase of a crisis is characterized by *attempts to reorganize*. With or without assistance, the individual or family attempts to bring previously used coping mechanisms to bear on the current situation. At this point the mechanisms used are likely to be short-range in nature and directed specifically at the immediate problem. For example, the homemaker who has not been able to mobilize sufficient energy to do the dishes for the last 3 days may wheel the portable television into the kitchen in an attempt to divert her mind sufficiently to get through the increasingly large stack of dirty dishes. The mechanism the woman in this example is using is suppression. If attempts at reorganization are successful at this point, they tend to build on one another and lead to general reorganization, the ultimate goal of crisis resolution. The affected persons gradually resume their normal activities of daily living, becoming anxious and depressed only when specific stimuli are present to remind them of the crisis situation. The attempt at reorganization lasts for weeks, if successful.

A phase characterized by an *attempt to escape the problem* occurs within a matter of days if initial attempts to reorganize are unsuccessful. Without appropriate intervention, it is during this phase that blaming commonly occurs. The persons involved tend to "escape the problem" by projecting responsibility for its existence onto other people, societal institutions, or a supernatural phenomenon such as God or fate. Blaming behaviors, at the very least, create increased tension in a system already overwhelmed by stress, and at worst lead to actions that ultimately compound rather than relieve the problem. For example, the husband who blames his wife's lack of supervision for their son's juvenile delinquency may initiate divorce proceedings only to find himself totally alone and still highly anxious a year later when the divorce becomes final. A couple who blames the rigid narrow-mindedness of the community in which they live for their failure to be accepted into the local country club may decide to move to a distant state only to find that they have left behind their primary support system in the form of coworkers. A highly religious person in this phase of crisis may officially leave his church as a means of publicly rejecting the God whom he blames for his problems. In so doing, he may also cut himself off from the human social system whose support he has used in the past and could benefit from now.

Regardless of whether the persons involved in the crisis resort to blaming behaviors or whether they attempt to escape the problem by consciously pretending it does not exist (as opposed to denial, which is an unconscious defense mechanism), this phase rarely results in a successful resolution to the crisis.

After failing at attempts to escape the problem, the individual or family moves into the phase of *local reorganization*. This phase has characteristics similar to the phase, attempts to reorganize, previously described.

After the local reorganization phase, the final phase of *general reorganization* occurs. It may take up to a year before new patterns of behavior are sufficiently well integrated into the individual's personality organization or the family's interactional structure and communication system to withstand additional stress on the system. However, the acute phase of the crisis is usually over within the 6-week time period previously mentioned.

Unsuccessful resolution of a crisis state occurs when during any phase, the individual or family adopts pathological means of adaptation, which serve to obscure and compound the crisis. This is most likely to occur when the ego strength of the individual is already weakened or when the family has been using dysfunctional adaptations prior to the crisis. The outlook is particulary dim when skilled intervention is not sought or available and the persons involved resume functioning on a level lower than the one at which they had previously been functioning.

Pseudoresolution occurs when the crisis is repressed and the individual or family have learned nothing from the experience, returning to their former level of functioning. Although all may appear well, these people have missed a valuable opportunity to increase their repertoire of adaptive responses. Furthermore, future crises are likely to be compounded by the reemergence of the conflicts, surrounding the previously unresolved repressed one. See Fig. 22-1 for a schematic representation of the processes leading to successful, unsuccessful, or pseudoresolution of a crisis state.

TECHNIQUES OF CRISIS INTERVENTION

The goal of crisis intervention is to assist the individual to seek new and useful adaptive mechanisms within the context of his social support system. By so doing, the mental health worker aids involved persons to reorganize their individual personalities and their social system on a higher level of functioning than that which they had previously experienced. If this goal is achieved, these persons are better able to deal successfully with future developmental and situational events that inevitably will occur within their lifetimes.

It is important to note that many people who are in a state of crisis are not aware of this fact. They may come to, or telephone,

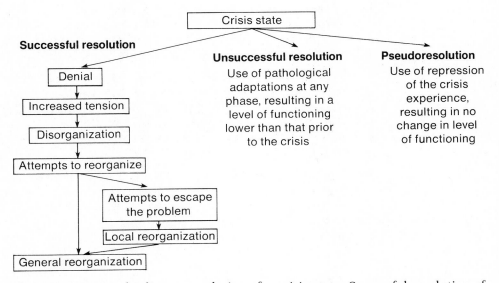

Fig. 22-1. Processes leading to resolution of a crisis state. Successful resolution of such a state follows a series of phases before culminating in the ultimate goal of general reorganization. The initial four phases are experienced by all persons. Some persons may then move directly from attempts to reorganize to general reorganization. Others may need to take a temporary detour and attempt to escape the problem. When this attempt fails, they proceed to local reorganization, eventually reaching the goal of general reorganization. Successful resolution results in functioning at a level higher than that before the crisis.

a crisis intervention center with vague, diffuse complaints such as, "I can't sleep," "I'm afraid I'm losing my mind," or "I'm afraid that something dreadful is going to happen." On the other hand, friends or relatives may bring a person for treatment, stating that he is "not behaving like himself."

The initial step in intervention is to take the time to thoroughly assess the situation. Direct questions are appropriate, since the individual or family is likely to be in the phase of disorganization during which it is very difficult for them to focus their thoughts and feelings. In addition to collecting identifying data, it is important to ask specifically who else is involved in the problem. Rosenbaum and Beebe* describe this step as the identification of the protagonists.

The next step is to define the event. It is not unusual for the persons involved to initially state that nothing unusual has occurred. If they respond in this way, it is not because they are lying, but rather because they are truly unaware of the significance of the event in their lives. To elicit this information, it is helpful to ask the person to review in detail what has occurred in his life over the past 2 weeks. If this account indicates nothing unusual, even with specific questioning, the interviewer asks the clients to go back 1 week further. Rarely is it necessary to go back further than 4 weeks. In the course of the narrative, the precipitating event will probably become clear to the interviewer and sometimes to the client as well. If the client is still unaware of the hazardous event, the interviewer can repeat back the situation the client has identified from the narrative and suggest that many people would find this situation troublesome. This intervention almost always elicits a surprised emotional response on the part of the client. The following is an example:

Mrs. Curry received a regularly scheduled monthly visit from the public health nurse. Instead of finding her in the kitchen cleaning up after breakfast as was usually the case, the nurse found Mrs. Curry sitting on the living room couch, still in her nightgown and robe, crying and wringing her hands. The nurse sat down next to her and asked what was wrong. Mrs. Curry replied, "I don't know. I don't know. I just feel

*Rosenbaum, C. Peter, and Beebe, John E., III: Psychiatric treatment, New York, 1975, McGraw-Hill Book Co.

awful—as if something horrible is happening to me. Please help me." The nurse then asked if something unusual had happened since her last visit. Mrs. Curry replied, "No, nothing except I am going crazy." The nurse asked Mrs. Curry to tell her what the days had been like for her starting with 2 weeks ago. Although Mrs. Curry protested mildly at having to go through the last 2 weeks in such detail, she complied with gentle questioning from the nurse. The nurse was not surprised to hear that Mrs. Curry's mother-in-law had moved into the home 6 days ago. After 1 or 2 days of settling-in activities, the mother-in-law requested to cook the meals "for my son" so that she would feel useful. Mrs. Curry stated that she felt resentful about turning over the meal preparation to her husband's mother but in turn felt guilty about her reaction, since she would now have more free time. As a result, she dismissed her feelings as "unreasonable," agreed to her mother-in-law's request, and made arrangements to go clothes shopping with a friend late the following afternoon. When the following afternoon arrived, Mrs. Curry could not meet her friend because she was immobilized by anxiety, the source of which was unknown to her. Since that time she had been relatively sleepless and decreasingly involved in the household activities. The above narrative was related by Mrs. Curry in a matter-of-fact way and with no particular emotion until the nurse said, "Many people find that when a new member of the family moves in, there is a major adjustment to make. I wonder if that's what could be troubling you?" At that point, Mrs. Curry began to sob but stopped wringing her hands.

Once the protagonists and the event had been identified the involved persons are helped to develop a plan for coping with the crisis situation. To be effective in this step, the mental health worker needs to explore with the clients the resources that are available and known to them as well as to suggest resources available in the community about which they might not know. Most mentally healthy people have numerous interpersonal, social, and community resources available to them but may need help to identify the appropriate ones to use and to accept aid from. For clients to benefit from this step they need to be encouraged to make as many arrangements for help as possible by themselves. However, the wise mental health worker realizes that high levels of anxiety often interfere with cognitive comprehension and retention of information, so information is best written out. For example, if it is decided that the clients could benefit from a talk with a representative of a social service agency, the name and telephone number of the agency and a suggested day and time for the clients to call for an appointment should be clearly written out.

These steps in crisis intervention are designed to help the clients achieve a correct cognitive perception of the situation, which is enhanced by the worker's seeking the facts surrounding the situation and by her helping the clients to keep the problem in their consciousness.

Another vital aspect of crisis intervention is assisting the clients in managing their feelings. To achieve this goal, the clients need to develop an awareness of their feelings. Appropriate verbalization of them, assisted by the reflection of the mental health worker, leads to desensitization and mastery of the feelings that seem overwhelming. In helping clients deal with their feelings, it is important not to give them false reassurance, although it is helpful to tell them that they are likely to feel better in 1 or 2 months despite the fact that it may seem impossible at this point. As previously stated it is also important not to encourage them to blame others. If the worker falls into this trap, the result is to support the clients' natural avoidance of looking at their own behavior, thereby decreasing their opportunities to develop more mature patterns of coping.

All these steps are usually gone through in the initial contact with persons in a crisis. Obviously such an interview may take longer than the traditional 50-minute therapy hour. Since the best results in crisis situations seem to be achieved through intensive but short-term intervention, it is advisable to spend as much time as is necessary, as often as is necessary, with the clients without engendering unwarranted dependency. At the end of the first visit the mental health worker will make a specific appointment to see the clients again, preferably in a few days but no longer than a week later. In the meantime the clients should know how they can contact the worker and should be encouraged to do so if they feel it is necessary. Often the knowledge that help is readily available is sufficient to enable the clients to manage without a telephone call until the next appointment.

During subsequent contacts the clients are assisted to go through the same steps all over again. In addition, the plan that was made in the previous session needs to be evaluated in terms of its effectiveness. If it seems to be working, it should be reinforced by supporting the clients' efforts at implementation. If the plan is not working or if new factors have altered the situation, the plan needs to be revised accordingly, but always with the mutual agreement of those involved.

In summary, crisis intervention is designed to help essentially healthy persons who are in a state of disequilibrium to help themselves. This goal is facilitated by assisting them to achieve correct cognitive perception of the situation and to gain effective management of their emotions. Successful resolution of crisis situations results in the clients' developing a larger repertoire of adaptive mechanisms, which in turn enables them to function on a level higher than the level on which they were functioning prior to the crisis state. In this way, effective crisis intervention prevents mental illness and promotes mental health.

CONCLUDING STATEMENTS

1. Crisis is defined by mental health authorities as *a state of disequilibrium resulting from the interaction of an event with the individual's or family's coping mechanisms, which are inadequate to meet the demands of the situation, combined with the individual's or family's perception of the meaning of the event.*
2. Interest in crisis intervention is great because more people are seeking mental health care, because of the realization that formerly unresolved crises emerge and can be treated in conjunction with the present crisis, and because crisis intervention provides a specific opportunity to promote mental health and prevent mental illness.
3. Three possible outcomes of a crisis state are: (a) the client may reintegrate at a lower or less healthy level of functioning, (b) the client may reintegrate at the same level of functioning as previously, or (c) the client may reintegrate at a higher, healthier level of functioning. This last possible outcome has great potential for increasing the level of mental health in a large population and is most likely to occur with intervention.
4. Events that are likely to precipitate crises are developmental or situational.
5. Developmental crises can be prevented through the use of anticipatory guidance, which is primarily an educative process that helps prepare the individual and family for behavioral changes that are likely to occur in the near future.

6. A crisis state is not seen as an illness, but rather as an upset in the steady state of the system, which is characterized by massive amounts of free-floating anxiety.

7. A state of crisis is self-limiting, usually from 4 to 6 weeks' duration.

8. A crisis state seems to be a response to an event that is perceived as hazardous. Hazardous events may represent a threat, a loss, or a challenge.

9. A crisis state rarely affects an individual without also affecting those significant others who comprise the individual's social support system.

10. Successful resolution of a crisis state follows a series of phases before culminating in the ultimate goal of general reorganization. The initial four phases of denial, increased tension, disorganization, and attempts to reorganize are experienced by all persons. Some persons may then move directly to general reorganization. Others may need to take a temporary detour and attempt to escape the problem. When this attempt fails they proceed to local reorganization, eventually reaching the goal of general reorganization.

11. Unsuccessful resolution of a crisis state occurs when pathological adaptations are used at any phase of the crisis state. Unsuccessful resolution is manifested when the person is functioning at a level lower than that prior to the crisis.

12. Pseudoresolution of a crisis state occurs when the crisis experience is repressed and leads to no change in the level of functioning.

13. The goal of crisis intervention is to assist the individual to seek new and useful adaptive mechanisms within the context of his social support system.

14. The initial step in intervention is to thoroughly assess the situation, identifying the protagonists and the event.

15. Once the protagonists and the event have been identified a plan for coping with the crisis situation is developed. To be effective, this plan must include awareness of available resources.

16. It is important to help the client to achieve a correct cognitive perception of the situation and to assist him in managing his feelings.

17. When engaging in crisis intervention, the mental health

worker is well advised to spend as much time as is necessary, as often as is necessary, with the clients without engendering unwarranted dependency.

18. The plan for coping with the crisis situation should be continuously evaluated as to its effectiveness and relevance.

19. Successful resolution of crisis situations results in the clients' developing a larger repertoire of adaptive mechanisms, which in turn enables them to function on a level higher than the level on which they were functioning prior to the crisis state.

SUGGESTED SOURCES OF ADDITIONAL INFORMATION

Classical

Coles, Robert: Children of crisis (all volumes), Boston, 1967, 1970, Little, Brown & Co.

DeYoung, Carol D.: Nursing's contribution in family crisis treatment, Nurs. Outlook **16**:60-62, Feb., 1968.

Joint Commission on Mental Health of Children: Crisis in child mental health: challenge for the 1970's, New York, 1970, Harper & Row, Publishers.

Parad, Howard J., editor: Crisis intervention: selected readings, New York, 1965, Family Service Association of America.

Contemporary

Berliner, Beverly S.: Nursing a patient in crisis, Am. J. Nurs. **70**:2154-2157, 1970.

Burgess, Ann Wolbert, and Holmstrom, Lynda Lytle: The rape victim in the emergency ward, Am. J. Nurs. **73**:1741-1745, 1973.

Carter, A.B.: Rural emergency psychiatric services, Am. J. Nurs. **73**:868-869, 1973.

Chesler, Phyllis: With child, New York, 1980, Harper & Row, Publishers.

Ching, J., Gordon, R., and O'Mahoney, M.: Crisis intervention following severe psychological trauma in late pregnancy, Hosp. Community Psychiatry **32**:53-56, Jan., 1981.

Donner, Gail, J.: Parenthood as a crisis, Perspect. Psychiatr. Care **10**:84-87, April-June, 1972.

Eisler, Richard M., and Hersen, Michel: Behavioral techniques in family-oriented crisis intervention, Arch. Gen. Psychiatry **28**:111-116, 1973.

Flomenhaft, Kalman, and Langsley, Donald G.: After crisis, Ment. Hyg. **55**:473-477, 1971.

Gallese, Lucille, and Treuting, Edna: Help for the rape victims through group therapy, J. Psychosoc. Nurs. Ment. Health Serv. **19**:20-21, Aug., 1981.

Gaston, Susan: Death and midlife crisis, J. Psychosoc. Nurs. Ment. Health Serv. **18**:31-35, Jan., 1980.

Germain, Carol: Sheltering abused women: a nursing perspective, J. Psychosoc. Nurs. Ment. Health Serv. **22:**24-31, Sept., 1984.

Greany, Geraldine: Is she a battered woman? A guide for emergency response, Am. J. Nurs. **84:**724-727, 1984.

Grier, Anne M., and Aldrich, C. Knight: The growth of a crisis intervention unit under the direction of a clinical specialist in psychiatric nursing, Perspect. Psychiatr. Care **10:**73-83, April-June, 1972.

Grollman, Earl A.: When your loved one is dying, Boston, 1980, Beacon Press.

Hall, Joanne E., and Weaver, Barbara R., editors: Nursing of families in crisis, Philadelphia, 1974, J.B. Lippincott Co.

Hargreaves, Anne: Coping with disasters, Am. J. Nurs. **80:**683-684, 1980.

Harrison, D.F.: Nurses and disasters, J. Psychosoc. Nurs. Ment. Health Serv. **19:**34-36, Dec., 1981.

Hatch, Christine, and Schut, Lydia: Description of a crisis-oriented psychiatric home visiting service, J. Psychosoc. Nurs. Ment. Health Serv. **18:**31-35, April, 1980.

Hauser, Marilyn J.: Bereavement outcome for widows, J. Psychosoc. Nurs. Ment. Health Serv. **21:**22-31, Sept., 1983.

Hurwitz, Arlene: Child abuse: a program for intervention, Downstate Medical Center, College of Nursing, Brooklyn, N.Y., Nurs. Outlook **25:**575-577, Sept., 1977.

Huppenbauer, Sandra: PTSD: a portrait of the problem, Am. J. Nurs. **82;**1699-1703, Nov., 1982.

King, Joan M.: The initial interview: basis for assessment in crisis intervention, Perspect. Psychiatr. Care **9:**247-256, Nov.-Dec., 1971.

Kuenzi, Sandra Hicks, and Fenton, Mary V.: Crisis intervention in acute areas, Am. J. Nurs. **75:**830-834, 1975.

Lieb, Julian, Lipsitch, Ian I., and Slaby, Edmund Andrew: The crisis team, a handbook for the mental health professional, New York, 1973, Harper & Row, Publishers.

McGill, Michael E.: The 40 to 60 year old male, New York, 1980, Simon & Schuster, Inc.

Marszalek, Ellen Jean, and Solomen, Janet S.: A breast counseling service, Am. J. Nurs. **81:**1658-1659, 1981.

Mims, Fern, and Chang, Audrey: Unwanted sexual experiences of young women, J. Psychosoc. Nurs. Ment. Health Serv. **22:**6-14, June, 1984.

Murphy, Shirley: After Mount St. Helens: disaster stress research, J. Psychosoc. Nurs. Ment. Health Serv. **22:**8-18, July, 1984.

Norman, Elizabeth: PTSD: the victims who survived, Am. J. Nurs. **82:**1696-1698, 1982.

Pisarcik, Gail, et al.: Psychiatric nurses in the emergency room, Am. J. Nurs. **79:**1264-1266, 1979.

Reese, Mary Ellen: Moving on, New York, 1980, Peter H. Wyden/Publisher.

Rueveni, Uri: Networking families in crisis, New York, 1979, Human Sciences Press.

Salerno, Elizabeth Meehan: A family in crisis, Am. J. Nurs. **73:**100-103, 1973.

Sheehy, Gail: Passages: predictable crises of adult life, New York, 1976, E.P. Dutton & Co., Inc.

Tatelbaum, Judy: The courage to grieve, New York, 1980, Lippincott & Crowell.

Toth, Susan, and Toth, Andre: Empathic intervention with the widow, Am. J. Nurs. **80:**1652-1654, 1980.

Twiname, Gayle: No-suicide contract for nurses, J. Psychosoc. Nurs. Ment. Health Serv. **19:**11-12, July, 1981.

Walker, Paula, and Brook, Bryan: Community homes as an alternative for youth in crisis, J. Psychosoc. Nurs. Ment. Health Serv. **19:**17-19, March, 1981.

Wise, Doreen James: Crisis intervention before cardiac surgery, Am. J. Nurs. **75:**1316-1318, 1975.

Of particular interest

Aguilera, Donna C., and Messick, Janice M.: Crisis intervention, theory and methodology, ed. 4, St. Louis, 1981, The C.V. Mosby Co.
This book is one of the most concise, comprehensive texts available in crisis intervention theory and practice. It is clearly organized and meaningful to the practitioner.

Mitchell, C.E.: Identifying the hazard: the key to crisis intervention, Am. J. Nurs. **77:**1194, 1977.
In this article the author underlines the importance of identifying a precipitant in the state of crisis. Included are assessment criteria and intervention strategies.

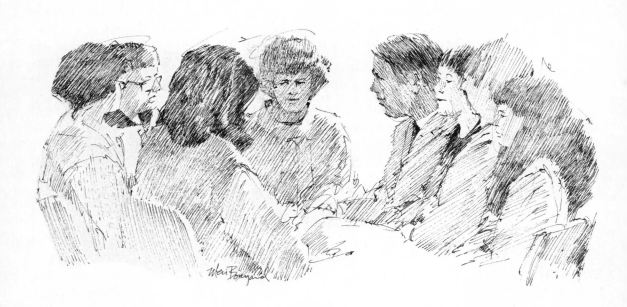

What do the rest of you think
about what Mary said?

LEARNING OBJECTIVES

After studying this chapter the student will be able to:

1 Discuss the characteristics of groups.

2 State the goal of a therapeutic group

3 Discuss the developmental phases of a therapeutic group.

4 State examples of the role of the leader in each phase of group development.

5 Discuss the characteristics of socialization groups.

6 Describe psychodrama, transactional analysis, and gestalt therapy as group interventions.

Human beings spend most of their time in group situations. They live, work, play, learn, and worship in groups. Group association is a prominent part of everyone's life because human beings are inherently social and because in complex, technological societies individuals are interdependent and must rely on each other for services. Therefore the nature of our humanness and the nature of the society in which we live dictate the necessity for a social structure organized around groups.

The individual's first experience with groups occurs in infancy when he is incorporated into his family—a specialized type of natural group. The second major group situation most people experience is school. In fact, significant group associations continue throughout the entire life span. Despite the pervasiveness of groups in our society, however, few persons give any thought to the nature and function of groups.

HISTORICAL PERSPECTIVE

Interestingly, the intervention known as group therapy did not originate within the mental health delivery system. Rather, it began in 1905 as a technique to assist tuberculosis patients to learn about their illness and to receive emotional support from each other. The success of these groups soon led to their use with patients suffering from "nervous disorders." It was not until World War II that group therapy became a standard intervention for the treatment of mentally ill persons.

During World War II many members of the civilian population as well as large numbers of Armed Forces personnel required psychiatric help. It became obvious that the traditional treatment methods utilized at that time could not provide the help required by the large population of mentally ill individuals. To make maximum use of psychiatrically trained personnel a plan was initiated through which patients were encouraged to talk out their problems in groups. As psychiatrists worked with this method and developed an effective technique that could be taught to others, it became obvious not only that group therapy was a more efficient means by which relatively few personnel could treat a large number of patients but, more importantly, that this mode of therapy had effects that could not be achieved through individual, one-to-one therapy. Some theorists believe that one reason for this positive effect is that groups tend to simulate the familial situation, wherein the leaders are seen in the role of parent figures and group members are seen as siblings. Therefore it becomes possible for persons who have had difficulty in their early family relationships to experientially work through many problems as a result of their interaction with other group members. Group members also find support and reassurance in the realization that others have problems that are similar to theirs. Consequently, group intervention is seen as the treatment of choice for some individuals.

CHARACTERISTICS OF GROUPS

A group is not a mere collection of individuals. Rather, a group is an identifiable system composed of three or more individuals who engage in certain tasks to achieve a common goal. Furthermore, to be a group the members must relate to each other, usually around the tasks and goals of the group. The individuals who ride the elevator in a skyscraper office building to get to their offices may share the common goal of getting to work but they rarely relate to each other about this goal. Therefore they would not be considered a group. If, on the other hand, the elevator stalled between floors and its occupants expressed their fears to each other, offered each other emotional support, made plans to get themselves out of their predicament, or otherwise began relating to each other, they would quickly become a group in the technical sense of the word.

As identifiable systems, groups share certain characteristics regardless of their differences in size, task, or goal. Since nursing care is often rendered in group situations, it is important for the nurse to develop an understanding of these characteristics.

Groups can be composed of as few as 3 or as many as 20 members. The upper limit of membership size is determined by the number of individuals who can easily relate to each other at the same time. In most group situations it is not possible for more than 20 people to meet this criterion and even then difficulty is encountered. When a group is larger than the number of individuals who can comfortably relate to one another simultaneously, *subgroups* are formed. For example, the 100-member senior class at the local high school cannot possibly function as a total group but is likely to be an aggregate of subgroups. Groups that are very small (3 or 4 members) also are not likely to be the most effective since there may be insufficient membership to fulfill all the roles necessary for the achievement of the group's goal.

All groups have goals. These may be multiple or single. Multiple goals may have equivalent importance, or they may be prioritized according to their value. Group members may or may not be equally aware of and supportive of the goals of the group. However, the group's effectiveness is strongly related to the degree to which the members are aware of and supportive of the goals. When the goals have been achieved, the group either disbands or determines new goals. Natural groups, such as families, tend to remain as groups by redefining their goals. Groups that have been formed around a single goal tend to disband after achievement of that goal. An example of such a group is the aforementioned senior high school class. The graduating seniors commonly feel a strong group association and promise to maintain contact with each other after graduation, but because the group has achieved its goal and disbands, the group members rarely follow through on their promise.

A group is a system and as such functions in a manner designed to maintain its equilibrium. Therefore the behavior of any one member affects and is affected by all other group members and must be seen as reflective of group behavior. Learning to view group behavior from a holistic perspective, rather than as a summation of individual interactions, is a difficult task for most students. A commonly used example that may be helpful in this regard is that of a symphony orchestra. If the listener attends to only the music played by each individual, he will have a distorted impression of what the finished piece sounds like, because each musician contributes only a part of what is necessary to the completed piece. However, when the listener attends to the contributions of all the musicians put together, a synchronized, harmonious piece is heard. This example not only illustrates the concept that the whole is different from and greater than the sum of its parts but it also implies that each part is necessary and of great value. In a group individuals have great value, but the result of their interactions is a product that can be best appreciated only when viewed from a group perspective.

The interactional behavior of the group's members has a great deal to do with the group's ability to achieve its goal. The term used to designate the behavior of group members is *role*. A role is the characteristic behavorial pattern employed by a group member and is determined by the personality of the individual and the needs of the group. At any point in time the group has a need to address the tasks necessary to achieve its goal, while simultaneously maintaining its life. Addressing the task is achieved through roles that have a content orientation, and group maintenance is achieved through roles that have a process orientation.

The content of a group is the overt verbal exchange, while the process is the underlying meaning the content has to the group, not to the individual. For example, Mr. Jones might say, "I'm not sure how to proceed." If Mr. Jones is viewed as an individual rather than as a group member, the content of his statement could lead one to believe that he feels insecure, a somewhat negative assessment. If this same content is viewed within the context of a group, it would be more appropriate to interpret the process as a need of the group for orientation and Mr. Jones as fulfilling the role of orienter. This interpretation not only conveys a positive tone, but is more accurate than the individually based one.

The roles assumed by group members relate to either the content or to the process of the group. Task- or content-oriented roles as suggested by Robert Bales* include coordinator, orienter, recorder, observer and commentator, opinion seeker or giver, elaborator, information seeker or giver, and initiator. Roles related to group maintenance or a process orientation include energizer,

---

*Bales, Robert: Interaction process analysis: a method for the study of small groups, Reading, Mass., 1950, Addison-Wesley Publishing Co., Inc.

encourager, dominator, aggressor, compromiser, blocker, harmonizer, and rejecter.

These lists of roles are not intended to be reflective of all the possible roles a group member could assume. However, they do represent the most commonly seen behaviors of group members and they also illustrate the reciprocal nature of content and process interactions (for example, information seeker or giver, encourager or blocker).

Since human beings have numerous experiences in many groups, by the time they reach adulthood most have developed a large repertoire of group behaviors. Therefore any one individual may assume different roles in different groups and different roles at different times in the same group, dependent in part on the needs of the group. Consequently, it is impossible to predict with complete assurance the role any individual will assume in a group. Furthermore, since the behavior of any group member affects and is affected by all other group members, it is not unusual for an individual to behave in a group in a way that is quite different from the way he behaves when relating to only one other individual.

To function effectively, groups develop rules or *norms* that govern their operation. Some norms may be externally imposed, but the norms that have the most meaning are those that have emerged from within the group. For example, group members are much more likely not to smoke if that norm was established by themselves rather than by the superintendent of the building in which they meet. Norms are sometimes fully known to all members and therefore can be explicitly stated. Other norms are not consciously formulated by the group, but rather have evolved as a result of the group's experience. Whether the group norms are explicit or implicit, their purpose is to influence the behavior of the group. Since implicit norms cannot be overtly conveyed, individuals who join an established group may be in a precarious position because they may unknowingly violate an implicit norm and receive a negative, nonverbal reaction from the others. The violation of implicit group norms is the basis of many social faux pas. The power of implicit norms is attested to by the excruciating embarrassment experienced by the person who has committed a social error, even when the reality of his error does not warrant such a reaction.

Another characteristic of groups is that each group has a unique identity, while at the same time sharing much in common with all other groups. The student will recognize this characteristic as also being true of individuals. The uniqueness of each group is based on the specific interactional combination of its size, its goals and the tasks designed to achieve its goals, the roles its members characteristically assume, and the norms the members establish to govern its operation. On the other hand, all groups share enough in common that an individual is able to apply that which he has learned in previous group associations to new group experiences. When a group is first formed, its members tend to behave in the ways they found to be successful in previous groups. As the group develops its own unique characteristics its members modify their behavior to a greater or lesser degree to adapt to the group's uniqueness, thereby further enlarging their repertoire of group behaviors.

The unique identity of a group is often recognized by both members and nonmembers. The reader is familiar with the "in-group, out-group" phenomenon where two superficially identical groups are valued very differently by their members. The group term for the value placed on a group by both its members and nonmembers is *attractiveness.* An in-group is seen as being attractive, an out-group unattractive. The degree of attractiveness a group has is determined to a large extent by its unique identity, and the mere altering of a few members, goals, or norms does not succeed in altering the group's identity or resultant attractiveness.

Finally, all groups, just like individuals, go through predictable developmental phases. However, the time at which the group moves from one phase to another is not as uniform as it is with individual development. Rather, the speed of group development is determined by a number of factors unique to the group, such as the anticipated duration of the group's life, the developmental strengths and weaknesses of its members, the importance the group places on its goal, the relevance of its norms to its goals, and the group's attractiveness. In addition, groups may skip developmental phases for a variety of reasons. However all groups must go through a beginning and ending phase. These and the intermediate phases of group development are described in conjunction with the discussion of group therapy in this chapter.

GROUP THERAPY
Considerations in establishing a therapy group

Group psychotherapists differ in their approach when establishing a therapeutic group. Questions involving the size of the membership, the frequency of meetings, and the characteristics of the participants must be decided. As might be expected, authorities answer these questions according to their personal treatment philosophies.

Some group psychotherapists insist on a balanced group, which means that only individuals of the same age, sex, and diagnostic category should be included. Others do not believe that a balanced group is necessary or even conducive to the best possible group interaction. Another consideration is whether to include persons with different levels of intelligence or verbal skills. Since group therapy depends on effective communication skills this may be an important consideration.

Certainly a decision must be made as to how large the group will be. Most authorities agree that a group should not be larger than 10, but many group leaders prefer a group no larger than 6. They also agree that the membership of a group should be stable.

A definite place in which to hold the group meeting must be identified. It should be quiet, comfortable, and private. The frequency and time of meeting must be decided as well as the date when group meetings will begin and end. When these decisions have been made and the group has come together for the first time, these norms should be shared with the members so that they will understand the nature of the contract they have with each other and with the group leader.

Some group leaders prefer to talk with potential group members before the actual group meetings begin. In this way each individual is acquainted with the nature of the sessions prior to the first meeting.

Characteristics of group therapy

The therapeutic group, like other groups, has a specific goal. It differs from a social group because its goal is to assist individuals to alter their behavioral patterns and to develop new and more effective ways of dealing with the stresses of daily living. To achieve this goal, individuals meet together regularly for a stated period of time to express their ideas, feelings, and concerns; to examine their current ways of behaving; and to develop new patterns of behavior.

The group leader works to develop among the group members a sense of trust in her as an individual and as a group leader. She avoids being critical or judgmental of the behavior of individual members of the group and relies on group action to control unacceptable behavior. The group leader strives to convey to the group members her acceptance of them as individuals and her respect for them as people. She avoids exerting undue control over the group or being the authority in the situation.

For a group to have maximum therapeutic effect it is essential that members learn to know and trust not only the leader but also each other. Therefore this becomes an important goal, the achievement of which is facilitated by the leader when she refers questions to the group, encourages participation from all members, and shows acceptance and respect for each individual. By engaging in these behaviors, the nurse leader acts as a role model for the members. The inexperienced group leader will be surprised at how quickly the group members learn to act toward each other in the manner suggested by her behavior.

Group development

Every group, like every individual, progresses through several developmental phases. The first developmental phase of a group is the *preaffiliation* or *getting acquainted phase*. During this time group members behave toward each other as strangers and are obviously distrustful of each other and of the leader. Their expectations of the group activity are, of necessity, determined by experiences they have had in other groups. Although members are likely to be overtly polite to each other, their behavior also indicates an approach-avoidance dilemma. That is, most members are eager to become involved with each other but simultaneously fear the risks that such involvement may entail. It is during this stage that the leader is most effective when she provides structure, protects members from embarrassment by not allowing them to prematurely reveal highly personal information, and gently invites trust.

The second developmental period is the *phase of experiencing intragroup conflict* and is characterized by power and control issues. Unavoidably, conflict will emerge during this time, since the members are in the process of establishing their positions in the group relative to the positions of other members and the leader. Often group members look to the leader for sanction or condemnation of another member. If the leader falls into this trap, she is likely to find the group critical of her because of her decision. In this instance it is always wise to deflect the question about a member's behavior back to the group by a comment such as, "I wonder what the rest of you think about Mr. Jones's question?" It is during this second phase of group development that the group attempts to formalize relationships through the establishment of explicit norms. These attempts should be supported as long as they do not infringe on the rights or safety of one or more members. Throughout the group process the leader has the responsibility of protecting the safety of individuals and property, but the necessity for doing so becomes greatest during this second phase of group development. It is during the second phase that group sessions may seem nonproductive in that the members alternate competitive, aggressive behavior with apathetic withdrawal. Interrelated with this phenomenon is the great danger of membership dropout.

If the leader can help the group safely navigate through this phase, characteristics of the third phase will emerge. This is called the *working phase* or the *phase of intimacy and differentiation*. During this phase the work of the group is achieved. It is a period of relatively high communication in which members appropriately share personal feelings and concerns about emotional problems.

It is during the working phase of the group that the members' sense of belonging, or group *cohesiveness*, is at its highest. When a group is cohesive, its members tend to feel emotionally close to one another, and individuals respond well to advice offered by other members. Consequently during this period there is an opportunity for emotional reeducation and relearning. The members discover through the reactions of the other group members that there are many different reactions to their feelings and behavior. They come to realize how universal their problems are and that they are not as unique in their difficulties as they may have believed.

The last developmental phase is precipitated by the approaching time for the group to conclude its meetings. Thus it is the *termination phase* and may require a number of meetings to work through the feelings of the individuals involved. The goal of the termination phase is to help group members integrate what they have learned about themselves and the behavioral changes they have made so that they can use these in the future. If the termination phase is not handled skillfully, not only will this goal not be achieved, but the group members may leave the group feeling that the only thing to be gained by group association is more emotional pain. During this period the members relive previous periods when they experienced personal loss of someone very close to them. They may express feelings of being abandoned, rejected, or forsaken. The expression of these feelings provides an excellent opportunity to help individual members of the group deal with these feelings and work through them.

Four phases of group development have been described. It should be noted, however, that these phases overlap one another and that only the first and the last phases are seen in all groups. Groups that meet for only a few sessions or groups whose members have a great deal of difficulty in trusting others are not likely to be able to move through the phase of experiencing intragroup conflict and the working phase. Consequently, the termination phase will not be as meaningful and therefore not as difficult as when the group has traveled successfully through all developmental phases.

Role of the leader

The group leader is the key to a successful group therapy experience. The leader needs to be aware of her own behavior and its effect on others. The effectiveness of the getting acquainted phase for the group is largely dependent on the way in which the leader orients the members to the group process, to each other, and to herself. The phase of experiencing intragroup conflict can be successfully resolved if the group leader is able to be supportive to the members and successfully establishes a feeling of acceptance and respect for all. As the group moves into the working phase, it is the leader who is able to involve the less verbal members by redirecting questions to them or by asking them how a situation seems to them. The leader sometimes provides essential factual information that is important in the resolution of an issue that has arisen. On occasion the leader may help a member learn exactly what others think about his behavior or his responses. The leader assists members in exploring situations they bring to the group from the outside and helps them to think through and test out more appropriate ways of responding.

As the group develops the leader will be confronted with a variety of specific problems in group interaction that will necessitate her intervention. Problems such as silence, monopolizing behavior, tardiness, and acting out on the part of members are common and require the skill of the leader if the group session is to be effective. It is beyond the scope of this text to discuss these problems and possible appropriate interventions, but the student should be aware that a number of excellent references are available that will provide specific direction. It should be noted, however, that the most effective group leader is one who is able to vary her style of intervention based on her assessment of the needs of the group.

Skillful termination of a group requires first and foremost that the leader recognize her own feelings of loss. If she recognizes her own feelings she is less likely to act them out by doing such things as "forgetting" the final meeting, acting punitively to members who express a sense of loss, or promising members that she will continue to contact them when this is not possible or desirable. The skillful group leader will understand that the anger at her and other members commonly expressed during this phase is a reflection of the severity of the loss the members are experiencing. She will not respond to anger with anger but will help the group members to acknowledge their sadness about the disbanding of the group.

Finally, the skillful group leader will help the group members to identify what they have gained through their association. If they conceptualize these gains the members will be able to take away something concrete that helps to offset the emotional loss.

Many group therapists believe that it is most beneficial to the group if two staff members act as co-therapists. In this situation one therapist is able to concentrate on the content being expressed while the other therapist focuses primarily on the group process. Although the co-therapists may change their function from one group session to another, it is believed that co-leaders who are experienced and comfortable with each other can view the group more comprehensively and therefore provide the group with helpful direction in regard to both content and process.

SOCIALIZATION GROUPS: A REMOTIVATION TECHNIQUE

Psychiatric hospitals are frequently heavily populated with mentally ill persons who appear to have lost interest in reality, to have lost a sense of personal value, and who seem to be unaware of other persons with whom they come in daily contact. Group interaction is one of the most successful ways of stimulating these people to rekindle their interest in their surroundings.

The nurse may be the only professional worker who is available or interested in developing some form of group experience that will encourage these individuals to begin to communicate with each other and with the staff. The primary goal of these group activities is to facilitate socialization and is most easily achieved by focusing on a task. If several persons come together as a group and carry on an activity for a few sessions, the initial attempt has been successful.

The focus of the group activity depends almost entirely on the individuals who are to be included as members. Their age, educational backgrounds, and physical health will greatly influence the choice of activities that can be suggested.

Some individuals might be interested in a current events discussion group. Others who evidence no interest in reading the newspaper or listening to the television news reports would not be interested in such a group activity. Some might be interested in forming a poetry reading group, whereas others would abhor such an activity. Some might enjoy sewing or knitting while they visit together; others would not.

In view of this wide variation in personal abilities and taste the first rule to follow in initiating any recreational or motivational activity is to be well acquainted with the individuals who will form the group membership. The nurse will find that it is wise to encourage the members to participate in selecting the focus for the group meetings. The wise group leader will formulate some tentative plans for the first meeting, but these need to be flexible and easily changed in case there are suggestions from the members.

The nurse leader will find that at first many persons will be reluctant to participate. Some individuals may require more than one friendly invitation to attend. Some who have lost interest in reality carry on an active fantasy life. Any group activity must compete with these fantasies for the individual's attention and enjoyment. Thus it is wise to offer the group members refreshments during the initial group meetings. As the group becomes cohesive, the members' interest in the group activity may become great enough to overshadow the food as the major enjoyment of the meeting.

It is wise to vary the focus of the group activity from time to time to maintain the interest of the group members. As the members become acquainted with one another, they themselves will suggest changes in the focus or the format of the meeting.

The following are some concrete suggestions for planning an effective socialization group experience*:

1. Develop a flexible plan that provides for change and spontaneity.
2. Encourage all group members to participate in planning.
3. Keep the plan practical and within achievable limits.
4. Initiate activities that group members are able to handle.
5. Provide something specific such as refreshments that will give each group member some tangible satisfaction.
6. Avoid monotony by varying the focus of group activity.
7. Maintain consistency in the feeling tone of each meeting so that group member's expectations will be fulfilled.

PSYCHODRAMA

Another type of therapeutic experience sometimes provided for a group of clients is called psychodrama. This technique was developed by J. L. Moreno, a psychiatrist who began working with emotionally disturbed individuals in a theater in Vienna as early as 1941. Psychodrama is usually conducted by a leader who has been especially prepared to direct this type of activity. Although a variety of methods may be used, one of the more frequent techniques places the leader on a stage in front of an audience of clients and staff members. The leader identifies a situation in which interpersonal conflict is involved. He invites members of the audience to come to the stage to act out this human relations problem.

When members of the audience agree to accept parts in the drama they are told the essential facts about the roles they are to play. The chosen situation frequently focuses on a conversation with the significant members of a family. In the role of an actor, the individual is given a specially selected part that affords him an opportunity to express his inner conflicts freely as a situation is acted out with other performers who symbolize or represent persons who are the real objects of his love or hate. For example, a son who normally represses his hostility toward his father may freely express it as an actor and may even reveal the cause. On the other hand, if he is induced to take the father role he may

*Brown, Martha, and Fowler, Grace R.: Psychodynamic nursing—a biosocial orientation, ed. 4, Philadelphia, 1972, W.B. Saunders Co.

then be more objective and understanding about his own father's point of view. It is surprising how effectively individuals fill the roles to which they are assigned and how realistically feelings are expressed. The leader stops the action when he believes the enactment has progressed far enough to provide the audience with a basis for a fruitful discussion.

Another method that has been used productively in psychodrama is for the leader to request a volunteer from the audience to come forward and set up a situation that he wishes to portray. This person is also asked to select individuals from the audience to play the parts required and to provide the role players with the necessary data about the roles they will enact. This technique focuses specially on some personal concern of the individual who volunteered to develop the psychodramatic situation. With either of these methods individuals from the audience may be asked to come forward to play the role of alter ego for the major characters in the psychodrama.

After the role playing is completed the people in the audience are given an opportunity to discuss the situation they have witnessed and experienced vicariously. The participants from the audience may focus attention on various aspects of the situation and frequently present similar life experiences.

Psychodrama provides individuals with an opportunity to express feelings and concerns that relate to a personal human relations situation that is like, but not identical to, a personal problem of their own. Thus psychodrama has somewhat the same therapeutic effect as *abreaction,* the lessening of emotional trauma by reenacting the situation. It also furnishes individuals with an opportunity for *catharsis,* an opportunity to freely express feelings. As in other group therapy situations, the individual is helped by the group to express feelings and consider them objectively.

The nurse is frequently involved in psychodrama as a role player or as a discussant. Skill and understanding of psychodrama are developed through continued participation in this treatment modality. Eventually the nurse may accept the role of the leader of the psychodrama sessions.

TRANSACTIONAL ANALYSIS

Transactional analysis is both a theoretical framework and a treatment method developed by Eric Berne. Its popularity and utility is attested to by the amount of literature available to lay persons on the subject. As a theory transactional analysis postulates that each person has three elements of his personality in greater or lesser operation at any given point in time. These elements are (1) the immature, need-gratifying aspect, referred to as the Child, (2) the moralistic, rigid standard-setting aspect, referred to as the Parent, (3) and the mature, reality-based aspect, referred to as the Adult. The student will notice the similarity between this theoretical formulation and Freud's conception of the id, superego, and ego, respectively. Unlike Freudian theory, however, Berne's construct does not imply a judgment about the existence of these personality elements. Rather, he states that problems arise only when there is an incongruency between the elements that are operating when people relate with each other. This belief is the foundation for his use of the term *transactional*. The emphasis on dysfunctional interpersonal relationships as the crux of emotional problems is reminiscent of Sullivan's theories. Consequently, Berne's theory of transactional analysis is seen by many as effectively combining the salient intrapsychic features of Freudian theory and the aspects of Sullivanian theory that provide direction for therapeutic intervention.

When persons communicate and the adult elements of their personalities are operative, it is likely that they will be effective in hearing and responding to each other. In addition, the nonverbal aspects of the process will be congruent with the verbal content and no hidden messages will be perceived by either person. Each will reality test on the basis of feedback received and each is likely to feel that the interaction has been satisfying. This is not to imply that no differences of opinion will arise during such an interaction but the individuals will probably feel that any differences are based on content issues, rather than on covert attempts to dominate, control, or otherwise minimize the value of the other person. Adult-Adult interactions are effective and therefore desirable interactional processes when the participants are engaged in problem-solving or task-oriented activities.

Another effective and desirable interactional process occurs when two or more chonological adults simultaneously have the child element of their personalities in preeminence. It is at these times they have fun "playing." Many adults have had the experience of spontaneously engaging in what appear to be foolish or childlike activities with another adult, such as frolicking through a park on a beautiful autumn day instead of attending a scheduled meeting. As long as this behavior does not have major irreversible consequences and does not become a persistent pattern it can enhance the individual's feelings of well-being and strengthen the relationship.

Problems arise when two persons characteristically relate to each other through divergent elements of their personalities. For example, a husband who relates to his wife through the parent element of his personality will feel continuously dissatisfied with their interactions unless she responds with the child element of her personality. If she does respond in this way, there may be little initial conflict because both their needs are superficially being met. However, it should be noted that neither is engaged in reality-testing behaviors and neither can change interactional elements without open conflict emerging. Therefore this pattern is growth-stifling for both partners.

The previous situation is merely one example of a common interactional problem. The reader can speculate as to the large variety of interactional problems that can occur when two or more people interact from the basis of incongruent personality elements. For more detailed explanations of transactional analysis the student is referred to the many excellent books on the subject.

Transactional analysis as a method of treatment is most effective as a form of family therapy. When this is not possible, it can be effectively implemented as a method of group therapy, in which the group members consciously and unconsciously assume characteristic familial roles. In either the family or group setting the participants can analyze their reactions and subsequent behavior in light of the Child-Parent-Adult framework and experience how they affect others and are affected by them. They also can experiment with using other elements of their personality and can receive immediate feedback.

Transactional analysis is also used for individual treatment. The effectiveness of this treatment modality is limited, however, since the client has only one other person with whom to interact, and feedback about behavioral changes in life situations is delayed. Nevertheless many therapists successfully adopt some of the concepts of transactional analysis in their treatment of individuals because these concepts are seen by many clients as easy to understand and relevant to their life situations.

Regardless of setting, the primary role of the transactional therapist is to observe and tactfully comment on the discrepancies between the personality elements of those engaged in the interactional process. The therapist often suggests and supports role playing with another personality element so that the person can experience its effects. The dynamics that underlie the person's use of one personality element as opposed to the other two are not always explored. If they are discussed it is usually done in the context of the present rather than in terms of childhood experiences.

GESTALT THERAPY

Gestalt therapy is as much a philosophy as it is an intervention technique. Its developer is Frederic S. Perls, who has trained many others in its use. The emphasis in gestalt therapy is on treatment of the person as a holistic being, placing as much importance on somatic responses as on emotional responses. Proponents of gestalt therapy believe that many persons' problems emanate from the fact that individuals have lost touch with their feelings, both physical and emotional. If one is unaware of what one is feeling, the likelihood of being able to express these feelings is greatly diminished and therefore one is unlikely to have one's needs met. Therefore treatment consists primarily of helping the individual increase sensory awareness of his present state. Once the individual begins the process of getting in touch with himself, his current relationships with others and with his environment are explored. The configuration of the holistic being in interaction with others and with the environment is referred to as the *gestalt* and is heavily based on systems theory. Although it is acknowledged that multiple causative factors produced the individual's current responses, the understanding of these factors is not believed to alleviate the present problems and they are therefore not explored.

As with transactional analysis, the principles of gestalt therapy can be used in a one-to-one psychotherapeutic relationship but are most commonly practiced as a form of group therapy. Eight to 10 participants are seen as an ideal number for a gestalt group. The environment in which the group meets is viewed as instrumental in facilitating self-awareness. Therefore factors such as comfortable chairs, a pleasing decor, and adequate space are seen as essential. Techniques such as role playing and ventilation are used frequently. The ultimate goal of gestalt therapy is to assist the client to fulfill his potential, and therefore it is appropriately used with individuals interested in self-growth as well as with persons who are emotionally disturbed.

SELECTION OF A THERAPEUTIC GROUP

It is important to note that the type of group activity that is most appropriate for the mentally ill person depends on a number of variables including his degree of ego strength and his current insight into his problems. It is likely that a person whose contact with reality is tenuous would benefit most from a socialization group rather than from a more formal group psychotherapy session. As the client gains more ego strength, he may be introduced into a group whose primary goal is that of supportive therapy. As members progress in this type of group, the focus of the group may very well change to that of insight therapy. This is not to say that socialization groups do not have therapeutic effects, but rather that the degree of stress the person is able to tolerate should be a major determining factor in the decision as to the type of group in which he will participate. Furthermore, this determination should be made jointly by the interdisciplinary health care team, which is able to view the client from a variety of perspectives.

GROWTH AND SELF-ACTUALIZATION GROUPS

Other types of groups such as sensitivity, encounter, and self-help groups are well known in our society. The nature of these groups will not be discussed here, because expert leaders or facilitators of these groups believe that their primary goal is not and should not be therapeutic in nature, but rather educative, in the sense of self-growth, self-actualization, and increased self-awareness. Therefore these types of groups are rarely, if ever, used with mentally ill persons, and the nurse is not likely to be involved with them in a professional capacity. Nevertheless, there is much available literature about these groups that the reader may be interested in exploring.

CONCLUDING STATEMENTS

1. The nature of our humanness and the nature of the society in which we live dictate the necessity for a social structure organized around groups.

2. A group is an identifiable system composed of three or more individuals who engage in certain tasks to achieve a common goal. In addition, group members relate to each other, usually around the tasks and goals of the group.

3. The size of an effective group is one that is large enough to fulfill all the roles necessary for the achievement of the group's goals, while being small enough so that its members can comfortably relate to one another at the same time.

4. All groups have goals. In effective groups the members are aware of and support the group's goals.

5. Since a group is a system, group interactions need to be viewed from a holistic perspective rather than as a summation of individual interactions.

6. *Role* is the term used to designate the behavior of group members. The role assumed by any group member is determined by his personality combined with the needs of the group.

7. At any point in time the group has a need to address the tasks necessary to achieve its goal while simultaneously maintaining its life. Addressing the task is achieved through roles that have a content orientation, and group maintenance is achieved through roles that have a process orientation.

8. To function effectively, groups develop norms that govern their operation. Norms that have the most meaning are those that have emerged from within the group. Norms may be explicit or implicit.

9. Each group has a unique identity, while at the same time sharing much in common with all other groups. The group's uniqueness is based on the specific interactional combination of a number of factors, such as its size and its goals.

10. The therapeutic group has as its goal the alteraton of the behavioral patterns of the group members through the development of new and more effective ways of coping with stressful situations.

11. Before group meetings are initiated decisions must be made about the size of membership, the frequency of meetings, the place and time of meetings, and the characteristics of members.

12. Each group progresses through several developmental phases including the getting acquainted phase, the phase of experi-

encing intragroup conflict, the working phase, and the termination phase.

13. Group interaction is one of the most successful ways of stimulating persons who have lost interest in their surroundings.

14. Psychodrama is a form of group therapy that allows individuals to role play problem situations by alternating various roles and to receive feedback from observers in the audience.

15. Transactional analysis uses the Child-Parent-Adult framework to analyze and improve interactional patterns.

16. Gestalt therapy focuses on helping persons fulfill their potential through increased sensory awareness of themselves and their relationships with others and with the environment within the context of the present.

17. The type of group activity most appropriate for mentally ill persons should be determined after consideration of a number of variables. In addition, as each individual progresses in treatment, the type of group activity appropriate to meet his needs will change.

SUGGESTED SOURCES OF ADDITIONAL INFORMATION

Classical

Armstrong, Shirley W., and Rouslin, Sheila: Group psychotherapy in nursing practice, New York, 1963, Macmillan Publishing Co., Inc.

Baker, Joan M., and Estes, Nada J.: Anger in group therapy, Am. J. Nurs. **65**:96-100, July, 1965.

Bales, Robert: Interaction process analysis: a method for the study of small groups, Reading, Mass., 1950, Addison-Wesley Publishing Co., Inc.

Brown, Donald I.: Nurses participate in group therapy, Am. J. Nurs. **62**:68-69, Jan., 1962.

Bueker, Kathleen, and Warrick, Annette: Can nurses be group therapists? Am. J. Nurs. **64**:114-116, May, 1964.

Fagin, Claire M.: Psychotherapeutic nursing, Am. J. Nurs. **67**:298-304, 1967.

Getty, Cathleen, and Shannon, Anna M.: Co-therapy as an egalitarian relationship, Am. J. Nurs. **69**:767-771, 1969.

Glover, B.H.: A new nurse therapist, Am. J. Nurs. **67**:1003-1005, 1967.

Hargreaves, Anne G.: The group culture and nursing practice, Am. J. Nurs. **67**:1840-1846, 1967.

Pullinger, Walter F.: Remotivation, Am. J. Nurs. **60**:682-685, 1960.

Sink, Susan Mary: Remotivation; toward reality for the aged, Nurs. Outlook **14**:26-28, Aug., 1966.

Von Mering, Otto, and King, Stanley H.: Remotivating the mental patient, New York, 1957, Russell Sage Foundation.

Contemporary

Adrian, Sarah: A systematic approach to selecting group participants, J. Psychosoc. Nurs. Ment. Health Serv. **18**:37-41, Feb., 1980.

Benton, Denise W.: The significance of the absent member in milieu therapy, Perspect. Psychiatr. Care **18**:21-25, Jan.-Feb., 1980.

Birckhead, Loretta: The nurse as leader: group psychotherapy with psychiatric patients, J. Psychosoc. Nurs. Ment. Serv. **22**:24-30, June, 1984.

Britnell, J., and Mitchell, K.: Inpatient group psychotherapy for the elderly, J. Psychosoc. Nurs. Ment. Health Serv. **19**:19-24, May, 1981.

Cohen, Marcia, and Amdur, Mark: Medication group for psychiatric patients, Am. J. Nurs. **81**:343-345, Feb., 1981.

Collison, Carol: Grappling with group resistance, J. Psychosoc. Nurs. Ment. Health Serv. **22**:6-12, Aug., 1984.

Dinnauer, L., Miller, M., and Frankforter, M.: Implementation strategies for an inpatient women's support group, J. Psychosoc. Nurs. Ment. Health Serv. **19**:13-16, Aug., 1981.

Echternacht, Marcy Rea: Day treatment groups: helping patients stay out, J. Psychosoc. Nurs. Ment. Health Serv. **22**:11-16, Oct., 1984.

Ernst, C., Vanderzyl, S., and Salinger, R.: Preparation of psychiatric inpatients for group therapy, J. Psychosoc. Nurs. Ment. Health Serv. **19**:28-33, July, 1981.

Fochtman, Grace A.: Therapeutic factors of the informal group, Am. J. Nurs. **75**:238, 1976.

Gallese, Lucille, and Teuting, Edna: Helping rape victims through group psychotherapy, J. Psychosoc. Nurs. Ment. Health Serv. **19**:2-21, Aug., 1981.

Gauron, Eugene F., et al.: The orientation group in pre-therapy training, Perspect. Psychiatr. Care **15**(1):32-37, 1977.

Gerace, Laina, and Rosenberg, Lisa: The use of art prints in group therapy with aftercare patients, Perspect. Psychiatr. Care **17**:83-86, March-April, 1979.

Gluck, Miriam Mandsager: Group therapy in a pain management program, J. Psychosoc. Nurs. Ment. Health Serv. **18**:21-24, Nov., 1980.

Hankins-McNary, Lulu: The use of humor in group therapy, Perspect. Psychiatr. Care **17**:228-231, Sept.-Oct., 1979.

Hoover, Robert, and Parnell, Pam: An inpatient educational group on stress and coping, J. Psychosoc. Nurs. Ment. Health Serv. **22**:16-22, June, 1984.

Johnson-Soderberg, Sherry: The theory and practice of scapegoating, Perspect. Psychiatr. Care **15**:153-159, 1977.

Joyce, Carol: The religious as group therapists: attitudes and conflicts, Perspect. Psychiatr. Care **15**(3):112-117, 1977.

Kahn, Alice N.: Group education for the overweight, Am. J. Nurs. **78**:254, 1978.

Lancaster, Jeanette: Activity groups as therapy, Am. J. Nurs. **76**:947-949, 1976.

Larkin, Anne: What's a medication group? J. Psychosoc. Nurs. Ment. Health Serv. **20**:35-37, Feb., 1982.

Mealy, Anne R.: Sculpting as a group technique for increasing awareness, Perspect. Psychiatr. Care **15**(3):118-121, 1977.

Neizo, B., and Murphy, M.: Medication groups on an acute psychiatric unit, Perspect. Psychiatr. Care **21**:70-73, April-June, 1983.

Newton, Geraldine: Self-help groups: can they help? J. Psychosoc. Nurs. Ment. Health Serv. **22**:27-31, July, 1984.

Pelletier, Luc: Interpersonal communications task group, J. Psychosoc. Nurs. Ment. Health Serv. **21**:32-36, Sept., 1983.

Rogers, Carl: On encounter groups, New York, 1970, Harper & Row, Publishers.

Rogers, Carl: Facilitating encounter groups, Am. J. Nurs. **71**:275-279, 1971.

Rogers, Joanna, and Grubb, Pearl: The V.A. psychiatric patient: re-socialization and community living, Perspect. Psychiatr. Care **17**:72-76, March-April, 1979.

Rouslin, Shiela: Relatedness in group psychotherapy, Perspect. Psychiatr. Care **11**(4):165-171, 1973.

Sanderson, Marilynn R., and Blackley, Judith J.: Problems displayed "in vitro"—a particular advantage of group therapy, Perspect. Psychiatr. Care **17**:176-186, July-Aug., 1979.

Shaw, Dale, et al.: Multiple impact therapy, Am. J. Nurs. **77**:246-248, 1977.

Silbert, Denise: Human sexuality growth groups, J. Psychosoc. Nurs. Ment. Health Serv. **19**:31-34, Feb., 1981.

Spetz, Henry: Contemporary trends in group psychotherapy: a literature survey, Hosp. Community Psychiatry **35**(2):132-142, 1984.

van Servellen, Gwen M., and Vohs Dull, Lynn: Group psychotherapy for depressed women: a model, J. Psychosoc. Nurs. Ment. Health Serv. **19**:25-31, Aug., 1981.

Ward, Judy Trowbridge: The sounds of silence: group psychotherapy with nonverbal patients, Perspect. Psychiatr. Care **12**:13-19, Jan.-March, 1974.

White, Eleanor, and Kahn, E. Michael: Use and modifications in group psychotherapy with chronic schizophrenic outpatients, J. Psychosoc. Nurs. Ment. Health Serv. **20**:14-20, Feb., 1982.

Witt, Jimmie: Transference and countertransference in group therapy settings, J. Psychosoc. Nurs. Ment. Health Serv. **20**:31-34, Feb., 1982.

Yalom, Irvin D.: The theory and practice of group psychotherapy, New York, 1975, Basic-Books, Inc., Publishers.

Of particular interest

Marram, Gwen D.: The group approach in nursing practice, ed. 2, St. Louis, 1978, The C.V. Mosby Co.

This text introduces the reader to group work through a review of various group concepts and applications. It is especially relevant for the student of psychiatric nursing.

Whitaker, D., and Lieberman, M.: Psychotherapy through the group process, Chicago, 1964, Aldine Publishing Co.

This book is one of the classics in group therapy literature. It is easily read, and the clinical examples assist the reader in application of the concepts.

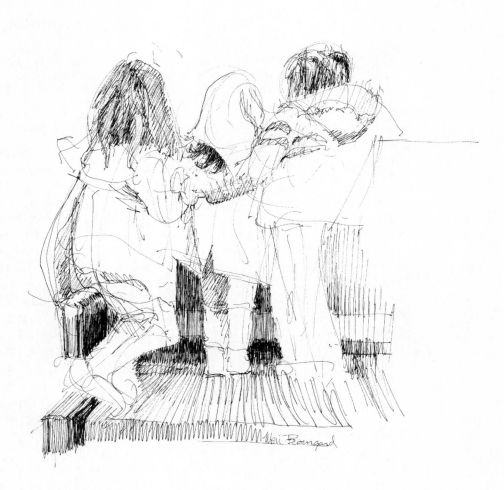

*Even though our individual needs
are different, we sure enjoy each other.*

LEARNING OBJECTIVES

After studying this chapter the student will be able to:

1 Define the term *family*.

2 Discuss the functions of the family.

3 Discuss the developmental stages of the family according to Duvall.

4 Discuss the patterns of behavior characteristic of the effective family.

5 Describe the characteristics of the child-abusing family as an example of the ineffective family.

6 Explain the rationale underlying the use of family therapy as a treatment modality.

It is commonly asserted that the family is the most basic of all societal institutions. This assertion stems from two factors. The first is the universal tendency of human beings to organize themselves around the structure of the family. Second, it is believed that the experiences a child has as a family member have the most powerful influence on the kind of adult he will become. Therefore the society as a whole is very much affected by the family, both directly and indirectly, in both the present and future. Other societal institutions, such as the school and the church, are certainly fundamental to the society but are believed to be organizational structures that fulfill functions that historically have been delegated by the family. These societal institutions have developed in the belief that the collective society can fulfill certain functions more efficiently than can the singular family. However, the question of whether the society can fulfill these functions more effectively than the family is the subject of continuous debate, and dynamic fluctuations of functions between the family and other societal institutions can be observed over the course of generations.

The nurse often deals not just with an individual but also with a family. This contact may be direct and formalized as when engaged in family therapy or direct but informal as when seeking information from or supplying information to family members. Some family theorists believe that even when the nurse is dealing only with an individual it is impossible for the interaction not to affect and be affected by that individual's family. Therefore interactions with an individual are seen as indirect interactions with that individual's family. This view stems from the belief that the family is a system. The behavior of an individual is greatly influenced by his family, and in turn, any alterations in his behavior invariably affect his family. Whether one agrees with this view or not, it is hard to deny the fact that to be effective the nurse needs to understand the family.

HISTORICAL PERSPECTIVE

Awareness of the family as a significant social institution has been present throughout history. However, it was not until the twentieth century that the family was recognized as a system and studied as such. Prior to that time the family unit was understood to be a summation of the characteristics of its members. This view resulted in ascribing praise or blame to one or more family members for the effectiveness of the family's functioning. When a member was diagnosed as being mentally ill it was often thought to be the fault of the parents, particularly the mother.

The family unit was not studied as a system until the escalating divorce rate after World War II created national concern about the future of the family in this country. In retrospect it seems clear that the large number of divorces that occurred after World War II resulted from the fact that while husbands were serving in the Armed Forces wives were working in factories, both evolving adaptations in the absence of the other. When the husband returned the lifestyles that each had evolved were not necessarily compatible and no help was available to assist the marriage partners to regain system homeokinesis.

Three of the earliest proponents of family therapy were Nathan W. Ackerman at Columbia University, Gerald Caplan at Harvard, and Don Jackson at the University of California. Their earliest work was done in the 1950s. Since that time many theorists have studied the family as a system and currently there is general agreement that effective promotion of mental health and prevention and treatment of mental illness must take place within a family context. What remains as an unresolved dilemma is how to deliver this type of care within a health delivery system designed to focus on the individual.

FAMILY STRUCTURE

In nonindustrial societies the family pattern most commonly observed is the *extended family*, where several generations live together and leave only for the purpose of joining another extended family through marriage. Before the industrial revolution families in the United States often consisted of children, parents, and grandparents and perhaps one or more unmarried aunts or uncles. This pattern of family life provided the work force necessary for the productive management of the family business, usually the farm. When daughters married, they often left their family to join the family of their husband, while the sons' wives were incorporated into their family. This traditional family structure was also the mechanism whereby family resources, primarily land, were passed from generation to generation. The advantages of the extended family structure were many—physical and emotional resources were shared among a large group, and a broad division of labor was possible.

However there were also many disadvantages. Families whose offspring were all female had to face the possibility of all the children leaving, thereby placing the elderly parents in a very vulnerable economic and social position. Furthermore although the prescribed roles of each family member provided stability and continuity, this prescription also thwarted individuality. The eldest boy was expected to continue the family business, leaving the younger brother, who might have been more interested and capable of so doing, the choice of either striking out on his own or working at the behest of his older sibling. The image we now have of the "good old days" as characterized by close-knit, warm, loving families is believed by most authorities to be a distortion of the reality of intense sibling rivalry and parental frustration.

The settlement of the Western frontier, which placed great value on rugged individualism, and the industrial revolution both contributed greatly to a dramatic change in the typical family structure. Individuals moved from settled rural areas to the unsettled West or to industrialized urban areas with the goal of making their own fortune. A pervasive belief in both instances was that more money could be earned with less labor. Initially that belief proved to be false as evidenced by the hardships of Western settlement and the horrors of the urban sweatshop. The mobility of American citizens along with waves of European immigrants combined to create cities where people lived in dense concentration. Population density and mobility mitigated against the perpetuation of the extended family, and the nuclear family structure became the norm.

The *nuclear family* is defined as a two-generational family where it is understood that the children will leave once they have achieved maturity. Therefore the nuclear family, as a family, is only a temporary arrangement. Although the nuclear family has the disadvantages of potential alienation from the family of origin and fewer emotional supports from within the family it has the major advantage of facilitating upward social mobility because it tends not to predetermine the children's roles as inheritors of the family business.

DEFINITION OF FAMILY

A family is traditionally defined as two or more people who are related by blood or by legal ties such as marriage or adoption. However, a family also has the characteristic of identifying itself and being identified by others as such. Sharing a common surname is a manifestation of this characteristic, although it is not requisite to being a family as evidenced by the increasing number of young women in our society who retain the surname of their family of origin after marriage. Another characteristic of a family is that it is a relatively permanent human affiliation. A family, therefore, has a history and a future.

In the complex, highly mobile, technological society in which we live, there are an increasing number of human groups that identify themselves as a family and that exist over a period of time, but whose members do not meet the traditional criteria of being related by blood or by legal ties. Therefore a more accurate and relevant definition of family may be one that reflects the functions of a family.

FUNCTIONS OF THE FAMILY

A family is a specialized group that bands together in pursuit of the common goal of growth and development of its members. This goal is achieved through certain functions. Although none of these functions are unique to the family, the combination of them is unique to this institution. The following is a list of functions considered by most authorities to belong to the family.

Regulation of sexual activity and reproduction. The family structure provides for socially sanctioned sexual activity between spouses, while at the same time enforcing the societal taboo against incest by defining parental and sibling relationships. Survival of the culture is ensured by systematizing reproduction within a context that is capable of providing for children who in turn become the vehicle for the transmission of cultural values and practices. Therefore a family conveys to its children its cultural heritage as a means of ensuring the culture's future.

Physical maintenance. The family structure provides a vehicle through which the physical needs of its members can be met. It provides an efficient means of organizing responsibility for meeting the needs of the individual for food, clothing, shelter, and health care. In this regard the family can be seen as an economic unit.

Protection. The family structure is designed to provide both literal and figurative protection of its members by providing a model for interacting with the society in a way that protects the family members from undesirable outside influences.

Education and socialization. Some authorities believe that the family's function of providing education and socialization is the most fundamental one in that it is through the family that children learn how to function in and relate to the world in which they live.

Recreation. Traditionally the family has been the structure in which the individual has engaged in leisure time activities that are a source of personal and group refreshment and renewal, leading to increased family cohesion. Unlike the last function of education and socialization, the function of recreation is seen as rapidly waning with the advent of television and other passive or nonparticipant forms of recreation.

Status conferring. Another traditional function of the family that seems to be undergoing fundamental alteration is that of status conferring. Before the advent of industrialization in a democratic society with the emphasis placed on individualism, the individual was conferred social status by virtue of the family into which he was born. Although this is no longer strictly the case today social status is still somewhat determined by the socioeconomic level of one's family of origin.

Affection giving. Only within the family can an individual be guaranteed unconditional acceptance by the mere fact of his relationship to that family. In all other societal interactions, the value placed on an individual is determined by such things as the quality or speed of his performance, his appearance, his social class, or his occupation. In functional families acceptance is conveyed by a deep, enduring affection among the members.

• • •

A perusal of these family functions reveals that the family unit provides services that are essential to the survival and stability of the society. For example, by regulating sexual activity within the family society is protected from the consequences of wanton mating. Simultaneously, the family unit provides essential services to its members, such as physical maintenance and affection giving.

All functions of a family are not equally prominent at any given time. Each function is more specific to certain stages of family development than others and as such become developmental tasks of the family.

Family sociologist Evelyn Duvall* has outlined a series of developmental stages of the family. This concept is not without problems but nevertheless provides a useful frame of reference from which many traditional families can be viewed.

DEVELOPMENTAL STAGES OF THE FAMILY

The first stage of family development is divided into two phases and is represented by the childless newly married couple. The initial phase begins at the time of marriage and consists of two persons (a dyad) who have made a major commitment to each other and therefore have the task of adjusting to living together as a married pair. This period of family life is filled with great stress as the two persons negotiate to effect a union while at the same time attempting to maintain their individuality. In other words these two individuals are learning to assume the roles of husband and wife. The divorce rate during this stage is very high, probably due to the shattering of the romantic illusion fostered during the preceding courtship period. The second phase of this stage commences with the wife's pregnancy. The family goal during this phase is to adjust to the pregnancy, which often means a change in affective focus. Prior to pregnancy both the husband and wife are focused on each other but during preg-

*Duvall, Evelyn M.: Family development, Philadelphia, 1962, J.B. Lippincott Co.

nancy the wife becomes increasingly self-absorbed as she emotionally prepares for the birth of the child. In addition the husband may feel an increase in responsibility, especially if the couple decides that the wife should leave an income-producing job.

The second stage of family development begins when the first child is born and generally is believed to last until this eldest child enters school. The major change experienced by the husband and wife is the expansion of their roles to include those of father and mother. The family unit is reorganized around the needs of infants and preschool children, which often require dramatic shifts in priorities and activities.

The third stage of family development begins when the eldest child enters school and ends when this child becomes an adolescent. If there are younger siblings, the family unit needs to reorganize to fit into the expanding world of school-aged children, while still meeting the needs of the preschoolers. Through the school-aged child the family is often confronted for the first time with societal values that may conflict with family values. The goal of this stage is for the family to protect school-aged children from undesirable influences while still enabling them to fit into the larger social world.

The fourth stage of a family's development begins when the oldest child becomes an adolescent. The family goal during this very tumultuous time is to loosen family ties to permit greater freedom and heavier responsibility of the members. This task is not easy because the children have a history of dependence on their parents and often overreact to their newfound independence, resulting in an increase rather than the desired decrease, in the control behaviors of the parents.

The fifth stage is referred to as the "launching" stage because it is during this time that the children are preparing to or are actually leaving home. This developmental task requires the reorganization of the family into an equalitarian unit as opposed to the earlier superior and subordinate structure. At this time the family needs to be able to release its members. It superficially appears that parents would have the most difficulty with this task, but it often is equally difficult for children to assume adult responsibility and leave the family to start their own family.

The next stage is termed the *postparental family* and is characterized by the parents having to subsume their parental roles into their marital roles. In other words, the father and mother are left with no children to parent and find themselves with only each other to relate to. This stage is commonly referred to as the "empty nest syndrome" and is successfully navigated only if the parents were able to satisfactorily maintain their marital relationship during the childbearing and childrearing years. During this stage parents often become grandparents, an event that requires once again learning a new role. Although the grandparent role has similarities to the parent role, it is fundamentally different because the ultimate responsibility for children rests with the parents, not the grandparents.

The last stage of family development is the retirement and postretirement years. During this time the couple prepares for the dissolution of the family by the death of one of the spouses. Couples who have satisfactorily achieved the earlier tasks and are able to view their families as satisfactory are able to thoughtfully prepare for this eventuality without undue anxiety.

THE CHANGING FAMILY

The structure, size, functions, and developmental stages of the family are undergoing many changes in today's society. For example, it is not uncommon for a family to consist of only one parent who is raising one or more children and fulfilling both roles of mother and father. Increasingly common are *blended* or *reconstituted families* that consist of a parent who had been previously married and has children. This parent is married to another parent who also has children from a previous marriage. Such a couple may also have children of their own so that the family's task in this instance is to "blend" together three different sets of children into a functional family structure.

Finally we are seeing an increase in the number of people who are joining together to form a family group based on mutual respect and common interests rather than for the purpose of procreation. These persons may or may not be related by blood or by law but tend to reside in the same household. The household concept, or living under the same roof, has been the criterion used by the U.S. Census Bureau to define a family. With the multiplicity of family structures apparent in the society this criterion may prove to be the most applicable. In any event, it is important for the nurse to extend her view of family beyond the traditional nuclear or extended family structure when dealing with individuals who do not live in these structures, if she is to accurately assess the individual's familial associations and dynamics. An example is the instance in which an adult woman was admitted to the hospital for surgery and was asked to supply the name of her next of kin. She responded by stating that her only blood relative lived at a great distance and was not involved in her day-to-day affairs, and that she preferred to have her housemate of 5 years listed as the person to be notified in an emergency. The admitting clerk replied that the person listed on the chart had to be related by blood or law. This situation reflects the legal and societal lag so often apparent in our society that put this woman in jeopardy by forcing her to either lie to get her needs met or to tell the truth but forego gratification of her needs—all at a time when she was already under the stress of ill health and impending surgery.

THE EFFECTIVE FAMILY*

The effective family is one that is able to facilitate the growth and development of its members while still maintaining cohesion as an identifiable system. This definition implies that the following patterns of behavior are characteristic of an effective family:

1. The family places the emotional, physical, and social needs of its members over other concerns, such as acquisition of possessions or status.
2. The family recognizes, values, and accommodates to differences among its members.
3. The family is sufficiently flexible so that changes stemming from within and outside the system can be accommodated without loss of family stability.
4. The family seeks and uses information from relevant outside sources, simultaneously maintaining its autonomy.
5. The family makes and carries out decisions, taking into accounts its goals and the age and experience of its members.

An effective family is not necessarily a family without problems. Rather, an effective family is one that has developed a structure and pattern of functioning that enables it to deal with its problems productively as they arise. Just as is true of individ-

*Adapted from Sedwick, Rae: Family mental health, St. Louis, 1981, The C.V. Mosby Co., pp. 20-24.

uals, families must learn these processes, and many authorities believe that helping young families to develop effective patterns of functioning is the crux of promoting mental health.

Most young people receive no preparation for establishing an effective family. Therefore they unconsciously perpetuate the only patterns of familial functioning they know—the patterns they experienced in their families of origin. If fortuitously such learned patterns of behavior are conducive to effective family functioning, effective families will perpetuate. If ineffective patterns are learned, the probability of perpetuating ineffective family patterns is greatly enhanced.

THE INEFFECTIVE FAMILY

Families that are unable to establish and maintain a structure and patterns of behavior conductive to effective functioning often show signs of continuous and irresolvable stress. Such stress may be manifested by the entire system as in instances where there is overt tension and hostility among members, or the stress may be focused on only one member who is covertly designated to assume and act out the family problems. In this instance the family member is often, although not always, a child. This phenomenon occurs because children are likely to be the most vulnerable since they are so highly dependent on the family and their behavioral patterns are less firmly entrenched. Bed-wetting, learning difficulties, antisocial behaviors, and profound fears in a child are all seen to be symptoms of an ineffective family.

It is beyond the scope of this text to discuss the many types of family dysfunction. The following discussion of child abuse is presented as an example of one increasingly common and very serious form of ineffective family functioning.

THE CHILD-ABUSING FAMILY

The incidence of reported child abuse appears to be dramatically increasing. However, accurate statistics are difficult to obtain because the phenomenon is poorly defined. Child abusers often go to extraordinary lengths to conceal their actions and friends, relatives, and health care workers are hesitant to get involved. Nevertheless, it is known that the neglect or abuse of children occurs often enough to be of major concern to the legal and health care professions.

Child abuse can range from violent, physical attacks that result in severe injury, to passive neglect that results in insidious malnutrition. Child abuse is not limited to physical maltreatment; it also includes emotional maltreatment such as continual yelling at and berating the child.

Children are the usual victims of family violence because they are relatively powerless and, until they reach adolescence are certainly physically weaker than adults. The pattern of the powerless becoming victims of violence is seen not only in child abuse but also in wife battering and the tyrannization of the elderly in their homes and on the street.

The concept of powerlessness includes not only physical weakness but also social subordination. Children, women and the elderly are all persons who traditionally have had less power in our society than has the young adult male. This situation is gradually changing. The values, needs, and rights of children, women, and the elderly are being recognized and becoming protected by law. These persons, therefore, are achieving a modicum of social power. Ironically some authorities believe that the very amelioration of this problem is contributing to its intensification, a phenomenon that is not socially unusual. In other words, individuals who have no power and do not assert themselves are often not overtly abused. An example is the benevolent plantation owner who had a patronizingly paternal attitude toward his compliant slaves. Once the slaves began to assert themselves, however, much more systematic and spontaneous abuse occurred. Likewise, as children, women, and the elderly achieve more power they are more likely to constitute a threat and therefore be abused more often.

Table 24-1 lists physical and behavioral indicators of child abuse and neglect. It should be noted that the laws of most states require that health care personnel report to legal authorities situations in which child abuse or maltreatment is suspected; most state laws do not require proof before reporting child abuse or maltreatment. After a report is made the child protective agency is responsible for the actual determination of the situation.

Many health care workers, including nurses are very hesitant to report incidents of suspected child abuse. Commonly expressed reservations include a fear of becoming involved in legal processes and a desire to protect the familial integrity. By not reporting suspected instances of child abuse the health care worker is not only *not* protecting the family, but is indirectly con-

TABLE 24-1   physical and behavioral indictors of child abuse and neglect*

type of abuse/neglect	physical indicators	behavioral indicators
Physical abuse	Unexplained bruises and welts: —on face, lips, mouth —on torso, back, buttocks, thighs —in various stages of healing —clustered, forming regular patterns —reflecting shape of article used to inflict (electric cord, belt buckle) —on several different surface areas —regularly appear after absence, weekend, or vacation Unexplained burns: —cigar, cigarette burns, especially on soles, palms, back, or buttocks —immersion burns (socklike, glovelike, doughnut shaped on buttocks or genitalia) —patterned like electric burner, iron, etc. —rope burns on arms, legs, neck, or torso —infected burns, indicating delay in seeking treatment Unexplained fractures/dislocations —to skull, nose, facial structure —in various stages of healing —multiple or spiral fractures Unexplained lacerations or abrasions: —to mouth, lips, gums, eyes —to external genitalia —in various stages of healing Bald patches on the scalp	Feels deserving of punishment Wary of adult contacts Apprehensive when other children cry Behavioral extremes: —aggressiveness —withdrawal Frightened of parents Afraid to go home Reports injury by parents Vacant or frozen stare Lies very still while surveying surroundings Will not cry when approached by examiner Responds to questions in monosyllables Inappropriate or precocious maturity Manipulative behavior to get attention Capable of only superficial relationships Indiscriminately seeks affection Poor self-concept
Physical neglect	Underweight, poor growth pattern, failure to thrive Consistent hunger, poor hygiene, inappropriate dress	Begging, stealing food Extended stays at school (early arrival and late departure) Rare attendance at school

*Heindl, Cathy, and others: The nurse's role in the prevention and treatment of child abuse and neglect. DHEW Publication No. (OHDS) 79-30202, Washington, D.C., 1979, U.S. Government Printing Office, p. 10.

TABLE 24-1 **physical and behavioral indictors of child abuse and neglect—cont'd**

type of abuse/neglect	physical indicators	behavioral indicators
	Consistent lack of supervision, especially in dangerous activities or for long periods	Constant fatigue, listlessness, or falling asleep in class
	Wasting of subcutaneous tissue	Inappropriate seeking of affection
	Unattended physical problems or medical needs	Assuming adult responsibilities and concerns
	Abandonment	Alcohol or drug abuse
	Abdominal distention	Delinquency (e.g., thefts)
	Bald patches on the scalp	States there is no caretaker
Sexual abuse	Difficulty in walking or sitting	Unwilling to change for gym or participate in physical education class
	Torn, stained, or bloody underclothing	Withdrawal, fantasy, or infantile behavior
	Pain, swelling, or itching in genital area	Bizarre, sophisticated, or unusual sexual behavior or knowledge
	Pain on urination	Poor peer relationships
	Bruises, bleeding, or lacerations in external genitalia, vaginal, or anal areas	Delinquent or runaway
	Vaginal/penile discharge	Reports sexual assault by caretaker
	Venereal disease, especially in preteens	Change in performance in school
	Poor sphincter tone	
	Pregnancy	
Emotional maltreatment	Speech disorders	Habit disorders (sucking, biting, rocking, etc.)
	Lags in physical development	Conduct/learning disorders (antisocial, destructive, etc.)
	Failure-to-thrive	Neurotic traits (sleep disorders, inhibition of play, unusual fearfulness)
	Hyperactive/disruptive behavior	Psychoneurotic reactions (hysteria, obsession, compulsion, phobias, hypochondria)
		Behavior extremes: —compliant, passive —aggressive, demanding
		Overly adaptive behavior: —inappropriately adult —inappropriately infantile
		Developmental lags (mental, emotional)
		Attempted suicide

**Dynamics
underlying child
abuse**

tributing to the perpetuation of physical and emotionally dangerous family patterns.

An understanding of the dynamics underlying child abuse includes societal, familial, and individual factors.

Societal factors. Dr. Harold Feldman, an expert on domestic
violence at Cornell University, believes the family violence is a
reflection of a society that endorses violence as a means of dealing with frustration and achieving goals. There has been a great
deal of publicity regarding the amount of violence on television
and in the movies. It is interesting to note that in our society a
movie is more likely to be rated "X" if it portrays explicit sexual
acts than if it depicts graphic details of a murder. More subtle
forms of violence are socially sanctioned by the national preoccupation with such sports as football and boxing. In this way
children learn that violent acts are socially acceptable outlets for
anger and frustration.

Familial factors. It is a well-known fact that child abusers are
people who have themselves been abused as children. Therefore
there is a multigenerational pattern of child abuse. In addition
many authorities believe that the nuclear family structure contributes to the incidence of child abuse. In this family structure
a small group of persons, the nuclear family, is often isolated
from other sources of concerned support. Therefore an intensity
of demands develops within the nuclear family, and there are few
outlets to meet these needs. This leads to increased tension that
may explode in the form of violence or neglect directed at the
most powerless member of the family—the child.

Individual factors. Whether or not ineffective family functioning will manifest itself by child abuse is largely determined by
the dynamics of the family members and how these interact with
each other. Table 24-2 lists behavorial indicators of abusive parents. These indicators, however, fail to reflect the very real human pain that many child-abusing parents experience. As previously stated, these individuals are most likely to have been
abused children themselves. Therefore they have many unmet
needs, are emotionally immature, and have limited control of
their impulses. Many abusing parents, especially mothers, unconsciously look to their child as a vehicle through which their own
needs can be met. When it becomes obvious that an infant or
young child takes more than it can give, these parents may react

with almost uncontrollable rage at once again being disappointed and deprived. In other words, these parents have many fundamental, unmet needs themselves that they look to their children to meet. When this need fulfillment is not forthcoming, they tend to react with violence, reflecting a primitive expression of frustration.

TABLE 24-2 behavioral indicators of abusive parents*

parents of abused children may

lack family supports such as friends, relatives, neighbors, and community groups; consistently fail to keep appointments, discourage social contact, and never participate in school activities or events

seem to trust no one

have a childhood history of abuse or neglect

be reluctant to give information about the child's injuries or condition. When questioned, are unable to explain or offer farfetched or contradictory explanations

respond inappropriately to the seriousness of the child's condition either by overreacting, seeming hostile or antagonistic when questioned even casually, or by underreacting, showing little concern or awareness and seeming more preoccupied with their own problems than those of the child

refuse to consent to diagnostic studies

fail or delay to take the child for medical care, for routine checkups, for optometric or dental care, or for treatment of injury or illness. In taking an injured child for medical care they may choose a different hospital or doctor each time

be overcritical of the child; seldom if ever discuss the child in positive terms

have unrealistic expectations of the child, expecting or demanding behavior that is beyond the child's years or ability

believe in the necessity of harsh punishment for children

seldom touch or look at the child; ignore the child's crying or react with impatience

keep the child confined, perhaps in a crib or playpen, for overlong periods of time

seem to lack understanding of children's physical, emotional, and psychological needs

appear to be misusing alcohol or drugs

be difficult or impossible to locate

appear to lack control or fear losing control

be of borderline intelligence, psychotic, psychopathic. While such diagnoses are the responsibility of mental health professionals, even the lay observer can note whether the parent seems intellectually capable of childrearing, exhibits generally irrational behavior, or seems excessively cruel and sadistic.

*Child abuse and neglect: vol 1, an overview of the problem; vol. 2, the problem and its management, DHEW Publication, Washington, D.C., 1975, U.S. Goverment Printing Office.

Why is it that one child in a family is consistently abused, while others develop unscathed? This question has no definitive answer, but some hypotheses can be stated. The abused child often has characteristics that set him apart from others in the family. These include birth order (youngest or oldest), physical characteristics (resembles paternal or maternal side of the family), particular skills or deficits, and identifiable personality characteristics (more or less intelligent, more or less assertive, likes solitary activities or activities involving others). In any event, the abused child seems to have particular significance not only to the parents but also to his siblings. The question arises as to why the abused child characteristically colludes with his family in concealing the events surrounding his injuries. Many social scientists believe the answer to this question lies in the fact that children so desperately need attention from significant adults that they are willing to submit to abuse if this appears to be the only way they can gain this attention. Family therapists postulate that the child knowingly assumes a role that is necessary for the survival of the family system. Regardless of why it occurs, it is well known that abused children block attempts to divulge the reality of the situation.

Role of the nurse   Because of the multifaceted dynamics operating in the ineffective family that abuses its children, treatment is very complex. Needless to say the physical needs of the injured or neglected child must be met before attempts are made to alter the family's pattern of functioning. During the time the child is receiving treatment the parents need a great deal of support and understanding. Health care personnel including nurses, often have great difficulty avoiding the tendency to blame one or both parents. This attitude, which may be conveyed overtly or covertly, is counterproductive, since it reinforces the guilt and sense of worthlessness the parents already feel. It also reflects a lack of understanding that family units function as a system where each member contributes to the function or dysfunction of the unit.

The treatment of choice for the abusive family, as for all ineffective families, is family therapy. As nurses become more educationally prepared, they increasingly become responsible for using this treatment modality.

FAMILY THERAPY

Family therapy as such is a relatively new treatment modality, although it has been unknowingly practiced in the past by the family physician and the public health nurse. These professional workers realized that the effectiveness of treatment of an individual was either enhanced or impeded by the attitudes of his family. In addition, these professionals often became quasi-family members and were consulted and included during family crises. With the explosion of medical knowledge and the increase in medical specialization, the intimate knowledge of the family history and dynamics became unknown to the physician. Simultaneously, public health nurses assumed a greater number of technical functions that consumed a larger part of their role, giving them less time to act as family confidants. Until recently it has seemed most expeditious of time and resources for the individual to be treated by professionals who were specialists. This approach has not only relegated the family to a position of second-class citizens but has deprived the individual of a valuable resource. Nowhere is this more dramatically illustrated than in the instance of emotional disorders.

The concept of family therapy is based on the belief that the family is a social system with its own characteristic structure and pattern of communication. Although this structure and communication pattern are certainly related to the personalities of the family members, they cannot be explained by a mere summation of the traits of the individuals who comprise the family. In other words, the family as a unit is seen as a system, and the family members as components of that system who influence it and are in turn influenced by it. If one accepts this concept, it becomes inappropriate to refer to one member as being emotionally ill without looking at the family constellation, which, it is believed, has sanctioned the deviant behavior of one member and in turn is affected by it. In other words, the behavior of the "sick" member serves a function within the family. This belief is supported by two observations. First it is not unusual for a person to be successfully treated for an emotional illness on an individual basis and for another member of the family to become ill, sometimes with very similar symptoms. This phenomenon suggests that the family structure and communication pattern, if they are to be maintained, require one member to be deviant. A second observation that supports the systems theory approach is the frequency with which family members bring one member for treatment with the statement that all is well within the family except for the stress-producing behavior of the one member. When that member is removed from the family, either through prolonged hospitalization or by geographical relocation, it is not uncommon for the family to enter into a state of acute disequilibrium that may manifest itself by such actions as divorce of the parents. This phenomenon is equally well documented in families in which a chronically physically ill person has died.

Lately there is a growing number of mental health professionals who believe that any attempt to treat individuals in isolation from their families is either futile or, if helpful to the individual is at the expense of the equilibrium of his family system. Proponents of family therapy maintain that major strides in the promotion of mental health and the prevention and treatment of mental illness will occur only when the needs of the individual are considered within the context of the family system, which still remains as the fundamental social unit of our society. Although this may seem an extreme view, there is no doubt that family therapy is the treatment of choice when the identified client is a child or adolescent, and this treatment modality should be used in other situations when possible.

The goals of family therapy are to assist in resolving pathological conflicts and anxiety, to strengthen the individual member against destructive forces both within himself and within the family environment, to strengthen the family against critical upsets, and to influence the orientation of the family identity and values toward health. When therapy commences the therapist assembles all family members, regardless of age and pays as much attention to their behavior with each other as to the content of what they say. For example, the husband and wife may vehemently state how emotionally close they are while at the same time sit as far as possible from each other. It is important for the therapist to avoid blaming one or the other member, and this pitfall will be avoided if the role of each member is seen in relation to the total family functioning. In one family therapy situation the identified client was a 20-year-old daughter who had made numerous suicidal attempts. This girl was hospitalized, and the entire family came to the hospital once a week for family therapy. The parents maintained that they had an unusually good relationship and could not understand why their daughter tormented them so with her life-threatening gestures. Several times during the course of therapy, their adolescent son took the risk of contradicting his parents by observing that the parents' relationship was highly tension-laden, at which point the daughter would begin crying. This behavior on her part diverted the participants' attention to her, and successfully prevented the parents from having to face, much less talk about, their differences. The therapist interpreted this behavior not as being sick, but rather as the daughter's role in maintaining the family equilibrium.

It is the prerogative of the family to determine their own destiny, and often the major role of the therapist is to comment on the interactional process as it is observed. Bringing this process to a level of consciousness allows the family to evaluate its purpose and outcome. If the family desires a change the therapist can be instrumental in modeling behaviors that can initiate such change.

Some family therapy sessions have been held in the home. As this trend develops it appears likely that the role of family therapist will become increasingly identified with the prepared psychiatric nurse, because she is comfortable in the role of family visitor, is knowledgeable about family dynamics, and is becoming skillful in family therapy.

CONJOINT THERAPY

Conjoint therapy usually refers to therapy in which marriage partners engage in a therapeutic endeavor with a therapist. The importance of this technique is supported not only by the well-being that can be attained by the marriage partners but also because these persons are seen by family theorists as the architects of the future family system. That is, treatment of the marital couple can have a profound effect on the promotion of mental health and prevention of mental illness of the growing family. Often it is found that couples who have marital conflict have incongruent expectations of each other, the most common being the expectation that each will have their dependency needs met by the other. When these expectations are simultaneously operationalized, both are disappointed. Frequently the mutual realization of these expectations moves the couple ahead to understand that both can have their needs met if they are willing to compromise. Several experts have written excellent texts about conjoint therapy, which the student is encouraged to read for additional information. Particularly recommended is *Conjoint Family Therapy* by Virginia Satir.

CONCLUDING STATEMENTS

1. The family is the most basic of all societal institutions, affecting and affected by the society.
2. Some family theorists believe that even when the nurse is dealing only with an individual it is impossible for the interaction not to affect and be affected by that individual's family. This view stems from the belief that the family is a system.
3. The extended family is a type of family structure seen in nonindustrial soceieties and consists of several generations living together.
4. The nuclear family is a type of family structure seen in industrialized societies and consists of two generations.
5. A family is traditionally defined as two or more people who are related by blood or legal ties, although an increasing number of nonrelated groups are identifying themselves as families.
6. The functions of the family include
   a. Regulation of sexual activity and reproduction
   b. Physical maintenance
   c. Protection
   d. Education and socialization
   e. Recreation
   f. Status conferring
   g. Affection giving
7. Traditional families progress through a series of developmental stages that are primarily related to role changes of their members.
8. The structure, size, functions, and developmental stages of the family are undergoing many changes in today's society. A common change is the blended or reconstituted family structure. It is important for the nurse to extend her view of the family beyond the traditional nuclear or extended family structure when dealing with individuals who do not live in these structures.
9. The effective family is one that is able to facilitate the growth

and development of its members while still maintaining cohesion as an identifiable system. This goal is achieved by patterns of behavior characteristic of effective families.

10. Most young people receive no preparation for establishing an effective family and therefore perpetuate the behavioral patterns they learned in their families of origin.

11. Ineffective families show signs of continuous and irresolvable stress manifested by either the entire system or by one of its members.

12. The child-abusing family is an increasingly common type of ineffective family.

13. Child abuse ranges from violent, physical attacks to passive neglect. Maltreatment may be physical or emotional.

14. Children are the usual victims of family violence because they are relatively powerless, a concept that implies not only physical weakness but also social subordination.

15. The laws of most states require that health care personnel report to legal authorities situations in which child abuse or maltreatment is suspected.

16. The dynamics underlying child abuse include societal, familial, and individual factors.

17. Child-abusing parents need a great deal of support and understanding that many health care workers find difficult to give.

18. Family therapy is the treatment of choice for child-abusing families as well as for all other ineffective families.

19. Family therapy is based on the belief that the behavior of any one family member affects and is affected by the entire family system. The family members are treated as a unit with the goal of assisting them to strengthen their identity so as to be better able to cope with both internal and external stressors.

20. Conjoint therapy usually involves only marital partners who are helped to become aware of their expectations of each other and of their marital relationship.

SUGGESTED SOURCES OF ADDITIONAL INFORMATION

Classical

Bowlby, John: Maternal care and mental health, ed. 2, World Health Organization Monograph Series No. 2, Geneva, 1965, World Health Organization.

Bulbuylan, Ann Agavni: The psychiatric nurse as family therapist, Perspect. Psychiatr. Care **7:**58-68, March-April, 1969.

Gerrish, Madalene J.: The family therapist is a nurse, Am. J. Nurs. **68:**320-323, 1968.

Getty, Cathleen, and Shannon, Anna M.: Nurses as co-therapists in a family-therapy setting, Perspect. Psychiatr. Care **5:**36-48, Jan.-Feb., 1967.

Hitchens, Emily Wurster: Denial: an identified theme in marital relationships of sex offenders, Perspect. Psychiatr. Care **10:**153-159, Oct.-Nov., 1972.

Rohde, Ildaura Murillo: The nurse as a family therapist, Nurs. Outlook **16:**49-52, May, 1968.

Sager, Clifford J., and Kaplan, Helen S., editors: Progress in group and family therapy, New York, 1972, Brunner/Mazel, Inc.

Satir, Virginia: Conjoint family therapy, ed. 2, Palo Alto, Calif., 1967, Science and Behavior Books, Inc.

Smith, Lois Elaine, and Mills, Bernadine L.: Intervention techniques and unhealthy family patterns, Perspect. Psychiatr. Care **7:**112-119, May-June, 1969.

Contemporary

Auerbach, Stevanne: Confronting the childcare crisis, Boston, 1980, Beacon Press.

Barash, Dorothy A.: Dynamics of the pathological family system, Perspect. Psychiatr. Care **17**(1):17-24, Jan.-Feb., 1979.

Battered women: issues of public policy, Washington, D.C., 1978, U.S. Commission on Civil Rights.

Beavers, W. Robert: Psychotherapy and growth: a family systems perspective, New York, 1970, Brunner/Mazel, Inc.

Bowlby, John: Loss, New York, 1980, Basic Books, Inc., Publishers.

Braxton, Earl T.: Structuring the black family for survival and growth, Perspect. Psychiatr. Care **14**(4):165-173, 1976.

Bumagin, Victoria E., and Hirn, Kathryn F.: Aging is a family affair, New York, 1980, Lippincott & Crowell.

Carter, Elizabeth A., and Orfanidis, Monica M.: The family life cycle: a framework for family therapy, New York, 1980, Halsted Press.

Child abuse and neglect: vol. 1, an overview of the problem, DHEW Publication, Washington, D.C., 1975, U.S. Government Printing Office.

Child abuse and neglect: vol. 2, the problem and its management, DHEW Publication, Washington, D.C., 1975, U.S. Government Printing Office.

Collison, Carol, and Futrell, Jo Ann: Family therapy for the single-parent family system, J. Psychosoc. Nurs. Ment. Health Serv. **20:**16-20, July, 1982.

Danziger, Sharon: Major treatment issues and techniques in family therapy with the borderline adolescent, J. Psychosoc. Nurs. Ment. Health Serv. **20:**27-34, Jan., 1982.

deChesnay, Mary: Father-daughter incest, J. Psychosoc. Nurs. Ment. Health Serv. **22:**24-31, Sept., 1984.

deYoung, Mary: Incest victims and offenders: myths and realities, J. Psychosoc. Nurs. Ment. Health Serv. **19:**37-39, Oct., 1981.

Duffy, Mary: When a woman heads the household, Nurs. Outlook **30:**468-473, Sept./Oct., 1982.

Erickson, G.D., and Hogan, T.P., editors: Family therapy: introduction to theory and technique, Monterey, Calif., 1972, Brooks/Cole Publishing Co.

Fife, Betsy: Childhood cancer is a family crisis, J. Psychosoc. Nurs. Ment. Health Serv. **18:**29-34, Oct., 1980.

Fife, Betsy, and Gant, Barbara: The resolution of school phobia through family therapy, J. Psychosoc. Nurs. Ment. Health Serv. **18:**13-16, Feb., 1980.

Fleming, Jennifer Baker: Stopping wife abuse, Garden City, N.Y., 1979, Anchor Press.

Fontana, Vincent J., and Esther Rovison: A multidisciplinary approach to the treatment of child abuse, Pediatrics **57**(5):760-764, May, 1979.

Friedman, Allison L., Juntti, M. Jeanette, and Scoblic, Mary A.: Nursing responsibility in child abuse, Nursing Forum **15**(1):95-112, 1976.

Geiser, Robert L.: The sexual abuse of children, Boston, 1980, Beacon Press.

Gemmill, Francine: A family approach to the battered woman, J. Psychosoc. Nurs. Ment. Health Serv. **20:**22-39, Sept., 1982.

Gerace, Laina: Phenomenon of early engagement in family therapy, J. Psychosoc. Nurs. Ment. Health Serv. **19:**25-28, April, 1981.

Grossman, J., Pozanski, E., and Bonegas, M.: Lunch: time to study family interactions, J. Psychosoc. Nurs. Ment. Health Serv. **21:**19-23, July, 1983.

Gunderson, Sandra S.: Advocacy in family therapy, J. Psychosoc. Nurs. Ment. Health Serv. **18:**24-28, Sept., 1980.

Haller, Linda Lacey: Family systems theory in psychiatric intervention, Am. J. Nurs. **74:**462-463, 1974.

Heindl, Cathy, and others: The nurse's role in the prevention and treatment of child abuse and neglect, DHEW Publication No. (OHDS) 79-30202, Washington, D.C., 1979, U.S. Government Printing Office.

Hickey, Brian: Bowen's family projection process and Tennessee William's "The Glass Menagerie," Perspect. Psychiatr. Care **22:**26-32, Jan.-March, 1984.

Hill, Martha: When the patient is the family, Am. J. Nurs. **81:**536-538, 1981.

Holfing, Charles K., and Lewis, Jerry M., editors: The family: evaluation and treatment, New York, 1980, Brunne/Mazel, Inc.

Jones, Susan, and Dimond, Margaret: Family theory and family therapy models: comparative review with implications for nursing practice, J. Psychosoc. Nurs. Ment. Health Serv. **20:**12-19, Oct., 1982.

Kjervik, Diane: The contemporary American family: romanticism vs.

reality, J. Psychosoc. Nurs. Ment. Health Serv. **20:**9-12, March, 1982.

Lantz, James, and Treece, Nancy: Identity operations and family treatment, J. Psychosoc. Nurs. Ment. Health Serv. **20:**20-23, Oct., 1982.

Leaman, Karen: Ambulatory nursing: recognizing and helping the abused child, Nursing (Horsham) **9**(2):64-67, Feb., 1979.

Lewis, Jerry, et al.: No single thread: psychological health in family systems, New York, 1980, Brunner/Mazel, Inc.

Lieske, Anna M.: Incest: an overview, Perspect. Psychiatr. Care **19:**59-63, March/April, 1981.

Light, Nada: Counterpoint: family treatment for the disturbed child? Perspect. Psychiatr. Care **19:**79-83, March-April, 1981.

List, Julie Autumn: The day the loving stopped, New York, 1980, Seaview Books.

Lusky, Karen F.: A death in the family, Perspect. Psychiatr. Care **21:**28-30, Jan.-March, 1983.

McDermott, John F.: Raising Cain—and Abel, too, New York, 1980, Peter H. Wyden/Publisher.

McKeel, Nancy L.: Child abuse can be prevented, Am. J. Nurs. **78:**1478-1482, Sept., 1978.

Miller, Alice: Prisoners of childhood, New York, 1980, Basic Books, Inc., Publishers.

Miller, Jean: Cognitive dissonance in modifying families' perceptions, Am. J. Nurs. **74:**1468-1470, 1974.

Miller, Virginia, and Mansfield, Elaine: Family therapy for the multiple incest family, J. Psychosoc. Nurs. Ment. Health Serv. **19:**29-32, April, 1984.

Moore, Judith Ann, and Wallen, Andrea: The intake decision—individual psychotherapy or family therapy? In Kneisl, Carol Ren, and Wilson, Holly Skodol, editors: Current perspectives in psychiatric nursing: issues and trends, vol. 2, St. Louis, 1978, The C.V. Mosby Co.

Moore, Judith, and Coulman, Mary: Anorexia nervosa: the patient, her family and key family therapy in interventions, J. Psychosoc. Nurs. Ment. Health Serv. **19:**9-14, May, 1981.

Napier, Augustus, Y., and Whitaker, Carl: The family crucible, New York, 1980, Harper & Row, Publishers.

Nix, Helen: Why parents anonymous? J. Psychosoc. Nurs. Ment. Health Serv. **18:**23-28, Oct., 1980.

Northouse, Laurel L.: Who supports the support system? J. Psychosoc. Nurs. Ment. Health Serv. **18:**11-15, May, 1980.

Olson, Robert J.: Index of suspicion: screening for child abusers, Am. J. Nurs. **76:**108-110, 1976.

Padberg, Joan: Bargaining to improve communications in conjoint family therapy, Perspect. Psychiatr. Care **75:**68-75, April-June, 1975.

Palermo, Eleanor: Remarriage: parental perceptions of step-relations with children and adolescents, J. Psychosoc. Nurs. Ment. Health Serv. **18:**9-13, April, 1980.

Pincus, Lily, and Dare, Christopher: Secrets in the family, New York, 1980, Harper & Row, Publishers.

Rapoport, Robert and Rhona, and Bumstead, Janice, editors: Working couples, New York, 1980, Harper & Row, Publishers.

Reuveni, Uri: Networking families in crisis, New York, 1979, Human Sciences Press.

Rubinelli, Jackie: Incest: it's time we face reality, J. Psychosoc. Nurs. Ment. Health Serv. **18:**17-18, April, 1980.

Scharer, Kathleen M.: Rescue fantasies: professional impediments in working with abused families, Am. J. Nurs. **78:**1483-1444, 1978.

Sedgwick, Rae: Family mental health: theory and practice, St. Louis, 1981, The C.V. Mosby Co.

Shapshay, Ruth, and Vines, Diane W.: Father-daughter incest: detection of cases, J. Psychosoc. Nurs. Ment. Health Serv. **20:**23-26, Jan., 1982.

Shaw, Dale, et al.: Multiple impact therapy: University of Texas Medical Branch in Galveston, Am. J. Nurs. **77:**246-248, Feb., 1977.

Sideleau, Barbara F.: Point: Family treatment for the disturbed child? Perspect. Psychiatr. Care **19:**78-86, March-April, 1981.

Smoyak, Shirley, editor: The psychiatric nurse as a family therapist, New York, 1975, John Wiley & Sons, Inc.

Starkey, P.: Genograms: a guide to understanding one's own family system, Perspect. Psychiatr. Care **19:**164-173, Sept.-Dec., 1982.

Steiner, Patricia: The well child and the hospitalized disabled sibling, J. Psychosoc. Nurs. Ment. Health Serv. **22:**23-26, March, 1984.

Stern, Phyllis N.: Conflicting family culture: an impediment to integration in stepfather families, J. Psychosoc. Nurs. Ment. Health Serv. **20:**27-33, Oct., 1982.

Swanson, Ardes, and Hurley, Patricia: Family systems: values and value conflicts, J. Psychosoc. Nurs. Ment. Health Serv. **21:**24-30, July, 1983.

Tamex, Eloisa: Familism, machismo and child rearing practices among Mexican Americans, J. Psychosoc. Nurs. Ment. Health Serv. **19:**21-25, Sept., 1981.

Taylor, John: The hyperactive child and the family: the complete what-to-do handbook, New York, 1980, Everest House.

Tousley, Martha: The use of family therapy in terminal illness and death, J. Psychosoc. Nurs. Ment. Health Serv. **20:**17-22, Jan., 1982.

Walker, Lenore: The battered woman, New York, 1980, Harper & Row, Publishers.

Wallerstein, Judith S., and Kelly, Joan Berlin: Surviving the breakup, New York, 1980, Basic Books, Inc., Publishers.

Weil, Susan: The unspoken needs of families during high-risk pregnancies, Am. J. Nurs. **81:**2047-2049, 1981.

Weiss, Robert S.: Going it alone, New York, 1980, Basic Books, Inc., Publishers.

Weiss, Robert S.: Marital separation, New York, 1980, Basic Books, Inc., Publishers.

Whall, A.: Nursing theory and the assessment of families, J. Psychosoc. Nurs. Ment. Health Serv. **19:**30-36, Jan., 1981.

White, Jane: Bulimia: utilizing individual and family therapy, J. Psychosoc. Nurs. Ment. Health Serv. **22:**22-28, April, 1984.

Of particular interest

Minuchin, S.: Families and family therapy, Cambridge Mass., 1974, Harvard University Press.

Structural family therapy is described in this important text. Theory is highlighted throughout by relevant clinical examples.

Smoyak, S.: Family therapy. In Psychiatric nursing 1946 to 1974: a report on the state of the art, New York, 1975, American Journal of Nursing Co.

This extensive literature review outlines the role of the nurse in family therapies as it has developed historically.

section VI

legal and other issues affecting psychiatric nursing practice

chapter twenty-five

impact of the law on the current practice of psychiatric nursing

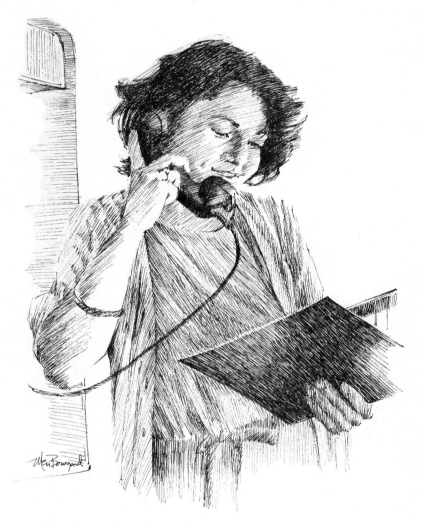

Yes, Mr. Benzel's commitment papers are in order.

**LEARNING
OBJECTIVES**

After studying this
chapter the student
will be able to:

1 Differentiate between voluntary and involuntary admission for the treatment of mental illness.

2 Describe the usual procedure for involuntary admission.

3 Discuss the following client rights:
   a. The right to habeas corpus.
   b. The right to treatment.
   c. The right to informed consent.
   d. The right to confidentiality—privacy.
   e. The right to an independent psychiatric examination.
   f. The right to refuse treatment.
   g. The right to least restrictive treatment.

4 Discuss the professional accountability of the nurse as defined by law.

5 Discuss the medical speciality of forensic psychiatry.

Psychiatric nursing and the law both are primarily concerned with the behavior of human beings. Psychiatric nursing is concerned with assisting individuals, families, and community groups to achieve satisfying and productive patterns of living. The law provides rules for behavioral conduct to facilitate orderly social functioning while simultaneously protecting the rights of the individual. Thus psychiatric nursing and the law affect each other greatly. The nurse can practice effectively only if she is knowledgeable about the rudimentary principles of the law that concern the mentally ill, since she is accountable for providing care that is not only clinically sound but also protects both the society and the client. Many authorities believe that the nurse can best fulfill this responsibility by assuming the role of client advocate. Thorner* states that the primary responsibility of the client advocate is to assist the client to learn about his rights and to protect and assert those rights within the health care system.

This chapter addresses those legal issues most likely to be encountered in the practice of psychiatric nursing in the hope that the nurse can satisfactorily fulfill the client advocate role.

*Thorner, Nancy: Nurses violate their patients' rights, J. Psychiatr. Nurs. **14**(1):7-12, Jan., 1976.

METHODS OF PSYCHIATRIC ADMISSION

The detention of persons considered to be mentally ill is permitted by law although the specifics of the law differ from state to state. However, all states assume the responsibility of segregating from society those persons whom psychiatrists deem dangerous or incompetent because of mental illness.

In 1953 the United States Public Health Service published the Draft Act Governing Hospitalization of the Mentally Ill. The following distinctions were suggested:

1. Voluntary admission is to be characterized by the individual's admission and discharge via his own signature.
2. Involuntary admission is undertaken by someone other than the client.

The least restrictive manner of obtaining treatment for mental illness is voluntary admission. Since many mentally ill individuals lack insight concerning their behavior and will not seek hospitalization of their own will, voluntary hospitalization is not always possible. The nurse must realize that it is a combination of overt behaviors and legal status, not a diagnostic category, that determines whether an individual can be treated voluntarily or involuntarily. Suicidal, violent, acute psychotic, and antisocial behaviors in persons unwilling to be treated are the usual reasons for a person to be involuntarily admitted to a psychiatric treatment center.

Two types of involuntary admissions result in commitment. One is an *emergency commitment* for observation. The length of this hospitalization is limited, usually for 10 to 60 days. The other type of commitment is called *indefinite* or *regular* commitment and extends for an unspecified period of time, usually subject to periodic judicial review. *Criminal commitment* is a form of indefinite commitment allowing involuntary hospitalization of persons charged with crimes who are awaiting trial or who have been acquitted of a crime by reason of insanity.

Generally only state facilities and some private psychiatric institutions admit persons on an involuntary status. Psychiatric units in general hospitals usually accept only persons who voluntarily choose to be treated. These units have often excluded individuals who have such poor impulse control that attempts to treat them on an unlocked unit would be dangerous for them and others. Such an admission policy permits treatment to be adapted to the needs of a select client population, defined largely on behavioral grounds and on the basis of willingness to accept treatment and hospitalization.

There is no uniformity of commitment methods among the states, but no one can be deprived of his liberty without due process of law. In general commitment proceedings consist of (1) application, (2) examination, (3) determination, and (4) detention if indicated. The action is usually initiated by relatives or friends, although any legally appointed officer of the law, members of charitable organizations, a public health official, or a private citizen may make the application, which will bring the matter to the attention of the proper court. In most states the court that settles matters of psychiatric commitment is the common pleas court or the probate court. Here the application is submitted, statements by interested parties are heard under oath, and all available information about the individual and his behavior is recorded.

Frequently the application must be accompanied by the certificates of one or more physicians or the judge may appoint one or two physicians to conduct a psychiatric examination. Some states require that at least one physician must be a psychiatrist. The testimony of lay witnesses and of the examining physicians must be sufficient to convince a judge or jury that the person in question is potentially dangerous to himself or others and needs to be segregated and treated. If the court finds that the need for hospitalization exists, the individual is generally committed to a publicly supported psychiatric treatment center.

The issue of commitment is more than simply a legal and psychiatric question. Ideally, it is an issue of freedom of choice. Each nurse must decide whether to take a stand for or against commitment. It is imperative that nurses know and understand the commitment procedures in the states in which they practice. Furthermore they must work for the necessary legislative amendments that would facilitate appropriate reforms so as to fulfill the dictum *primum nil nocere*—we must minimize harm.

CLIENTS' RIGHTS

A right is the enjoyment of a privilege that is secured by law to a person. Mentally ill persons who are hospitalized may experience a double limitation on their rights—one created by the organization of the hospital system and the other created by their illness. While the individual's illness may limit him to some extent the prejudging of his competency by the staff may be a greater obstacle to his exercising his rights. For example, a simple request to make a telephone call to his home is subject to interpretation, evaluation, and possible denial if it is not deemed to be in the best interest of the client and the hospital organization. Thus a tension exists in all psychiatric institutions between the client's need to exercise his civil rights and the hospital's need to provide care in an effective and efficient manner. When the hospital's organizational needs take precedence over the client's treatment needs or his civil rights, dehumanization, frustration, resignation, and despair occur.

If it is proved that the individual is incapable of conducting his affairs a guardian may be appointed by the court or by state authorities to protect the individual's rights and property. In some states this property guardian is called a conservator. If the amount of the client's property warrants the expense of guardianship or if business involving such property must be transacted, the guardian's responsibilities are not trivial. A guardian is one who has direct responsibility for the individual's personal welfare. He is generally a near relative. He cannot confine the individual in an institution without permission or approval of the court but can dictate, within certain limits, the nature of the treatment and can sign a permit for a major operation. He may also have custody of the minor children of the individual if the other parent is absent or incapable of accepting this responsibility.

The wife or husband of a client rather than the parents is regarded as the natural guardian. Every guardian must give bond for the proper performance of his duties. At regular intervals the guardian is required to make an accounting of expenses and income. His first consideration must be the comfort of the client. The guardian is required to protect the client's welfare judiciously.

The law has defined certain rules for the control of human conduct, including protection from injury-producing situations. These rules have been developed from rights that pertain to each individual and may not be violated without legal repercussion, unless the individual consents to their invasion. The first 10 amendments to the U.S. Constitution, adopted in 1791, deal with human rights. Some of the rights included in these amendments are the freedom of speech, the right of protection from unreasonable search and seizure, the right to a speedy trial, and the right to due process of law before being denied life, liberty, or property.

A serious loss of civil rights was often the consequence of involuntary commitment to a psychiatric hospital. As a result in many states the committed person was not able to make valid contracts, vote, marry, or divorce. However, in almost all legal jurisdictions legally committed individuals presently retain their constitutional and human rights, particularly those pertaining to their person, property, and civil liberties. Various rights have been listed in recent legislation, such as the following:

1. The right to keep clothing and personal effects
2. The right to communicate by telephone, to correspond, and to visit with persons outside the institution
3. The right to vote
4. The right to religious freedom
5. The right to enter contractual relationships
6. The right to make purchases
7. The right to make wills
8. The right to education
9. The right to habeas corpus
10. The right to be employed
11. The right to independent psychiatric examinations
12. The right to civil service status
13. The right to marry
14. The right to sue and to be sued
15. The right to retain licenses or permits established by law
16. The right not to be subjected to unnecessary mechanical restraint

In 1973 the American Hospital Association published a Patient's Bill of Rights (see Appendix D). The rights of clients are only as secure as the dedication of nurses and physicians who have the authority to protect them. These professionals must realize that most judges believe that personal freedom takes priority over endeavors to promote mental health that limit this freedom.

In 1976 the American Nurses' Association (ANA) developed a Code for Nurses (see Appendix C). The code deals with issues of ethical nursing conduct. In developing the code the ANA recognized that the recipients of health care have basic rights that must not be intruded on by those who provide service. It is the responsibility of the nurse to recognize and respect the client's dignity as a human being by protecting his rights.

In 1977 the President's Commission on Mental Health recommended that each state have a bill of rights for all mentally ill individuals. A copy of these rights must be displayed in all psychiatric settings, be given to each client using the facilities, and be explained in an easily understandable manner.

Statements regarding clients' rights have been developed because of judicial disillusionment with the basic assumptions underlying the way mental health professionals have traditionally dealt with mentally ill individuals. It is imperative that judges and legislators continually reexamine fundamental assumptions that have gone unchallenged throughout the years. However, it is important to recognize that the mere enactment of legislation designed to protect clients' rights does not ensure enforcement. Nurses seeking employment in psychiatric institutions must be certain that these facilities have the proper internal structure to protect the client's rights. Facilities with no internal structure to enforce clients' rights are in a vulnerable position because clients may be forced to go outside the institution, possibly to court, to see that their rights are protected.

The right to habeas corpus. The object of the right to habeas corpus is to ensure the speedy release of any individual who claims that he is being deprived of his liberty and being detained illegally. This fundamental right has not always been respected. Kenneth Donaldson, a client in a civil commitment case decided by the Supreme Court, was refused writs of habeas corpus 18 times during his 15 years of hospitalization before he finally won his chance to have a court hear his case.

The right to treatment. In 1960 Morton Birnbaum advocated the enforcement and recognition of the legal right of a mentally ill individual hospitalized in a public psychiatric institution to adequate medical treatment for psychiatric illness. Adequate treatment for the institutionalized mentally ill and mentally retarded is a constitutional right. The U.S. Second Federal Appeals Court and the Alabama Federal District Court have elaborated the following legal doctrines: (1) persons in custody for mental illness have a right to treatment, (2) they may not be held without treatment, and (3) treatment can be legally defined.

In 1971 the guardians of civily committed patients and some employees of Bryce State Mental Hospital filed a class action suit against the Commissioner of Mental Health, members of the Alabama Mental Health Board, and others *(Wyatt vs Stickney)*. The defendants were charged with providing inadequate treatment to approximately 5000 mentally ill persons. The court based its decision on the constitutional guarantee of a right to treatment. In 1972 the court issued an order that detailed criteria for adequate treatment: (1) a humane psychological and physical environment, (2) qualified staff in sufficient numbers to administer adequate treatment, and (3) individualized treatment plans.

The right to informed consent. If clients consent to treatment, their consent must be informed by staff explanation. It is important to understand what consent means. For a consent to be valid it must be based on adequate knowledge and information and must be given by a person who has the legal capacity to consent. Furthermore it must be voluntarily given. A rapidly growing mental health doctrine requires that clients be given specific and adequate information about the proposed treatment procedure. This is to include the administration of the treatment, its probability of success or failure, its risks and side effects, alternative treatment procedures, and the probable consequences of not receiving treatment.

It is the duty of the mental health professional to provide the necessary information whether or not the client requests it. The precise information given will depend on the nature, severity, and consequences of the proposed treatment. The mental health professional misleads the client when the beneficial effects of a treatment are exaggerated, while the dangers of the treatment are minimized or withheld. If the client is injured the mental health professional could be held responsible via malpractice or negligence claims.

The right of confidentiality-privacy. Confidentiality and privacy of information about the client must be respected at all times. The frequent necessity to exchange information about the client between health care centers does not alter the legal requirements to protect the client's privacy. The individual revealing information about the client's condition without authorization could be subject to legal difficulties. A lawsuit for invasion of privacy, liability, or slander is possible, depending on the facts of the situation and the type of information revealed.

Statutes that pertain to the confidentiality of psychiatric hospital records vary greatly among the states. Some statutes only prohibit disclosure of information about the client's diagnosis and treatment while others prohibit disclosure of the fact of hospitalization. Most statutes permit disclosure to private physicians, welfare officials, police, and insurance companies. Some may permit disclosure to prospective employers. Other statutes prohibit disclosure to almost everyone unless the person consents to disclosure.

The client should be told of the need to share information with other persons and agencies. He should be asked to sign the appropriate consent form.

Some states consider mental health professional-client communication, including nurse-client communication, as privileged. Four criteria are used for judging whether communication is privileged:

1. The communication is given with confidence in its nondisclosure.
2. Confidentiality is essential to the maintenance of the relationship.
3. The relationship is one that in the opinion of the community ought to be zealously fostered.
4. The injury that would result to the relationship by disclosure of the communication is greater than the benefit gained in winning litigation.

The unnecessary disclosure of confidential information is considered improper by law. A breach of confidence is considered to be the discussion of the client's confidential information with a third party. This type of unlawful disclosure may provide the client with a cause for action against the party revealing such information.

The right to an independent psychiatric examination. Fairness or due process requires that a client have an opportunity to secure a psychiatric examination by a physician of his choice. The provision of this independent judgment in commitment proceedings is designed to protect the client from the judgment of mental health professionals appointed by the court who may have motivations other than the client's interests. If the state is allowed to use such testimony, the client should have the same right. Furthermore the constitutional right to present witnesses may also necessitate that clients be allowed to choose expert witnesses. Some authorities believe that the state should provide the client with sufficient funds to retain at least one expert witness.

The right to refuse treatment. An important basis of the right to refuse treatment is the constitutional right to privacy and personal autonomy. As long as the public health, safety, or morals remain unharmed, the courts will respect a client's decision to refuse treatment. Ford* states that "The constitutional origins of the right to refuse medication stem from a long-standing recognition by the courts that each person has a strong interest in being free from nonconsensual invasion of his bodily integrity. . . ."

In 1976 the Third Circuit Court of Appeals found at least three constitutional deprivations that may accompany the involuntary administration of medication *(Scott vs Plante)*. The first involves the involuntary administration of psychotropic drugs, which affect mental processes and which may interfere with a person's First Amendment rights to freedom of speech and association.

The second deprivation incurred when medication is administered against the client's will is the violation of his right to consent to medical treatment. In the third, the court considered that the administration of involuntary medication may raise an Eighth Amendment issue concerning cruel and unusual punishment. The nurse must be knowledgable about these issues before forcefully administering medication that the client refuses. The consequence of such an action on the nurse's part could result in a charge of assault.

The right to least restrictive treatment. During his hospital stay the client may become violent and the hospital is obliged to control him so that he does not harm others or himself. If a delirious postoperative patient were left unattended by an open window and jumped from it the hospital would be considered negligent.

However, the right to restrain a client is a right limited only

---

*Ford, Maurice D.: The psychiatrist's double bind: the right to refuse medication, Am. J. Psychiatry **137**(3):332-339, March, 1980.

to the duration of real necessity. Although no one would dispute the right of hospital personnel to prevent a delirious individual from pulling out a catheter in most situations the hospital personnel cannot interfere with the actions of a client. If, for example, he shouts obscenities but is not a threat to himself or others, hospital personnel cannot tie him down or lock him up. To commit such an act invites a suit for false imprisonment.

Some state laws have specified the type of physical restraints that may be used, including the consistency of the actual material from which the restraint is made. Nurses must be mindful of such regulations. The restraint need not be physical; threats of force are sufficient cause for legal action. One who is physically restrained may have cause to file an action for battery. Alternatives for restraining clients must be considered. One such alternative is the provision of constant observation by nursing personnel. Nurses must also be aware that understaffing is not a suitable justification for the use of chemical or physical restraints. The issue of safety is the primary concern.

PROFESSIONAL ACCOUNTABILITY

Creighton* defines negligence as the omission to do something that a reasonable person guided by ordinary considerations that regulate human affairs would do, and the commission of an act as doing something that a wise and reasonable person would not do. Nursing malpractice has been defined by a California court as the nurse's neglect to apply a degree of learning and skill in treating and caring for a client, that is customarily practiced in caring for and treating the sick. This definition also includes acting outside the realm of authorized nursing practice.

A *tort* is a legal wrong, injury, or damage committed on a person or property independent of a contract. A *contract* is an agreement between two or more parties, although not every agreement is a contract. In general, moral agreements, agreements of conscience, or agreements involving social obligations are not classified as contracts.

When an individual becomes a psychiatric patient he automatically contracts with licensed health care personnel, includ-

*Creighton, Helen: Law every nurse should know, Philadelphia, 1981, W.B. Saunders Co.

ing the nurse, for treatment. In such a contract both parties implicitly agree that the nurse will provide reasonable and prudent care for the client.

If this contract is violated the client may initiate action to obtain a remedy for an injury to his rights. In this instance the client is referred to as the *plaintiff*. The nurse, or *defendant*, is then required to answer and defend her action or be judged by default. A nurse may be a defendant in a negligent tort. Under the law of negligent tort, the plantiff must prove the following:

1. A legal duty of care existed.
2. The nurse performed her duty negligently.
3. Damages were suffered by him as a result.
4. The damages were substantial.

The majority of lawsuits in psychiatric nursing involve negligence in the observation of suicidal precautions, assistance in the administration of electroconvulsive therapy, and the reporting of information or lack of such reporting in regard to medications.

COMMUNITY ACCOUNTABILITY

By providing rules of behavioral conduct to facilitate orderly social functioning, the law not only protects the individual from society but also society from the individual. Forensic psychiatry, which is a specialty within psychiatry, is involved in the criminal justice system. Forensic psychiatrists are concerned with determinations of dangerousness, mental incompetency, and insanity.

Dangerousness

The body of law dealing with various crimes and their legal penalties, the Model Penal Code, encourages extended sentences for those persons deemed to be dangerous. Numerous legal definitions of dangerousness have been used for the care and treatment of offenders. Rubin* believes that if fear of bodily harm from violent behavior could be reduced by being able to define, predict, and modify such behavior, the quality of life in the United States would be greatly improved.

To be judged dangerous the Moral Penal Code requires that a psychiatrist demonstrate that a person:

1. Possesses a gravely abnormal mental illness.
2. Has engaged in criminal conduct characterized by a pat-

*Rubin, Bernard: Psychiatry and the law. In Arieti, Silvano, editor: American handbook of psychiatry, vol. 5, New York, 1974, Basic Books, Inc., Publishers.

tern of repetitive behavior or by persistent aggressive behavior with indifference to consequences.

3. Is a serious danger to others as a result of the two above conditions.

Sentences of up to 25 years may be imposed on a number of special categories of persons, including the dangerous, mentally ill offender. This category requires the demonstration of the following:

1. The offender possesses a mental illness.
2. Such a mental condition makes the offender a serious danger to others' safety.
3. The offender committed a major crime such as murder, treason, a felony, or other crime as an instance of aggressive behavior without heed to the consequences.

It is exceedingly difficult to define and predict dangerousness. The psychiatrist is often in a dilemma when he must determine dangerousness since the process of making such a determination is often contrary to the physician-client relationship.

The doctrine of mental incompetency

Mental incompetency exists when the defendant, because of mental illness or other reasons does not understand the object and nature of the proceedings against him. It may also mean that the defendant cannot comprehend his own condition in relation to the proceedings or for some other reason is unable to assist his lawyer in his own defense. If the defendant is deemed incompetent, all criminal proceedings are suspended and the state is denied the power to proceed against him. To prosecute an incompetent is to deny his right to due process of law. Psychiatrists are often given the responsibility for making decisions regarding competency.

The defense of insanity

In the seventeenth century, Sir Matthew Hale, Chief Justice of the Court of King's Bench, wrote, "Human beings are naturally endowed with these two great faculties, understanding and liberty of will. . . . The consent of the will is that which renders human actions commendable or culpable. . . ."* Hale elaborated that the choice of will or liberty presupposes an act of under-

*Rubin, Bernard: Psychiatry and the law. In Aireti, Silvano, editor: American handbook of psychiatry, vol. 5, New York, 1974, Basic Books, Inc., Publishers, p. 872.

standing to the knowledge of a thing or an action chosen by the will. Where there is a total defect in understanding there is no free act of will. As a result judges began to charge juries that a defendant was not to be held responsible for his actions unless he had the capacity to distinguish evil from good.

In May 1800, believing that he was commanded by God to sacrifice himself for the world's salvation, Manes Hatfield fired a shot at George III. Hatfield's counsel argued that although the defendant was not mentally ill, his delusion was truly characteristic of mental illness. The trial was stopped and the jury returned a verdict of not guilty by reason of insanity. In 1843 Daniel M'Naghten shot Daniel Drummond, Secretary to Prime Minister Robert Peel. The M'Naghten rule, a test of the defendant's knowledge of right and wrong, was developed as a result of the arguments and testimony in this case.

Most American jurisdictions accepted the M'Naghten rule and began to supplement it with the "irresistible impulse test." This test states that the defendant must have had a mental disease that kept him from controlling his behavior. In 1962 the American Law Institute developed the Model Penal Code, which states that "a person is not responsible for criminal conduct if at the time of such conduct, as a result of disease or defect, he lacked substantial capacity either to appreciate the wrongfulness of his conduct or to conform his conduct to the requirements of law."* This modification in the M'Naghten rule is accepted in most jurisdictions. The American Psychiatric Association favors the American Law Institute test because it allows psychiatric testimony to clearly describe the history, adaptation, development, and function of patients' behavioral processes and the results of other medical tests to evaluate the clinical symptoms of mental illness in relation to alleged criminal acts.

CONCLUDING STATEMENTS

1. The nurse can practice effectively only if she is knowledgeable about the rudimentary principles of law that concern the mentally ill.
2. A combination of overt behaviors and legal status, not a diagnostic category, determines whether an individual can be treated voluntarily or involuntarily.
3. There is no uniformity of commitment methods among the

states, but no one can be deprived of his liberty without due process of law.

4. Nurses must work for the necessary legislative amendments that would facilitate appropriate reforms so as to fulfill the dictum *primum nil nocere*—we must minimize harm.

5. Involuntary admission usually consists of (1) application, (2) examination, (3) determination, and (4) detention, if indicated.

6. As a client advocate the nurse's primary responsibility is to assist the client to learn about his rights and to protect and assert those rights within the health care system.

7. A right is the enjoyment of a privilege that is secured by law to a person.

8. Mentally ill persons who are hospitalized may experience a double limitation on their rights—one created by the organization of the hospital system and the other created by their illness.

9. The nurse must be knowledgeable about the Patient's Bill of Rights published by the American Hospital Association in 1973.

10. The Code for Nurses developed in 1976 by the American Nurses' Association (ANA) deals with issues of ethical nursing conduct.

11. Nurses seeking employment in psychiatric institutions must be certain that these facilities have the proper internal structure to protect clients' rights.

12. The following client rights have particular applicability in the practice of psychiatric nursing.
    a. The right to habeas corpus
    b. The right to treatment
    c. The right to informed consent
    d. The right to confidentiality-privacy
    e. The right to independent psychiatric examination
    f. The right to refuse treatment
    g. The right to least restrictive treatment

13. By virtue of the psychiatric client being in need of nursing care, the client and the nurse have a contract in which both parties agree that the nurse will provide reasonable and prudent care to the client.

14. The law not only protects the individual from society, but also the society from the individual.
15. Forensic psychiatry is concerned with determinations of dangerousness, mental incompetency, and insanity to promote orderly social functioning.

SUGGESTED SOURCES OF ADDITIONAL INFORMATION

Classical

Ginsberg, Leon H.: Civil rights of the mentally ill—a review of the issues, Community Ment. Health J. **4:**244-250, June, 1968.

Szasz, Thomas: Law, liberty, and psychiatry, New York, 1968, Collier Books.

Zilboorg, Gregory: The psychology of the criminal act and punishment, Westport, Conn., 1968, Greenwood Press, Inc.

Contemporary

Applebaum, Paul S., and Gutheil, Thomas G.: Drug refusal: a study of psychiatric inpatients, Am. J. Psychiatry **137:**340-346, March, 1980.

Appelbaum, P., and Reiser, S.: Ethics rounds: a model for teaching ethics in a psychiatric setting, Hosp. Community Psychiatry **32**(8):555-560, 1981.

Benoliel, Jeanne: Ethics in nursing practice and education, Nurs. Outlook **31:**210-215, July-Aug., 1983.

Cohen, R.J.: Malpractice: a guide for mental health professionals, New York, 1979, The Free Press.

Creighton, Helen: Law every nurse should know, Philadelphia, 1981, W.B. Saunders Co.

Crowder, John E., and Klatte, Ernest W.: Involuntary admission to general hospitals: legal status is not the same issue, Hosp. Community Psychiatry **31:**325-327, May, 1980.

Curtin, Leah: Is there a right to health care?, Am. J. Nurs. **80:**462-465, 1980.

Davis, A., and Aroskar, M.: Ethical dilemmas and nursing practice, New York, 1978, Appleton-Century-Crofts.

Ennis, Bruce J.: Emerging legal rights of the mentally handicapped. In Issac Ray Symposium: Human rights, the law and psychiatric treatment, Pittsburgh, 1974, University of Pittsburgh School of Law.

Ennis, Bruce J., and Emery, Richard D.: The rights of mental patients, New York, 1978, Avon Books.

Ennis, Bruce J., and Friedman, Paul R., editors: Legal rights of the mentally handicapped, vol 1, Pittsburgh, 1973, Practicing Law Institute, The Mental Health Law Project-University of Pittsburgh School of Law.

Ford, Maurice D.: The psychiatrist's double bind: the right to refuse medication, Am. J. Psychiatry **137:**332-339, March, 1980.

Garritson, Susan, and Davis, Ann: Least restrictive alternatives: ethical considerations, J. Psychosoc. Nurs. Ment. Health Serv. **21:**17-23, Dec., 1983.

Gonzalez, H.: The consumer movement: the implications for psychiatric care, Perspect. Psychiatr. Care **14:**186, Oct.-Dec., 1976.

Greenblatt, Milton: Class action and the right to treatment, Hosp. Community Psychiatry **25:**449-452, 1974.

Griffith, E., and Etkin, K.: Legal rights and involuntary transfer following a voluntary admission, Hosp. Community Psychiatry **32:**319-322, 1981.

Gutheil, Thomas, Shapiro, Robert, and St. Clair, R. Lawrence: Legal guardianship in drug refusal: an illusory solution, Am. J. Psychiatry **137:**347-352, March, 1980.

Kaimowitz vs Michigan Department of Mental Health Civil Action, 73-19434-AW (Mich Cir Ct, July 10, 1973).

Knecht vs Gillman, 4882d 1136 (8th Cir 1973).

Leeman, Cavin: Involuntary admissions to general hospitals: progress or threat? Hosp. Community Psychiatry **31:**315-317, May, 1980.

Leeman, Cavin, and Berger, Howard S.: The Massachusetts psychiatric society's position paper on voluntary psychiatric admissions to general hospitals, Hosp. Community Psychiatry **31:**318-324, May, 1980.

Mackey vs Procunier, 477F2d 877 (9th Cir 1973).

Mancini, Marguerite: Nursing, minors and the law, Am. J. Nurs. **78:**124, Jan., 1978.

National Association of Mental Health Position Statement: Civil rights of mental patients, Ment. Hyg. **56:**67-69, Spring, 1972.

O'Connor vs Donaldson, 422 U.S. 563 (1975).

Padberg, Joan: Nursing and forensic psychiatry, Perspect. Psychiatr. Care **10:**163-167, Nov., 1972.

President's Commission on Mental Health: report to the president, vol. 1, Washington, D.C., 1978.

Reiser, Stanely J.: Refusing treatment for mental illness: historical ethical dimensions, Am. J. Psychiatry **137:**329-331, March, 1980.

Report of the task panel on legal and ethical issues: task panel reports submitted to the President's Commission on Mental Health, vol. 4, Washington, D.C., 1978, U.S. Government Printing Office.

Robitscher, Jonas B.: Medical, moral and legal issues in mental health care, Hosp. Community Psychiatry **25:**446-448, 1974.

Robitscher, Jonas B.: The powers of psychiatry, Boston, 1980, Houghton Mifflin Co.

Rosner, S. Steven: The rights of mental patients—the new Massachusetts law, Ment. Hyg. **56:**117-119, Winter, 1972.

Rubin, Bernard: Psychiatry and the law. In Arieti, Silvano, editor: American handbook of psychiatry, vol. 5, New York, 1974, Basic Books, Inc., Publishers.

Scott vs Plante, 532F2d 939, 946 (3rd Cir 1976).

Smith, S., and Davis, A.: Ethical dilemmas: conflict among rights, duties, obligations, Am. J. Nurs. **80:**1462-1466, 1980.

Stone, A.A.: Informed consent: special problems for psychiatry, Hosp. Community Psychiatry **30:**321-327, May, 1978.

Swan, Marlene, and Dipert, Dennis: A survey of the impact of a patients' rights law on state facilities in Indiana, Hosp. Community Psychiatry **30**(4):234-237, April, 1979.

Tancredi, Laurence R., Lieb, Julian, and Slaby, Andrew E.: Legal issues in psychiatric care, New York, 1975, Harper & Row, Publishers.

Thorner, Nancy: Nurses violate their patients' rights, J. Psychiatr. Nurs. **14:**(1):7-12, Jan., 1976.

Weihofen, Henry, and Usdin, Gene L.: Who is competent to make a will? Ment. Hyg. **54:**37-43, Jan., 1970.

Weiner, Barbara: Supreme court decisions on mental health: a review, Hosp. Community Psychiatry **33:**461-464, 1982.

Wilhelm, Yvonne M.: A look at psychiatric commitment, Perspect. Psychiatr. Care **10:**49-86, March-April, 1971.

Of particular interest

Nations, Wanda C.: Nurse-lawyer is patient advocate, Am. J. Nurs. **73:**1039-1041, 1973.
This is an excellent article depicting the innovative role of nurse-lawyer. It is relevant for the beginning nurse in outlining pertinent legal issues in nursing and providing direction toward patient advocacy.

Stachyra, M.: Nurses, psychotherapy, and the law, Perspect. Psychiatr. Care **2:**200, Sept.-Oct., 1969.
This article addresses specific issues related to nurses practicing psychotherapy. It discusses various practice acts and suggests direction for changes in existing laws.

chapter twenty-six

issues affecting
the future of
psychiatric nursing

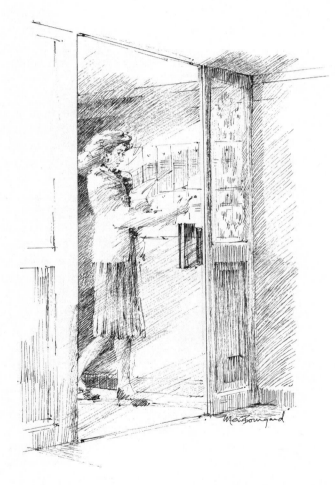

*Who would have thought
I'd be making house calls!*

LEARNING OBJECTIVES
After studying this chapter the student will be able to:

1 Identify one issue affecting the future of psychiatric nursing from each of the following categories: economic, social, professional, clinical, delivery system, and educational.

2 Discuss how each identified issue is likely to affect the future of psychiatric nursing.

The final years of the twentieth century will be times of challenge for psychiatric nursing. The very existence of this health care specialty is in question, while simultaneously the potential for it to make a valuable and unique contribution to the welfare of society has never been so great. Today's students of nursing will be practicing well into the twenty-first century and will be the nursing leaders of tomorrow. Since it is their nursing practice that will be affected by the way in which current issues are resolved, it is imperative that nursing students become aware of those factors which will shape the nature and scope of psychiatric nursing in the future.

This chapter is designed to highlight some of the major issues that confront psychiatric nursing. The nature of any issue is that solutions are not readily discernible. If they were, issues would not be present. Another characteristic of issues is the multiplicity of factors that interrelate to create an issue. However, whenever a discussion of issues is attempted, it becomes necessary to artificially separate each factor to facilitate discussion. Consequently, this chapter presents my view of those issues facing psychiatric nursing and does not purport to supply solutions. It is hoped that the reader's awareness of these issues will be increased whether or not the reader agrees with my analysis of them. As a result of an increased awareness, it is further hoped that the reader will be motivated to formulate her own concerns and develop a plan to address them.

ECONOMIC ISSUES

Not since the Great Depression of the 1930s has the U.S. economy been as influential a factor in shaping daily events as it is today. Unlike the depression when there was too little money available, we are currently living in a period where, in a sense, there is too much money available. The tragedy, however, is that despite the abundance of money, most persons are unable to attain or maintain the standard of living they desire because the cost of goods and services is also very high. Consequently, many individuals and families find themselves in a position where they have more income than ever before, but their expenses are also higher than ever before.

The effect of the economy is all pervasive. It is a direct or indirect factor that influences all other issues in psychiatric nursing. For example, the consumer who is faced with expenses equal to or greater than his income must establish priorities for the expenditure of the available funds. Often health care takes a low priority, particularly health care designed to promote health and prevent illness. Furthermore, health care providers are being called to ever greater accountability for the expenditure of their time. Unfortunately, it is not usually possible to demonstrate that time spent in crisis intervention with an individual or family has prevented costly mental illness. At least, this expenditure of time cannot be compared to the administration of a parenteral diuretic, the results of which are quickly visible in the improved cardiopulmonary function of the recipient.

Nurses who care for the mentally ill, by their very function, are highly vulnerable to the economic issue. As the reader is well aware, the crux of psychiatric nursing is believed to be the provision of corrective emotional experiences for clients. This process often manifests itself by the nurse and client engaging in such activities as walking or talking together, playing cards, or sitting silently with each other. It is understandable that the casual observer of these activities would raise questions as to their value. Nurses must assume the initiative and responsibility for engaging in research that documents the efficacy of such approaches.

Economic constraints that result in demands for increased accountability also inevitably result in increased paperwork. Unfortunately, the persons required to do this paperwork are often those who least wish to do so—people prepared to function as clinicians. In addition, events that can be quantified, that is, reduced to numbers, are more easily accounted for than events that are not quantifiable. Take, for example, the difference between health counseling, which may take 30 minutes, and changing a Foley catheter, which may take 15 minutes. The latter intervention can be easily documented as to need, action taken, and results achieved, while the former may prove difficult to justify in terms of these criteria. Therefore the necessity for accountability has increased the value of activities that can be quantified and has devalued activities that cannot be easily translated into numerical values.

The development of Diagnosis-Related Groups (DRGs) is a prominent example of the influence of the economy on health care. In the late 1960s the increasing complexity of medical care and its spiraling cost resulted in research designed to create a framework through which the quality and efficiency of institutional health care could be monitored. Continuous efforts have been mounted to refine this schema and it is now being used in some states and proposed in many others as a means of stabilizing health care costs through prospective payment. In other words, the amount of payment an institution will receive through third party reimbursement is determined by such variables as the patient's diagnosis, his age, and the medical procedures performed. If in a specific instance the costs exceed the coverage, these costs must be borne by the institution. The converse is true as well and provides a powerful incentive to discharge patients as quickly as possible.

The impact of the use of DRGs on the quality of health care in general is not yet known; their impact on nursing is even less predictable because nursing care is not a variable factored into the formula. What is known, however, is that the use of DRGs as the basis for third party reimbursement increases the accountability of all members of the health care team. Unfortunately, paperwork is also increased.

In regard to psychiatric nursing it is generally believed that the use of the DRGs will lead to early discharge of clients, resulting in an increased number of acutely ill clients being treated in the community. This in turn will require nurses who work with the mentally ill in the community to become expert in monitoring the effects of prescribed psychotropic medications. Although this function is certainly within the scope of nursing practice, it is feared that it will become the nurse's primary function to the neglect of other equally necessary roles such as counselor, teacher, and socializing agent.

It is also feared that hospitals will cope with decreased budgets by eliminating or curtailing inservice education programs for nurses. Although this would be a serious development for any area of nursing, it is potentially lethal for psychiatric nursing because such limited time is spent studying this subject in formal educational programs. This issue is discussed further in this chapter under the heading "Educational Issues."

SOCIAL ISSUES

A major social trend that has had a direct impact on psychiatric nursing is the continued, organized effort of women to achieve social and economic equality. Since nursing is primarily a women's profession, changes in the status of women are closely intertwined with changes in the profession. No longer are women content to be dependent on men; no longer are nurses willing to be handmaidens to physicians. Women are demanding more education; nurses are becoming increasingly better educated. Women are demanding financial remuneration commensurate with their preparation and responsibilities; nurses are organizing and striking to receive salaries more closely reflective of their preparation and responsibilities.

An unfortunate but, it is hoped, temporary result of the women's movement is the tendency of young women to choose careers other than those traditionally associated with women, namely, teaching and nursing. While it is certainly desirable for all young people, both men and women, to have the opportunity to pursue careers for which they are best suited, it is unfortunate that many young women are dismissing nursing as a career merely because it has been historically associated with women. Compounding this problem is the fact that the number of persons, both male and female, in the 18- to 24-year age group is dropping steadily and will continue to do so well into the twenty-first century. Consequently, the pool of persons from which students of nursing are traditionally recruited is smaller than ever before and subject to the increased recruitment efforts of other occupational groups.

A social phenomenon that is unprecedented is the self-help phenomenon. Consumers no longer believe that professionals necessarily know best. Popular magazines regularly feature articles about health issues, ranging from diet to human behavior. Self-help books on a wide range of subjects are readily available, and some that deal with human emotions have been best-sellers.

The result of this phenomenon is a citizenry that is well educated about health matters and that consequently demands quality care at reasonable cost. The field of psychiatry, which less than a century ago was scorned, has now become demystified. The implications of this trend is that all mental health care professionals, including nurses, are increasingly held accountable by consumers and cannot hide behind professional jargon and unexplained actions.

PROFESSIONAL ISSUES

A major issue is the question of whether the nurse who cares for the mentally ill is really a nurse like any other or whether by virtue of her specialty she has forfeited her identity as a nurse. This issue affects medicine as well as nursing and stems from two factors.

One factor underlying this issue is that, despite knowledge and verbalizations to the contrary, health care professionals still practice in a manner that perpetuates a dichotomy between the mind and the body. In addition, knowledge and care of the body seem to be more valued by lay persons and professionals alike than knowledge and care of the mind. Perhaps this is the case because physiological functioning is better understood and more predictable than psychological functioning. Whatever the reason, the result is that when nurses or physicians choose to specialize in the care of the mentally ill they run the risk of divorcing themselves from the mainstream of health care delivery. Some persons have suggested that mental illness, as currently defined, is not an illness at all but rather a reflection of societal problems. Therefore, it is argued, preparation for the care of these persons should not be within the health care disciplines. When this issue is exacerbated by economic constraints, it is logical for the system to attempt to replace the nurse with less expensive attendants or aides who can be trained in a short period of time to focus only on behavior and engage in many of the activities performed by a nurse.

Research continues to document the fact that humans are holistic beings; the whole of the person is greater than the sum of his parts. Therefore health care directed only to the body or only to the mind is bound to be ultimately ineffective and at worst harmful. All health care professionals must have an in-depth knowledge of both the biophysical and the psychosocial sciences to practice effectively. Consequently, it is necessary for nurses who give care to the mentally ill to remain knowledgeable about physiological as well as psychological processes and to document the difference that this knowledge makes in the nursing care they give.

Another professional issue facing psychiatric nursing is role blurring. Before the advent of the phenothiazine derivatives the roles of mental health care workers were more clearly defined. The nurse was primarily concerned with the client's activities of daily living, the psychiatrist focused on diagnosing and prescribing, the psychologist focused on testing and research, and the social worker had the client's family as her domain. Very little treatment occurred. When psychotropic drugs made clients more accessible to therapeutic interventions all mental health disciplines began to claim these interventions as being within their scope of practice. The result was role blurring, where members of all disciplines engage in individual, family, and group therapy. The question then arises as to what, if anything, differentiates the nurse from the physician, the psychologist, or the social worker? Psychiatric nursing must convincingly answer this question or run the risk of extinction.

CLINICAL ISSUES

The incidence of mental illness in our society is clearly on the increase. Factors such as economic pressures, changing moral values, and an increase in violent crimes all result from and contribute to a stress-laden life-style to which individuals and families must adapt. Intervention measures designed to promote mental health and to prevent mental illness are needed in addition to measures designed to treat those who are already mentally ill. Meeting the mental health needs of the citizenry constitutes an enormous challenge to society.

Most authorities acknowledge that the most cost-effective and best way to meet these needs is through programs geared to prevention. These programs are designed to alter the environment in a way that is conducive to better mental health or to helping individuals, families, and communities to increase and diversify their coping mechanisms. An example of the former is efforts directed toward decreasing violence on the streets; examples of the latter are Head Start programs, victim assistance programs, and self-help groups such as Recovery, Inc.

Although there is almost universal agreement that prevention of mental illness and promotion of mental health are the best routes in terms of long-term goals, it is exceedingly difficult to document the effects of such programs in the short term. With a scarcity of resources, government and private agencies are less likely to allocate funds to such programs, feeling a need to concentrate limited resources on short-term, obvious problems, namely, the treatment of those already mentally ill.

Most major forms of mental illness are now viewed as chronic in the sense that the individual will always need a greater or lesser degree of supervision and care. With the advent of community mental health centers there was concomitantly great hope that the bulk of those persons requiring mental health care could be maintained in and benefit from care in the community. This hope was short-lived, however, as the "revolving door" syndrome developed. This syndrome is a phenomenon whereby persons receive intensive care through hospitalization, are discharged to the community where they may or may not continue to receive care, and shortly require hospitalization again wherein the cycle is repeated. The response to the revolving door syndrome was initially a sense of failure on the part of mental health care workers and the system. That attitude has gradually shifted from a sense of failure to an acceptance of the chronicity of mental illness.

Major changes need to take place in the mental health care delivery system. Because of the enormity and severity of the problem, there is a need for the development of treatment modalities and intervention techniques that address large population groups. Traditional one-to-one, family, and even group, interpersonally based treatment modalities are no longer viable as the main forms of intervention. These techniques have proved to be costly and, at worst, not necessarily therapeutically effective. In addition these modalities clearly benefit only those who value feelings and thoughts, are verbally fluent, have financial resources, are highly motivated, and have the intelligence necessary to deal with the abstractions inherent in these treatment modalities. Obviously these criteria rule out large numbers of individuals as well as certain population groups such as cultural minorities, children, the elderly, and the poor. It is these groups in which there is the greatest incidence of mental illness and for whom we have the least understanding of its cause and the fewest effective means of treatment. Although the need for change is well accepted by most mental health disciplines, there seems to be a paucity of ideas as to what changes can and should occur. Consequently, mental health workers are still being educationally and experientially prepared in the traditional modes of treatment while being told that in most instances their developing skills will be to no avail in solving the larger issues of the day.

What then is required? First and foremost, research must be instituted if reliable answers to these problems are to be found. Research needs to focus on the cause, prevention, and treatment of mental illness. This is easier said than done. Research regarding human behavior is substantively different from pure laboratory research in a variety of ways. First, there is a multiplicity of variables that are difficult if not impossible to control. In a laboratory, chemical elements can be isolated and then systematically combined with other elements one by one and the effects clearly observed. When dealing with human beings it is impossible to isolate a subject's personality from his intelligence or from his culture. Second, many laboratory experiments yield results in a relatively short period of time, at least within the lifetime of the researcher. In contrast, much behavioral science research is longitudinal in nature, requiring the observation and study of the subjects over a generation or two. In addition to the time and money involved, longitudinal research also runs the risk of incurring environmental changes that may affect the outcome, for example, a war.

A prime concern in behavioral research, perhaps the seminal issue, is the necessity felt in a democratic society to protect the rights of each individual. Therefore procedures involved in research as well as treatment are subjected to vigorous scrutiny and are not approved if there is any potential for harm to the persons involved. It is clearly unethical, for example, to create situations that are believed to produce schizophrenia in an effort to determine the cause of this tragic illness. Consequently, the best that behavioral research can show is a relationship between and among variables after the fact. Despite these obstacles, however, it is mandatory that society continue to support behavioral science research directed toward understanding the cause of mental illness and developing effective treatment modalities.

DELIVERY SYSTEM ISSUES

The philosophical basis of the community mental health movement was and still is seen as desirable. Not only is it more humane, but also it is more cost effective to maintain persons outside of institutions. While the society and the health care professions endorse the end result, it appears that little thought has been given to the changes that this would require in treatment methods and, therefore, in educational preparation of health care workers. Unfortunately, in too many instances the community mental health movement has meant little more than a change of setting: the same treatment philosophy and modalities have been moved from the institution to a decentralized center in the community.

Rather than solving any problems this short-sighted approach has in many instances compounded existent problems and created new ones. Chief among these are the revolving door syndrome, the community disorganization resulting from scores of mentally ill persons with few or no resources being thrust into the streets, and the inadequate treatment received by the mentally ill. Another irony or paradox of the community mental health movement is the fact that the best prepared health care workers, including nurses, are slowly but steadily moving into the community as a result, in part, of a powerful attitudinal shift elevating the status of those working in the community and denigrating those who choose to work in institutions. Consequently, some authorities fear that the care of institutionalized, chronically and acutely ill persons will be left to the least well-prepared health care workers. This situation, it is feared, will result in such terrible treatment that the "back wards" of the late nineteenth and early twentieth centuries will be seen as model treatment settings in comparison. This view may be an overstatement of the reality, but there is no doubt that the potential for this situation to occur is great enough to warrant grave concern.

Another major delivery system issue is the geographical maldistribution of mental health care workers and treatment centers that tend to be clustered together in large urban areas, particularly on the East and West coasts of the United States. It is in these areas that professionals can receive not only appropriate financial remuneration, but also the intellectual, cultural, and social stimulation they desire. As a result large groups of consumers do not have geographical access to continuous mental health care.

As previously stated, mental health professionals continue to be educationally prepared in the traditional treatment modalities, so it is understandable that they choose to work with those clients who can benefit from these measures. Therefore, in addition to geographical maldistribution, there is also a disproportionately small number of mental health care workers who choose to work with the poor, including the inner-city poor, the educationally and culturally disadvantaged, minority groups, children, and the elderly. Since these groups represent the largest number of mentally ill, it should be clear that the mental health needs of this country are not being met. This situation is so serious that the U.S. Congress has directed the National Institute of Mental Health to fund only those training programs that address one or more of these target populations.

EDUCATIONAL ISSUES

The cost of higher education in this country is skyrocketing daily and therefore placing postsecondary education out of the reach of more and more people at a time when scientific and technological advances require increasingly more educational preparation for those who wish to make a societal contribution. This situation is particularly true for women and members of cultural minorities who are attempting to achieve equality, in part, through education. Consequently, a smaller proportion of black and Hispanic people and women are able to afford the cost of higher education, which in turn results in fewer health care workers from those populations that require the most health care.

Of great concern is the fact that fewer and fewer nurses are choosing to work in psychiatric settings or to pursue graduate education in this field. It is believed that the reasons for this are multiple and complex. Many psychiatric nurse educators, however, believe that a major contributing factor is the trend in undergraduate nursing programs to integrate content. This trend is a result of nursing's attempt to teach in a way that helps the student view the client holistically and to move away from the medical model that tends to segment clients according to the disease or illness from which they are suffering. While these goals are commendable, one unanticipated effect has been that some students of nursing do not have a specific learning experience with the mentally ill. Consequently, it becomes understandable that graduates of these programs are unlikely to choose psychiatric nursing as a field in which to work, and therefore the pool of persons who are interested in and qualified to pursue graduate education in psychiatric nursing is lessened. As with all other issues, the cyclical nature of this problem is evident in the fact that as fewer nurses become prepared at the graduate level there ultimately will be fewer psychiatric nurses prepared to teach, which in turn results in poorer preparation of beginning practitioners in psychiatric nursing, ending with fewer choosing to work in the area. Thus the cycle is complete and is set to repeat itself. Unless efforts are made to recruit qualified persons into psychiatric nursing, this health care specialty will die a natural death and need not fear extinction from external forces.

CONCLUDING STATEMENTS

1. The final years of the twentieth century are times of challenge for psychiatric nursing.
2. Economic issues directly or indirectly affect all other issues in psychiatric nursing.
3. Nurses must assume the initiative and responsibility for engaging in research that documents the efficacy of nurse-client activities that are designed to provide corrective emotional experiences for clients.
4. Economic constraints lead to demands for increased accountability, which leads to increased paperwork, which in turn leads to a valuing of activities that are quantifiable in nature. The use of Diagnosis-Related Groups (DRGs) as a basis for third party reimbursement is a prominent example of this phenomenon.
5. Nurses who provide care to the mentally ill, by the very virtue of their function, are vulnerable to the economic issue.
6. The women's movement, the decreased pool of potential nursing students, and the self-help movement are social issues that have direct relevance for psychiatric nursing.
7. Professional issues that affect psychiatric nursing include the nurse's identity as a nurse like all others and the role blurring among mental health professionals.
8. The incidence of mental illness in our society is clearly on the increase, and meeting the mental health needs of the citizenry constitutes an enormous challenge to society.
9. Major changes need to take place in the mental health care

delivery system so that the treatment needs of large population groups can be met.

10. Despite the difficulties involved in behavioral research, it is mandatory that society continue to support behavioral science research that is directed toward understanding the cause of mental illness and developing effective treatment modalities.

11. Delivery system issues include the need for changes in treatment methods and in the educational preparation of health care workers. In addition, the trend toward the best prepared health care workers leaving the care of a hospitalized person to less well-prepared workers raises grave concern.

12. Geographical maldistribution of mental health care workers and treatment centers results in large groups of consumers who do not have geographical access to continuous mental health care.

13. Fewer and fewer nurses are choosing to work in psychiatric settings or to pursue graduate education in this field.

14. Efforts must be made to recruit qualified persons into psychiatric nursing.

SUGGESTED SOURCES OF ADDITIONAL INFORMATION

Classical

Leininger, Madeleine M.: Trends, issues and problems, Perspect. Psychiatr. Care **10**:11-20, Jan.-Feb., 1969.

Mereness, Dorothy: Problems and issues in contemporary psychiatric nursing, Perspect. Psychiatr. Care **2**(1):14-16, 1964.

Ramshorn, Mary T.: The major thrust in American psychiatry: past, present, and future, Perspect. Psychiatr. Care **9**:145-153, July-Aug., 1971.

Ujhely, G.: The nurse as psychotherapist: what are the issues? Perspect. Psychiatr. Care **11**(4):155-160, 1973.

Contemporary

Adams, G., Cheney, C., Gomez, E., Stafford, L., and Tristan, M.: Primary mental health care: an innovative model, J. Psychosoc. Nurs. Ment. Health Serv. **18**:26-30, Jan., 1980.

Ahmed, Mary Cooke: Taking charge of change in hospital nursing practice, Am. J. Nurs. **81**:540-543, 1981.

Ames, David: The limits of general hospital care: a continuing role for state hospitals, Hosp. Community Psychiatry **34**(2):145-150, 1983.

Amesbury, William: The comprehensive mental health system: is it achievable? Perspect. Psychiatr. Care **21**:31-33, Jan.-March, 1983.

Andrulis, Dennis, and Mazade, Noel: American mental health policy:

changing direction in the 80's, Hosp. Community Psychiatry. **34**(7):601-606, 1983.

Bachrach, Leona: Research on services for the homeless mentally ill, Hosp. Community Psychiatry **35**(9):910-913, 1984.

Ball, F.L. Jessica, and Havassy, Barbara: A survey of the problems and needs of homeless consumers of acute psychiatric services, Hosp. Community Psychiatry **35**(9):917-921, 1984.

Biegel, Allan: The community mental health centers: a look ahead, Hosp. Community Psychiatry **33**(9):741-745, 1982.

Bloom, Bernard: The logic and urgency of primary prevention, Hosp. Community Psychiatry **32**(12):839-843, 1981.

Boyle, Kathleen: Power in nursing: a collaborative approach, Nurs. Outlook **32**:164-167, May-June, 1984.

Brewer, Carol: Variable billing: is it viable? Nurs. Outlook **32**:38-41, Jan.-Feb., 1984.

Caton, Carol: The new chronic patient and the system of community care, Hosp. Community Psychiatry **32**(7):475-478, 1981.

Craig, Thomas, and Laska, Eugene: Deinstitutionalization and the survival of the state hospital, Hosp. Community Psychiatry **34**(7):616-622, 1983.

Cohen, N., Putnam, J., and Sullivan, Ann: The mentally ill homeless: isolation and adaptation, Hosp. Community Psychiatry **35**(9):922-924, 1984.

Dorwart, Robert: Deinstitutionalization: who is left behind? Hosp. Community Psychiatry **31**(5):336-338, 1980.

Dumas, Rhetaugh: Social, economic, and political factors and mental illness, J. Psychosoc. Nurs. Ment. Health Serv. **21**:31-35, March, 1983.

Ellison, Edythe: Social networks and the mental health caregiving system: implications for psychiatric nursing practice, J. Psychosoc. Nurs. Ment. Health Serv. **21**:18-24, Feb., 1983.

Fagin, Claire: Nursing as an alternative to high-cost care, Am. J. Nurs. **82**:56-60, 1982.

Fink, Edward: Encouraging third-party coverage of partial hospitals, Hosp. Community Psychiatry **33**(1):38-41, 1982.

Gardner, Harold, and Fiske, Marilyn: Pluralism and competition: a possibility for primary care, Am. J. Nurs. **81**:2152-2157, 1981.

Goldman, H., Adams, N., and Taube, C.: Deinstitutionalization: the data demythologized, Hosp. Community Psychiatry **34**(2):129-134, 1983.

Goldman, H., Pincers, H., Taube, C., and Regier, D.: Prospective payment for psychiatric hospitalization: questions and issues, Hosp. Community Psychiatry **35**:460-464, May, 1984.

Griffith, H.: Strategies for direct third party re-imbursement for nurses, Am. J. Nurs. **82**:408-411, 1982.

Griffin, Hurdis: Competition in health care, Nurs. Outlook **31**:262-266, Sept.-Oct., 1983.

Hagar, Lorraine, and Kincheloe, Marsha: The disintegration of a community mental health outpatient program or, off the back wards into the streets, Pespect. Psychiatr. Care **21**:102-107, July-Sept., 1983.

Hassett, Mary: Computers and nursing education in the 1980's, Nurs. Outlook **32**:34-36, Jan.-Feb., 1984.

Hoeffer, Beverly: The private practice model: an ethical perspective, J. Psychosoc. Nurs. Ment. Health Serv. **21**:31-37, July, 1983.

Huey, Karen: Conference report—patient re-entry into the community, Hosp. Community Psychiatry **31**(1):52-56, 1980.

Joel, Lucille: DRGs and RIMs: implications for nursing, Nurs. Outlook **32**:42-49, Jan.-Feb., 1984.

Jones, Robert: Street people and psychiatry: an introduction, Hosp. Community Psychiatry **34**(9):807-812, 1983.

Kelly, Gerard: Minimizing the adverse effects of mass relocation among chronic psychiatric patients, Hosp. Community Psychiatry **34**(2):150-154, 1983.

Lamb, H. Richard: Deinstitutionalization and the homeless mentally ill, Hosp. Community Psychiatry **35**(9):899-907, 1984.

Lamb, H. Richard: What did we really expect from deinstitutionalization? Hosp. Community Psychiatry **32**(2):105-109, 1981.

Lamb, H. Richard: Young adult chronic patients: the new drifters, Hosp. Community Psychiatry **33**(6):465-468, 1982.

Lamb, H. Richard, and Peele, R.: The need for continuing asylum and sanctuary, Hosp. Community Psychiatry **35**(8):798-802, 1984.

Lang, Norma: Nurse-managed centers: will they thrive? Am. J. Nurs. **83**:1290-1293, 1983.

Lewis, Edith: Challenges and choices: a special report on the 1984 ANA convention, Nurs. Outlook **32**:278-282, Sept.-Oct., 1984.

Lipton, F., Sabatani, A., and Katz, S.: Down and out in the city: the homeless mentally ill, Hosp. Community Psychiatry **34**(9):817-822, 1983.

McCloskey, J.C., and Grace, H., editors: Current issues in nursing, Boston, 1982, Blackwell Scientific Publications, Inc.

Mann, Louise, and Whall, Ann: Informed consent and the deinstitutionalized patient, J. Psychosoc. Nurs. Ment. Health Serv. **22**:22-27, Jan., 1984.

Miller, Robert: Beyond the old state hospital: new opportunities ahead, Hosp. Community Psychiatry **32**(1):27-31, 1981.

Mitsunaga, Betty: Designing psychiatric/mental health nursing for the future: problems and prospects, J. Psychosoc. Nurs. Ment. Serv. **20**:15-21, Dec., 1982.

Okin, Robert: State hospitals in the 1980's, Hosp. Community Psychiatry **33**(9):717-721, 1982.

Polk, Glenda: The socialization and utilization of nurse consultants, J. Psychosoc. Nurs. Ment. Health Serv. **18**:33-36, Feb., 1980.

Ramshorn, Mary: Community mental health nursing revisited, Perspect. Psychiatr. Care **21**:120-123, Oct.-Dec., 1983.

Rose, Michael: Laying seige to hospital privileges, Am. J. Nurs. **84**:612-615, 1984.

Ruch, Michael: The multidisciplinary approach: when too many is too much, J. Psychosoc. Nurs. Ment. Health Serv. **22**:18-23, Sept., 1984.

Samter, J., Schirer, M., and Shulman, D.: Interface of psychiatric clinical specialists in a community hospital setting, J. Psychosoc. Nurs. Ment. Health Serv. **19**:20-29, Jan., 1981.

Stickey, S., Morr, G., and Gardner, E.: Psychiatric nurse consultation: who calls and why, J. Psychosoc. Nurs. Ment. Health Serv. **19**(10):22-26, Oct., 1981.

Stockdill, James, and Pardes, Herbert: Survival strategies for community mental health services in the 1980s, Hosp. Community Psychiatry **35**(2):127-132, 1984.

Sweeney, D., Garrison, J., Dabrowski, C., and McGettigan, P.: Mapping urban hotels: life space of the chronic mental patient, J. Psychosoc. Nurs. Ment. Health Serv. **20**:9-14, May, 1982.

Talbott, John: The national plan for the chronically mentally ill: a programmatic analysis, Hosp. Community Psychiatry **32**(10):699-704, 1981.

Taube, C., Lee, E., and Forthofer, R.: Diagnostic-related groups for mental disorders, alcoholism, and drug abuse: evaluation and alternatives, Hosp. Community Psychiatry **35**:452-455, May, 1984.

Watson, Jean: Professional identity crisis—is nursing finally growing up? Am. J. Nurs. **81**:1488-1490, 1981.

Of particular interest

Fagin, Claire: Psychiatric nursing at the crossroads: quo vadis, Perspect. Psychiatr. Care **19**:99-106, May-Aug., 1981.
This paper was delivered by Dr. Fagin at the 1981 Perspectives in Psychiatric Care Conference, in honor of Dr. Hildegard Peplau's contributions to the specialty of psychiatric nursing. Dr. Fagin explores the past three decades of psychiatric nursing and discusses the opportunities and tasks for the future.

Hoeffer, Beverly, and Murphy, Shirley: The unfinished task: development of nursing theory for psychiatric and mental health nursing, J. Psychosoc. Nurs. Ment. Health Serv. **20**:8-14, Dec., 1982.
This paper, originally presented at the Fourth National Symposium on Psychiatric/Mental Health Nursing in San Francisco, is an intriguing discussion that defines theory development as an urgent task for psychiatric nursing.

glossary

The following words are frequently used by the psychiatric nurse. Many of the definitions were taken from *A Psychiatric Glossary.** A larger and equally useful book is the *Psychiatric Dictionary.*†

acting out Expression of unconscious emotional conflicts or feelings of hostility or love in actions that the protagonist does not consciously know are related to such conflicts or feelings.

addiction Strong emotional and physiological dependence on alcohol or a drug that has progressed beyond voluntary control.

affect Emotional feeling tone; affect and emotional response are commonly used interchangeably.

affective psychosis Psychotic reaction in which the predominant feature is a severe disorder of mood or emotional feelings.

aggression In psychiatry, a forceful attacking action (physical, verbal, or symbolic).

agitation State of chronic restlessness; psychomotor expression of emotional tension.

agoraphobia Fear of open spaces.

Alzheimer's disease Degenerative brain disease of unknown cause marked by insidious onset and uniformly progressive deterioration: the disorder occurs most commonly in those over 65, but may occur as early as age 40.

ambivalence Coexistence of two opposing drives, desires, feelings, or emotions toward the same person, object, or goal; may be conscious or partially conscious.

anal stage Second stage of psychosexual development, immediately following the oral stage, marked by a shift of libidinal energy to the anus and urethra; includes both anal-expulsive and anal-retentive phases. Many adult traits, such as stinginess, hoarding, and collecting find their prototypes here.

anorexia nervosa Psychiatric disorder found predominantly in young females, marked by extreme weight loss, an intense fear of fat, a distorted body image, and peculiar patterns of eating and handling food.

antisocial personality Personality disorder marked by a history of chronic antisocial behavior in which the rights of others are violated, with persistence into adult life of a pattern of antisocial behavior that

*American Psychiatric Association, Diagnostic and Statistical Manual of Mental Disorders, Third Edition, Washington, D.C., APA, 1980.
†Campbell, Robert J.: Psychiatric dictionary, ed. 5, New York, 1981, Oxford University Press, Inc.

began in adolescence, and a failure to sustain good job performance over several years. Lying, stealing, fighting, and truancy are typical early signs.

anxiety Apprehension, tension, or uneasiness that stems from the anticipation of danger, the source of which is largely unknown or unrecognized; primarily of intrapsychic origin, in distinction to fear, which is the emotional response to a consciously recognized and usually external threat or danger.

apathy Used by H.S. Sullivan to describe the security operation whereby the individual defends against anxiety by not experiencing the emotion associated with an anxiety-producing event; there is a manifestation of extreme indifference.

autonomy Quality or state of being self-governing. The living organism does not represent merely an inactive element but is, to a large extent, a self-governing entity.

autism (autistic thinking) Form of thinking that attempts to gratify unfulfilled desires without due regard for reality; objective facts are distorted, obscured, or excluded in varying degrees.

blocking Difficulty in recollection or interruption of a train of thought or speech due to emotional factors that are usually unconscious.

body image Concept that each person has of his own body as an object in space, independently and apart from all other objects.

brain syndrome Group of symptoms resulting from impaired function of the brain; may be acute (reversible) or chronic (irreversible).

bulimia Psychiatric disorder, occurring primarily in females, marked by episodic uncontrolled, and rapid consumption of food over a short period of time (binges), inconspicuous eating during a binge, and termination of the binge by abdominal pain, social interruption, sleep, or self-induced vomiting.

cathexis Investment of an object or idea with special significance or value to the individual.

cerea flexibilitas "Waxy flexibility" often present in catatonic schizophrenia, in which the person's arm or leg remains passively in the position in which it is placed.

cognitive Refers to mental processes of comprehension, judgment, memory, and reasoning.

compensation (1) Mental mechanism, operating unconsciously, by which the individual attempts to make up for real or fancied deficiencies; (2) conscious process by which the individual strives to make up for real or imagined defects in such areas as physique, performance, skills, or psychological attributes—the two types frequently merge.

complex Group of associated ideas that have a common strong emotional tone; these may be in part unconscious and may significantly influence attitudes and associations.

compulsion Insistent, repetitive, intrusive, and unwanted urge to perform an act that is contrary to the person's ordinary conscious wishes or standards; a defensive substitute for hidden and still more unacceptable ideas and wishes (anxiety results from failure to perform the compulsive act).

concept Mental image.

condensation Psychological process often present in dreams in which two or more concepts are fused so that a single symbol represents the multiple components.

confabulation Unconscious, defensive "filling in" of actual memory gaps by imaginary or fantastic experiences, often complex, that are recounted in a detailed and plausible way as though they were factual.

conflict Clash, conscious or unconscious, between two opposing emotional forces; if unconscious, an internal (instinctual) wish or striving is opposed by another internal and contradictory wish.

confusion Disturbed orientation in respect to time, place, or person; sometimes accompanied by disturbances of consciousness.

conscience Psychic organizations that stand in opposition to the expression of instinctual actions; the function of conscience is to warn the ego to avoid the pain of intense guilt feelings.

consciousness Clear awareness of self and the environment.

conversion disorder Psychiatric disorder characterized by a loss of or alteration in physical functioning that is apparently an expression of an unconscious psychological conflict or need. The disturbance cannot be explained by any physical disorder or pathophysiological mechanism.

coping mechanism Adaptation to anxiety based on conscious acknowledgement of a problem; the individual engages in reality-oriented problem-solving activities designed to reduce tension.

countertransference Therapist's conscious or unconscious emotional reaction to her client.

crisis State of disequilibrium resulting from the interaction of an event with the individual's or family's coping mechanisms, which are inadequate to meet the demands of the situation, combined with the individual's or family's perception of the meaning of the event.

defense mechanism Means by which the organism protects itself against danger arising from impulses or affects.

delirium Disturbance in thinking with disorientation and confusion; illusions, delusions, or hallucinations may be present.

delusion False belief out of keeping with the individual's level of knowledge and his cultural group; the belief is maintained against logical argument and despite objective contradictory evidence.

delusions of grandeur Exaggerated, unrealistic ideas of one's importance or identity.

delusions of persecution Unrealistic ideas that one has been singled out for persecution.

delusions of reference Incorrect assumption that certain casual or unrelated remarks or the behavior of others applies to oneself.

dementia Old term denoting madness or insanity; now used to describe organic mental disorders marked by a deterioration of intellectual abilities, impaired memory, abstract thinking, cognition, judgment, and impulse control.

dementia praecox Obsolescent descriptive term for schizophrenia.

denial Mental mechanism, operating unconsciously, used to resolve emotional conflict and to allay consequent anxiety by denying some of the important elements; the feelings denied may be thoughts, wishes, needs, or external reality factors; what is consciously intolerable is simply disowned by the protectively automatic and unconscious denial of its existence.

dependency needs Vital infantile needs for mothering, love, affection, shelter, protection, security, food, and warmth; these needs may continue beyond infancy in overt or hidden forms or be increased in the adult as a regressive manifestation.

depersonalization Feelings of unreality or strangeness concerning either the environment or the self.

depression In the psychiatric sense, a morbid sadness, dejection, or melancholy; may vary in depth from neurosis to psychosis; to be differentiated from grief that is realistic and proportionate to what has been lost.

derailment Pattern of speech seen most commonly in schizophrenic disorders, in which incomprehensible, disconnected, and unrelated ideas replace logical and orderly thought.

dereistic Describes mental activity that is not in accordance with reality, logic, or experience; similar to autistic.

deviant Any person differing markedly from what is accepted as the norm, the average, or the usual.

disorientation Loss of awareness of the position of self in relation to space, time, or persons.

displacement Mental mechanism, operating unconsciously, by which an emotion is transferred or "displaced" from its original object to a more acceptable substitute object.

dissociation Psychological separation or splitting off; an intrapsychic defensive process, which operates automatically and unconsciously, through which emotional significance and affect are separated and detached from an idea, situation, or object.

dynamic psychiatry Psychiatry stressing the existence of mental forces that energetically demand expression; dynamic psychiatry implies the study of the active, energy-laden, and changing factors in human behavior, as opposed to the older, more static, and descriptive study of clinical patterns, symptoms, and classification.

dysarthria Impaired, difficult speech, usually due to organic disorders of the nervous system; sometimes applied to emotional speech difficulties such as stammering and stuttering.

ego Refers to the conscious self, the "I"; in Freudian theory, the central part of the personality that deals with reality and is influenced by social forces; the ego modifies behavior by largely unconscious compromise between the primitive instinctual drives (the id) and the conscience (the superego).

ego ideal That part of the personality which comprises the aims and goals of the self; usually refers to the conscious or unconscious emulation of significant persons with whom it has identified.

elation Affect consisting of feelings of euphoria, triumph, intense self-satisfaction, optimism; an elated though unstable mood is characteristic of mania.

emotion Subjective feeling such as fear, anger, grief, joy, or love.

empathic linkage H.S. Sullivan's term for the relationship unique to infant and mother, whereby each is highly sensitive to the other's feeling states.

empathy Objective and insightful awareness of the feelings, emotions, and behavior of another person and their meaning and significance; to be distinguished from sympathy, which is nonobjective and usually noncritical.

euphoria Exaggerated feeling of physical and emotional well-being not consonant with apparent stimuli or events; usually of psychological origin, but also seen in organic brain disorders and toxic states.

exhibitionism Commonly, showing off; psychiatrically, body exposure, usually of the male genitals to females; sexual stimulation or gratification usually accompanies the act.

expansive Lacking restraint in feelings and actions; the overvaluation of one's own work.

extroversion State in which attention and energies are largely directed outward from the self, as opposed to interest primarily directed toward the self as in introversion.

fabrication Relating imaginary events as true, not in the sense of lying but to cover up gaps in memory.

fetishism Sexual deviation manifested by the attachment of sexual feeling to an inanimate object (fetish); contact with the object usually leads to orgasm.

fixation Arrest of psychosexual maturation at an immature level; depending on degree, may be either normal or pathological.

flight of ideas Verbal skipping from one idea to another before the preceding one has been concluded; the ideas appear to be continuous but are fragmentary and determined by chance associations.

free association In psychoanalytic therapy, unselected verbalization by the person of whatever comes to mind.

free-floating anxiety Pervasive anxiety that the individual cannot explain to his own satisfaction.

functional mental illness Illness of emotional origin in which organic or structural changes are either absent or are developed secondarily to prolonged emotional stress.

general paresis Psychosis associated with organic disease of the central nervous system resulting from chronic syphilitic infection.

genital stage Period of psychosexual development from the age of about 12 to 18 years old, marked by a reactivation of libidinal energy and the focusing of this energy on the genital area.

grandiose In psychiatry, refers to delusions of great wealth, power, and fame.

hallucination False sensory perception in the absence of an actual external stimulus; may be of emotional or chemical (drugs, alcohol, etc.) origin and may occur in any of the five senses.

holism Thesis that the study of parts cannot explain the whole, because the whole is something different from the summation of its parts. From a holistic point of view the human being is more than a mere aggregation of physiological, psychological, and social functions; the person as a whole has attributes that cannot be explained by the attributes of the parts.

homosexual panic Acute and severe attack of anxiety based on unconscious conflicts involving homosexuality.

homosexuality Sexual attraction or relationship between members of the same sex; active homosexuality is marked by overt activity, whereas latent homosexuality is marked by unconscious homosexual desires or conscious desires consistently denied expression.

hypnosis Altered state of conscious awareness induced in a suggestible subject; under hypnosis a person manifests increased receptivity to suggestion and direction.

hysteria Illness resulting from emotional conflict and generally characterized by immaturity, impulsiveness, attention seeking, dependency, and use of the mental mechanisms of conversion and dissociation.

id In Freudian theory, that part of the personality structure that harbors the unconscious instinctive desires and strivings of the individual.

ideas of reference Incorrect interpretation of casual incidents and external events as having direct reference to oneself; may reach sufficient intensity to constitute delusions.

identification Mental mechanism, operating unconsciously, by which an individual endeavors to pattern himself after another; plays a major role in the development of one's personality and specifically of one's superego (conscience).

idiopathic Term applied to diseases of unknown cause, for example, idiopathic epilepsy.

illusion Misinterpretation of a real external sensory experience.

incorporation Primitive mental mechanism, operating unconsciously, by which a person or parts of another person are symbolically ingested and assimilated; for example, infantile fantasy that the mother's breast has been ingested and is a part of oneself.

infantilism Term applied to adults who are childish or mentally or physically immature.

inhibition Unconscious interference with or restriction of instinctual drives.

insight Self-understanding; a major goal of psychotherapy; the extent of the individual's understanding of the origin, nature, and mechanisms of his attitudes and behavior.

instinct Inborn drive; human instincts include those of self-preservation, sexuality, and (according to some authorities) the ego instincts and the herd or social instincts.

integration Useful organization of both new and old data, experience, and emotional capacities incorporated into the personality; also refers to the organization and amalgamation of functions at various levels of psychosexual development.

interpersonal psychiatry Theory of psychiatry developed by H.S. Sullivan, stressing the nature and quality of relationships with significant others as the most critical factor in personality development.

intrapsychic Situated, originating, or taking place in the psyche.

introjection Mental mechanism, operating unconsciously, whereby loved or hated external objects are taken within oneself symbolically; the converse of projection; may serve as a defense against conscious recognition of intolerable hostile impulses; for example, in severe depression the individual may unconsciously direct unacceptable hatred or aggression toward himself, that is, toward the introjected object within himself; related to the more primitive mechanisms of incorporation.

introversion Preoccupation with oneself, with accompanying reduction of interest in the outside world; roughly the reverse of extroversion.

involutional psychosis Psychotic reaction taking place during the involutional period, climacteric or menopause, characterized most commonly by depression and occasionally by paranoid thinking; the course tends to be prolonged, and the condition may be manifested by feelings of guilt, anxiety, agitation, delusional ideas, insomnia, and somatic preoccupation.

isolation Mental mechanism whereby the feeling is detached from the event in an individual's memory, thus enabling the event to be recalled without its attendant anxiety.

kleptomania Compulsive stealing, largely with any apparent material need for the stolen objects.

Korsakoff's psychosis (Korsakoff's syndrome) Disorder marked by disturbance of attention and memory, as evidenced by confabulation and by involvement of the peripheral nerves; may be due to alcohol, certain poisons, or infections.

labile Rapidly shifting emotions.

latency period In psychoanalysis, a phase between the phallic (or oedipal) and adolescent periods of psychosexual development; characterized by a marked decrease of sexual behavior and interest in sex.

libido Psychic drive or energy usually associated with the sexual instinct (sexual is used here in the broad sense to include pleasure and love-object seeking); also used broadly to connote the psychic energy associated with instincts in general.

life review Process of thinking about the meaning of one's life, believed to be a universal occurrence in older person as they face the prospect of impending death.

lucid interval Period during which there is a remission of symptoms in a psychosis.

lust H.S. Sullivan's term for the sexual urges first erupting in early adolescence.

malingerer Individual who consciously simulates illness to avoid a personally unpleasant or intolerable alternative.

manic-depressive psychosis Major emotional illness marked by severe mood swings alternating from elation to depression and a tendency toward remission and recurrence; depressed type is characterized by depression of mood with retardation and inhibition of thinking and physical activity; manic type is characterized by elation, overtalkativeness, extremely rapid ideation, and increased motor activity.

megalomania Syndrome marked by delusions of great self-importance, wealth, or power.

melancholia Pathological dejection, usually of psychotic depth.

mental mechanisms Also called defense mechanisms and mental dynamisms; specific intrapsychic defensive processes, operating unconsciously, that are employed to seek resolution of emotional conflict and freedom from anxiety; conscious efforts are frequently made for the same reasons, but true mental mechanisms are out of awareness (unconscious).

milieu Environment; the people and objects with which the individual deals.

mood Pervasive and sustained emotion that in the extreme markedly colors the person's perception of the world. Mood is to affect as climate is to weather. Common examples of mood include depression, elation, anger, and anxiety.

mysophobia Morbid fear of dirt, germs, or contamination.

narcissism Self-love; in a broader sense indicates a degree of self-interest normal in early childhood but pathological when seen in similar degree in adulthood.

narcolepsy Condition in which the individual is overcome by short irresistible periods of sleep.

negative feelings As used in psychiatry, refers to hostile, unfriendly feelings.

negativism Perverse opposition and resistance to suggestions or advice; often observed in people who subjectively feel "pushed around."

neologism In psychiatry, new word or condensed combination of several words coined by a client to express a highly complex meaning related to his conflicts; not readily understood by others; common in schizophrenia.

nihilism In psychiatry, refers to the delusion of nonexistence of the self or part of self.

object That through which an instinct can achieve its aim; object relations theory is the psychoanalytic description of the internalization of interpersonal relations and the organizing effects of internalized human object relationships on the structure of the psyche.

obsession Persistent, unwanted idea or impulse that cannot be eliminated by usual logic or reasoning.

obsessive-compulsive disorder Psychiatric disorder characterized by disturbing, unwanted, intruding thoughts and ideas, and repetitive impulses to perform acts that the person may consider abnormal, undesirable, or distasteful.

Oedipus complex Situation occurring during the phallic stage of psychosexual development (approximate ages 3 to 6) in which the child shifts energies into sexual interest in parents. The child normally becomes attached to the parent of the opposite sex, and develops competitive feelings toward the same sex parent. Eventually, through identification with the same sex parent, the child relinquishes oedipal strivings.

omnipotence Infantile perception that the outside world is part of the organism and within it, which leads to a primitive feeling of all-powerfulness. This feeling gradually becomes limited as the ego and a sense of reality develop. Similar phenomena are found in disturbed individuals who lose contact with reality.

oral stage Includes both the oral-erotic and oral-sadistic phases of infantile psychosexual development, lasting from birth to 12 months or longer; oral-erotic phase is the initial pleasurable experience of nursing; oral-sadistic phase is the subsequent aggressive (biting) phase; both eroticism and sadism normally continue to later life in disguised or sublimated forms.

orientation Awareness of oneself in relation to time, place, and person.

panic In psychiatry, refers to an attack of acute, intense, and overwhelming anxiety, accompanied by a considerable degree of personality disorganization.

paranoia Psychotic disorder that develops slowly and becomes chronic; characterized by an intricate and internally logical system of persecutory or grandiose delusions, or both; stands by itself and does not interfere with the remainder of the personality, which continues essentially normal and apparently intact; to be distinguished from paranoid schizophrenic reactions and paranoid states.

pedophilia Term used to describe adults who demonstrate a pathological sexual interest in children.

penis envy Literally, envy by the female of the penis of the male; more generally, the female's wish for male attributes, position, or advantages; believed by many to be a significant factor in female character development.

personality Aggregate of the physical and mental qualities of the individual as these interact in characteristic fashion with the environment.

perversion Substitution of another aim for the usual aim in any activity; usually related to sexual activity when a component of sex or an earlier stage of sexual development is substituted for normal coitus.

phallus In psychoanalysis, the penis during the period of infantile sexuality when it is intensely charged with narcissistic love. When the narcissistic qualities associated with one's own genital organ are directed outwardly upon a love-object, it is said that the stage of genital love has been reached. Thus genital love in the male may be called penile love, in contrast to phallic love.

phallic stage Period of psychosexual development from the age of about 3 to 6 years during which sexual interest, curiosity, and pleasurable experience center about the penis and, in girls, to a lesser extent, the clitoris.

phobia Obsessive, persistent, unrealistic fear of an external object or situation such as heights, open spaces, dirt, and animals; fear believed to arise through a process of displacing an internal (unconscious) conflict to an external object symbolically related to the conflict.

phobic disorder Psychiatric disorder characterized by persistent and irrational fear of a specific object, activity, or situation resulting in a compelling desire to avoid the object, activity, or situation.

physiological dependence Need for agents that modify mood, behavior and cognition, characterized by physiological adaptation to the agent so that the body must have it to function asymptomatically. In addition, tolerance to the substance occurs so that the individual must increase the dosage to achieve the same effects. The symptoms of withdrawal can be demonstrated when the agent is withheld.

pleasure principle Basic psychoanalytic concept that humans instinctually seek to avoid pain and discomfort and strive for gratification and pleasure; in personality development theories, the pleasure principle antedates and subsequently comes into conflict with the reality principle.

preconscious Thoughts not in immediate awareness but that can be recalled by conscious effort.

preoccupation State of being self-absorbed or engrossed in one's own thoughts, typically to a degree that hinders effective contact with or relationship to external reality.

projection Mental mechanism, operating unconsciously, whereby that which is emotionally unacceptable in the self is unconsciously rejected and attributed (projected) to others.

psyche Mind, in distinction to the soma, or body.

psychodynamics Systematized knowledge and theory of human behavior and its motivation, the study of which depends largely on the functional significance of emotion; psychodynamics recognizes the role of unconscious motivation in human behavior; a predictive science, based on the assumption that a person's total makeup and probable reactions at any given moment are the product of past interactions between his specific genetic endowment and the environment in which he has lived from conception onward.

psychogenesis Production or causation of a symptom or illness by mental or psychic factors as opposed to organic ones.

psychological dependence Need for agents that modify mood, behavior and cognition, marked by a felt need for the agent and the belief of the individual that he cannot function without it; the idea of a potential unavailability of the agent causes high anxiety and unremitting efforts to obtain it.

psychosexual development Changes and stages that characterize the development of the psychological aspect of sexuality during the period from birth to adult life.

psychotherapy Any form of treatment for mental illness, behavioral dysfunctions, and other problems that are assumed to be of an emotional nature, in which a trained person deliberately establishes a professional relationship with a client for the purpose of removing, modifying, or retarding existing symptoms, of attenuating or reversing disturbed patterns of behavior, and of promoting positive personality development and growth.

rapport Confidential relationships between the client and the professional person who is in a helping relationship with him.

rationalization Mental mechanism, operating unconsciously, by which the individual attempts to justify or make consciously tolerable by plausible means those feelings, behaviors, and motives that would otherwise be intolerable (not to be confused with conscious evasion or dissimulation).

reaction formation Mental mechanism, operating unconsciously, wherein attitudes and behavior are adopted that are the opposite of impulses the individual disowns either consciously or unconsciously—for example, excessive moral zeal may be the product of strong but repressed antisocial impulses.

reality principle In Freudian theory, the concept that the pleasure principle in personality development in infancy is normally modified by the inescapable demands and requirements of external reality; the process by which this compromise is effected is technically known as reality testing, both in normal development and in psychiatric treatment.

regression Partial or symbolic return to more infantile ways of gratification; most clearly seen in severe psychoses.

repression Mental mechanism, operating unconsciously; the common denominator and unconscious precursor of all mental mechanisms in which there is involuntary relegation of unbearable ideas and impulses into the unconscious from whence they are not ordinarily subject to voluntary recall but may emerge in disguised form through use of the various mental mechanisms; particularly operative in early years.

resistance In psychiatry, an individual's massive psychological defense against bringing repressed (unconscious) thoughts or impulses into awareness, thus avoiding anxiety.

Rorschach test Psychological test developed by the Swiss psychiatrist

Hermann Rorschach (1884-1922), which seeks to disclose conscious and unconscious personality traits and emotional conflicts through eliciting the person's associations to a standard set of inkblots.

sadism Pleasure derived from inflicting physical or psychological pain on others; the sexual significance of sadistic wishes or behavior may be conscious or unconscious; the reverse of masochism.

schizoid Adjective describing traits of shyness, introspection, and introversion.

schizophrenia, catatonic Type of schizophrenia characterized by immobility with muscular rigidity or inflexibility; alternating periods of physical hyperactivity and excitability may occur; generally there is marked inaccessibility to ordinary methods of communication.

schizophrenia, disorganized Type of schizophrenia characterized by incoherence and flat, incongruous, or silly affect, with no systematized delusions.

schizophrenia, paranoid Type of schizophrenia marked by a feeling that external reality has altered; suspiciousness; ideas of reference; hallucinations; delusions of persecution or grandiosity.

schizophrenia, residual Condition of being without gross psychotic symptoms following a psychotic schizophrenic episode.

schizophrenia, undifferentiated Type of schizophrenia characterized by prominent delusions, hallucinations, incoherence, or grossly disorganized behavior that cannot be classified in one of the other categories.

security operations H.S. Sullivan's term for mechanisms such as apathy and selective inattention that, no matter how rational at first glance, are defenses against recognizing or experiencing anxiety.

selective inattention Term for a security operation identified by H.S. Sullivan, whereby anxiety-producing aspects of a situation are not allowed into awareness.

senile dementia Term used to describe dementias occurring after age 65 that are irreversible in nature.

sensorium Roughly approximates consciousness; includes the special sensory perceptive powers and their central correlation and integration in the brain; a clear sensorium conveys the presence of a reasonably accurate memory together with a correct orientation for time, place, and person.

soma Body; the physical aspect of a human as distinguished from the psyche.

somatic Bodily; having reference to the body or its organs.

somatoform disorder Group of disorders characterized by physical symptoms for which there are no demonstrable organic findings or known physical mechanisms and for which there is positive evidence or strong presumption that the symptoms are linked to psychological factors.

somnolent detachment H.S. Sullivan's term for the security operation with its origin in infancy, whereby the individual falls asleep when confronted by a highly-threatening, anxiety-producing experience.

stereotypy Persistent, mechanical repetition of an activity; common in schizophrenia.

stressor In terms of stress and adaptation theory, the stressor is any system input, which may have either positive or negative effects, depending on the way it is processed; may be classified as situational (untoward events) or developmental (anticipated events related to growth and maturation).

subconscious Psychiatrically obsolescent term that refers in general to both that which is not subject to recall and to that which may, with independent effort, be recalled.

sublimation Mental mechanism, operating unconsciously, through which consciously unacceptable instinctual drives are diverted into personally and socially acceptable channels.

substance abuse Pathological use of agents modifying mood, behavior, and cognition, creating an impairment in social or occupational functioning.

substitution Mental mechanism, operating unconsciously, by which an unattainable or unacceptable goal, emotion, or object is replaced by one that is more attainable or acceptable.

suggestibility Referring to a person's susceptibility to having his ideas or actions changed by the influence of others.

superego In Freudian theory, that part of the mind that unconsciously identifies itself with important and esteemed persons from early life, particularly parents; the supposed or actual wishes of these significant persons are taken over as part of one's own personal standards to help form the "conscience."

suppression Conscious effort to overcome unacceptable thoughts or desires by forcing them out of the conscious mind.

symbolization Mental mechanism, operating unconsciously, in which a person forms an abstract representation of a particular object, idea, or constellation. The symbol carries, in more or less disguised form, the emotional feelings vested in the initial object or ideas.

tardive dyskinesia A serious side effect of antipsychotic medication characterized by grimacing, choreiform, or athetoid movements of the arms, fingers, ankles, and toes, and tonic contractions of the neck and back muscles. At the present time it is irreversible.

toxic psychosis Psychosis resulting from the toxic effect of chemicals and drugs, including those produced in the body.

transference Unconscious attachment to others of feelings and attitudes that were originally associated with important figures (parents, siblings, etc.) in one's early life. The transference relationship follows roughly the pattern of its prototype; the therapist uses the phenomenon as a therapeutic tool to help the client understand his emotional problems and their origin; in the client-therapist relationship the transference may be negative (hostile) or positive (affectionate).

transvestism Sexual pleasure derived from dressing or masquerading in the clothing of the opposite sex; the sexual origins of transvestism may be unconscious.

unconscious In Freudian theory, that part of the mind or mental functioning the content of which is only rarely subject to awareness; a repository for data that have never been conscious (primary repression) or that may have become conscious briefly and were then repressed (secondary repression).

undoing Primitive defense mechanism, operating unconsciously, by which something unacceptable and already done is symbolically acted out in reverse, usually repetitiously, in the hope of "undoing" it and thus relieving anxiety.

volition Will.

word salad Voluble speech in which words and phrases have no logical connection or meaning.

zones, erotic Regions such as the lips, breasts, and genitoanal area, stimulation of which causes erotic excitement.

DSM-III multiaxial evaluation

AXIS I: **Clinical syndromes**
Conditions not attributable to a mental disorder that are a
focus of attention or treatment
Additional codes

AXIS II: **Personality disorders**
Specific developmental disorders

All official DSM-III codes and terms are included in ICD-9-CM. However, to differentiate those DSM-III categories that use the same ICD-9-CM codes, unofficial non-ICD-9-CM codes are provided in parentheses for use when greater specificity is necessary. The long dashes indicate the need for fifth-digit subtype or other qualifying term.

DISORDERS USUALLY FIRST EVIDENT IN INFANCY, CHILDHOOD OR ADOLESCENCE

Mental retardation

(Code in fifth digit: 1 = with other behavioral symptoms [requiring attention or treatment and that are not part of another disorder], 0 = without other behavioral symptoms.)

317.0(×) Mild mental retardation, _____
318.0(×) Moderate mental retardation, _____
318.1(×) Severe mental retardation, _____
318.2(×) Profound mental retardation, _____
319.0(×) Unspecified mental retardation, _____

Attention deficit disorder

314.01   with hyperactivity
314.00   without hyperactivity
314.80   residual type

From American Psychiatric Association: Diagnostic and statistical manual of mental disorders, ed. 3, Washington, D.C., 1980, pp. 15-19, 27, 29-30. Reprinted with permission from the American Psychiatric Association.

Conduct disorder

312.00 undersocialized, aggressive
312.10 undersocialized, nonaggressive
312.23 socialized, aggressive
312.21 socialized, nonaggressive
312.90 atypical

Anxiety disorders of childhood or adolescence

309.21 Separation anxiety disorder
313.21 Avoidant disorder of childhood or adolescence
313.00 Overanxious disorder

Other disorders of infancy, childhood or adolescence

313.89 Reactive attachment disorder of infancy
313.22 Schizoid disorder of childhood or adolescence
313.23 Elective mutism
313.81 Oppositional disorder
313.82 Identity disorder

Eating disorders

307.10 Anorexia nervosa
307.51 Bulimia
307.52 Pica
307.53 Rumination disorder of infancy
307.50 Atypical eating disorder

Stereotyped movement disorders

307.21 Transient tic disorder
307.22 Chronic motor tic disorder
307.23 Tourette's disorder
307.20 Atypical tic disorder
307.30 Atypical stereotyped movement disorder

Other disorders with physical manifestations

307.00 Stuttering
307.60 Functional enuresis
307.70 Functional encopresis
307.46 Sleepwalking disorder
307.46 Sleep terror disorder (307.49)

Pervasive developmental disorders

Code in fifth digit: 0 = full syndrome
present, 1 = residual state.
299.0×   Infantile autism, _____
299.9×   Childhood onset pervasive developmental disorder,
_____
299.8×   Atypical, _____

> **Specific developmental disorders**
> **Note: These are coded on Axis II.**
>
> 315.00   Developmental reading disorder
> 315.10   Developmental arithmetic disorder
> 315.31   Developmental language disorder
> 315.39   Developmental articulation disorder
> 315.50   Mixed specific developmental disorder
> 315.90   Atypical specific developmental disorder

ORGANIC MENTAL DISORDERS
Section 1

Organic mental disorders whose etiology or pathophysiological process is listed below (taken from the mental disorders section of ICD-9-CM).

Dementias arising in the senium and presenium

Primary degenerative dementia, senile onset,

290.30   with delirium
290.20   with delusions
290.21   with depression
290.00   uncomplicated

Code in fifth digit:
1 = with delirium, 2 = with delusions, 3 = with depression,
0 = uncomplicated.
290.1×   Primary degenerative dementia, presenile onset,
_____
290.4×   Multi-infarct dementia, _____

Substance-induced

Alcohol

303.00   intoxication
291.40   idiosyncratic intoxication

291.80   withdrawal
291.00   withdrawal delirium
291.30   hallucinosis
291.10   amnestic disorder

Code severity of dementia in fifth digit: 1 = mild, 2 = moderate, 3 = severe, 0 = unspecified.

291.2×   Dementia associated with alcoholism, ————

Barbiturate or similarly acting sedative or hypnotic

305.40   intoxication (327.00)
292.00   withdrawal (327.01)
292.00   withdrawal delirium (327.02)
292.83   amnestic disorder (327.04)

Opioid

305.50   intoxication (327.10)
292.00   withdrawal (327.11)

Cocaine

305.60   intoxication (327.20)

Amphetamine or similar acting sympathomimetic

305.70   intoxication (327.30)
292.81   delirium (327.32)
292.11   delusional disorder (327.35)
292.00   withdrawal (327.31)

Phencyclidine (PCP) or similarly acting arylcyclohexylamine

305.90   intoxication (327.40)
292.81   delirium (327.42)
292.90   mixed organic mental disorder (327.49)

Hallucinogen

305.30   hallucinosis (327.56)
292.11   delusional disorder (327.55)
292.84   affective disorder (327.57)

Cannabis

305.20   intoxication (327.60)
292.11   delusional disorder (327.65)

Tobacco

292.00   withdrawal (327.71)

Caffeine

305.90   intoxication (327.80)

Other or unspecified substance

305.90   intoxication (327.90)
292.00   withdrawal (327.91)
292.81   delirium (327.92)
292.82   dementia (327.93)
292.83   amnestic disorder (327.94)
292.11   delusional disorder (327.95)
292.12   hallucinosis (327.96)
292.84   affective disorder (327.97)
292.89   personality disorder (327.98)
292.90   atypical or mixed organic mental disorder (327.99)

Section 2

Organic brain syndromes whose etiology or pathophysiological process is either noted as an additional diagnosis from outside the mental disorders section of ICD-9-CM or is unknown.

293.00   Delirium
294.10   Dementia
294.00   Amnestic syndrome
293.81   Organic delusional syndrome
293.82   Organic hallucinosis
293.83   Organic affective syndrome
310.10   Organic personality syndrome
294.80   Atypical or mixed organic brain syndrome

SUBSTANCE USE DISORDERS

Code in fifth digit: 1 = continuous, 2 = episodic, 3 = in remission, 0 = unspecified

305.0×   Alcohol abuse, _____
303.9×   Alcohol dependence (Alcoholism), _____
305.4×   Barbiturate or similarly acting sedative or hypnotic abuse, _____
304.1×   Barbiturate or similarly acting sedative or hypnotic dependence, _____
305.5×   Opioid abuse, _____

304.0× Opioid dependence, _____
305.6× Cocaine abuse, _____
305.7× Amphetamine or similarly acting sympathomimetic abuse, _____
304.4× Amphetamine or similarly acting sympathomimetic dependence, _____
305.9× Phencyclidine (PCP) or similarly acting arylcyclohexylamine abuse, _____ (328.4×)
305.3× Hallucinogen abuse, _____
305.2× Cannabis abuse, _____
304.3× Cannabis dependence, _____
305.1× Tobacco dependence, _____
305.9× Other, mixed or unspecified substance abuse, _____
304.6× Other specified substance dependence, _____
304.9× Unspecified substance dependence _____
304.7× Dependence on combination of opioid and other non-alcoholic substance, _____
304.8× Dependence on combination of substances, excluding opioids and alcohol, _____

SCHIZOPHRENIC DISORDERS

Code in fifth digit: 1 = subchronic, 2 = chronic, 3 = subchronic with acute exacerbation, 4 = chronic with acute exacerbation, 5 = in remission, 0 = unspecified.

Schizophrenia
295.1× disorganized, _____
295.2× catatonic, _____
295.3× paranoid, _____
295.9× undifferentiated, _____
295.6× residual, _____

PARANOID DISORDERS
297.10 Paranoia
297.30 Shared paranoid disorder
298.30 Acute paranoid disorder
297.30 Atypical paranoid disorder

PSYCHOTIC DISORDERS NOT ELSEWHERE CLASSIFIED
295.40 Schizophreniform disorder
298.80 Brief reactive psychosis
295.70 Schizoaffective disorder
298.90 Atypical psychosis

NEUROTIC DISORDERS

These are included in Affective, Anxiety, Somatoform, Dissociative, and Psychosexual Disorders. To facilitate the identification of the categories that in DSM-II were grouped together in the class of Neuroses, the DMS-II terms are included separately in parentheses after the corresponding categories. These DSM-II terms are included in ICD-9-CM and therefore are acceptable as alternatives to the recommended DSM-III terms that precede them.

AFFECTIVE DISORDERS

Major affective disorders

Code major depressive episode in fifth digit: 6 = in remission, 4 = with psychotic features (the unofficial non-ICD-9-CM fifth digit 7 may be used instead to indicate that the psychotic features are mood-incongruent), 3 = with melancholia, 2 = without melancholia, 0 = unspecified.

Code manic episode in fifth digit: 6 = in remission, 4 = with psychotic features (the unofficial non-ICD-9-CM fifth digit 7 may be used instead to indicate that the psychotic features are mood-incongruent), 2 = without psychotic features, 0 = unspecified.

Bipolar disorder

296.6×	mixed,	_____
296.4×	manic,	_____
296.5×	depressed,	_____

Major depression

296.2×	single episode,	_____
296.3×	recurrent,	_____

Other specific affective disorders

301.13	Cyclothymic disorder
300.40	Dysthymic disorder (or Depressive neurosis)

Atypical affective disorders

296.70	Atypical bipolar disorder
296.82	Atypical depression

ANXIETY DISORDERS

Phobic disorders (or Phobic neuroses)

300.21	Agoraphobia with panic attacks
300.22	Agoraphobia without panic attacks
300.23	Social phobia
300.29	Simple phobia

Anxiety states (or Anxiety neuroses)

300.01   Panic disorder
300.02   Generalized anxiety disorder
300.30   Obsessive compulsive disorder (or Obsessive compulsive neurosis)

Post-traumatic stress disorder

308.30   acute
309.81   chronic or delayed
300.00   Atypical anxiety disorder

SOMATOFORM DISORDERS

300.81   Somatization disorder
300.11   Conversion disorder (or Hysterical neurosis, conversion type)
307.80   Psychogenic pain disorder
300.70   Hypochondriasis (or Hypochondriacal neurosis)
300.70   Atypical somatoform disorder (300.71)

DISSOCIATIVE DISORDERS (OR HYSTERICAL NEUROSES, DISSOCIATIVE TYPE)

300.12   Psychogenic amnesia
300.13   Psychogenic fugue
300.14   Multiple personality
300.60   Depersonalization disorder (or Depersonalization neurosis)
300.15   Atypical dissociative disorder

PSYCHOSEXUAL DISORDERS

Gender identity disorders

Indicate sexual history in the fifth digit of Transsexualism code: 1 = asexual, 2 = homosexual, 3 = heterosexual, 0 = unspecified.

302.5×   Transsexualism, _____
302.60   Gender identity disorder of childhood
302.85   Atypical gender identity disorder

Paraphilias

302.81   Fetishism
302.30   Transvestism
302.10   Zoophilia
302.20   Pedophilia
302.40   Exhibitionism
302.82   Voyeurism

302.83	Sexual masochism
302.84	Sexual sadism
302.90	Atypical paraphilia

Psychosexual dysfunctions

302.71	Inhibited sexual desire
302.72	Inhibited sexual excitement
302.73	Inhibited female orgasm
302.74	Inhibited male orgasm
302.75	Premature ejaculation
302.76	Functional dyspareunia
306.51	Functional vaginismus
302.70	Atypical psychosexual dysfunction

Other psychosexual disorders

302.00	Ego-dystonic homosexuality
302.89	Psychosexual disorder not elsewhere classified

FACTITIOUS DISORDERS

300.16	Factitious disorder with psychological symptoms
301.51	Chronic factitious disorder with physical symptoms
300.19	Atypical factitious disorder with physical symptoms

DISORDERS OF IMPULSE CONTROL NOT ELSEWHERE CLASSIFIED

312.31	Pathological gambling
312.32	Kleptomania
312.33	Pyromania
312.34	Intermittent explosive disorder
312.35	Isolated explosive disorder
312.39	Atypical impulse control disorder

ADJUSTMENT DISORDER

309.00	with depressed mood
309.24	with anxious mood
309.28	with mixed emotional features
309.30	with disturbance of conduct
309.40	with mixed disturbance of emotions and conduct
309.23	with work (or academic) inhibition
309.83	with withdrawal
309.90	with atypical features

PSYCHOLOGICAL FACTORS AFFECTING PHYSICAL CONDITION

Specify physical condition on Axis III.

316.00 Psychological factors affecting physical condition

PERSONALITY DISORDERS
Note: These are coded on Axis II.

301.00	Paranoid	301.82	Avoidant
301.20	Schizoid	301.60	Dependent
301.22	Schizotypal	301.40	Compulsive
301.50	Histrionic	301.84	Passive-Aggressive
301.81	Narcissistic	301.89	Atypical, mixed or
301.70	Antisocial		other personality
301.83	Borderline		disorder

V CODES FOR CONDITIONS NOT ATTRIBUTABLE TO A MENTAL DISORDER THAT ARE A FOCUS OF ATTENTION OR TREATMENT

V65.20	Malingering
V62.89	Borderline intellectual functioning (V62.88)
V71.01	Adult antisocial behavior
V71.02	Childhood or adolescent antisocial behavior
V62.30	Academic problem
V62.20	Occupational problem
V62.82	Uncomplicated bereavement
V15.81	Noncompliance with medical treatment
V62.89	Phase of life problem or other life circumstance problem
V61.10	Marital problem
V61.20	Parent-child problem
V61.80	Other specified family circumstances
V62.81	Other interpersonal problem

ADDITIONAL CODES

300.90	Unspecified mental disorder (nonpsychotic)
V71.09	No diagnosis or condition on Axis I
799.90	Diagnosis or condition deferred on Axis I

V71.09	No diagnosis on Axis II
799.90	Diagnosis deferred on Axis II

AXIS III: Physical disorders and conditions
AXIS IV: Severity of psychosocial stressors

code	term	adult examples	child or adolescent examples
1	None	No apparent psychosocial stressor	No apparent psychosocial stressor
2	Minimal	Minor violation of the law, small bank loan	Vacation with family
3	Mild	Argument with neighbor; change in work hours	Change in schoolteacher; new school year
4	Moderate	New career; death of close friend; pregnancy	Chronic parental fighting; change to new school; illness of close relative; birth of sibling
5	Severe	Serious illness in self or family; major financial loss; marital separation; birth of child	Death of peer; divorce of parents; arrest; hospitalization; persistent and harsh parental discipline
6	Extreme	Death of close relative; divorce	Death of parent or sibling; repeated physical or sexual abuse
7	Catastrophic	Concentration camp experience; devastating natural disaster	Multiple family deaths
0	Unspecified	No information, or not applicable	No information; or not applicable

AXIS V: Highest level of adaptive functioning during the past year

levels	adult examples	child or adolescent examples
1 SUPERIOR—Unusually effective functioning in social relations, occupational functioning and use of leisure time.	Single parent living in deteriorating neighborhood takes excellent care of children and home, has warm relations with friends, and finds time for pursuit of hobby.	A 12-year-old girl gets superior grades in school, is extremely popular among her peers, and excels in many sports. She does all of this with apparent ease and comfort.
2 VERY GOOD—Better than average functioning in social relations, occupational functioning, and use of leisure time.	A 65-year-old retired widower does some volunteer work, often sees old friends, and pursues hobbies.	An adolescent boy gets excellent grades, works part time, has several close friends, and plays banjo in a jazz band. He admits to some distress in "keeping up with everything."
3 GOOD—No more than slight impairment in either social or occupational functioning.	A woman with many friends functions extremely well at a difficult job, but says "the strain is too much."	An 8-eight-old boy does well in school, has several friends, but bullies younger children.
4 FAIR—Moderate impairment in either social relations or occupational functioning, or some impairment in both.	A lawyer has trouble carrying through assignments; has several acquaintances, but hardly any close friends.	A 10-year-old girl does poorly in school, but has adequate peer and family relations.

Continued.

AXIS V: **Highest level of adaptive functioning during the past year—cont'd**

levels	adult examples	child or adolescent examples
5 POOR—Marked impairment in either social relations or occupational functioning, or moderate impairment in both.	A man with one or two friends has trouble keeping a job for more than a few weeks.	A 14-year-old boy almost fails in school and has trouble getting along with his peers.
6 VERY POOR—Marked impairment in both social relations and occupational functioning.	A woman is unable to do any of her housework and has violent outbursts toward family and neighbors.	A 6-year-old girl needs special help in all subjects and has virtually no peer relationships.
7 GROSSLY IMPAIRED— Gross impairment in virtually all areas of functioning.	An elderly man needs supervision to maintain minimal personal hygiene and is usually incoherent.	A 4-year-old boy needs constant restraint to avoid hurting himself and is almost totally lacking in skills.
0 UNSPECIFIED	No information	No information

ANA standards of psychiatric and mental health nursing practice

Standard I—Theory

The nurse applies appropriate theory that is scientifically sound as a basis for decisions regarding nursing practice.

Standard II—Data collection

The nurse continuously collects data that are comprehensive, accurate, and systematic.

Standard III—Diagnosis

The nurse utilizes nursing diagnoses and standard classification of mental disorders to express conclusions supported by recorded assessment data and current scientific premises.

Standard IV—Planning

The nurse develops a nursing care plan with specific goals and interventions delineating nursing actions unique to each client's needs.

Standard V—Intervention

The nurse intervenes as guided by the nursing care plan to implement nursing actions that promote, maintain, or restore physical and mental health, prevent illness, and effect rehabilitation.

Standard V-A—Psychotherapeutic interventions

The nurse (generalist) uses psychotherapeutic interventions to assist clients to regain or improve their previous coping abilities and to prevent further disability.

Reprinted with permission of the American Nurses' Association, Kansas City, 1982.

649

Standard V-B—Health teaching

The nurse assists clients, families, and groups to achieve satisfying and productive patterns of living through health teaching.

Standard V-C—Self-care activities

The nurse uses the activities of daily living in a goal-directed way to foster adequate self-care and physical and mental well-being of clients.

Standard V-D—Somatic therapies

The nurse uses knowledge of somatic therapies and applies related client skills in working with clients.

Standard V-E—Therapeutic environment

The nurse provides, structures, and maintains a therapeutic environment in collaboration with the client and other health care providers.

Standard V-F—Psychotherapy

The nurse (specialist) utilizes advanced clinical expertise in individual, group, and family psychotherapy, child psychotherapy, and other treatment modalities to function as a psychotherapist and recognizes professional accountability for nursing practice.

Standard VI—Evaluation

The nurse evaluates clients' responses to nursing actions in order to revise the data base, nursing diagnoses, and nursing care plan.

Standard VII—Peer review

The nurse participates in peer review and other means of evaluation to assure quality of nursing care provided for clients.

Standard VIII—Continuing education

The nurse assumes responsibility for continuing education and professional development and contributes to the professional growth of others.

Standard IX—Interdisciplinary collaboration

The nurse collaborates with interdisciplinary teams in assessing, planning, implementing, and evaluating programs and other mental health activities.

Standard X—Utilization of community health systems

The nurse (specialist) participates with other members of the community in assessing, planning, implementing, and evaluating mental health services and community systems that include the promotion of the broad continuum of primary, secondary, and tertiary prevention of mental illness.

Standard XI—Research

The nurse contributes to nursing and the mental health field through innovations in theory and practice and participation in research.

appendix C

the code for nurses

1. The nurse provides services with respect for human dignity and the uniqueness of the client unrestricted by considerations of social or economic status, personal attributes, or the nature of health problems.
2. The nurse safeguards the client's right to privacy by judiciously protecting information of a confidential nature.
3. The nurse acts to safeguard the client and the public when health care and safety are affected by the incompetent, unethical, or illegal practice of any person.
4. The nurse assumes responsibility and accountability for individual nursing judgments and actions.
5. The nurse maintains competence in nursing.
6. The nurse exercises informed judgment and uses individual competence and qualifications as criteria in seeking consultation, accepting responsibilities, and delegating nursing activities to others.
7. The nurse participates in activities that contribute to the ongoing development of the profession's body of knowledge.
8. The nurse participates in the profession's efforts to implement and improve standards of nursing.
9. The nurse participates in the profession's efforts to establish and maintain conditions of employment conducive to high quality nursing care.
10. The nurse participates in the profession's effort to protect the public from misinformation and misrepresentation and to maintain the integrity of nursing.
11. The nurse collaborates with members of the health professions and other citizens in promoting community and national efforts to meet the health needs of the public.

From American Nurses' Association: Code for nurses (with interpretive statements), Kansas City, Mo., 1976. Reprinted with permission from the American Nurses' Association.

a patient's bill of rights

1. The patient has the right to considerate and respectful care.
2. The patient has the right to obtain from his physician complete current information concerning his diagnosis, treatment, and prognosis in terms the patient can be reasonably expected to understand. When it is not medically advisable to give such information to the patient, the information should be made available to an appropriate person in his behalf. He has the right to know, by name, the physician responsible for coordinating his care.
3. The patient has the right to receive from his physician information necessary to give informed consent prior to the start of any procedure and/or treatment. Except in emergencies, such information for informed consent should include but not necessarily be limited to the specific procedure and/or treatment, the medically significant risks involved, and the probable duration of incapacitation. Where medically significant alternatives for care or treatment exist, or when the patient requests information concerning medical alternatives, the patient has the right to such information. The patient also has the right to know the name of the person responsible for the procedures and/or treatment.
4. The patient has the right to refuse treatment to the extent permitted by law and to be informed of the medical consequences of his action.
5. The patient has the right to every consideration of his privacy concerning his own medical care program. Case discussion, consultation, examination, and treatment are confidential and should be conducted discreetly. Those not directly involved in his care must have the permission of the patient to be present.

Reprinted with the permission of the American Hospital Association, copyright 1972.

6. The patient has the right to expect that all communications and records pertaining to his care should be treated as confidential.

7. The patient has the right to expect that within its capacity a hospital must make reasonable response to the request of a patient for services. The hospital must provide evaluation, service, and/or referral as indicated by the urgency of the case. When medically permissible, a patient may be transferred to another facility only after he has received complete information and explanation concerning the needs for and alternatives to such a transfer. The institution to which the patient is to be transferred must first have accepted the patient for transfer.

8. The patient has the right to obtain information as to any relationship of his hospital to other heath care and educational institutions insofar as his care is concerned. The patient has the right to obtain information as to the existence of any professional relationships among individuals, by name, who are treating him.

9. The patient has the right to be advised if the hospital proposes to engage in or perform human experimentation affecting his care or treatment. The patient has the right to refuse to participate in such research projects.

10. The patient has the right to expect reasonable continuity of care. He has the right to know in advance what appointment times and physicians are available and where. The patient has the right to expect that the hospital will provide a mechanism whereby he is informed by his physician or a delegate of the physician of the patient's continuing health care requirements following discharge.

11. The patient has the right to examine and receive an explanation of his bill regardless of source of payment.

12. The patient has the right to know what hospital rules and regulations apply to his conduct as a patient.

index

655